THE DIABETES ANNUAL/1

THE DIABETES ANNUAL/1

Edited by

K.G.M.M. ALBERTI
Department of Clinical Biochemistry and Metabolic Medicine,
The Royal Victoria Infirmary, Newcastle upon Tyne, U.K.

L.P. KRALL
Joslin Diabetes Center, Boston,
MA, U.S.A.

ELSEVIER
Amsterdam – New York – Oxford

ISBN 0 444 90343 7

Notice The editors and publisher of this work have made every effort to ensure that the drug dosage schedules herein are accurate and in accord with the standards accepted at the time of publication. Readers are advised, however, to check the product information sheet included in the package of each drug prior to administration to be certain that changes have not been made in either the recommended dose or contra-indications. Such verification is especially important in regard to new or infrequently used drugs.

Published by:
Elsevier Science Publishers B.V.
P.O. Box 1126
1000 BC Amsterdam

Sole distributors for the USA and Canada:
Elsevier Science Publishing Co. Inc.
52 Vanderbilt Avenue
New York, NY 10017

Printed in The Netherlands by Casparie – Amsterdam

List of contributors

N.N. ABUMRAD,
Department of Physiology and Surgery,
Vanderbilt University Medical School,
Nashville, TN 37232
U.S.A.

D.W. BEAVEN,
Department of Medicine,
Christchurch Clinical School of Medicine,
The Princess Margaret Hospital,
Christchurch,
New Zealand

M. BERGER,
Department of Medicine E,
Düsseldorf University,
Moorenstrasse 5,
4000 Düsseldorf,
Federal Republic of Germany

E. BIERMAN,
Division of Medicine and Endocrinology,
University of Washington,
Seattle, WA 98195,
U.S.A.

C. BINDER,
Steno Memorial Hospital,
DK-2820 Gentofte,
Denmark

G.F. BOTTAZZO,
Department of Immunology,
Arthur Stanley House,
Middlesex Hospital Medical School,
London, W1P 9PG,
U.K.

C. BRADLEY,
Department of Psychology,
University of Sheffield,
Sheffield, S10 2TN,
U.K.

J.D. BRUNZELL,
Division of Medicine and Endocrinology,
University of Washington,
Seattle, WA 98195,
U.S.A.

A. CHAIT,
Division of Metabolism and Endocrinology,
Department of Medicine,
University of Washington,
Seattle, WA 98195,
U.S.A.

A.D. CHERRINGTON,
Department of Physiology and Surgery,
Vanderbilt University Medical School,
Nashville, TN 37232
U.S.A.

J. DUPRE
University Hospital,
339 Windermere Road,
P.O. Box 5339,
Postal Station A,
London, Ont., N6A 5A5,
Canada

R.P. EATON,
Department of Medicine,
University of New Mexico,
School of Medicine,
Albuquerque, NM 87131,
U.S.A.

E.N. ELLIS,
Department of Pediatrics,
University of Minnesota,
420 Delaware Street S.E.,
Minneapolis, MN 55455,
U.S.A.

D.D. ETZWILER,
International Diabetes Center,
4959 Excelsior Boulevard,
Minneapolis, MN 55416,
U.S.A.

O. FABER,
Steno Memorial Hospital,
DK-2820 Gentofte,
Denmark

B. FORMBY,
Sansum Medical Research Foundation,
2219 Bath Street,
Santa Barbara, CA 93105,
U.S.A.

E. GALE,
Department of Immunology,
Arthur Stanley House,
Middlesex Hospital Medical School,
London, W1P 9PG,
U.K.

F.C. GOETZ,
Department of Surgery and Medicine,
University of Minnesota Hospitals,
420 Delaware Street S.E.
Minneapolis, MN 55455,
U.S.A.

J.-Cl. HENQUIN,
Unité de Diabétologie et Nutrition,
University of Louvain,
Faculty of Medicine, UCL 54.74,
B-1200 Brussels,
Belgium

C.R. KAHN,
Joslin Diabetes Center and Department of Medicine,
Brigham and Women's Hospital,
Boston, MA 02215,
U.S.A.

D. KENDALL,
Department of Surgery and Medicine,
University of Minnesota Hospitals,
420 Delaware Street S.E.
Minneapolis, MN 55455,
U.S.A.

H. KING,
WHO Collaboration Centre for the Epidemiology of Diabetes Mellitus,
Royal Southern Memorial Hospital,
260 Kooyong Road,
Caulfield, 3162 Victoria
Australia

E.M. KOHNER,
Department of Medicine
Hammersmith Hospital,
Du Cane Road,
London, W12 0HS
U.K.

H. LEBOVITZ,
Downstate Medical Center,
450 Clarkson Avenue, Box 21,
Brooklyn, NY 11203,
U.S.A.

R.D.G. LESLIE,
Diabetic Clinic,
King's College Hospital,
Denmark Hill,
London, SE5 9RS,
U.K.

S.M. MAUER,
Department of Pediatrics,
University of Minnesota,
420 Delaware Street S.E.,
Minneapolis, MN 55455
U.S.A.

D.E. McMILLAN,
Hal B. Wallis Research Facility
Eisenhower Medical Center,
39000 Bob Hope Drive,
Rancho Mirage, CA 92270,
U.S.A.

L. MØLSTED-PEDERSEN,
Department of Obstetrics and Gynecology,
Rigshospitalet,
University of Copenhagen,
DK-2100 Copenhagen Ø
Denmark

V. MOHAN,
Hammersmith Hospital,
Du Cane Road,
London, W12 0HS,
U.K.

J.S. NAJARIAN,
Department of Surgery and Medicine,
University of Minnesota Hospitals,
420 Delaware Street S.E.
Minneapolis, MN 55455,
U.S.A.

C.M. PETERSON,
Sansum Medical Research Foundation,
2219 Bath Street,
Santa Barbara, CA 93105,
U.S.A.

R. PUJOL-BORRELL,
Department of Immunology,
Arthur Stanley House,
Middlesex Hospital Medical School,
London, W1P 9PG,
U.K.

D.A. PYKE,
Diabetic Clinic,
King's College Hospital,
Denmark Hill,
London, SE5 9RS,
U.K.

A. RAMACHANDRAN,
Diabetes Research Centre,
5, Main Road,
Royapuram,
Madras, 600013,
India

W.G. REEVES,
Department of Immunology,
University Hospital,
Queen's Medical Centre,
Nottingham, NG7 2UH,
U.K.

A.E. RENOLD,
Institut de Biochimie Clinique,
University of Geneva,
Sentier de la Roseraie,
1211 Geneva 4,
Switzerland

D.S. SCHADE,
Department of Medicine,
University of New Mexico,
School of Medicine,
Albuquerque, NM 87131,
U.S.A.

K.E. STEINER,
Department of Physiology and Surgery,
Vanderbilt University Medical School,
Nashville, TN 37232
U.S.A.

R.W. STEVENSON,
Department of Physiology and Surgery,
Vanderbilt University Medical School,
Nashville, TN 37232
U.S.A.

D.E.R. SUTHERLAND,
Department of Surgery and Medicine,
University of Minnesota Hospitals,
420 Delaware Street S.E.
Minneapolis, MN 55455
U.S.A.

R. TATTERSALL,
Department of Medicine,
Queen's Medical Centre,
Nottingham, NG7 2UH,
U.K.

R.H. UNGER,
Veterans Administration Medical Center
and University of Texas Health Science
Center,
Dallas, TX 75246
U.S.A.

M. VISWANATHAN,
Diabetes Research Centre,
5, Main Road,
Royapuram,
Madras, 600013,
India

J.D. WARD,
Royal Hallamshire Hospital,
Sheffield, S10 2JF,
U.K.

P. ZIMMET,
WHO Collaboration Centre for the Epidemiology of Diabetes Mellitus,
Royal Southern Memorial Hospital,
260 Kooyong Road,
Caulfield, 3162 Victoria,
Australia

Preface

In recent years there has been a profusion of new books and journals in the general area of diabetes. It is therefore encumbent on the originators of any new tome to produce cogent reasons for further flooding the market. Financial gain is certainly not a motive – Saturday night moonlighting as a short-order cook would be more profitable. More is it the very profusion of literature that has led to the present volume.

The specialist research worker is likely to keep up to date – more or less – in his or her own area. Even then there may be problems if one considers, for example, the number of papers published each year on the mechanism of insulin secretion. The specialist wishing to maintain contact in other areas and the generalist, as many diabetes-orientated physicians have to be, can obtain at best a patchy knowledge of recent developments in the field – and then only with assiduous and disciplined reading. Important papers in journals outside of the few major ones will be missed altogether. Reviews are relied upon more and more heavily. Too often, however, these do not only reflect the bias of the author but give reference only to the author's works. To read these may often be worse than not reading at all.

Several solutions to these problems have been promoted. 'Current Contents' provides a list of all articles published in the majority of journals on a weekly basis. One of us (KGMMA) finds this frustrating as he ends up with lists of journal titles on his desk but never looks them up whilst the other (LPK) never looks at all. Selected title lists and abstract journals are also on the increase but again fall short of providing the real information or any sort of attempt to place it in context.

Our solution has been to follow the time-honoured principle of providing up-to-date reviews in diabetes, covering as much of the current literature as possible. For this volume, authors of chapters have been provided with abstracts of all relevant articles published in 1982, 1983, and early 1984. They have been asked to concentrate on the more important articles and to produce a synthesis and critique of this recent literature thereby producing, we hope, up-to-date reviews of a wide range of topics in clinical and experimental diabetes.

On this occasion certain topics have been omitted but will be included in Annual 2. Future Annuals will concentrate only on recent advances in the areas. A particular topic will not necessarily be covered every year – this will depend on progress and publications in that area in the preceding 12 months. Inevitably, chapters are longer in this volume than in future volumes because of the need to provide background information. However, the intention, the philosophy, and we hope, the reality is that the Diabetes Annual will provide up-to-date accounts of recent developments in diabetes placed in their appropriate context, and of value to all those with an interest in the subject.

K.G.M.M. Alberti
L.P. Krall

Contents

The Diabetes Annual/1
K.G.M.M. Alberti and L.P. Krall, editors

ISBN 0444 90 343 7
$0.85 per article per page (transactional system)
$0.20 per article per page (licensing system)

1 The epidemiology of diabetes mellitus: recent developments

P. ZIMMET AND H. KING

One of the earliest definitions of epidemiology was that of Parkin (1873) – 'That branch of medical science which treats epidemics'. A recent definition of epidemiology is that it is the study of the occurrence, distribution, and determinants of health-related states and events in populations, and the application of this study to the control of diseases (1).

Over the past two to three decades there has been a slow but definite upsurge in studies on diabetes epidemiology. Unquestionably the most significant milestone in the study of the epidemiology of diabetes was the publication, in 1978, of the book *Epidemiology of Diabetes and its Vascular Lesions* (2). Its author, the late Dr Kelly West, left his own unique memorial in a book that critically reviewed over 2300 papers that contributed, in one form or another, to the subject.

Since 1978, there has been an explosion of interest in diabetes epidemiology as reflected by contributions to the literature. Thus the selection of studies for a review such as this is difficult. We have chosen *three major themes* and feel that the progress in these areas has or will have a major impact on our understanding of the natural history of, and risk factors for, both insulin-dependent (IDDM) and non-insulin-dependent diabetes mellitus (NIDDM) and their complications.

Major geographic and ethnic differences exist in the prevalence and incidence of both IDDM and NIDDM. There is a greater than 35-fold difference in risk between countries having the highest and lowest incidence of IDDM. Similarly, there are major variations in the prevalence and incidence of micro- and macrovascular complications of diabetes between countries.

These facts raise important questions as to the influence of different genetic and environmental factors in the etiology of both forms of diabetes, as well as the natural history of the disease. For this reason, we have chosen as major themes of this review: (1) Genetic and environmental determinants in the etiology of NIDDM. (2) Longitudinal studies of the natural history of NIDDM, IDDM and impaired glucose tolerance (IGT). (3) Studies of the morbidity and mortality associated with diabetes, including multinational studies e.g. the World Health Organization (WHO) Multinational Study of Vascular Disease in Diabetes.

In accordance with basic epidemiological principles, we have confined this review to those studies which are population-based. In addition, as the subject of tropical diabetes is addressed elsewhere in this volume, we have not reviewed the literature on this topic.

Genetic and environmental determinants for NIDDM

Genetic susceptibility to NIDDM

The classification of diabetes into the two major categories of IDDM and NIDDM gains considerable support both from clinical and laboratory based investigations (3, 4). One of the most striking contrasts between IDDM and NIDDM is in the association between certain antigens in the histocompatibility leukocyte antigen (HLA) system and IDDM and the lack of such a strong association with NIDDM (5).

In all populations, NIDDM is far more prevalent than IDDM (6). Among Europeans, the former is about 10 times as prevalent as the latter. In India and many parts of Asia and the Pacific, the disparity is even greater (6). Although NIDDM appears to be increasing in prevalence in many of these populations, IDDM is encountered relatively rarely.

While the search for a specific genetic marker(s) for NIDDM still continues, two recent studies relating foreign genetic admixture to NIDDM prevalence are of great interest and confirm the important role of genetic factors in this form of diabetes.

Serjeantson et al. (7) have reported that Nauruans with Caucasoid genetic admixture had a lower prevalence of diabetes than full-blood Nauruans suggesting that ancestral foreign genes had a protective effect against the disease. In the generation aged 60 years and over, 83% of full-blooded Nauruans in the HLA subsample had DM, compared with only 17% of part-Nauruans. That this difference was due to genetic influences seems indisputable, since there was no evidence to suggest differences in diet or lifestyle between part- and full-blooded Nauruans. In addition, body mass index did not differ between part- and full-blooded men or women, so that differences in obesity could not explain these findings. While a more severe form of diabetes in subjects with Caucasoid admixture could account for the findings of this study through excess mortality, this is extremely unlikely and is not supported by a study of microvascular disease in Nauruan diabetics (8).

Gardner et al. (9) have reported similar findings in Mexican-Americans in San Antonio. NIDDM rates showed a relationship with the proportion of native American genes.

Diabetes prevalence in Mexican-Americans was intermediate between Pimas (100% native American) and the Anglo Hanes II population (0%

native American genes) (see Fig. 1). Diabetes prevalence in Mexican-Americans was highest in those assessed to have 46% native American genes and lowest in those with 18%. The Nauru and Mexican-American studies provide further evidence of the strong influence of genetic factors in NIDDM as has been suggested by studies of identical twins (10).

At present, there is considerable interest in the role of environmental factors which may precipitate NIDDM in genetically susceptible individuals, e.g. Pimas, Nauruans, Mexican-Americans etc. Factors under investigation include lack of exercise, both quantitative (caloric intake) and qualitative (fiber, simple sugar, etc.) aspects of diet, obesity, and psycho-social stress. These are reviewed in detail elsewhere (2, 5, 6).

The rural vs urban and migrant vs non-migrant group gradients noted in studies in Pacific and other countries suggest a combination of genetic and environmental factors in the causation of NIDDM (6, 11). As little can be

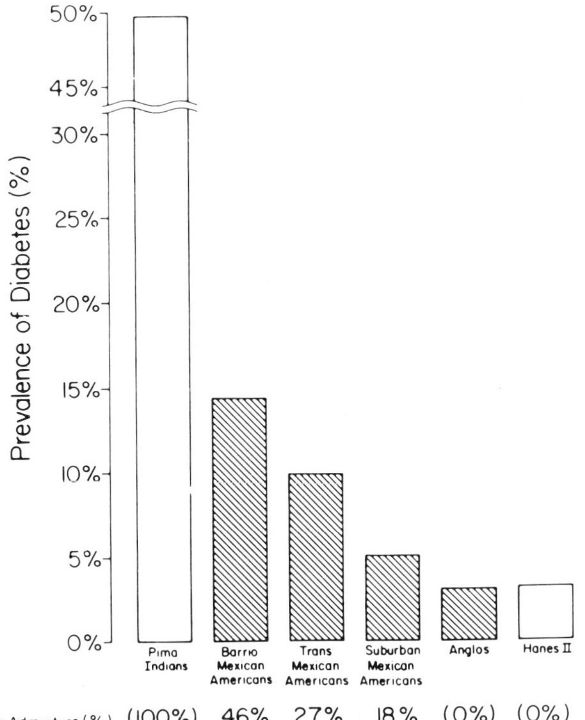

FIG. 1. *Age-adjusted NIDDM prevalence and native American admixture estimates of Pima Indians, San Antonio Mexican-Americans and Anglos, and Hanes II subjects. The hatched bars represent the San Antonio sub-populations.*
Reproduced from Gardner et al. (9) by courtesy of Dr Michael Stern and The Editors of Diabetes.

done to change genetic susceptibility, one of the major challenges in diabetes research today is the identification of environmental risk factors to try to halt the escalating problem of DM in these developing populations.

Environmental risk factors for NIDDM

A key activity in the planning of any diabetes prevention program is to define the environmental risk factors for DM in a given population. The striking emergence of NIDDM as a major health problem in populations undergoing modernization of lifestyle strongly suggests the importance of environmental factors (2, 5). However, the major problem is to ascertain which factor or combination of factors is operative. This becomes a difficult task as many environmental changes are likely to occur simultaneously with modernization.

The development of prevention programs for diabetes in any community is very dependent on accurate data as to the environmental risk factors for the disease. Thus, it is clearly pointless to concentrate on elimination of obesity when obesity may not be a major risk factor in that community.

Just as diabetes is a heterogeneous disorder, so also is obesity, and this confounds studies of the inter-relationship of the two. Furthermore, the variety of populations, diagnostic methods and criteria in earlier studies cause problems in interpreting the literature. We have reviewed this subject in detail elsewhere (12).

The case for obesity as a risk factor for NIDDM is not unequivocal. Several recent studies have raised questions as to the strength of the relationship between obesity and glucose intolerance (13, 14). However, as these were cross-sectional studies, there are inherent limitations in their interpretation.

Identical twin studies indicate that the genetic component of NIDDM acts independently of obesity. Twin pairs are concordant for NIDDM, even when their weight differs considerably, and when neither twin is overweight (10). These findings suggest that other factors, in addition to obesity, are responsible for increased risk at least in identical twins.

Studies of the Pima Indians have continued to provide a wealth of information about the natural history of NIDDM and there is a more clear-cut relationship between incidence of NIDDM and obesity in this population. While diabetes prevalence and obesity showed no relationschip, NIDDM incidence was strongly related to obesity (15). However, this relationship was interactive with history of parental diabetes. Adjusted for age and obesity, incidence was 2.3 times as high in subjects with one diabetic parent, and 3.9 times as high in those with two diabetic parents as in those with two non-diabetic parents.

Of considerable interest is a recent study by Stern et al. in Mexican-Americans (14). They compared diabetes prevalence between Mexican-

Americans and Anglo-Americans in 3 categories of obesity. The prevalence of NIDDM was significantly greater in the former even when comparisons were made within the 3 obesity categories. They concluded that, although obesity contributes to NIDDM in Mexican-Americans, it does not by itself explain the excess in prevalence.

Studies of three Pacific populations recently undertaken by King et al. (13), which were performed using standardized methodology, have demonstrated marked differences in the association between NIDDM and obesity, physical inactivity and urbanization. Although these studies were cross-sectional, the limitations imposed by this constraint might be expected to exert a similar effect upon the three populations, in which marked differences in the natural history of the disease, or in therapy, are unlikely.

The findings suggested that risk variables for NIDDM differed between populations, and between sexes within populations. In some cases, obesity had a strong association with risk; in others the principal risk variable appeared to be physical inactivity. More than one factor was associated with increased risk in Micronesians. In Micronesian males, there was evidence of interaction between obesity and urbanization.

The studies discussed above highlight the need to study the relationship of obesity and diabetes in much more depth. Studies are also needed to demonstrate whether prevention of obesity can prevent NIDDM in subjects with genetic predisposition. In addition, the question arises as to the stage of life at which obesity may have a maximal diabetogenic effect.

Because the third trimester of pregnancy is a critical period for adipose cell hyperplasia in man, Pettitt et al. (16) have studied the relationship between obesity in children and diabetes in pregnancy in their mothers in Pima Indians. Obesity in Pima children was directly related to maternal obesity. These workers suggested that the prenatal environment of the offspring of diabetic women results in the development of obesity, not only in childhood, but up to at least 19 years of age. They felt that the most likely explanation of their findings was that excessive severity and frequency of obesity in the children of diabetic mothers was largely due to the abnormal intrauterine environment, and fetal overnutrition. They further suggested that one cause of obesity, which might subsequently lead to diabetes in the offspring, may be maternal diabetes during gestation. If this were the case, controlling diabetes during pregnancy could be a first step in the prevention of obesity and subsequent diabetes in the offspring.

Not all obese Pimas (17) or Nauruans (18) develop diabetes and it could be postulated that there are either genetic or environmental protective factors operating. West suggested that duration of obesity may be a major determinant for the development of diabetes (2). Longitudinal epidemiological studies such as those underway in the Pima Indian population may provide the final answer to some of the paradoxes that presently exist.

Longitudinal studies of the natural history of NIDDM, IDDM and IGT

Evidence of growing sophistication in the design of studies in diabetes epidemiology is provided by the increasing number of longitudinal studies which have recently appeared in the literature. These have made important contributions to our knowledge of the natural history of both NIDDM and IDDM, and of the newly defined category of IGT.

Longitudinal studies of NIDDM

The need for a population-based approach to diabetes epidemiological studies was recently highlighted by Bender et al. (19), who determined that only 47% of diabetics identified in a population-based study in Wadena, Minnesota, would have been identified from hospital sources alone. They also demonstrated that the cases identified from hospital records differed from those identified from other sources in several important respects – severity of disease, presence of major health problems and sex ratio. Bias due to the use of hospital-based data is likely to be greater in the case of a disease such as NIDDM, which commonly remains undetected in the community, than in IDDM. In IDDM, onset is usually of sufficient severity to lead cases to seek hospital treatment.

Bender et al. (19) also demonstrated an incidence of NIDDM of 101 per 100,000 person-years in the Wadena population. Another large cohort, also in Minnesota, has been followed by Melton et al. in Rochester (20). They reported an incidence of 80 per 100,000 person-years for obese NIDDM and 46 per 100,000 person-years for non-obese NIDDM, both lower than the Wadena rates. Melton et al. also noted that the separation of NIDDM into obese and non-obese subtypes achieved little in the way of defining more homogeneous subgroups.

Tan (21) has reported an all-ages estimate of diabetes incidence of 189 per 100,000 person-years in Prince Edward Island, Canada. Assuming that the majority of cases were NIDDM, this estimate is surprisingly high. The design of this study would tend toward an under-ascertainment of cases of NIDDM, as patients were recruited by means of a register based upon a state-supported treatment program. Thus a proportion of NIDDM cases might be expected to be untreated, or unknown.

In a recent study in the United Kingdom, Barker et al. (22) described a lower incidence than those of the above studies. The overall incidence in nine British towns of differing social and economic conditions was 24 per 100,000 person-years. Of note was a higher incidence in the towns with 'worse' socio-economic conditions. It is not clear to what extent the low estimates of incidence may be due to the study design which only included cases referred for hospital treatment.

Butler et al. (23) used a longitudinal study design to assess predictors of future diabetes in the adult population of Tecumseh. They found that whilst age, adiposity and baseline blood glucose concentration were the principal predictors, family history of diabetes was only a significant predictor among middle-aged, overweight men. This finding is at variance with longitudinal studies in the Pima Indians (15) which have demonstrated a strong familial tendency for NIDDM.

The only recent study of the incidence of NIDDM in a non-Caucasoid population was that of Zimmet et al. (24), who demonstrated an incidence of 1540 per 100,000 person-years in the Micronesian population of Nauru. Such a high figure is in keeping with the very high prevalence of NIDDM reported in this population (17), and with an earlier incidence study in the Pima Indians (25), which demonstrated a nineteenfold excess in the incidence of NIDDM over the population of Rochester, Minnesota.

Longitudinal studies of IDDM

A number of population-based estimates of incidence of IDDM have appeared in the literature during the period covered by this review. Some of these are summarized in Table 1. The lowest estimate was from Kuwait where Taha et al. (26) found an incidence of 4 per 100,000 person-years in subjects 0–14 years of age, and 6 per 100,000 person-years in subjects aged 0–19 years. By contrast, the highest estimate was from North Sweden and was 38 per 100,000 person-years (27). The second highest rate reported was from Finland and was 29 per 100,000 person-years (28). Intermediate rates were reported from the Netherlands (29), Scotland (30), Pittsburgh (31), Rhode Island (32) and Toronto (33). These data suggest an association between geographic latitude and incidence of IDDM, though the basis for the association remains unclear.

Diabetes registers

An important development in diabetes epidemiology has been the recent interest in, and establishment of, ongoing registers of diabetics. Such registers are particularly suitable for insulin-treated subjects, as complete or almost complete ascertainment by routine methods is feasible in this group.

In an attempt to foster collaboration between research workers developing diabetes registers, and to focus upon the need for standardization of methodology, an International Workshop on Diabetes was held in Philadelphia, USA in October 1983 (34). Although studies of IDDM incidence may be performed by ad hoc techniques (either prospective or retrospective), the registry system is perceived as a valuable tool in the study of the natural history of insulin-treated diabetes, by virtue of access to cases soon after diagnosis, and maintenance of close contact with patients over an extended period of time.

TABLE 1. *Some estimates of incidence of IDDM from studies published 1982–4.*

First author*		Location	Period of study	Age criteria	Incidence per 100,000
Taha	(26)	Kuwait	1980–1	0–14	4
Taha	(26)	Kuwait	1980–1	0–19	6
Hagglof	(27)	North Sweden	1973–7	0–14	38
Reunanen	(28)	Finland	1970–9	0–14	29
Reunanen	(28)	Finland	1970–9	0–19	27
Vaandrager	(29)	Netherlands	1978–80	0–14	11
Vaandrager	(29)	Netherlands	1978–80	0–19	11
Patterson	(30)	Scotland, UK	1968–76	0–18	14
LaPorte	(31)	Pittsburgh, USA	1965–76	0–19	10–16
Fishbein	(32)	Rhode Island, USA	1979–80	0–29	14
Ehrlich	(33)	Toronto, Canada	1976–80	0–18	9

* Reference number in parenthesis.

Among the recent contributions to the knowledge of the epidemiology of IDDM emanating from registry-based studies are those of Green et al. in Funen County, Denmark (35–38). These highlight the heterogeneity of insulin-treated diabetes, and demonstrate a similar trend in incidence, with a peak in the mid 1970s. There was also evidence of seasonality in the Danish incidence data, which was not observed in data obtained from the Pittsburgh IDDM Registry (39). In the latter, a lower incidence was observed in nonwhite than white subjects of both sexes.

Data from the Pittsburgh registry also demonstrated age-specific incidence of IDDM in siblings of pre-existing cases 6–18 times that of the general population (40). A recent report from the Danish registry (41) demonstrated an excess mortality in male as against female IDDM cases in all categories studied, although the excess was greatest for diabetes mellitus itself and for cardiovascular diseases. This report also highlighted under-reporting of diabetes mellitus on death certificates. A further recent report from this registry (42) examined the use of hospital services amongst insulin-treated diabetic patients, and showed that hospital bed-day occupancy was five times that of the general population. Data from the Rhode Island Registry (32) indicate that hospitalization of IDDM cases is associated with poor control of disease, infection and poor socio-economic status.

The natural history of impaired glucose tolerance

The category of IGT was introduced by the National Diabetes Data Group in 1979 (3) and adopted by WHO in the following year (4). A substantial number of individuals who showed abnormal glucose tolerance after an oral glucose challenge which was insufficient to classify them as diabetic, were nevertheless known to be at increased risk of macrovascular disease (3, 4). Furthermore, preliminary studies suggested that such subjects had an unpredictable prognosis. The risk of diabetes appeared to be greater in those with IGT than in normal subjects yet a substantial proportion of the former were subsequently shown to revert to normoglycemia (3, 4).

Findings from longitudinal studies of IGT have recently appeared in the literature. Of these studies, two were from the United Kingdom (43, 44), one from Denmark (45), two from Japan (46, 47) and one from Nauru (48).

In all the studies which examined determinants of future diabetes, baseline blood glucose concentration was the most powerful and consistent predictor (43, 44, 46–48). Obesity was a further independent predictor in the two Japanese studies (46, 47), but was inconsistent in its effect in the studies in the United Kingdom (43, 44) and Nauru (48). Both the Bedford (47) and Danish (45) studies confirmed an excess in mortality in IGT, as compared with normal subjects.

Studies to date therefore support the recognition of IGT as an independent category of glucose tolerance. However, much work is still required to determine its full significance, and to identify the subset of IGT subjects who will eventually progress to overt diabetes.

Studies of the morbidity and mortality associated with diabetes

The importance of inter-ethnic comparisons of diabetes complications and their risk factors has been underlined by the WHO Multinational Study for Vascular Disease in Diabetes (49). While marked differences in prevalence of macrovascular disease were noted between the 14 national samples, prevalence of microvascular complications were very similar. West et al. (50) reported on risk factors for microangiopathy in 3583 diabetics from 9 of the 14 populations. The most consistent relationship was found with fasting plasma glucose (two-hour concentrations were not measured) and duration of diabetes.

In a separate study, King et al. (8) also studied risk factors for diabetic retinopathy in the diabetes-prone Nauruans. Although increasing two-hour plasma glucose significantly increased the risk of retinopathy, duration of disease was the strongest predictor variable. Rate et al. (51) found diabetic retinopathy to be strongly correlated with duration of diabetes in Hopi and Navajo Indians. However, in this study plasma glucose was not included in the analysis.

All of the above studies were cross-sectional in nature and it will only be with prospective studies that the importance of various risk factors can be assessed with confidence.

The WHO Multinational Study provided the opportunity to compare the prevalence of macrovascular disease in diabetics of different ethnic groups living in a variety of environments (52). The major variations in the prevalence of arterial disease between the populations (the lowest rates were in Oriental diabetics) could be accounted for in part by the risk factors studied i.e. fasting plasma glucose, systolic blood pressure, serum lipids, adiposity, duration of diabetes, smoking and treatment. The authors concluded that cultural and/or ethnic factors are more likely to contribute to the variation in arterial disease susceptibility than the diabetic state per se. They found that despite the major variation in arterial disease prevalence, the risk for diabetic women appeared to equal that for diabetic men.

This latter finding has some relevance, as in Western societies, non-diabetic women appear to have a favored status compared to men with regard to mortality attributable to ischemic heart disease (53). Jarrett et al. (54) studied mortality from coronary heart disease and all causes over 10 years in participants in the Bedford Survey (UK). Age corrected mortality rates from all causes and coronary heart disease were highest in diabetics and intermediate in subjects with IGT, and female IGT subjects showed a greater increase in mortality risk than men. During the 10 year follow-up of the Bedford IGT subjects, coronary heart disease morbidity and mortality rates were similar in men and women. These studies suggest that diabetes causes a loss of natural protection against cardiovascular disease in Western women.

The first population based study for diabetes was carried out in 1946–47 in Oxford, Massachussets, USA (55). Recently, O'Sullivan and Mahan have provided data on a case-control analysis of mortality relating to diabetes during a 29-year prospective study of this population (56). Mortality rates were significantly higher for diabetics than for age- and sex-matched controls, and disproportionately higher for women largely due to the advantageous mortality experience of non-diabetic women compared with non-diabetic men. The cardiovascular death rate among women with known diabetes was higher.

Barrett-Connor and Winegrad (57) confirmed the excess risk of fatal ischemic heart disease in diabetic women, after adjustment for cardiovascular disease risk factors, in Rancho Bernardo, USA (the relative risk was 2.5 for men and 3.4 for women). A possible explanation for this was provided in an earlier report by the same authors (53). They investigated the frequency and clustering of five heart disease risk factors – cholesterol, triglycerides, systolic blood pressure, obesity and cigarette smoking. Diabetics were more likely than non-diabetics to have high risk factor levels, although excess clustering of risk factors was statistically significant only in women.

Bender et al. (19) and Melton et al. (58) have assessed the bias produced by the study of clinic or hospital-based subjects. Both reports demonstrated that clinic or hospital-based studies produce a distortion in the apparent clinical spectrum of diabetes and its complications observed at different settings in the medical care system. They noted an overestimate of the relative frequency of IDDM and of the vascular complications of diabetes among hospital and diabetes clinic patients.

One of the few recent epidemiological reports on diabetes from Africa provides a good example of this problem. Lester has recently reported on the clinical pattern of diabetes in a clinic population in Ethiopia (59). Of the 847 subjects studied, 20% were classified as IDDM and 79% as NIDDM. Microvascular complications were common but macrovascular complications were rare.

The situation in Ethiopia is akin to that in many under-developed countries where malnutrition and infectious diseases are still the major problems confronting health services. Thus, while we call for more population studies from these nations, we must also be cognizant of international variation in health priorities.

The future of diabetes epidemiology

The many reports reviewed above are a testament to the recent activity and progress in diabetes epidemiology. From the relatively simple descriptive studies which dominated the diabetes literature a few years ago, we are now witnessing a shift towards increasing sophistication in study design and analytic techniques, incorporating longitudinal data and multicentre collaboration. These developments augur favorably for the future of diabetes epidemiology – both as a scientific discipline, and as a public health tool in the fight against this heterogeneous chronic disease which represents a major health burden worldwide.

References

1. Last JM (1983): *A Dictionary of Epidemiology, 1st ed*, p. 33. Oxford Medical Publications, Oxford.
2. West K (1978): *Epidemiology of Diabetes and its Vascular Lesions, 1st ed.* Elsevier, New York.
3. National Diabetes Data Group (1979): Classification and diagnosis of diabetes mellitus and other categories of glucose intolerance. *Diabetes*, *28*, 1038.
4. WHO Expert Committee on Diabetes Mellitus (1980): *Second Report, Technical Series 646*. WHO, Geneva.
5. Zimmet P (1982): Type 2 (non-insulin-dependent) diabetes – an epidemiological overview. *Diabetologia*, *22*, 399.
6. Zimmet P (1983): Epidemiology of diabetes mellitus. In: *Diabetes Mellitus – Theory and Practice*, *3rd ed.*, pp 451–468. Editors: M. Ellenberg and H. Rifkin. Medical Examination Publishing Co., Inc., New York.

7. Serjeantson SW, Owerbach D, Zimmet P, Nerup J, Thoma K (1983): Genetics of diabetes in Nauru: Effects of foreign admixture, HLA antigens and the insulin-gene-linked polymorphism. *Diabetologia, 25*, 13.
8. King H, Balkau B, Zimmet P, Taylor R, Raper LR, Borger J and Heriot W (1983): Diabetic retinopathy in Nauruans. *Am. J. Epidemiol. 117*, 659.
9. Gardner LI, Stern MP, Haffner SM, Gaskill SP, Hazuda HP, Relethford JH, Eifler CW (1984): Prevalence of diabetes in Mexican Americans: relationship to percent of gene pool derived from native American sources. *Diabetes, 33*, 86.
10. Barnett AH, Eff C, Leslie RDG, Pyke DA (1981): Diabetes in identical twins. A study in 200 pairs. *Diabetologia, 20*, 87.
11. Taylor R, Zimmet P (1983): Migrant studies in diabetes epidemiology. In: *Diabetes in Epidemiological Perspective*, pp 58–77. Editors: J.I. Mann, K. Pyörälä, A. Teuscher. Churchill/Livingstone, Edinburgh.
12. Zimmet P, King H (1982): The role of obesity in the high prevalence of diabetes in Pacific populations. In: *Proceedings of the Nutrition Society of Australia, Vol. 7*, pp 69–75. Nutrition Society of Australia. Brown Prior Anderson Pty Ltd, Melbourne.
13. King H, Zimmet P, Raper LR, Balkau B (1984): Risk factors for diabetes in three Pacific populations. *Am. J. Epidemiol.*, 119, 396.
14. Stern, MP, Gaskill SP, Hazuda HP, Gardner LI, Haffner SM (1983): Does obesity explain excess prevalence of diabetes among Mexican Americans? Results of the San Antonio Heart Study. *Diabetologia, 14*, 272.
15. Knowler WC, Bennett PH, Pettit PJ, Savage PJ (1981): Diabetes incidence in Pima Indians: Contributions of obesity and parental diabetes. *Am. J. Epidemiol., 113*, 144.
16. Pettitt DJ, Baird HR, Kirk MS, Aleck KA, Bennett PH, Knowler WC (1983): Excessive obesity in offspring of Pima Indian women with diabetes during pregnancy. *N. Engl. J. Med., 308*, 242.
17. Knowler WC, Savage PJ, Nagulesparan M, Howar BV, Pettit DJ, Lisse JR, Aronoff SL, Bennett PH (1982): Obesity, insulin resistance and diabetes mellitus in the Pima Indians. In: *The Genetics of Diabetes Mellitus, Proceedings of the Serono Symposia, Vol. 47*, pp 243–50. Editors: J. Köbberling and R. Tattersall. Academic Press, London.
18. Zimmet P, King H, Taylor R, Raper LR, Balkau B, Borger J, Heriot W, Thoma K (1984). The high prevalence of diabetes mellitus, impaired glucose tolerance and diabetec retinopathy in Nauru – The 1982 Survey. *Diabetes Res., 1*, 13.
19. Bender AP, Sprafka JM, Jagger H, Wannamaker J, Muckala KH (1983): Incidence, prevalence, mortality and population-based profile of diabetes mellitus in Wadena, Minnesota, 1981. *Minnesota Med., 66*, 383.
20. Melton LJ, Palumbo PJ, Chu CP (1983): Incidence of Diabetes Mellitus by clinical type. *Diabetes Care, 6*, 75.
21. Tan MH, Wornell MC, Beck AW (1981): Epidemiology of diabetes mellitus in Prince Edward Island. *Diabetes Care, 4*, 519.
22. Barker DJP, Gardner MJ, Power C (1982): Incidence of diabetes amongst people aged 18–50 years in nine British towns: a collaborative study. *Diabetologia, 22*, 421.

23. Butler W, Ostrander LD, Carman WJ, Lamphiear DE (1982): Diabetes mellitus in Tecumseh, Michigan. Prevalence, incidence and associated conditions. *Am. J. Epidemol.*, *116*, 971.
24. Zimmet P, Pinkstone G, Whitehouse S, Thoma K (1982): The high incidence of diabetes mellitus in the Micronesian population of Nauru. *Acta Diabetol. Lat.*, *19*, 75.
25. Knowler WC, Bennett PH, Hamman RF, Miller M (1978): Diabetes incidence and prevalence in Pima Indians: A 19-fold greater incidence than in Rochester, Minnesota. *Am. J. Epidemiol.*, *108*, 497.
26. Taha TH, Moussa MAA, Rashid AR, Fenech FF (1983): Diabetes Mellitus in Kuwait – Incidence in the first 29 years of life. *Diabetologia*, *25*, 206.
27. Hägglöf B, Holmgren G, Wall S (1982): Incidence of insulin-dependent diabetes mellitus among children in a North-Swedish population 1938–1977. *Hum. Hered.*, *32*, 408.
28. Reunanen A, Åkerblom HK, Käär M-L (1982): Prevalence and ten-year (1970–1979) incidence of insulin-dependent diabetes mellitus in children and adolescents in Finland. *Acta Paediatr. Scand.*, *71*, 892.
29. Vaandrager GJ, Bruining GJ, Veenhof FJ, Drayer NM (1983): The incidence of insulin-dependent diabetes mellitus in the young (0–19 years) during 1978–1980 in the Netherlands. *Ned. Tijdschr. Geneeskd.*, *127*, 2344.
30. Patterson CC, Thorogood M, Smith PG, Heasman MA, Clarke JA, Mann JI (1983): Epidemiology of Type 1 (insulin-dependent) diabetes in Scotland 1968–1976: Evidence of an increasing incidence. *Diabetologia*, *24*, 238.
31. LaPorte RE, Fishbein HA, Drash AL, Kuller LH, Schneider BB, Orchard TJ, Wagener DR (1981): The Pittsburgh insulin-dependent diabetes mellitus (IDDM) registry: The incidence of insulin-dependent diabetes in Allegheny County, Pennsylvania (1965–1976). *Diabetes*, *30*, 279.
32. Fishbein HA, Faich GA, Ellis SE (1982): Incidence and hospitalization patterns of insulin-dependent diabetes mellitus. *Diabetes Care*, *5*, 630.
33. Ehrlich RM, Walsh LJ, Falk JA, Middleton PJ, Simpson NE (1982): The incidence of Type 1 (insulin-dependent) diabetes in Toronto. *Diabetologia*, *22*, 289.
34. LaPorte R, Tajima N, Åkerblom HR et al. (1984): Geographic differences in the risk of insulin-dependent diabetes mellitus. Thc importance of registries. Unpublished manuscript.
35. Green A, Hauge M, Holm NV, Rasch LL (1980): Epidemiological studies of diabetes mellitus in Denmark. 1. A case finding method based on the National Service Conscript Registry. *Diabetologia*, *19*, 355.
36. Green A, Hauge M, Holm NV, Rasch LL (1981): Epidemiological studies of diabetes mellitus in Denmark. 2. A prevalence study based on insulin prescriptions. *Diabetologia*, *20*, 468.
37. Green A, Andersen PK (1983): Epidemiological studies of diabetes mellitus in Denmark: 3. Clinical characteristics and incidence of diabetes among males aged 0 to 19 years. *Diabetologia*, *25*, 226.
38. Green A, Hougaard P (1983): Epidemiological studies of diabetes mellitus in Denmark: 4. Clinical characteristics of insulin-treated diabetes. *Diabetologia*, *25*, 231.

39. Fishbein HA, LaPorte RE, Orchard TJ, Drash AL, Kuller LH, Wagener DK (1982): The Pittsburgh Insulin-Dependent Diabetes Mellitus Registry: seasonal incidence. *Diabetologia*, *23*, 83.
40. Wagener D, Kuller L, Orchard T, LaPorte R, Rabin B, Drash A (1982): Pittsburgh Diabetes Mellitus Study – II. Secondary attack rates in families with insulin-dependent diabetes mellitus. *Am. J. Epidemiol.*, *115*, 868.
41. Green A, Hougaard P (1984): Epidemiological studies of diabetes mellitus in Denmark. 5. Mortality and causes of death among insulin-treated diabetics. *Diabetologia*, *26*, 190.
42. Green A, Solander F (1984): Epidemiological studies of diabetes mellitus in Denmark. 6. Use of hospital services by insulin-treated diabetics. *Diabetologia*, *26*, 195.
43. Jarrett RJ, Keen H, Fuller JH, McCartney M (1979): Worsening to diabetes in men with impaired glucose tolerance ('borderline diabetes'). *Diabetologia*, *16*, 25.
44. Keen H, Jarrett RJ, McCartney P (1982): The ten-year follow-up of the Bedford survey (1962–1972): glucose tolerance and diabetes. *Diabetologia*, *22*, 73.
45. Agner E, Thorsteinsson B, Eriksen M (1982): Impaired glucose tolerance and diabetes mellitus in elderly subjects. *Diabetes Care*, *5*, 600.
46. Sasaki A, Suzuki T, Horiuchi N (1982): Development of diabetes in Japanese subjects with impaired glucose tolerance: a seven year follow-up study. *Diabetologia*, *22*, 154.
47. Kadowaki T, Miyake Y, Hagura R, Akanuma Y, Kajinuma H, Kuzuya N, Takaku F, Kosaka K (1984): Risk factors for worsening to diabetes in subjects with impaired glucose tolerance. *Diabetologia*, *26*, 44.
48. King H, Zimmet P, Raper LR, Balkau B (1984): The natural history of impaired glucose tolerance in the Micronesian population of Nauru: a six-year follow-up study. *Diabetologia*, *26*, 39.
49. Jarrett RJ, Keen H, Grabauskas V (1979): The WHO Multinational Study of Vascular Disease in Diabetes: 1. General Description. *Diabetes Care*, *2*, 175.
50. West KM, Ahuja MMS, Bennett PH, Czyzyk A, Mateo de Acosta O, Fuller JH, Arab B, Arabauskas V, Jarrett J, Kosaka K, Keen H, Krolewski AS, Miki E, Schliack V, Teuscher A, Watkins PJ, Stober JA (1983): The role of circulating glucose and triglyceride concentrations and their interactions with other 'risk factors' as determinants of arterial disease in nine diabetic population samples from the WHO Multinational Study. *Diabetes Care*, *6*, 361.
51. Rate RG, Knowler WC, Morse HG et al (1983): Diabetes Mellitus in Hopi and Navajo Indians – prevalence of microvascular complications. *Diabetes*, *32*, 894.
52. Keen H, Jarrett RJ (1979): The WHO Multinational Study of Vascular Disease in Diabetes: 2. Macrovascular disease prevalence. *Diabetes Care*, *2*, 187.
53. Wingard DL, Barrett-Connor E, Criqui MH, Suarez L (1983): Clustering of heart disease risk factors in diabetic compared to nondiabetic adults. *Am. J. Epidemiol.*, *117*, 19.

54. Jarrett RJ, McCartney P, Keen H (1982): The Bedford Survey: Ten year mortality rates in newly diagnosed diabetics, borderline diabetics and normoglycaemic controls and risk indices for coronary heart disease in borderline diabetics. *Diabetologia*, *22*, 79.
55. Wilkerson HLC, Krall LP (1947): Diabetes in a New England town: a study of 3516 persons in Oxford, Mass. *J. Am. Med. Assoc.*, *135*, 209.
56. O'Sullivan JB, Mahan CM (1982): Mortality related to diabetes and blood glucose levels in a community study. *Am. J. Epidemiol.*, *116*, 678.
57. Barrett-Connor E, Wingard DL (1983): Sex differential in ischaemic heart disease mortality in diabetics: a prospective population-based study. *Am. J. Epidemiol.*, *118*, 489.
58. Melton LJ, Ochi JW, Pasquale BA, Palumbo J, Chu CP (1984): Referral bias in diabetes research. *Diabetes Care*, *7*, 12.
59. Lester FT (1984): The clinical pattern of diabetes mellitus in Ethopians. *Diabetes Care*, *7*, 6.

The Diabetes Annual/1
K.G.M.M. Alberti and L.P. Krall, editors

ISBN 0444 90 343 7
$0.85 per article per page (transactional system)
$0.20 per article per page (licensing system)

2 Etiology of diabetes: the role of autoimmune mechanisms

GIAN FRANCO BOTTAZZO, RICARDO PUJOL-BORRELL AND EDWIN GALE

The past decade has witnessed tremendous advances in our understanding of the role that a variety of immunological processes may play in initiating and sustaining damage to pancreatic B-cells. An elegant description of the insulitis process, characterized by infiltration of the islets by mononuclear cells (1) was already available in the mid-sixties, and suggested the attractive hypothesis of an immune basis to Type 1 diabetes. In the early seventies specific cell-mediated immune phenomena (2) directed against pancreatic extracts were demonstrated, and cytoplasmic islet cell antibodies were described (3). The genetic connection of the disease with the HLA system (4, 5) then set the scene for a rapid expansion of interest. This is reflected in the number of symposia and workshops which have been organized since the first 'Immunology of Diabetes' meeting was held in Brussels in 1973 (6). There followed symposia in 1975 (7), 1978 (8) and 1982 (9). The workshop held in London in 1983 (10, 11) and the recent symposium in Rome have helped to bring the subject up to date and to serve as a common focus for workers in many different aspects of diabetes. A book was circulated during the latter symposium (12), and some of the more significant papers were published separately (13).

A process of slow destruction

The role of autoimmunity

The most exciting development in recent years has been the demonstration that, despite the acute onset of clinical symptoms, the disease results from long, slow and progressive damage to the pancreatic B-cells (14). This evidence was obtained primarily by the study of unaffected first degree

Research in the author's Departments is supported by the Juvenile Diabetes Foundation (USA), Medical Research Council, British Diabetic Association, Joint Research Board of St Bartholomew's Medical College, Wellcome Trust Foundation, and Novo Research Institute, Copenhagen.

relatives of patients with childhood diabetes (15). At the same time it was shown that siblings who shared one or two HLA-haplotypes with the diabetic proband had a greatly increased risk of developing the disease (16). These genetic markers and the presence of a variety of islet cell antibodies (ICA) identify potential candidates for Type 1 diabetes with a reasonably high degree of precision. Complement-fixing ICA (CF-ICA) (17) appears to be the most specific marker of incipient diabetes but islet cell surface antibodies (ICSA) (18) and cytotoxic ICA (19) have also been demonstrated years before the disease becomes manifest. Similar results have come from other prospective (20, 21, 22, 23) and cross-sectional (24–26) family studies. According to these reports, between 5 and 15% of unaffected relatives have one or more types of islet cell antibody. The variable frequency of ICA may be attributed to differences in techniques used for their determination (vide infra). The predictive value of ICA has also been confirmed by the study of monozygotic triplets (27) and twins (Johnston, personal communication) in whom one had diabetes while co-twins or triplets were discordant for diabetes for 5 years or more.

In patients with more than one autoimmune disease ICAs, and in particular CF-ICAs, also predict future dependence on insulin (28). Autoimmune disease is more likely to be present in families with 2 diabetic probands, and conversely diabetes is more common in families affected by autoimmune disorders (25). Prospective investigation of islet cell function in non-diabetic individuals carrying ICA has demonstrated significant impairment of the first phase insulin response to intravenous glucose, a change demonstrable as much as 7 years before onset of the clinical disorder (29). The earliest metabolic abnormalities coincided with the appearance of ICA in some individuals. In contrast, HLA-identical siblings negative for ICA showed an exaggerated first phase response to intravenous glucose or arginine (30), an observation that awaits confirmation.

All the prospective studies carried out to date indicate that individuals in whom cytoplasmic ICA persists will almost inevitably become diabetic. In the London family study, however, in which family members were followed at 3–5-month intervals over a period of 6 years, certain individuals with ICA at entry have as yet shown no sign of glucose intolerance. Retrospective analysis suggests that despite persistence of ICA detected with anti-IgG sera, the ability to fix complement has been lost (31). Other groups (32, 33) have pointed out that the negative results for CF-ICA might be due to declining titers of ICA (34). Titration experiments will be needed to settle this issue. In all other prospective studies conducted to date the persistence of a strong ICA reaction has ultimately led to the development of diabetes, but since November 1981, when the last of 7 family members developed diabetes, none of the remaining ICA-positive individuals in the London study have contracted the disease (up to August 1984).

These ICA-positive subjects were also monitored for possible variations in T-lymphocyte subsets in an 18-month prospective follow-up study (35). No significant changes were observed, and 'activated' T-lymphocytes (vide infra) were detected only occasionally. More 'high-risk' individuals need to be assessed over long periods before the relevance of these observations becomes apparent.

The role of the environment

The seasonal incidence of childhood diabetes and serological studies have suggested a viral etiology (36–38). The problem is to identify the point in the prediabetic period at which this attack is launched. Two case histories exemplify this difficulty. In one long-term prospective study (39), a girl became diabetic 3 years after entry. Retrospective analysis provided serological confirmation that she and other family members had experienced a Coxsackie B4 infection, but her serum was already positive for ICA when she contracted the viral infection. More recently, a young boy developed diabetes 3 months after an episode of mumps. Six months before the episode he had symptoms of a mild viral type of infection, and at that time his serum contained no anti-mumps antibodies but was already positive for ICA (40).

Another potential model of the interplay between viral infection and immunological factors is the association of diabetes with the congenital rubella syndrome. In a large retrospective study ICSA were demonstrated in a proportion of these individuals before the onset of diabetes, and in some, they were already present at birth (41). It is interesting to note that HLA-DR3 was more frequently present in these patients, while the frequency of HLA-DR2 was reduced – as in Type 1 diabetes (42). About half also had thyroid antibodies. The real question remains: is the B-cell damage due to direct viral attack, or to an autoimmune process superimposed on viral damage sustained early in life?

The theme of early damage crops up again with the startling suggestion that the initial B-cell damage might be programmed at the time of conception, due to the ingestion of toxic substances by the mother (43). While the hypothesis has its attractions, it has not been confirmed in other studies (44) although in a subsequent experimental model a typical pattern of insulitis was observed (45).

Cytoplasmic ICA: the state of the art

The first account of cytoplasmic islet cell antibodies was followed by the description of several other species of islet cell antibodies in the sera of patients with diabetes (Table 1). These findings reinforce the concept of a broad-based heterogenous response to several B-cell autoantigens.

ICA represents a polyclonal autoimmune response composed entirely of IgG predominantly of the IgG2 subclass. This is in contrast to a wider class and subclass distribution of autoantibodies in thyroid and gastric autoimmunity (46). There is still some disagreement as to whether IgG2 (46) or IgG1 (34) predominates when such restriction is less marked. This discrepancy could be due to differences in affinity and specificity of the anti-subclass antisera commercially available. It has been shown that the ability of

TABLE 1. *Varieties of islet cell antibodies*

Antigen	Method of detection	Abbreviation most commonly used
Cytoplasmic and common to all islet cell types	(a) Indirect immunofluorescence on cryostat sections (from snap-frozen blood group O) human pancreas	ICA-IgG ICA-c
Cytoplasmic, only B-cells?	(b) Complement fixation immuno-fluorescence technique on cryostat sections (from snap-frozen blood group O) human pancreas	CF-ICA
Islet cell membrane	(c) Immunofluorescence on viable islet cells from human-fetal, rat or mouse pancreas	ICSA
Islet cell membrane	(d) ^{125}I-staphylococcus protein A on dispersed rodent islet cells	ICSA
	^{53}Cr release/vital staining on rodent islet cells or rat insulinoma cell line cultures	Cytotoxic antibody
Detergent lysates from human islet cells	(e) Immunoprecipitation	64K
Detergent lysates from DR3 human islet cells	(e) Immunoprecipitation	38K
Pancreatic cells (glucagon cells)	(a) and (b) More emphasis on CF	GPCA (glucagon producing cell antibodies)
Pancreatic cells (somatostatin cells)	(a) and (b)	SPCA (somatostatin producing cell antibodies)

ICA to fix complement is independent of the titer or subclass composition (46), a result which has yet to be confirmed (34).

Unfixed Group O human pancreas is still the substrate of choice for routine screening of ICA. Pancreatic specimens need to be selected carefully for a high antigen content if reliable results are to be obtained, especially because of the known weak positive staining of ICA. It has been suggested that sera previously scored negative will become positive after repeated or prolonged (up to 24 hours) incubation (34, 47). The sensitivity of the test can vary widely depending on the age of the donor and the period of warm ischemia before the tissue is frozen (48). Variations between observers, laboratories, and commercial antihuman immunoglobulin preparations need to be taken into account if a standardized system is to be developed.

In some countries it is difficult to obtain fresh cadaveric pancreas from kidney donors and this has prompted a move to perform the ICA test on fixed tissues. Despite the enthusiasm with which the initial report (49) was received, several laboratories encountered problems in adapting the technique, especially with respect to interpretation of the ICA staining pattern (50, 51). Moreover, the test was rendered laborious by the need to pre-incubate all sera with insulin to remove insulin antibodies, since these would otherwise stain insulin-producing cells on sections of fixed pancreas. Normal human sera often stain the fixed islets non-specifically, and the CF-ICA test is not feasible because complement itself attaches to the islets (52). Although certain laboratories remain in favor of using fixed pancreas (53), the general opinion, now shared by the original proponents (54), is that this source of tissue is not ideal and should perhaps be abandoned.

Islet cell surface antibodies (ICSA): theoretical interest or practical use?

ICSA would certainly appear to have greater pathogenic significance than ICA, since they represent the initial attack on the plasma membrane of viable B-cells. At present, however, ICA retain their usefulness for routine screening.

ICSA are detected by fluorescence or *Staphylococcus aureus* protein A techniques on viable cultured human fetal (55) or adult animal pancreas (56). Since human sera contain heterophile antibodies which stain animal pancreas non-specifically, despite prolonged absorption with other animal tissues, human islets (although hard to obtain) remain the tissue of choice. In both human and animal tissues diabetic sera contain separate specificities for B- and to a lesser extent A- and D-cells. Using a cell sorter technique to separate the ICSA-positive cells (57) a small number of sera were identified containing surface reacting antibodies to pancreatic polypeptide (PP) cells. Antibodies to these cells have not as yet been detected on cryostat sections, probably because it is necessary to employ the mid-posterior portion of the head of the pancreas, which is known to be rich in PP-cells (58).

A high proportion of newly diagnosed diabetic sera contain ICSA, but about 30% give negative results on sections (56). This suggests the involvement of an additional antigen that is expressed entirely on the plasma membrane of B-cells.

ICSA have cytotoxic effects 'in vitro', when fresh complement is added to the culture medium. The lysing effect is preferentially against insulin cells as assessed using vital dyes (59) or the ^{51}Cr release assay (60). Newly diagnosed diabetic children undergoing treatment with plasmapheresis (61) show a rebound of complement-fixing ICSA cytotoxic for a rat insulinoma cell line when treatment is stopped. The presence of these antibodies at diagnosis does not correlate with residual B-cell function, and they tend to disappear in the course of time like other autoimmune phenomena in Type 1 diabetes.

Immunoglobulin preparations obtained from ICSA-positive sera produced significant inhibition of glucose-induced insulin release when isolated rat islet cells were incubated for a short period without the addition of complement (62). It has also been claimed that when islets from human (63) or animal (64) pancreas are incubated with diabetic sera, repeated addition of complement over 18 hours resulted in potent inhibition of insulin secretion. Arginine-stimulated glucagon release remained unchanged. The role of complement, either in exerting direct cytotoxic effects or enhancing blockade of secretion mechanisms by ICSA, has yet to be clarified (65). In all experiments of this type it is highly advisable to check islet cell viability when experiments are performed in the presence of complement.

In selected sera it has been found that certain ICSA do not exert complement dependent cytotoxicity, but rather have a potent lytic effect in an antibody-dependent cell-mediated cytotoxicity (ADCC) system. This primarily involves killer (K) lymphocytes (66). In these experiments a human fetal B-cell line was employed and the lack of complement-mediated cytotoxicity may be explained by the reduced number of surface autoantigen molecules recognized by ICSA. In this situation complement cannot effectively bridge and complete its cascade of lytic events, but cell interaction does permit this cytotoxic process to take place.

Successful passive transfer of ICSA to experimental animals has been described. Perfused pancreas from mice injected with immunoglobulin from newly diagnosed diabetic patients showed inhibition of insulin release in response to appropriate stimuli (67). Visual demonstration of immunoglobulin deposition within the islets has also been observed in similar passive transfer experiments (68).

Isolation and characterization of islet cell autoantigens

Only one set of islet cell antigens has so far been identified. This has a molecular weight of 64,000, as shown by immunoprecipitation methods using sera from recently diagnosed patients and a detergent lysate of isolated human islets labelled with 35S methionine (69). A possible second antigen with a molecular weight of 38,000 was also precipitated, but was only found to be present when an HLA-DR3 donor pancreas was used. The latter finding requires confirmation. It remains to be established whether the protein complex precipitated in the 64K band represents the full set of B-cell autoantigens expressed selectively in the cytoplasm, plasma membrane, or both, including all the specific epitopes recognized by the various circulating ICAs. No reports on the further purification and characterization of this target protein have as yet appeared. One approach is by analysis of the amino acid sequence of the 64K band and subsequent use of recombinant DNA techniques, which would permit in-vitro production of this autoantigen in large quantities.

A paramount problem for future research is that of obtaining islet cells in adequate numbers. A high yield of animal islet cells has been obtained from a radiation-induced rat insulinoma (70), but the problem with animal islets is that they express some autoantigens that are similar, but also some that are quite different from human islets. The recent description of a B-cell line derived from human fetal islets has brought new hopes that human material could soon be available in large amounts (66). Alternatively, isolation and subsequent purification of islet cell autoantigens might be achieved by fusion of lymphocytes from diabetic patients with appropriate myeloma cell lines. The results obtained so far with mouse or human myeloma cell partners have led to the production of monoclonal antibodies which do not resemble spontaneously produced human ICA. In diabetics cytoplasmic ICA react with all islet cells (71) are entirely organ-specific and exclusively of IgG class. The most relevant monoclonal antibodies to islet cells described to date are of the IgM class. One reacts with glucagon cells only (72) and a second stains the whole islet but with a linear pattern which differs from the granular diffuse cytoplasmic fluorescence of human ICA, and cross-reacts with a surface molecule on 'activated' T-lymphocytes (4F2) (73). A newer antibody gives an IFL pattern identical to the human antibodies, but cross-reacts with various endocrine organs and gastric parietal cells (74). The attempt to produce specific monoclonal islet cell antibodies is under way in several laboratories.

Clinical significance of ICA: relevance to practical management

It is now generally accepted that ICAs are organ-specific antibody markers closely related to Type 1 diabetes. They are present in 70-80% of patients at diagnosis and tend to disappear thereafter. Some series have identified a proportion of patients in whom ICAs are invariably negative, regardless of the methodology used. Such a group has been described in black diabetic patients (75) and it is of interest that these possess neither HLA-DR3 nor HLA-DR4. A subgroup of Finnish patients in whom ICA negativity is associated with the possession of HLA-B69 has also been described (76). It is worth bearing in mind that the incidence of diabetes in Finland is double that of the rest of the world. The reason for this is unknown, but could provide useful clues to the basic pathogenic mechanisms.

ICA determinations have been used in many studies of large populations with differing ethnic and genetic backgrounds (77–80). These studies have shown that the caucasoid diabetic population has the greatest prevalence of ICA. In addition, the pattern of persistence or disappearance of ICA in diabetic patients has greatly reinforced the concept of heterogeneity within Type 1 diabetes (81), already foreseen on genetic grounds in parallel studies (82). The best evidence in support of heterogeneity is offered by female patients carrying HLA-DR3, in whom persistence of islet cell antibodies is associated with serological and clinical evidence of other autoimmune endocrine manifestations.

Patients with overt polyendocrine disease and mild glucose intolerance show an increased frequency of ICA (83). When Type 2 patients with no evidence of other endocrine disorders are tested for ICA, a subgroup of ICA-positive individuals, forming about 10% of this population (84) has been demonstrated and they have an increased prevalence of HLA-DR3 (85). These patients also had a lower stimulated C-peptide response (86). The presence of ICA predicts a need for insulin therapy in these 'pseudo' Type 2 patients.

Should immunosuppressive drugs be used in the early treatment of Type 1 diabetes (87)? If so, the relevance of these immunological markers may need to be reassessed. Controlled trials would then compare patients in whom various islet cell antibodies and evidence of pancreatic cell mediated immunity were present with patients who do not possess these markers. Various unsuccessful attempts have been made to see whether the presence of ICA is of value in predicting the course of clinical diabetes. Prospective monitoring of ICA during the 'honeymoon' period has yet to clarify the obscure events underlying the remission phenomenon (88) but suggests an inverse relationship with residual B-cell function as measured by determination of C-peptide (89, 90), although conflicting results were obtained in another study (91), possibly owing to differences in patient selection.

Cell-mediated immunity (CMI)

Our understanding of the role of cell-mediated immunity in the pathogenesis of Type 1 diabetes has progressed slowly when compared with the rapidity of developments in the field of pancreatic humoral autoimmunity. There are several possible reasons for this. CMI techniques are much more laborious and lack the precision needed to dissect such an heterogenous cell population. Basic immunology is still struggling in its attempt to define the physiological mechanisms underlying this arm of the immune system. Even the monoclonal antibody revolution has not helped to clarify this issue. With these reagents it is now possible to identify various subsets of lymphocytes and other immune cells (92). Even so, as illustrated in Table 2, studies with the specific aim of detecting abnormalities of lymphocyte subpopulations at the time of diagnosis (93–106) and prospectively

TABLE 2. *Lymphocyte abnormalities in diabetes mellitus*

Lymphocyte population	Technique or monoclonal Ab	Alterations detected	Ref.
Total T-cells	E-rosettes	decrease	(93)
	OKT3	decrease	(94,95)
	UCHT1	no difference	(96, 97)
	Leu4	decrease	(98)
Helper/inducer	OKT4	decrease	(93, 94, 99)
		no difference	(100, 101)
		increase	(96, 102)
	Leu3A	no difference	(97)
		decrease	(99)
	3A1	no difference	(100)
		decrease	(95, 96, 101, 102)
Suppressor/cytotoxic	OKT8	decrease	(95, 96, 101, 102)
		no difference	(93, 100)
'Activated' T-lymphocytes	anti-DR, 4F2, TAC	increase	(35, 97, 100, 103**)
'Activated' T-helper	5/9	decrease	(104)
Natural killer cells (NK)	Leu7, Leu11a	decrease	(98,104)
Killer cells	low affinity rosettes	increase	(105)
Monocytes	OKM1	decrease	(95)
Helper/suppressor ratio	OKT4/OKT8	no difference	(100, 101)
		increase	(94, 95, 96, 106)
		decrease	(93*, 99, 106)

* Tested when good metabolic control was already achieved.

** Prospective and twin studies.

thereafter (97, 102) have failed to reach significant conclusions (107). Disagreement mainly concerns the total number of T-lymphocytes, helper and cytotoxic/suppressor lymphocytes. Several explanations can be found for these discrepancies. There is inter-laboratory and inter-observer variation, lack of standardization of reagents and, perhaps most important, a lack of very early cases, since we know that immunological abnormalities tend to disappear from the time symptoms appear. Another important factor, often underestimated, is the effect on the immune system of the profound metabolic derangement produced by the disease itself (93).

The most consistent results have been obtained by measurement of 'activated' T-cells at the time of diagnosis (97, 100). Here again, these tend to re-enter the normal range within months of starting on insulin therapy (103). T-cells, when stimulated by antigens, express new surface markers which are essential for an efficient participation in the immune response. The best characterized of these molecules are the HLA-DR series, T-cell growth factor receptor (interleukin 2, IL-2, defined as Tac^+ cells by monoclonal antibody), transferrin receptors and a less specific molecule known as 4F2. The present hypothesis is that T-cells are activated in diabetes because they have been stimulated specifically by pancreatic antigens, and not just triggered by environmental agents. One method to test this hypothesis is to clone autoreactive T-lymphocytes. This can be done by taking advantage of the expression of T-cell growth factor receptors, which in the presence of IL-2 allow T-cells to divide further and ultimately to be cloned by the limiting dilution technique (108). Using this approach, it has become possible to establish specific lines and clones which recognize acetylcholine receptors in myasthenia gravis (109) and autologous thyrocytes in autoimmune thyroid disease (110). A similar method has been applied in diabetes and Tac^+, i.e. 'activated' T-cells, which were shown to be elevated in about 6% of diabetic patients with a duration of less than 2 years, proliferated in the presence of IL-2. This was shown by measurement of increased thymidine uptake in a 6-day culture proliferating assay (111). Unfortunately, the expansion to a T-cell clone and the final characterization of the cell line was not possible because of lack of sufficient islet cell antigens. If this problem were overcome, it would allow the establishment of T-cell clones specifically recognizing pancreatic B-cells.

Decreased T-suppressor cell activity, as measured by non-specific functional assay, has been described in patients with a short duration of diabetes (112). In a similar population, suppressor cell function was found to be defective when islet cell antigens were used in the system (113). Evidence of an organ-specific suppressor T-cell defect in diabetes and other endocrine autoimmune diseases has been obtained using the direct leukocyte migration inhibition (LMI) test (114). Leukocytes from patients with Type 1 diabetes, previously shown to respond to an insulinoma extract, lost their MIF specificity when co-cultured with normal lymphocytes, and more significantly, with lymphocytes from patients with autoimmune thyroid disease. Conversely, T-lymphocytes from diabetic patients, thus sensitized to islet cell antigen but not to thyroid antigen, ameliorated the migration inhibition of T-lymphocytes from autoimmune thyroid disease in response to thyroid antigens. Interpretation of these results relied on the assumption that adding a small number of normally functioning T-suppressor cells is sufficient to compensate a selective suppressor T-cell defect in response to islet and other endocrine cell antigens. Even though these experiments are technically complicated, and interpretation is sometimes controversial, it is of interest that similar results have been obtained in autoimmune liver disease (115) and gluten enteropathy (116).

Killer lymphocytes have previously been found to be elevated in Type 1 diabetic patients at the time of diagnosis, using the low affinity E-rosette technique (105). Other studies have in contrast suggested that patients have a reduced number of these cells at the time of diagnosis. These results were obtained using monoclonal antibodies which define phenotypically distinct populations of killer cells (98). These include large granular lymphocytes or natural killer cells and lymphocytes with receptors for the Fc portion of IgG, the classic killer cells. In this context it is worth reporting that a non-T-cell enriched population separated from similar patients showed excessive cytotoxicity against rat islet cells (117) and mononuclear cell preparations were able to block insulin secretion from mouse islet cells in response to challenge with appropriate stimuli (118). Discrepancies in these results might be explained by the known heterogeneity of the immune response in diabetic patients, but it seems more likely that the enumeration of cells by phenotypic markers does not necessarily correspond to the functional state of these abnormal lymphoid cells (119).

Evidence of polyclonal B-lymphocyte activation by means of generation of antibody-secreting plaque-forming cells has also been shown in about 50% of newly diagnosed patients with diabetes (120). These data confirm previous findings in patients in whom diabetes was associated with Hashimoto thyroiditis (106). This suggests that B-lymphocytes in diabetic patients are under loose control, and are more likely to produce autoantibodies. The T-cell population with its different regulatory arms is failing to maintain control over the whole system. At present it is hard to identify the point at which such a defect, or defects, reside. Abnormal production of certain lymphokines such as IL-2 (121) and even insulin deficiency itself, which has important metabolic effects upon lymphocyte function and insulin receptor expression (122) may contribute to the fine dysregulation of T- or B-lymphocytes enabling them to mount an autoimmune response against pancreatic B-cells. Only one report has described lymphocyte homing into the pancreas in 2 out of 3 juvenile cases. Separated lymphocytes labelled with Indium III were reinjected into the patient and the distribution of tracer was increased in the pancreatic region (123) to monitor the insulitis process directly 'in vivo'. Experience in the use of this technique is still limited and these results should be interpreted with caution.

Other distinct autoimmune phenomena: new clues to the pathogenesis of Type 1 diabetes

The spontaneous development of insulin autoantibodies is becoming increasingly important within the context of pancreatic autoimmunity. The full 'insulin autoimmune syndrome' is mainly seen in Japan (124) but exists in other countries to a lesser extent (125). The patients, most of whom had thyrotoxicosis treated with methimazole, present with attacks of hypoglycemia which may recur over months but with a tendency to spontaneous remission. Insulin antibodies have also been described in newly diagnosed patients with Type 1 diabetes (126) and in some non-diabetic polyendocrine cases (127). Although criticisms have been raised on technical points related to measurement of these antibodies by RIA or ELISA, it is possible that previous failure to demonstrate spontaneous anti-insulin autoantibodies in diabetic patients could be because these specificities are in the form of immune complexes and need to be dissociated before being tested. Information is not yet available on the correlation of these specificities with classical ICA.

Related to this interesting finding is the description of insulin receptor antibodies of the IgM class in untreated young insulin-dependent diabetic patients (128). Until now IgG anti-insulin receptor antibodies were associated with a rare form of diabetes characterized by extreme insulin resistance and associated with acanthosis nigricans (129). The antibodies in the diabetic children were able to displace radioactive insulin from its receptors and also stimulated adipocyte metabolism. Although this work needs confirmation in view of the known effect of the Fc fragment from normal immunoglobulins on adipocyte function (130), these receptor antibodies could be secondary to spontaneous insulin autoimmunization. The presence of these two types of autoimmune reaction suggests that insulin may act as a powerful immunogen, especially if inappropriate secretion of immature molecules occurs during the slow process of autoimmune B-cell damage (131). The demonstration that insulin is an integral surface protein expressed on the plasma membrane of dispersed rat islet cells reinforces this possibility (132). T-cells could then 'see' insulin molecules in conjunction with major histocompatibility products (vide infra) and this mechanism could form another arm of the autoimmune process directed against B-cells (133). HLA-DR7 and HLA-DR4 positive individuals are more liable to produce insulin antibodies both to animal and human preparations (134, 135) and these patients may be the best candidates for spontaneous autoimmunization to their own insulin or proinsulin. The operation of the anti-idiotype network (vide infra) could then explain the appearance of insulin receptor antibodies as anti-idiotypes made in response to the idiotypic epitope present in the original anti-insulin antibody molecule (136). This anti-idiotype may possess an insulin-like configuration (so called 'internal image') which mimics the binding of the circulating hormone with its receptor. Alteɪnatively T-cell participation in insulin-receptor autoimmunization cannot be entirely excluded, especially in view of the latest finding that MHC Class I molecules seem to be closely associated to insulin receptors on the plasma membrane, possibly sharing common determinants between them (137).

Previous studies showed anterior pituitary antibodies in about 7% of Type 1 adult diabetics who also suffer from polyendocrine autoimmunity and most of these antibodies appear to react with prolactin cells (138). In family studies, predisposed relatives with CF-ICA also proved to have antibodies reacting with several pituitary cell types (139). The highest prevalence was in those who became diabetic during follow-up. In the pre-diabetic latency period, 36% of ICA-positive relatives have these antibodies; in newly diagnosed diabetes, 16% were positive by immunofluorescence on pituitary tissue and in long-standing diabetes only 2% were positive. The current view is that these antibodies may be markers of some as yet unknown stimulating immunoglobulins, similar to those found in patients with a variety of goiters, which exert potent activity on cell replication (140, 141). These hypothetical factors may act on pituitary receptors either directly or by increased secretion of as yet uncharacterized hypothalamic (142) or pituitary (143) hormones affecting insulin secretion and possibly cell division.

Antibodies to endocrine cells in the intestinal tract have also been described (144). The significance of these unexpected organ-specific reactions is that they indicate further heterogeneity in this complex syndrome, and suggest that in some cases the entero-insular axis is also involved in the final development of diabetes.

Separate autoantibodies to glucagon and somatostatin cells have been described in a small proportion of diabetic patients (145). No direct correlation with abnormalities of secretion of the corresponding hormone has been detected (146, 147) but a recent report has indicated (148) that antibodies to glucagon cells with strong complement-fixing ability may represent a more direct marker of subtle defects of glucagon secretion. Interestingly, a proportion of these patients also have antibodies reacting with adrenal medullary cells, possibly involving catecholamine abnormalities. Defects in secretion of these hormones might possibly explain, in part, defective counter-regulation against hypoglycemia in some diabetic patients (149).

The association between Type 1 diabetes and the presence of other organ-specific autoantibodies (thyroid, gastric and adrenal cortex) has long been recognized (150). For practical purposes it is advisable to screen longstanding diabetics with persistent ICA for the presence of other endocrine autoantibodies (151). This may alert the physician to sub-clinical abnormalities in other endocrine systems (152, 153). For similar reasons it may be advisable to screen for other organ-specific antibodies in newly diagnosed diabetic children (154).

Non-organ-specific autoantibodies (anti-nuclear, anti-smooth muscle contractile proteins, anti-mitochondrial, etc.) have also been found with increased frequency in Type 1 diabetic patients (see Table 3 and Refs 155 and 156). Their presence suggests the participation of environmental factors with which they are known to be associated. Anti-lymphocytic autoantibodies should be added to this list (98, 157). These occur throughout the spectrum of autoimmune conditions and are often found in non-organ-specific autoimmune disorders such as SLE and rheumatoid arthritis. Their role is still controversial, but they could be important in producing an imbalance in the T-cell compartment.

A new look at the insulitis process

Mononuclear cell infiltration, the characteristic feature of autoimmune insulitis, has mainly been seen in pancreatic specimens taken at autopsy from

TABLE 3. *Autoantibodies other than ICA in Type 1 diabetes*

	Reacting with:		Ref.
1. Organ-specific	Thyroid:	Thyroglobulin	
		Microsomal	(150, 152)
	Stomach:	Gastric parietal cell	(154)
		Intrinsic factor	(150)
	Adrenal:	Cortex	(153)
		Medulla	(148)
	Pituitary:	Prolactin cells	(138)
		Multiple cells	(139)
	Gut:	Secretin cells	(144)
		GIP cells	
2. Non-organ-specific	Single-stranded DNA		
	Double-stranded DNA		(155)
	Tubulin		(156)
	Lymphocytes		(157)
3. Other	Insulin		(126, 127)
	Insulin receptor		(128, 129)

newly diagnosed diabetic patients. Combining the published data (158–160), it appears that 20 out of 21 patients with demonstrable insulitis were under 13 years of age, while in 15 patients over that age insulitis was present only in 5. It is known that in the diabetic pancreas many islets are shrunken, insulin-deficient and separated by conspicuous bands of fibrous tissue (these have been termed 'pseudo-atrophic islets'), but large islets containing B-cells are also present (161). It has been pointed out (160) that severe exocrine acinar cell atrophy is present only around insulin-deficient islets. These changes may be related to islet-exocrine vascular connections and unbalanced effects of islet hormones on pancreatic acini.

Until now, histopathological studies of the insulitis process have been performed exclusively on formalin-fixed blocks. A direct demonstration and better definition of the various immune phenomena occurring in vivo has been achieved by examining fresh-frozen blocks of pancreas obtained from a newly diagnosed diabetic child who died 24 hours after diagnosis (162). Active insulitis and other classic histological features of the acute diabetic state were seen in this pancreas, and the availability of frozen blocks made evaluation of lymphocyte subsets possible using monoclonal antibodies. When these reagents were applied and located by the immunofluorescence technique, the majority of mononuclear cells were found to be T-lymphocytes. Cytotoxic-suppressor lymphocytes appear to constitute the main bulk of the infiltrate, but the other main lymphocyte subpopulations, including natural killer and killer lymphocytes, were also represented. A high proportion of autoreactive T-lymphocytes expressed HLA-DR molecules, indicating that they were 'activated' T-cells and suggesting a specific immune response directed against islet antigens.

When anti-IgG reagents were applied, several interesting phenomena could be observed, which were not previously described. Pre-plasma cells synthesizing IgG, as shown by the bright intracytoplasmic fluorescence produced, were seen emerging from pancreatic vessels, and converging on the islets. In other fields the cells were grouped around individual islets. Mature plasma cells are rarely seen by conventional histology in diabetic insulitis, a negative finding which has been confirmed in the latest histological report (160). One of the more striking features in the pancreas from this child was the presence of IgG deposition within some of the islets. Two main patterns of immunofluorescence were observed. In one, the islets appeared to be coated with a smooth layer of IgG on their outer membrane and in the other IgG could be detected inside the cytoplasm. The latter finding suggested penetration of the islet cells following injury to the plasma membrane. These findings were recently confirmed in a larger series of pancreatic autopsy specimens. Immunoglobulins were found to be deposited in the islets in 9 out of 15 blocks examined by the immunoperoxidase technique carried out on sections of Bouin-fixed paraffin-embedded pancreas (163). In this latter report immunoglobulin deposition was not confined to the

B-cells but was also present in other pancreatic endocrine cells identified by the double IFL technique with the corresponding hormone antisera. These findings parallel previous observations suggesting a wider cross-reactivity of ICSA when these cells were carefully characterized using a cell-sorting technique (57). Class I major histocompatibility antigens, or HLA-A,B,C molecules are known to be synthesized by and expressed on virtually all nucleated cells in the body. This was confirmed for pancreatic islet cells when monoclonal antibodies against the non-polymorphic portion of HLA-A,B,C molecules were applied to frozen sections of normal human pancreas. However, the same monoclonal reagents stained some of the islets of the diabetic child much more strongly, indicating an overproduction of these membrane glycoproteins in the diseased pancreas (164). These results suggest a more precise role for cytotoxic T-lymphocytes in the recognition of islet-surface autoantigens. As mentioned, these cells predominate in the insulitis process and are known to operate by recognition of Class I molecules, when involved in eliminating cells damaged by environmental agents such as viruses (165).

The Class II major histocompatibility antigens, HLA-DR molecules, are not expressed on resting endocrine cells under physiological conditions. However, since aberrant expression of HLA-DR molecules has recently been demonstrated in autoimmune thyroid disease (166), careful search with monoclonal antibodies to the non-polymorphic region of the HLA-DR molecule was performed on the same human diabetic pancreas (164). After scanning many sections from different portions of the gland it was found that in some islets the few remaining insulin-producing cells were also expressing HLA-DR molecules. Glucagon and somatostatin cells, known to be unaffected by the insulitis process, were consistently negative for DR staining. The precise identification of DR-positive insulin cells and differential staining of other pancreatic endocrine cells was made possible by using several combinations of monoclonal reagents, including those to pancreatic hormones, and observing these with different fluorochromes (Bottazzo, in preparation).

New and revised hypotheses on the etiology of Type 1 diabetes

The role of the environment remains elusive, but epidemiological studies and single case reports suggest that viruses or toxic factors might be directly implicated in about 2% of cases of diabetes. Another 10% of Type 1 patients may belong to the subgroup characterized by later onset, female preponderance and coexistence of other endocrine autoimmune abnormalities (167). The etiological agent which triggers the process remains unknown in the great majority of patients (168).

The total genetic contribution (see Chapter 3) cannot exceed 50%, since this is the maximum estimate of the rate of concordance in identical twins with Type 1 diabetes. Different haplotypes in the major histocompatibility complex are now implicated, involving HLA-DR3, DR4 and several 'complotypes', i.e. allotypes of the complement components C2, C4 and Bf. This entire set of genes on Chromosome 6 has been calculated to account for between 60 and 70% of the genetic susceptibility (82). This leaves another 30–40% of the risk to be accounted for by genes on other chromosomes (169). The present candidates include Chromosome 11 where DNA sequences flanking the insulin gene probably contribute to susceptibility (170, 171) and Chromosome 14 where the immunoglobulin heavy-chain genes are situated. There is controversy as to whether Ig heavy-chain genes do or do not contribute to Type 1 diabetes, but there is some evidence that they are involved in susceptibility to Graves' disease (172). Another candidate is Chromosome 2, which contains the kappa light chain immunoglobulin genes, and genes for the blood groups Lewis and Kidd (173).

The 'H' and 'V' genes theory

A hypothesis concerning the mechanism of autoimmune recognition based on Burnett's 'forbidden' clone theory (174) has been intermittently in vogue over several years (175). This hypothesis, and its adaption to the etiology of diabetes, has been postulated in two parts. The 'H-gene' theory ('H' stands for histocompatibility) relies on the proposition that during ontogeny there is clonal deletion of B-lymphocytes which recognize an individual's own major and minor histocompatibility antigens. Such deletions would influence, either directly or indirectly, the chance appearance by somatic mutation of autoreactive 'forbidden' clones from 'pre-forbidden' clones. The effect could be to diminish or enhance the risk of autoimmunity depending on which HLA pattern the individual possesses. Thus HLA-DR2 confers protection from diabetes: the 'H gene' theory argues that protection arises because the clones which recognize HLA-DR2, and were therefore deleted, were the clones which after somatic mutation could have reacted with islet cell autoantigens. In contrast HLA-DR3 predisposes to diabetes, and in this case an indirect mechanism has to be postulated. Clones of lymphocytes which are deleted during ontogeny because they recognized HLA-DR3 molecules are among those which also exert control on 'pre-forbidden' clones. After appropriate somatic mutation these cells would become 'forbidden' clones able to recognize islet cells (Fig. 1).

The 'H-gene' theory has now been extended to implicate immunoglobulin genes (i.e. genes coding for the variable (V) region of immunoglobulins) in addition to the histocompatibility genes predisposing to autoimmunity. Evidence that these genes are implicated in the pathogenesis of diabetes has been based on analysis of highly selected multiplex families in which members had diabetes or thyrotoxicosis (176). A larger family study

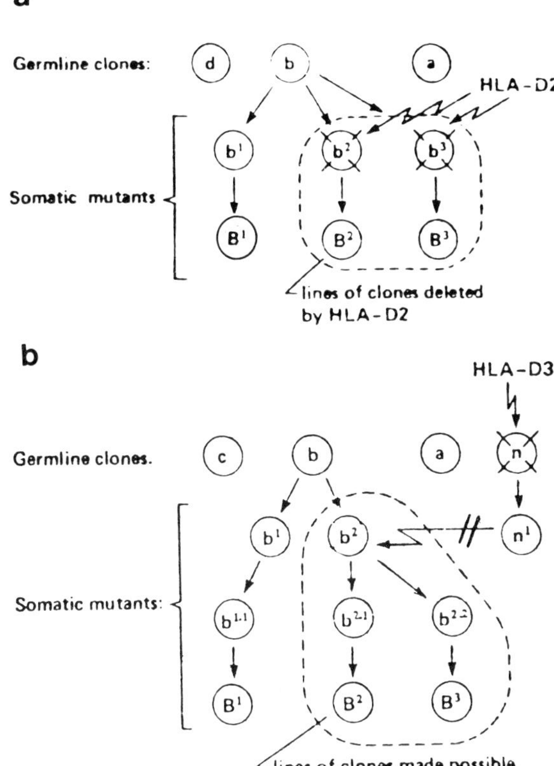

FIG. 1. *(a) Mechanism for the protective effect of HLA-D2 against Type 1 diabetes. Clonal deletion of b^2 and b^3 imposed by HLA-D2 could reduce the chance of occurrence of the anti-B-cell clones B^2 and B^3 that cause Type 1 diabetes. (b) Mechanism for the predisposing effect of HLA-D3 to Type 1 diabetes. HLA-D3 could facilitate the occurrence of clones B^2 and B^3 by deleting clone N, the precursor of anti-idiotypic clone N', which would otherwise have deleted potential precursors (e.g. b^2 of anti-B-cell clones). Thus anti-B-cell clones (B) in HLA-D3 = B^1, B^2, B^3 and in non-HLA-D3 = B^1. Modified from Adams et al. (176), by courtesy of the Editors of the Lancet.*

analysed by the same statistical methods yielded results which did not support an association between the Km allotype and susceptibility to Type 1 diabetes (177). Extension of the multiplex family study (178) together with direct analysis of the expressed IgV genes using hybridomas and V gene probes may help to resolve this issue.

The idiotype–anti-idiotype hypothesis

The theory of idiotype and anti-idiotype interactions, proposed as an alternative physiological means of regulating the immune system (179), has attracted considerable interest. This school of thought is based upon the fact that each immunoglobulin has a unique amino acid sequence in the variable region which confers specific antigenic properties ('the idiotype'). This implies that this particular configuration may in turn elicit an anti-idiotypic immunoglobulin response and the natural expansion of this phenomenon would ultimately lead to an amplified regulatory system.

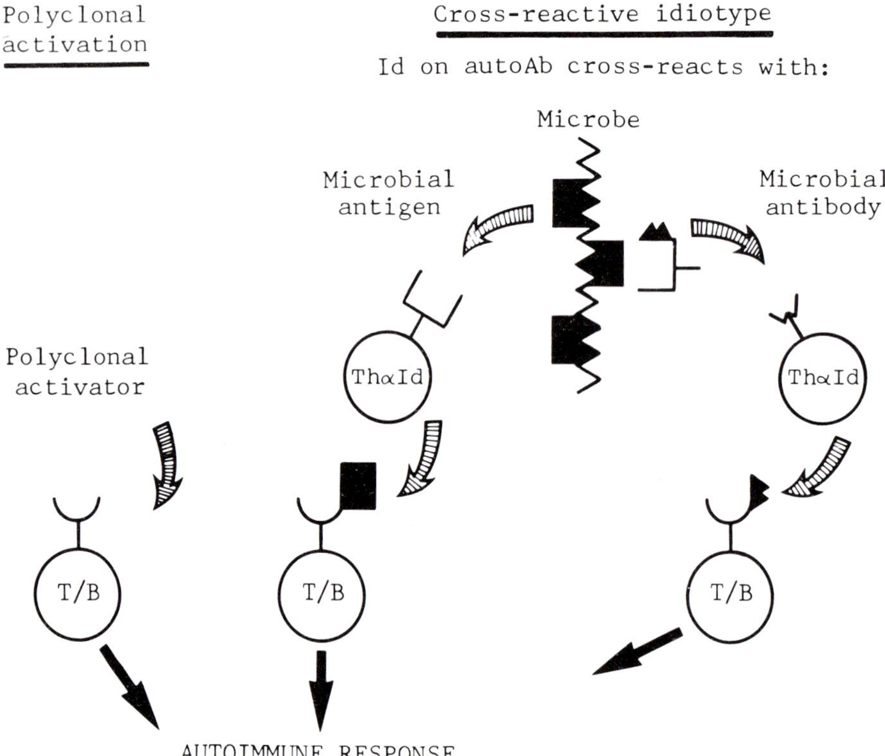

FIG. 2. *Bypass mechanisms for induction of autoimmunity where helper T-cells recognizing carrier determinants on autoantigens are suppressed or eliminated, autoreactive lymphocytes could be triggered by polyclonal activators, or by the presence on the receptor of an idiotype which cross-reacts with an idiotype on a microbial antibody or with an epitope on an infecting microorganism. Reproduced from Cooke et al. (180), by courtesy of the Editors of Immunology Today.*

The concept of the idiotype network has been used to explain autoimmunity. It has been suggested (180) that if an environmental agent such as a virus, bacteria or parasite triggered an antibody response this specificity could share similarities with idiotypes already expressed on potentially autoreactive T-helper lymphocytes. This cross-reactivity could augment a silent autoantibody response against, for example, endocrine cells (Fig. 2). In an expansion of this hypothesis it has been suggested that certain viral antibodies, directed at the viral structures which react with the corresponding cell surface viral receptor, may elicit an anti-idiotypic response. This new immunoglobulin could have a configuration complementary to the viral cell binding site and would react with the cell surface receptor for the virus, thus initiating cell injury (181) (Fig. 3). Arguments in favor of this concept include the fact that an anti-idiotype response to autoantibodies against circulating hormones may mimic the action of the hormone itself (182). One prediction arising from this hypothesis is that autoantibodies

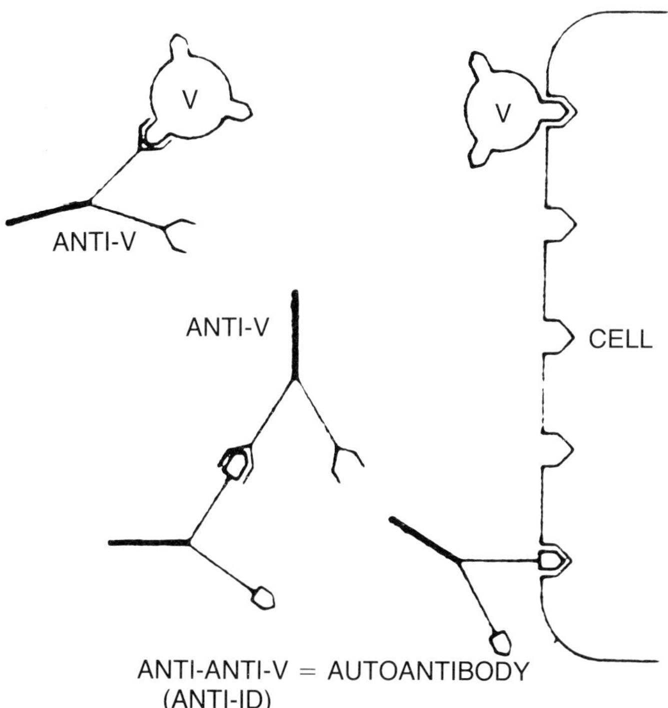

FIG. 3. *Autoantibodies seen as anti-idiotype antibodies to viral antibodies. An anti-idiotype against an antibody to the part of a virus which binds to a cell surface may itself act as an antibody against the cell surface receptor. Reproduced from Plotz (181), by courtesy of the Editors of the Lancet.*

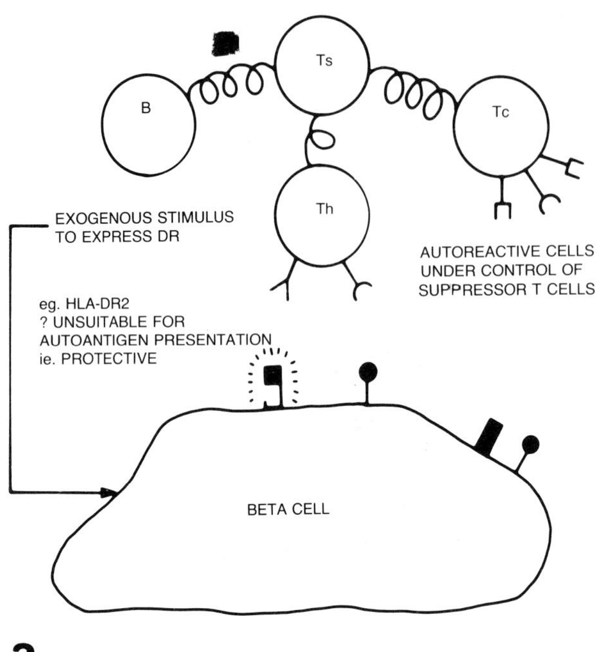
Ts
B
Tc
Th
EXOGENOUS STIMULUS
TO EXPRESS DR
AUTOREACTIVE CELLS
UNDER CONTROL OF
SUPPRESSOR T CELLS
eg. HLA-DR2
? UNSUITABLE FOR
AUTOANTIGEN PRESENTATION
ie. PROTECTIVE
BETA CELL

a

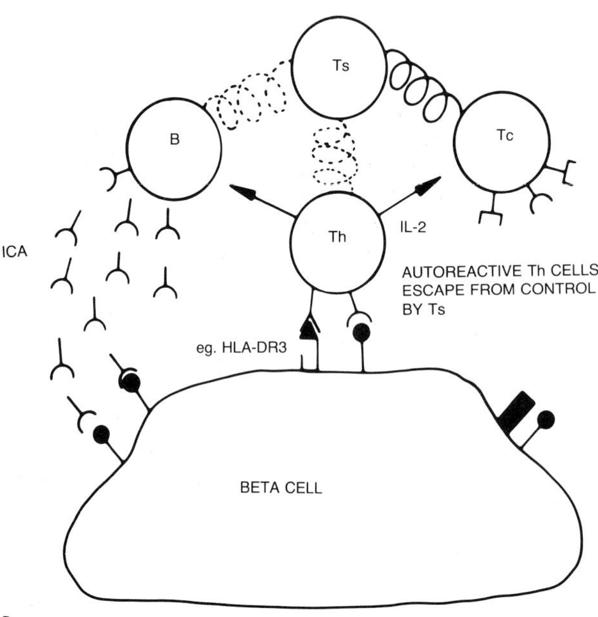
Ts
B
Tc
ICA
Th
IL-2
AUTOREACTIVE Th CELLS
ESCAPE FROM CONTROL
BY Ts
eg. HLA-DR3
BETA CELL

b

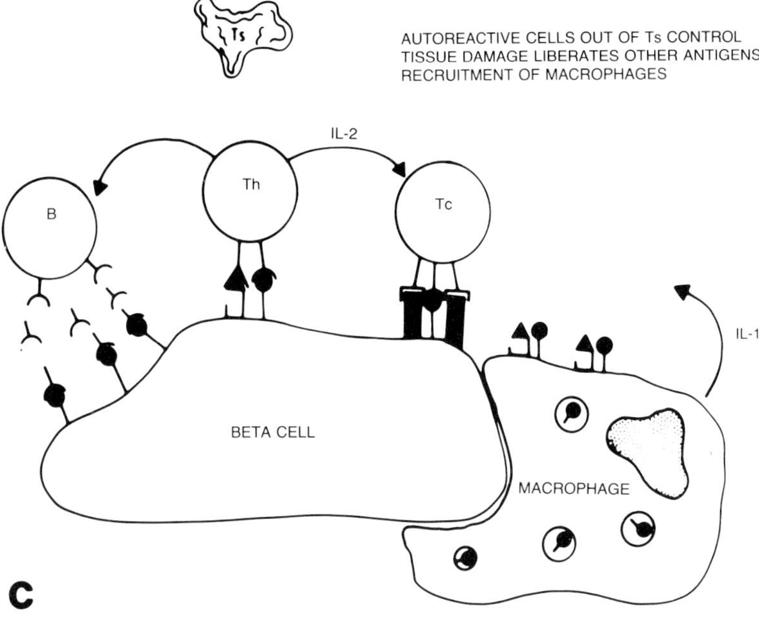

FIG. 4. *Diagram to illustrate a hypothesis regarding three stages in the induction of autoimmune disease, taking the pancreatic B-cell as an example. (a) In genetically non-susceptible individuals and in the absence of environmental stimuli there is a lack of HLA-DR expression and consequently no autoimmunity. Environmental agents may induce DR ( ) as illustrated, but the molecule has a particular configuration which is not ideal for presenting surface autoantigens ( ) efficiently, e.g. DR2 haplotypes protective for Type 1 diabetes. Suppressor T-cells (Ts) maintain other lymphocytes under tight control ( ). (b) In genetically predisposed individuals, environmental agents induce DR expression. The shape of this particular DR ( ) permits the correct presentation of autoantigen to helper-cells (Th). Th induce B-lymphocytes to generate autoantibodies ( ). During the long latency period which precedes the onset of clinical symptoms there is mild continuing damage. (c) With abnormality of Ts function (possibly specific to insulin-secreting cells in diabetes), organ damage becomes clinically manifest. The organ is infiltrated with cytotoxic T-cells (Tc) and macrophages. Tc have a receptor for Class I HLA-A, B, C molecules ( ). Their expression is increased in affected tissues. This type of damage leads to the release of many autoantigens and to the generation of new autoantibodies which perpetuate the disease. The role of organ-specific 'dendritic' APCs in these events is under investigation. Adapted from Bottazzo et al. (187).*

should commonly appear in the sera of some individuals following viral infection and that these should react with non-virally infected tissues. However, sera with high titers of antiviral antibodies do not stain normal human pancreas by the indirect immunofluorescence technique. This has been attempted unsuccessfully after incubation with sera containing high titers of Coxsackie antibodies (37). This suggests that these particular anti-idiotypic antibodies are not common, even though a more refined technique should be developed in case they are of low affinity and present at low titers.

Aberrant HLA-DR molecule expression: possible initiator

The Class II major histocompatibility molecules encoded by genes in the HLA-D region play a key role in the presentation of antigens and regulation of the immune response. The expression of these cell surface glycoproteins is normally restricted to B-lymphocytes, macrophages, dendritic and other antigen presenting cells and capillary endothelium (183). Modulation of HLA-DR expression has been observed only exceptionally outside the immune system. Thus, guinea pig mammary gland, duct and epithelium become Ia positive during pregnancy and lactation (184). Expression of Class II molecules can be induced during graft-versus-host disease (185) and in some forms of cancer (186).

Our own recent hypothesis concerning the generation of organ-specific autoimmunity (187) was based on the observation that DR antigen expression could be induced in normal thyroid cells (188) and that DR glycoproteins were spontaneously expressed on thyrocytes of glands from patients with thyrotoxicosis or Hashimoto's thyroiditis (166). These findings have been extended to the pancreatic B-cell in the context of diabetic insulitis (164). Similar data have recently been obtained in biopsies from patients with primary biliary cirrhosis (189) and alopecia areata (190), conditions thought to have an autoimmune etiology.

The new hypothesis envisages the following series of events. Viruses or other environmental agents present in the endocrine tissues of genetically predisposed individuals do not necessarily confer signs of overt infection; nor do they need to be strictly organ-specific. These factors could enhance the production of gamma-interferon, a known inducer of HLA-DR expression (191). The aberrant expression of DR molecules on endocrine glands leads to the correct presentation of surface autoantigens and subsequent induction of autoreactive T-cells (Fig 4). These T-cells would in turn produce more interferon, maintaining DR molecular production and expression on the target organ and activation of effector B- and T-lymphocytes. Whether the initial activation of autoreactive T-cells leads to autoimmune disease would depend on a variety of other factors such as selective abnormalities of the suppressor T-cell pathway reported to coexist with autoimmunity (114).

General considerations and future trends

Environmental factors responsible for the development of diabetes remain elusive. Suggested agents are in any case common in the population, and may have exerted their effects years before the onset of the clinical condition. We cannot rule out the possibility, however, that they may have a synergistic effect in genetically susceptible individuals in whom the process of B-cell destruction is already under way.

Autoimmunity appears to be more important in the slow process of B-cell destruction. Whether primary or secondary, autoimmune processes are at least demonstrable, subject to a variety of laboratory tests, and capable of careful dissection and characterization.

Effort should also be concentrated on developing techniques to 'immortalize' pancreatic B-cells. When available in large quantities these may prove an invaluable means of devising new methods (such as RIA and ELISA) for ICA determination. These could then be used to screen large populations. In addition the availability of islet cells in adequate numbers is an essential pre-requisite for expanding B-cell specific T-cell clones. This might open the way to selective therapeutic intervention (192). Levels of 'activated' T-cells need to be measured systematically at the time of diagnosis and, most important, prospectively in 'high-risk' individuals. T-cells expressing IL-2 will be the most suitable cells for subsequent cloning.

It is imperative to produce monoclonal antibodies recognizing relevant epitopes on islet cells. These reagents would offer another important tool for the purification of B-cell autoantigen(s). With this technique we would also be in an ideal position for fusing B-lymphocytes from ICA-positive prediabetic individuals in order to monitor the subsequent destruction of B-cells in a prospective manner, and to define those specificities more closely related to onset of the disease.

Most of the immunological phenomena demonstrated in Type 1 diabetes are detected in peripheral blood. It remains to be seen to what extent they mirror the attack launched locally against B-cells in the pancreas. Recent evidence obtained from detailed examination of a fresh diabetic pancreas needs to be confirmed and expanded in a larger series. There is hope that both clinicians and pathologists will become alert to the need for rapid autopsy and preparation of frozen blocks of pancreas in young diabetic patients who meet with misadventure soon after diagnosis. A computer search of deaths in the UK from recent diabetes in those under the age of 19 has indicated that 8 autopsies were performed in 1982, but that in only half were pancreatic blocks examined; none were frozen (Fowler, personal communication).

The proliferation of new hypotheses concerning the pathogenesis of autoimmune disease, including diabetes, has undoubtedly stimulated new ideas and novel lines of research. Individually none fully explains the observed phenomena, but each will provide elements, necessary for completion of this jigsaw puzzle. Despite the criticisms raised, the somatic mutation emphasized in the 'H'- and 'V-genes' theory may help us to understand the abrupt onset of diabetes in individuals who have had islet cell antibodies for months or years without clinical symptoms. Perhaps as the result of mutations occurring in the B-lymphocytes producing ICA, the antibodies become much more harmful to pancreatic B-cells. Against this background of shifting specificity, such antibodies could have an increased affinity for a particular B-cell antigen, facilitating the fixation of complement components which, in their turn, are influenced by the individual's particular 'complotype'. All these events might act in synergy with a 'mutated' T-cell clone repertoire. It seems unlikely that abnormalities of the idiotype network would be the *sole cause* of autoimmunity. The important observation that fine regulation of idiotypic interactions by the immune system is not restricted to the recognition of the major histocompatibility complex indicates that idiotypic dysregulation cannot by itself explain the known HLA-DR association with certain endocrine autoimmune diseases, in particular Type 1 diabetes. It seems more likely that they could play a major role in the generation of anti-hormone receptor antibodies in response to an initial antibody to the native hormone.

The hypothesis based on the observation that endocrine cells can spontaneously express HLA-DR molecules has been received with particular interest. It remains to be established whether this phenomenon constitutes the initial event or is secondary to environmental attack or immune dysregulation. However, its formulation may help to explain the vague association with viral infections, the long latency period and the HLA-DR associations of autoimmune diseases in man, including Type 1 diabetes.

Acknowledgements

We are indebted to Drs Ian Todd, Marco Londei and Marc Feldmann for stimulating discussion during the preparation of the manuscript. We thank Profs Deborah Doniach, Ivan Roitt, John Dickinson and Mike Besser for constant support and encouragement throughout the years. Mrs Mirtha Clarck patiently edited and typed the manuscript.

References

1. Gepts W (1965): Pathologic anatomy of the pancreas in juvenile diabetes mellitus. *Diabetes*, *14*, 619–633.
2. Nerup J, Andersen OO, Bendixen G, Egeverg J, Poulsen JE (1971): Antipancreatic cellular hypersensitivity in diabetes mellitus. *Diabetes*, *20*, 424–427.

3. Bottazzo GF, Florin-Christensen A, Doniach D (1974): Islet cell antibodies in diabetes mellitus with autoimmune polyendocrine deficiency. *Lancet, 2,* 1279–1283.
4. Nerup J, Platz P, Andersen OO, Christy M, Lyngsoe J, Poulsen JE, Ryder LP, Nielsen LS, Thomsen M, Svejgaard A (1974): HLA antigens and diabetes mellitus. *Lancet, 2,* 864–866.
5. Cudworth AG, Woodrow JC (1975): Evidence for HLA-linked genes in juvenile diabetes mellitus. *Br. Med. J., 3,* 133–135.
6. Bastenie PA, Gepts W (Eds.) (1974): *Immunity and Autoimmunity in Diabetes Mellitus.* Excerpta Medica, Amsterdam.
7. Andersen OO, Deckert T, Nerup J. (Eds) (1976): Immunological aspects of diabetes mellitus. *Acta Endocrinol. (Copenhagen), Suppl. 205.*
8. Irvine WJ, Teviot O (Eds) (1980): *Immunology of Diabetes.* Scientific Publications, Edinburgh.
9. Kolb H, Schernthaner G, Gries FA (Eds) (1983): *Diabetes and Immunology: Pathogenesis and Immunotherapy.* Hans Huber, Bern.
10. Woodrow JC (1983): Up-date on insulin-dependent diabetes. *Br. Med. J., 286,* 1683.
11. Reeves G (1983): The immunology of Beta cell failure: a case for immune response genes? *Immunol. Today, 4,* 207–208.
12. Andreani D, Di Mario U, Federlin KF, Heding LH (Eds) (1984): *Immunology in Diabetes.* Kimpton, London.
13. Andreani D, Berger M, Di Mario U, Eisenbarth G, Lernmark A, Rubinstein A (1984): Immunology in Diabetes '84. *Diabetologia, 27, Suppl. July.*
14. Bottazzo GF, Pozzilli P, Mirakian R, Dean BM, Doniach D (1984): Early immunological events in diabetes. In: *Immunology in Diabetes,* Chapter 7, pp. 95–104. Editors: D. Andreani, U. Di Mario, K.F. Federlin and L.G. Heding. Kimpton, London.
15. Gorsuch AN, Spencer KM, Lister J, McNally JM, Dean BM, Bottazzo GF, Cudworth AG (1981): The natural history of Type I (insulin-dependent) diabetes mellitus: evidence for a long pre-diabetic period. *Lancet, 2,* 1363–1365.
16. Gorsuch AN, Spencer KM, Lister J, Wolf E, Bottazzo GF, Cudworth AG (1982): Can future Type I diabetes be predicted? A prospective study in families of affected children. *Diabetes, 31,* 862–866.
17. Bottazzo GF, Dean BM, Gorsuch AN, Cudworth AG, Doniach D (1980): Complement-fixing islet cell antibodies in Type I Diabetes: Possible monitors of active beta-cell damage. *Lancet, 1,* 668–672.
18. Pujol-Borrell R, Hanafusa T, Cudworth AG, Bottazzo GF (1982): Islet cell surface antibodies and the natural history of Type I (insulin-dependent) diabetes mellitus. *Diabetologia, 23,* 194.
19. Dobersen MJ, Scharff J, Ginsberg-Fellner F, Notkins AL (1980): Cytotoxic antibodies to Beta cells in the serum of patients with insulin-dependent diabetes mellitus. *N. Engl. J. Med., 303,* 1493–1498.
20. Ginsberg-Fellner F, Dobersen MJ, Witt ME, Rayfield EJ, Rubinstein P, Notkins AL (1982): HLA-antigens, cytoplasmic islet cell antibodies and carbohydrate tolerance in families of children with insulin dependent diabetes mellitus. *Diabetes, 31,* 292–298.

21. Srikanta S, Ganda OP, Jackson RA, Brink SJ, Fleischnick E, Yunis E, Alper C, Soeldner JS, Eisenbarth GS (1984): Pre-type I diabetes: common endocrinological course despite immunological and immunogenetic heterogeneity. *Diabetologia, 27, Suppl.*, 146–148.
22. Riley W, Spillar R, Warltz J, Body B (1984): Predictive value of islet-cell autoantibodies (ICA): 6 year's experience. *Diabetes, 33*, 157A.
23. Winearls BC, Bodmer JG, Bodmer WF, Bottazzo GF, McNally J, Mann J, Thoroughgood M, Smith A, Baum D (1984): A family study of the association between insulin-dependent diabetes mellitus, autoantibodies and the HLA system. *Tissue Antigens* (in press).
24. Norden G, Jensen E, Stilbo I, Bottazzo GF, Lernmark A (1983): B-cell function and islet cell and other organ-specific autoantibodies in relatives of insulin-dependent diabetic patients. *Acta Med. Scand., 213*, 199–203.
25. Betterle C, Zanette F, Pedini B, Presotto F, Rapp LB, Monciotti CM, Rigon F (1984): Clinical and subclinical organ-specific autoimmune manifestations in Type I (insulin-dependent) diabetic patients, and their first degree relatives. *Diabetologia, 26*, 431–436.
26. Barbosa J, Chavers B, Dunsworth T, Michael A (1982): Islet cell antibodies and histocompatibility antigens in insulin-dependent diabetics and their first degree relatives. *Diabetes, 31*, 585–588.
27. Srikanta S, Ganda OP, Eisenbarth GS, Soeldner JS (1983): Islet cell antibodies and beta cell function in monozygotic triplets and twins initially discordant for Type I diabetes mellitus. *N. Engl. J. Med., 308*, 322–325.
28. Betterle C, Zanette F, Tiengo A, Trevison A (1982): Five year follow-up of non-diabetes with islet cell antibodies. (Letter to the Editor) *Lancet, 1*, 284–285.
29. Srikanta S, Ganda OP, Jackson RA, Gleason RE, Kaldany A, Garovoy MR, Milford EL, Carpenter CB, Soeldner JS, Eisenbarth GS (1983): Type I diabetes mellitus in monozygotic twins: chronic progressive Beta cell dysfunction. *Ann. Intern. Med., 99*, 320–326.
30. Hollander PH, Asplin CM, Kniaz D, Hansen JA, Palmer JP (1982): Beta-cell dysfunction in non-diabetic HLA-identical siblings of insulin-dependent diabetics. *Diabetes, 31*, 149–153.
31. Spencer KM, Tarn A, Dean BM, Lister J, Bottazzo GF (1984): Fluctuating islet-cell autoimmunity in unaffected relatives of patients with insulin-dependent diabetes. *Lancet, 1*, 764–766.
32. Srikanta S, Eisenbarth GS (1984): Disappearing anti-islet antibodies? (Letter to the Editor) *Lancet, 1*, 1176–1177.
33. Riley W, McLaren N (1984): Islet cell antibodies are seldom transient. (Letter to the Editor) *Lancet, 1*, 1351–1352.
34. Bruining GJ, Molenaar J, Tuk CW, Lindeman J, Bruining HA, Marner B (1984): Clinical time course and characteristics of islet cell cytoplasmic antibodies in childhood diabetes. *Diabetologia, 26*, 24–29.
35. Pozzilli P, Sensi M, Al-Sakkaf L, Tarn A, Zuccarini O, Bottazzo GF (1984): Prospective study of lymphocyte subsets in subjects genetically susceptible to Type I (insulin-dependent) diabetes. *Diabetologia, 27, Suppl.*, 132–135.
36. Palmer JP, Cooney MK, Ward RH, Hansen JA, Brodsky JB, Ray CG, Crossley JR, Asplin CM, Williams RH (1982): Reduced Coxsackie antibody

titres in Type I diabetic patients presenting during an outbreak of Coxsackie B3 and B4 injection. *Diabetologia*, *22*, 426–429.

37. King ML, Shaikh A, Bidwell D, Voller A, Banatvala JE (1983): Coxsackie-B-virus-specific IgM responses in children with insulin-dependent (juvenile-onset, Type I) diabetes mellitus. *Lancet*, *1*, 1397–1399.
38. Schernthaner G, Banatvala JE, Scherbaum W, Mayr WR, Borkenstein M, Schnober E (1984): Coxsackie B virus specific IgM responses, complement fixing islet cell antibodies, and HLA-DR antigens in newly diagnosed Type I diabetics: a one year follow-up study of C peptide secretion in 94 patients, pp 102–103. In: *Immunology in Diabetes '84*. Editor: M. Iavicoli. Novo Farmaceutica-Italia, Rome.
39. Asplin MS, Cooney MK, Crossley JR, Dornan TL, Raghu P, Palmer JP (1982): Coxsackie B4 infection and islet cell antibodies three years before overt diabetes. *J. Pediatr.*, *101*, 398–400.
40. Bodansky HJ, Littlewood JM, Bottazzo GF, Dean BM, Hambling MH (1984): Which virus causes the initial islets lesion in Type I diabetes? (Letter to the Editor) *Lancet*, *1*, 401–402.
41. Ginsberg-Fellner F, Witt ME, Yaginashi S, Dobersen MJ, Taub F, Fedun B, McEvoy RC, Roman SH, Davies TF, Cooper LZ, Rubinstein P, Notkins AL (1984): Congenital rubella syndrome as a model for Type I (insulin-dependent) diabetes mellitus: increased prevalence of islet cell surface antibodies. *Diabetologia*, *27*, *Suppl.*, 87–90.
42. Rubinstein P, Walker ME, Fedun N, Witt ME, Cooper LZ, Ginsberg-Fellner F (1982): The HLA system in congenital rubella syndrome with and without diabetes. *Diabetes*, *31*, 1088–1091.
43. Helgason T, Jonasson MR (1981): Evidence for a food additive as a cause of ketosis prone diabetes. *Lancet*, *2*, 716–720.
44. Spencer KM, Gorsuch AN, Cudworth AG, Bottazzo GF (1982): Diabetes and month of birth. (Letter to the Editor) *Lancet*, *1*, 449.
45. Helgason T, Ewen SWB, Ross IS, Stowers JM (1982): Diabetes produced in mice by smoke-cured mutton. *Lancet*, *2*, 1017–1024.
46. Dean BM, Bottazzo GF, Cudworth AG (1983): IgG subclass distribution in organ-specific autoantibodies. The relationship to complement fixing ability. *Clin. Exp. Immunol.*, *52*, 61–66.
47. Pilcher C, Elliot RB (1984): Improved sensitivity of islet cell cytoplasmic antibody assay in diabetics. (Letter to the Editor) *Lancet*, *1*, 1352.
48. Marner B, Lernmark D, Nerup J, Molenaar JL, Tuk CW, Bruining GJ (1983): Analysis of islet cell antibodies on frozen sections of human pancreas. *Diabetologia*, *25*, 93–96.
49. Dobersen MJ, Bell M, Jenson AB, Notkins AL, Ginsberg-Fellner F (1979): Detection of antibodies to islet cells and insulin with paraffin-embedded pancreas as antigen. (Letter to the Editor) *Lancet*, *2*, 1078.
50. Dean B, Pujol-Borrell R, Bottazzo GF (1982): Determination of islet cell antibodies by immunofluorescence. (Letter to the Editor) *Lancet*, *2*, 1343–1344.
51. Rosenbloom AL (1983): Autoantibodies to islet cells: comparison of methods. (Letter to the Editor) *Lancet*, *1*, 72–73.

52. Dean B, Pujol-Borrell R, Doniach D, Bottazzo GF (1983): Islet cell antibody determination: the essential message. (Letter to the Editor) *Lancet*, *1*, 654.
53. Clark A, Smith D, Chapel H (1983): Islet cell autoantibodies: which method? (Letter to the Editor) *Lancet*, *1*, 479–480.
54. Yagihashi S, Suzuki H, Dobersen MJ, Onedera T, Notkins AL, Ginsberg-Fellner F (1982): Autoantibodies to islet cells: comparison of methods. (Letter to the Editor) *Lancet*, *2*, 1218.
55. Pujol-Borrell R, Khoury EL, Bottazzo GF (1982): Islet cell surface antibodies in Type I (insulin-dependent) diabetes mellitus: use of human fetal pancreas cultures as substrate. *Diabetologia*, *22*, 89–95.
56. Papadopoulos GK, Lernmark A (1983): The spectrum of islet cell antibodies. In: *Autoimmune Endocrine Disease*, pp. 167–180. Editor: T.F. Davies. John Wiley, New York.
57. Van de Winkel M, Smets G, Gepts W, Pipeleers D (1982): Islet cell surface antibodies from insulin-dependent diabetics bind specifically to pancreatic B cells. *J. Clin. Invest.*, *70*, 41–49.
58. Orci L (1982): Macro- and micro-domains in the endocrine pancreas. *Diabetes*, *31*, 538–565.
59. Dobersen MJ, Schaff JE, Ginsberg-Fellner F, Notkins AL (1982): Preferential lysis of Beta cells by islet cell surface antibodies. *Diabetes*, *31*, 459–462.
60. Kanatsuna T, Freedman ZR, Rubenstein AH, Lernmark A (1982): Effect of islet cell surface antibodies and complement on the release of insulin and chromium from perifused Beta cells. *Clin. Exp. Immunol.*, *47*, 85–92.
61. Rabinovitch A, Mackay P, Ludvigsson J, Lernmark A (1984): A prospective analysis of islet cell cytotoxic antibodies in insulin-dependent diabetic children. Transient effects of plasmapheresis. *Diabetes*, *32*, 224–228.
62. Kanatsuna T, Baekkeskov S, Lernmark A, Ludvigsson J (1983): Immunoglobulin from insulin dependent diabetic children inhibits glucose induced insulin release. *Diabetes*, *32*, 520–524.
63. Sai P, Boitard Chr, Debray-Sachs M, Pouplard A, Assan R, Hamburger J (1981): Complement fixing islet cell antibodies from some diabetic patients alter insulin release in vitro. *Diabetes*, *30*, 1051–1057.
64. Boitard C, Sai P, Debray-Sachs M, Assan R, Hamburger J (1984): Anti-pancreatic immunity. In vitro studies of cellular and humoral immune reactions directed toward pancreatic islets. *Clin. Exp. Immunol.*, *55*, 571–580.
65. Debray-Sachs M, Quiniou MC, Assan R, Bach JF (1984): Correlation between complement dependent cytotoxic and insulin release inhibitory antibodies to Beta cells in the serum of patients with IDDM. In: *Immunology in Diabetes '84*, p. 33. Editor: M. Iavicoli. Novo Farmaceutica-Italia, Rome.
66. Marayuma T, Takei I, Matsuba I, Tsuruoka A, Taniyama M, Ikeda Y, Kataoka K, Abe M, Matsuki S (1984): Cell-mediated cytotoxic islet cell surface antibodies to human pancreatic Beta cell. *Diabetologia*, *26*, 30–33.
67. Svennigsen A, Dryberg T, Gerling I, Lernmark A, Mackay P, Rabinovitch A (1983): Inhibition of insulin release after passive transfer of immunoglobulin from insulin-dependent diabetic children to mice. *J. Clin. Endocrinol. Metab.*, *57*, 1301–1304.
68. Sai P, Clauser E, Boitard CL, Debray-Sachs M, Pouplard A, Assan R (1984): Passive transfer of glucose intolerance to mice by immunoglobulins from

insulin-dependent diabetic patients. *Diabetologia* (in press).

69. Baekkeskov S, Nielsen JH, Marner B, Bilde T, Ludvigsson J, Lernmark A (1982): Autoantibodies in newly diagnosed diabetic children immunoprecipitate human pancreatic islet cell proteins. *Nature (London)*, *298*, 167–169.
70. Gazdar AF, Chick WL, Oie HK, Sims HL, King DL, Weir GC, Lauritis V (1980): Continuous clonal insulin and somatostatin secreting cell lines established from transplantable rat islet cell tumour. *Proc. Natl Acad. Sci. USA*, *77*, 3519–3523.
71. Bottazzo GF, Doniach D (1978): Islet-cell antibodies in diabetes mellitus. Evidence of an autoantigen common to all cells in the islet of Langerhans. *Ric. Clin. Labor.*, *8*, 29–38.
72. Eisenbarth GS, Linnenbach A, Jackson R, Scearce R, Croce CM (1982): Human hybridomas secreting anti-islet autoantibodies. *Nature (London)*, *300*, 264–267.
73. Eisenbarth GS, Jackson R, Srikanta S, Powers A, Buse J, Mori H (1984): Utilization of monoclonal antibody techniques to study Type I (insulin-dependent) diabetes mellitus. In: *Immunology in Diabetes*, Chapter 11, pp. 143–157. Editors: D. Andreani, U. Di Mario, K.F. Federlin and L.G. Heding. Kimpton, London.
74. Satoh J, Prabhakar, Haspel MV, Ginsberg-Fellner F, Notkins AL (1983): Human monoclonal antibodies that react with multiple endocrine organs. *N. Engl. J. Med.*, *309*, 217–220.
75. MacLaren NK, Riley W, Rosenbloom E, Elder M, Spillar R, Cuddeback J (1982): The heterogeneity of black insulin-dependent diabetes. *Diabetes*, *31*, *Suppl.*, *2*, 65A.
76. Mustonen A, Ilonen J, Ackerblom HK, Tilikainen A (1982): An islet cell antibody negative form of insulin dependent diabetes mellitus associated with HLA antigens. A9, BW16. *Clin. Exp. Immunol.*, *48*, 213–217.
77. Neufeld M, McLaren NK, Riley WJ, Lezote P, McLaughlin JV, Silverstein J, Rosenbloom AL (1980): Islet-cell and other organ-specific antibodies in US caucasians and blacks with insulin-dependent diabetes mellitus. *Diabetes*, *29*, 589–592.
78. Knowler WC, Bennet PH, Bottazzo GF, Doniach D (1979): Islet cell antibodies and diabetes mellitus in Pima Indians. *Diabetologia*, *17*, 161–164.
79. Oli JM, Bottazzo GF, Doniach D (1981): Islet cell antibodies and diabetes. *Niger. Trop. Geogr. Med.*, *33*, 161–164.
80. Kanazawa Y (1984): Some genetic and immunological aspects of Type I (insulin-dependent) diabetes in Japan. In: *Immunology in Diabetes*, Chapter 12, pp 159–169. Editors: D. Andreani, U. Di Mario, K.F. Federlin and L.G. Heding. Kimpton, London.
81. Bottazzo GF, Mirakian R, Dean BM, McNally JM, Doniach D (1982): How immunology helps to define heterogeneity in diabetes mellitus. In: *The Genetics of Diabetes Mellitus*, pp 79–90. Editors: J. Kobberling and R. Tattersall. Academic Press, London.
82. Rimoin DL, Rotter JI (1984): Aspects of the genetics of insulin-dependent diabetes mellitus. In: *Immunology in Diabetes*, Chapter 5, pp 63–71. Editors: D. Andreani, U. Di Mario, K.F. Federlin and L.G. Heding. Kimpton, London.

83. Irvine WJ (1984): Classification of diabetes mellitus. In: *Immunology in Diabetes*, Chapter 25, pp 283–294. Editors: D. Andreani, U. Di Mario, K.F. Federlin and L.G. Heding. Kimpton, London.
84. Di Mario U, Irvine WJ, Borsey DQ, Kyner JL, Weston J, Galfo C (1983): Immunological phenomena in diabetics not requiring insulin at diagnosis. *Diabetologia*, *25*, 392–395.
85. Gleichman H, Zorcher B, Greulich B, Gries FA, Henrichs HR, Bertrams J, Kolb H (1984): Correlation of islet cell antibodies and HLA-DR phenotypes with diabetes mellitus in adults. *Diabetologia*, *27*, 90–92.
86. Groop L, Bottazzo GF, Doniach D (1984): Islet cell antibodies identify 'pseudo-type II' diabetes in patients aged 35-75 years at diagnosis. Submitted for publication.
87. Rossini A (1983): Immunotherapy for insulin-dependent diabetic? *N. Engl. J. Med.*, *308*, 333–335.
88. Coscelli C, Zavaroni I, Bernasconi S, Savi M, Dall'Aglio E, Dean BM, Bottazzo GF (1984): Time course of ICA and residual endogenous Beta cell function in newly diagnosed Type I diabetic patients with or without clinical remission. Submitted for publication.
89. Peig M, Pujol-Borrell R, Levy I, Casamitjana R, Figuerola D, McNally JM (1983): Correlation between C-peptide and islet cell antibodies in newly diagnosed Type I (insulin-dependent) diabetic patients: a follow-up study. *Diabetologia*, *25*, 186.
90. Marner B, Agner T, Binder C, Lernmark A, Nerup J (1983): Prospective analysis of islet cell antibody and C-peptide levels during the first 24 months of insulin dependent diabetes. *Diabetologia*, *25*, 179.
91. Mustonen A, Knip M, Akerblom K (1983): An association between complement fixing cytoplasmic islet cell antibodies and endogenous insulin secretion in children with insulin-dependent diabetes mellitus. *Diabetes*, *32*, 743–747.
92. Bernard A, Bounsell L, Dausset J, Milstein C, Schlossman SF (Eds) (1984): *Leucocyte Typing*. Springer-Verlag, Berlin.
93. Rodier M, Andary M, Richard JL, Mirouze J, Clot J (1984): Peripheral blood T-cell subsets studied by monoclonal antibodies in Type I (insulin-dependent) diabetes: effect of blood glucose control. *Diabetologia*, 27, *Suppl.*, 136–138.
94. Mascart-Lemone F, Delespesse G, Dorchy H, Lemiere B and Servais G (1982): Characterisation of immunoregulatory T lymphocytes in insulin-dependent diabetic children by means of monoclonal antibodies. *Clin. Exp. Immunol.*, *47*, 296–300.
95. Galluzzo A, Giordano C, Rubino G, Bompiani GD (1984): Immunoregulatory T-lymphocyte subset deficiency in newly diagnosed Type I (insulin-dependent) diabetes mellitus. *Diabetologia*, *26*, 426–430.
96. Buschard K, Ropke C, Madsbad S, Mehlsen J, Sorensen TB, Rygaard J (1983): Alterations of peripheral T lymphocyte subpopulations in patients with insulin-dependent (Type I) diabetes mellitus. *J. Clin. Lab. Immunol.*, *10*, 127–131.
97. Pozzilli P, Zuccarini O, Iavicoli M, Andreani D, Sensi M, Spencer KM, Bottazzo GF, Beverley PCL, Kyner JL, Cudworth AG (1983): Monoclonal

antibodies defined abnormalities of T lymphocytes in Type I (insulin-dependent) diabetes. *Diabetes*, *32*, 91–94.

98. Herold K, Huen A, Gould L, Traisman H, Rubenstein AH (1984): Alterations in lymphocyte subpopulations in Type I (insulin-dependent) diabetes mellitus: exploration of possible mechanisms and relationships to autoimmune phenomena. *Diabetologia*, *27*, *Suppl.*, 102–105.
99. Ilonen J, Surcel HM; Mustonen A, Kaar ML, Akerblom HK (1984): Lymphocyte subpopulations at the onset of Type I (insulin-dependent diabetes). *Diabetologia*, *27*, *Suppl.*, 106–108.
100. Jackson RA, Morris MA, Haynes BF, Eisenbarth GS (1982): Increased circulating Ia antigen-bearing T cells in Type I diabetes mellitus. *N. Engl. J. Med.*, *306*, 785–788.
101. Gupta S, Fiterig SM, Khanna S, Orti E (1982): Deficiency of suppressor T cells in insulin-dependent diabetes mellitus. *Immunol. Lett.*, *4*, 289–294.
102. Buschard K, Ropke C, Madsbad S, Mehlsem J, Rygaard J (1983): T-lymphocyte subsets in patients with newly diagnosed Type I (insulin-dependent) diabetes: a prospective study. *Diabetologia*, *25*, 247–251.
103. Alviggi L, Johnston C, Hoskins DJ, Tee DEH, Pyke D, Leslie RDG, Vergani D (1984): Pathogenesis of insulin-dependent diabetes: a role for activated T lymphocytes. *Lancet*, *2*, 4–6.
104. Nanni Costa A, Orsoni G, Bergnino L, Iannelli S, Ciaverello A, Vannini P, Bonomini V (1984): Lymphocyte subsets and responsiveness in insulin-dependent diabetes mellitus (IDDM). In: *Immunology in Diabetes '84*. Editor: M. Iavicoli. Novo Farmaceutica-Italia, Rome.
105. Pozzilli P, Sensi M, Dean B, Gorsuch AN, Cudworth AG (1979): Evidence for raised K cell levels in Type I diabetes. *Lancet*, *2*, 173–175.
106. Horita M, Suzuki H, Onodera T, Ginsberg-Fellner F, Fauci AS, Notkins AL (1982): Abnormalities of immunoregulatory subsets in patients with insulin-dependent diabetes mellitus. *J. Immunol.*, *129*, 1426–1429.
107. Lernmark A (1984): Cell-mediated immunity in Type I (insulin-dependent) diabetes: Update 84. In: *Immunology in Diabetes*, Chapter 9, pp 121-131. Editors: D. Andreani, U. di Mario, K.F. Federlin and L.H. Heding. Kimpton, London.
108. Lamb JR, Eckles DD, Lake D, Johnson AH, Hartzman RJ, Weedy JN (1982): Antigen-specific human T-lymphocyte clones: induction, antigen-specificity, and MHC restriction of influenza virus immune clones. *J. Immunol.*, *128*, 233–235.
109. Hohlfeld R, Tdyka KV, Heininger K, Gross-Wilde H, Kalies I (1984): Autoimmune human T lymphocytes specific for acetylcholine receptor. *Nature (London)*, *310*, 244–246.
110. Londei M, Bottazzo GF, Feldmann M (1984): Human T cell clones from thyroid autoimmune thyroid glands: specific recognition of autologous thyroid cells. Submitted for publication.
111. Hayward AR, Herberger M (1984): Culture and phenotype of activated T-cells from patients with Type I DM. *Diabetes*, *33*, 319–323.
112. Buschard K, Madsbad S, Rygaard J (1982): Suppressor cell activity in patients with newly diagnosed insulin-dependent diabetes mellitus: a prospective study. *J. Clin. Lab. Immunol.*, *8*, 19–29.

113. Fairchild RS, Kyner JL, Abdon NI (1982): Specific immunoregulation abnormality in insulin-dependent diabetes mellitus. *J. Lab. Clin. Med.*, *99*, 175–184.
114. Topliss D, How T, Lewis M, Row V, Volpe R (1983): Evidence for cell-mediated immunity and specific suppressor T-lymphocyte dysfunction in Graves' disease and diabetes mellitus. *J. Clin. Endocrinol. Metabol.*, *57*, 700–705.
115. Vento S, Hegarty JE, Bottazzo GF, Macchia E, Williams R, Eddleston ALWF (1984): Antigen specific suppressor cell function in autoimmune chronic active hepatitis. *Lancet*, *1*, 1200–1204.
116. Corazza GR, Sarchielli P, Frisoni M, Londei M, Gasbarrini G (1984): Gluten-specific suppressor T cell dysfunction in coeliac disease. Submitted for publication.
117. Charles MA, Suzuki M, Waldeck N, Dodson LE, Slater L, Ong K, Kershnar A, Buckingham B, Golden M (1983): Immune islet killing mechanisms associated with insulin-dependent diabetes: In vitro expression of cellular and antibody mediated islet cell cytotoxicity. *J. Immunol.*, *130*, 1189–1193.
118. Boitard Chr, Chatenoud L, Debray-Sachs M (1982): In vitro inhibition of pancreatic B cell function by lymphocytes from diabetics with associated autoimmune disease: a T cell phenomenon. *J. Immunol.*, *129*, 2529–2539.
119. Sensi M, Pozzilli P, Gorsuch AN, Bottazzo GF, Cudworth AG (1981): Increased K-cell activity in insulin-dependent (Type I) diabetes. *Diabetologia*, *20*, 106–109.
120. Papadopoulos GK, Petersen J, Andersen V, Lernmark A, Marner B, Nerup J, Binder C (1984): Increased plaque forming cells levels in peripheral blood of newly diagnosed insulin-dependent diabetic patients. *Acta Endocrinol. (Copenhagen)*, *105*, 521–527.
121. Zier KS, Leo MM, Spielman RS, Baker L (1984): Decreased synthesis of interleukin-2 (IL-2) in insulin-dependent diabetes mellitus. *Diabetes*, *33*, 552–555.
122. Helderman JH, Strom TB (1974): Specific insulin binding site on T and B lymphocytes as a marker of cell activation. *Nature (London)*, *274*, 62–63.
123. Kaldany A, Hill T, Wentworth S, Brink SJ, D'Elia JA, Clouse M, Soeldner JS (1982): Trapping of peripheral blood lymphocytes in the pancreas of patients with acute onset insulin-dependent diabetes mellitus. *Diabetes*, *31*, 463–466.
124. Hirata Y (1983): Methimazole and insulin autoimmune syndrome with hypoglycaemia. (Letter to the Editor) *Lancet*, *2*, 1037–1038.
125. Burden AC, Rosenthal FD (1983): Methimazole and insulin autoimmune syndrome. (Letter to the Editor) *Lancet*, *2*, 1311.
126. Palmer JP, Asplin CM, Clemons P, Lyen K, Tatpati O, Raghu PK, Paquette TL (1983): Insulin antibodies in insulin-dependent diabetics before insulin treatment. *Science*, *222*, 1337–1339.
127. Wilkin J, Nicholson S (1984): Autoantibodies against human insulin. *Br. Med. J.*, *288*, 349–352.
128. Maron R, Elias D, Jongh BM, Bruining GJ, Van Rood JJ, Schechter Y, Cohen IR (1983): Autoantibodies to the insulin receptor in juvenile onset of insulin dependent diabetes. *Nature (London)*, *303*, 817–818.

129. Kahn CR, Kasuga M, King GS, Grunfeld C (1982): Autoantibodies to insulin receptors in man: immunological determinants and mechanisms of action. In: *Receptor Antibodies and Disease*, Ciba Symposium 90, pp 91-106. Pitman, London.
130. Khoker MA, Dandona P (1983): Insulin-like stimulatory effect of Fc fragments of human immunoglobulin G on rat adipocyte lipogenesis: indirect evidence for Fc receptor on adipocytes. *J. Clin. Endocrinol. Metab.*, *56*, 393–396.
131. Rotter JI, Rimoin DL (1983): Genetics of Type I diabetes. *Acta Endocrinol. (Copenhagen)*, *103*, *Suppl. 256*, 26A.
132. Kaplan DR, Colca JR, McDaniel ML (1983): Insulin as a surface marker on isolated cells from the rat pancreatic islets. *J. Cell Biol.*, *97*, 433–437.
133. Kaplan DR (1984): Possible target antigens in autoimmune endocrine disease. *Immunol. Today*, *5*, 130–131.
134. Schernthaner G, Borkenstein M, Fink M, Mayr WR, Menzel J, Schuber E (1983): Immunogeneity of human insulin (Novo) or pork monocomponent insulin in HLA-DR typed insulin-dependent diabetic individuals. *Diabetes Care*, *6*, *Suppl. 1*, 43–48.
135. Reeves WG, Gelsthorpe K, Van der Minne R, Toresma R, Tattersall RB (1984): HLA phenotype and insulin antibody production. *Clin. Exp. Immunol.*, *57*, 443–448.
136. Cohen IR, Elias D, Maron R, Schechter Y (1983): Immunization to insulin generates anti-idiotypes that behaves as antibodies to insulin hormone receptor and cause diabetes mellitus. In: *Idiotypic Manipulations in Biological Systems*, pp 1–22. Editors: H. Kohler, P.A. Cazenave and J. Urbain. Academic Press, New York.
137. Brossette N, Van Obberghen E, Fehlmann M (1984): Interaction between insulin-receptors and major histocompatibility complex antigens in mouse liver membranes. *Diabetologia*, *27*, *Suppl.*, 74–76.
138. Bottazzo GF, Pouplard A, Florin-Christensen A, Doniach D (1975): Autoantibodies to prolactin-secreting cells of human pituitary. *Lancet*, *2*, 97–101.
139. Mirakian R, Cudworth AG, Bottazzo GF, Richardson CA, Doniach D (1982): Autoimmunity to anterior pituitary cells and the pathogenesis of Type I (insulin-dependent) diabetes mellitus. *Lancet*, *1*, 755–759.
140. Drexhage HA, Bottazzo GF, Doniach D, Bitensky L, Chayen J (1980): Evidence for thyroid-growth-stimulating immunoglobulins in some goitrous thyroid diseases. *Lancet*, *2*, 287–292.
141. Chiovato L, Van der Gaar RG, Hanafusa T, Drexhage HA, Doniach D, Bottazzo GF (1983): The growing importance of receptor antibodies for thyroidology. In: *Autoimmunity in Thyroid Disorders*. Editors: H. Schatz and D. Doniach. Georg Thieme Verlag, Stuttgart.
142. Bobbioni E, Jeanrenaud B (1982): Effect of rat hypothalamic extract administration on insulin secretion in vivo. *Endocrinology*, *110*, 631–636.
143. Beloff-Chain A, Morton J, Dunmore S, Taylor GW, Morris MR (1983): Evidence that the insulin secretagogue B-cell-tropin is ACTH 22-39. *Nature (London)*, *301*, 255–258.
144. Mirakian R, Richardson CA, Bottazzo GF, Doniach D (1981): Humoral autoimmunity to gut related endocrine cells. *Clin. Immunol. Newslett.*, *2*, 161–167.

145. Bottazzo GF, Vandelli C, Mirakian R (1980): The detection of autoantibodies to discrete endocrine cells in complex endocrine organs. In: *Autoimmune Aspects of Endocrine Disorders*, pp 367–377. Editors: A. Pinchera, D. Doniach, G.F. Fenzi and L. Baschien. Academic Press, London.
146. Winter WE, MacLaren NK, Riley WJ, Unger RH, Neufeld M, Ozand PT (1984): Pancreatic Alpha-cell autoantibodies and glucagon response to arginine. *Diabetes*, *33*, 435–437.
147. Betterle C, Zanette F, Trevisan A, Valerio A, Tessari P, Tiengo A (1982): Glucagon cell autoantibodies: a clinical and metabolic study. *Diabetologia*, *23*, 293A.
148. Shopfer K, Matter L, Tenschert R, Bauer S, Zuppinger K (1984): Anti-glucagon-cell and anti-adrenal-medullary-cell antibodies in islet autoantibody positive diabetic children. (Letter to the Editor) *N. Engl. J. Med.*, *310*, 1536–1537.
149. White NH, Skor DA, Cryer PE, Santiago JV (1984): Anti-glucagon and anti-adrenal medullary cell antibodies in islet cell autoantibody-positive diabetic children. (Letter to the Editor) *N. Engl. J. Med.*, *310*, 1537.
150. MacCuish AC, Irvine WJ (1975): Autoimmunological aspects of diabetes mellitus. *Clin. Endocrinol. Metab.*, *4*, 435–471.
151. Doniach D, Bottazzo GF (1983): Early detection of autoimmune endocrine disorders. *Hosp. Up-date*, *9*, 1145–1160.
152. Riley WJ, MacLaren NK, Lezotte DC, Spillar RP, Rosenbloom AL (1983): Thyroid autoimmunity in insulin-dependent diabetes mellitus: the case for routine screening. *J. Pediatr.*, *98*, 350–354.
153. Riley WJ, MacLaren NK, Neufeld M (1980): Adrenal autoantibodies and Addison's disease in insulin dependent diabetes mellitus. *J. Pediatr.*, *97*, 191–198.
154. Riley WJ, Toskes PP, MacLaren NK, Silverstein JS (1982): Predictive value of gastric parietal cell autoantibodies as a marker for gastric and hematological abnormalities associated with insulin-dependent diabetes. *Diabetes*, *31*, 1081–1088.
155. Huang SW, Hallquist-Haedt L, Rich S, Barbosa J (1981): Prevalence of antibodies to nucleic acids in insulin-dependent diabetics and their relatives. *Diabetes*, *30*, 873–874.
156. Vialettes B, Rousset B, Vague PH, Mornex R (1983): Tubulin antibodies in recent onset Type I (insulin-dependent) diabetes: A new serological marker separate from islet cell antibodies. *Diabetologia*, *25*, 202.
157. Serjeantson S, Theopilus J, Zimmet P, Court J, Crossley JR, Elliot RB (1981): Lymphocytotoxic antibodies and histocompatibility antigens in juvenile-onset diabetes mellitus. *Diabetes 30*, 26–29.
158. Junker K, Egeberg J, Kromann H, Nerup J (1977): An autopsy study of the islets of Langerhans in acute onset juvenile diabetes mellitus. *Acta Pathol. Microbiol. Scand.*, *85*, 699–706.
159. Gepts W, De Mey J (1978): Islet cell survival determined by morphology – an immunocytochemical study of the islets of Langerhans in juvenile diabetes mellitus. *Diabetes*, *27*, *Suppl.*, 251–261.
160. Foulis AK, Stewart JA (1984): The pancreas in recent-onset Type I (insulin-dependent) diabetes mellitus: insulin content of islets, insulitis and associated changes in the exocrine acinar tissue. *Diabetologia*, *26*, 456–461.

161. Gepts W (1984): The pathology of the pancreas in human diabetes. In: *Immunology in Diabetes*, Chapter 2, pp 21-34. Editors: D. Andreani, U. Di Mario, K.F. Federlin and L.G. Heding. Kimpton, London.
162. Bottazzo GF, Dean BM, McNally JM, Mackay EM (1983): Direct evidence of various immunological phenomena associated with the 'insulitis' process. *Diabetologia*, *25*, 142A.
163. Sai P, Kremer M, Nomballais MF, Dillet G (1984): Antibodies spontaneously bound to islet cells in Type I diabetes. (Letter to the Editor) *Lancet*, *2*, 233–234.
164. Bottazzo GF, Dean BM (1984): Evidence of the expression of Class II (HLA-DR) and increased presentation of Class I (HLA-A,B,C) molecules in pancreatic islets in Type I (insulin-dependent) diabetes. *Diabetologia*, *27*, 259A.
165. Zinkernagel RM, Doherty PC (1974): Immunological surveillance against altered self-components by sensitized T lymphocytes in lymphocytic choriomeningitis. *Nature (London)*, *251*, 547.
166. Hanafusa T, Pujol-Borrell R, Chiovato L, Russell RCG, Doniach D, Bottazzo GF (1983): Aberrant expression of HLA-DR antigen on thyrocytes in Graves' disease: relevance for autoimmunity. *Lancet*, *2*, 1111–1115.
167. Bottazzo GF, Doniach D (1984): Polyendocrine autoimmunity. In: *Autoimmunity and Endocrine Disease*. Editor: R. Volpe, M. Dekker, Inc., New York (In press).
168. Ratzman KP, Strese J, Witt S, Berling H, Keilacker H, Michaelis D (1984): Mumps infection and insulin-dependent diabetes mellitus. *Diabetes Care*, *7*, 170–173.
169. Bottazzo GF, Todd I, Pujol-Borrell R (1984): Hypothesis for the genetic contributions to the aetiology of diabetes mellitus. *Immunol. Today*, *5*, 230–231.
170. Bell GI, Horita S, Karam JN (1984): A polymorphic locus near the human insulin gene is associated with insulin-dependent diabetes mellitus. *Diabetes*, *33*, 176–183.
171. Hitman GA, Tarn AC, Drummond V, Williams LG, Joweti NI, Bottazzo GF, Galton DJ (1984): An association of insulin-dependent diabetes with a highly variable locus close to the insulin gene on chromosome 11. Submitted for publication.
172. Bothwell A (1983): Enhancement, translocation and the behavior of V genes. *Immunol. Today*, *4*, 315.
173. Hodge SE, Anderson OE, Neis-Wanger K, Spencer MA, Sparkes RS, Sparkes MC, Crist M, Terasaki PI, Rimoin DL, Rotter JL (1981): Close genetic linkage between diabetes mellitus and kidd blood group. *Lancet*, *2*, 893–895.
174. Burnet BM (1959): *The Clonal Selection Theory of Acquired Immunity*. Cambridge University Press, Cambridge.
175. Adams DD (1983): Autoimmune Mechanisms. In: *Autoimmune Endocrine Disease*, pp 1–39. Editor: T.F. Davies. John Wiley and Sons, New York.
176. Adams DD, Adams YJ, Knight JG, McCall J, White P, Horrocks R, Loghem E (1984): A solution to the genetic and environmental puzzles of insulin-dependent diabetes mellitus. *Lancet*, *1*, 420–423.
177. Field LL, Anderson CE, Rimoin DL (1984): Inheritance of immunoglobulin

light chain genes in pairs of siblings with insulin dependent diabetes mellitus. (Letter to the Editor) *Lancet*, *1*, 1132.
178. Adams DD (1984): V genes and autoimmune disease. (Letter to the Editor) *Lancet*, *2*, 463–464.
179. Jerne NK, Roland G, Cazenave PA (1982): *Embo J.*, *1*, 243–424.
180. Cooke A, Lydyard PM, Roitt IM (1983): Mechanisms of autoimmunity: a role for cross-reactive idiotypes. *Immunol. Today*, *4*, 170–175.
181. Plotz PH (1983): Autoantibodies are anti-idiotype antibodies to anti-viral antibodies. *Lancet*, *2*, 824–826.
182. Strosberg D, Courand PO, Schreiber A (1982): Immunological studies of hormone receptors, a two way approach. *Immunol. Today*, *2*, 1499–1507.
183. Barclay AN, Mason DW (1982): Induction of Ia antigen in rat epidermal cells and gut epithelium by immunological stimuli. *J. Exp. Med.*, *156*, 1665–1676.
184. Klareskog L, Forsum U, Peterson PA (1980): Hormonal regulation of the expression of I antigens on mammary gland epithelium. *Eur. J. Immunol.*, *10*, 958–963.
185. Barclay AN, Mason DW (1983): Graft rejection and Ia antigens – paradox resolved? *Nature (London)*, *303*, 382–383.
186. Lloyd KO, Ng J, Diffold WG (1981): Analysis of the biosynthesis of HLA-DR glycoproteins in human malignant melanoma cell lines. *J. Immunol.*, *126*, 2408–2413.
187. Bottazzo GF, Pujol-Borrell R, Hanafusa T, Feldmann M (1983): Hypothesis: role of aberrant HLA-DR expression and antigen presentation in the inductions of endocrine autoimmunity. *Lancet*, *2*, 1115–1119.
188. Pujol-Borrell R, Hanafusa T, Chiovato L, Bottazzo GF (1983): Lectin-induced expression of DR antigen on human cultured follicular thyroid cells. *Nature (London)*, *304*, 71–73.
189. Ballardini G, Bianchi F, Mirakian R, Pisi E, Doniach D, Bottazzo GF (1984): Aberrant expression of HLA-DR antigens on bile duct epithelium in primary biliary cirrhosis: relevance to pathogenesis. *Lancet* (in press).
190. Messenger AG, Bleehen SS, Slater DN, Rooney N (1984): Expression of HLA-DR in hair follicles in allopecia areata. *Lancet*, *2*, 287.
191. Todd I, Pujol-Borrell R, Hammond L, Bottazzo GF, Feldmann M (1984): Interferon-gamma induces HLA-DR expression by thyroid epithelium. Submitted for publication.
192. Bottazzo GF (1984): B-cell damage in diabetic insulitis: are we approaching the solution? *Diabetologia*, *26*, 241–249.

The Diabetes Annual/1
K.G.M.M. Alberti and L.P. Krall, editors

ISBN 0444 90 343 7
$0.85 per article per page (transactional system)
$0.20 per article per page (licensing system)

3 Genetics of diabetes

R.D.G. LESLIE AND D.A. PYKE

Our understanding of the genetics of diabetes has been revolutionized in the last decade by studies in identical twins and of HLA genes. These studies have proved that the two clinical types of the disorder, insulin-dependent diabetes (IDDM or Type 1 diabetes) and non-insulin-dependent diabetes (NIDDM or Type 2) are genetically distinct. IDDM is associated with genes in the HLA region of Chromosome 6, while NIDDM is not.

Insulin-dependent diabetes (IDDM)

Genetic influences are powerful in IDDM but the disease is in part determined by non-genetic factors. Studies of identical twins have shown that in approximately half of those with IDDM the co-twin is unaffected; as identical twins share the same genes, such differences must be due to environmental factors (1). Environmental agents are not entirely responsible for the development of IDDM since even those IDDM twins with an unaffected co-twin are themselves genetically susceptible to the disease through genes in the HLA region (2). The nature of the environmental agent is unclear though both viruses and toxins have been implicated.

The HLA association with IDDM is principally through alleles of the HLA-D/DR locus. The strongest positive association is between HLA-D/DR 3 and D/DR 4 and the strongest negative association is with HLA-D/DR 2 (3). The positive associations with HLA B8, 15 and 18 are due to linkage disequilibrium of these genes with D/DR 3 and D/DR 4; and in the same way, the negative association with HLA-B7 is due to this gene being in linkage disequilibrium with D/DR 2.

Population studies demonstrate that HLA-DR4 is positively and HLA-DR2 is negatively associated with IDDM in all ethnic groups. HLA-DR3 is associated with IDDM only in American black and Caucasian populations. The strength of these associations is expressed as a relative risk (RR), which is the factor by which disease risk is increased in those with as compared to those without a genetic marker. Thus an increased relative risk is carried by individuals with HLA-DR4 (RR = 7) and DR3 (RR = 5) and a decreased risk by HLA-DR2 (RR = 0.12). The most powerful evidence that IDDM is associated with an HLA-haplotype is provided by family studies. If IDDM is linked with an HLA-haplotype then the disease and the haplotype should segregate together in families such that similarly affected sibs will tend to share one or two haplotypes. This is indeed the case; about 95% of IDDMs share an HLA-haplotype with an affected sib (4).

One or two HLA genes?

The mode of inheritance of IDDM remains controversial. Autosomal dominant inheritance is unlikely. A simple autosomal recessive model can be rejected using a method devised by Rotter (5). This model rejects simple recessive inheritance when the number of DR3/DR4 heterozygotes exceeds the combined sum of DR3/3 and DR4/4 homozygotes in a diabetic population. The method does not depend on ratios or data from non-diabetic populations. Recessive inheritance was rejected since of 193 IDDMs the number of heterozygotes was 68 compared with a maximum number of 22 homozygotes ($P < 0.0001$). This method does not reject two alleles at a single locus acting in addition to increase gene penetrance. However, this single-locus gene dosage model can also be rejected since it cannot account for the consistent increase observed in the relative risk of DR3/4 heterozygotes (RR = 14) compared with DR3 or DR4 homozygotes. More strikingly it cannot account for the increased disease expression in identical co-twins of IDDMs heterozygous for HLA-DR3/DR4 as compared with co-twins of IDDMs with either DR3 or DR4 alone (2). A total of 106 pairs of identical twins were typed for HLA-DR of whom 56 were concordant and 50 discordant for IDDM. The heterozygous phenotype DR3/DR4 was more prevalent in concordant than discordant pairs (59 and 28% respectively). The discordant pairs were likely to remain discordant as at least 5 years had elapsed since the affected twin had been diagnosed. Phenotypes, not genotypes were studied – so the rate of homozygosity could not be established. However, if we assume that those twins in whom the second DR antigen could not be identified were actually homozygous for HLA-DR3 or 4 then 70% of HLA-DR3/4 heterozygotes were concordant for diabetes as compared with at the most 38% of both DR3 and DR4 homozygotes. This increase in disease expression in heterozygotes as compared with homozygotes has been confirmed in family studies (6) and is incompatible with a single-gene two-allele model in which there is a gene dosage effect. Current evidence therefore favors two susceptibility genes associated with HLA-DR3 and DR4, respectively.

Heterogeneity

If there are two or more genes causing diabetes, then each gene might be associated with a different disease pathogenesis. Hence IDDM has been divided into an autoimmune and a viral-induced type (7). Whilst there is no evidence to support the existence of the latter type there is substantial evidence that those patients with IDDM in whom islet cell antibodies persist have an increased prevalence of HLA-B8 and DR3 as compared with patients in whom the antibody does not persist (8). Genetic control of autoantibody production has been confirmed in a family study for complement-fixing but not non-complement-fixing islet cell antibodies (9). Of 323 sibs of 193 diabetics 42 had islet cell antibodies and these antibodies were distributed in a random fashion between HLA non-identical, haplo-identical and identical sibs. The distribution of those 13 with complement-fixing islet cell antibodies on the other hand favored an HLA association since none were found in HLA-non-identical sibs as against 7 in haplo-identical and 6 in HLA-identical sibs. It has been suggested that those diabetics with persistent islet cell antibodies have a strong autoimmune basis to their diabetes and tend to be diagnosed in middle age (8). However, there is no evidence that the frequency of HLA-DR3 increases with age at diagnosis of diabetes. In this it differs from HLA-DR4 which is found in some 77% of IDDMs diagnosed under the age of 10 but only 27% diagnosed over the age of 30 (8th International Tissue Typing Workshop). Nevertheless HLA-DR4 remains a high-risk antigen in Caucasians diagnosed in middle age (10). In 54 insulin-requiring, ketosis-prone, lean diabetics diagnosed after the age of 40 the frequency of HLA-DR4 was increased (RR = 4.6) and that of HLA-DR2 was decreased (RR = 0.18) even after correction for the number of antigens tested.

Susceptibility axes

The question arises as to whether the tendency for genes to co-exist in IDDM in the HLA B, C, D, DR and Bf and complement region of Chromosome 6 is due to linkage disequilibrium with HLA-D/DR genes or whether these other genes themselves play a role in the pathogenesis of the disease through gene interaction. There is no evidence that either complement or Bf genes confer genetic susceptibility independently of the HLA system. Thus in a study of HLA and Bf genotypes in 75 families with an IDDM proband the frequency of the rare allele BfF1 was increased but only in association with HLA-B18 and CW5 (11). All HLA-B8 subjects and 15 of 16 BW62 subjects had the BfS allele. If the association between IDDM and complement and Bf alleles is through linkage disequilibrium with the HLA-DR region then the alleles associated with HLA-DR3 and 4 should be the same in diabetics and non-diabetics. A study of genetic markers in 60 patients with IDDM and 169 control subjects indicated that the association between IDDM and HLA-DR3 is accounted for by the haplotype or susceptibility axis HLA B8 BfS C4AQO C4B1 DR3 (RR = 1.9) and B18 BfF1 C4A3 C4BQO DR3 (RR = 7.6) but not by other DR3 axes such as B8 BfS C4QO C4A1 DR3 (RR = 1) (12). Similarly the association between HLA-DR4 and IDDM is accounted by the axis HLA-B15 BfS C4A3 C4B2.9 DR4 (RR = 17.7) but not by other axes such as B4 BfS C4A3 C4QO DR4 (RR = 0.6). Thus certain susceptibility axes in some IDDM patients carry a greater risk than the HLA-DR allele alone suggesting gene interaction is important because linkage disequilibrium cannot of itself explain the association with complement and Bf alleles. This assumes that both HLA-DR3 and DR4 are single alleles each linked to a susceptibility gene. Recent evidence indicates that they are not. The human HLA-D region encodes Class 2 antigens each of which consists of two polypeptide chains (α and β) inserted into the plasma membrane. The β-chain is coded by several genes which show marked polymorphism. Differences may exist in hybridization patterns of DNA coding for the β-chain in patients positive for HLA DR4 with and without IDDM (13). A β-chain cDNA probe, pDR-β-1, has been prepared which contains DNA sequences complementary to both the coding region and 3′-non-translated sequences of Class 2 antigen β-chain messenger RNA. DNA from HLA-DR4 subjects was digested with endonucleases BamH1, EcoR1 and PstI; electrophoresed on agar gel; transferred to nitrocellulose sheets by Southern blotting; hybridized with the probe and autoradiographed. A 3.7 kb fragment following BamH1 digestion was absent in 29 diabetics but present in 3 of 9 HLA-DR4 non-diabetics. An 18 kb fragment following PstI digestion was found in all 15 diabetics with HLA-DR4 but only 6 of 9 non-diabetics with HLA-DR4. These genetic differences in the HLA-D region between diabetics and non-diabetics who are HLA-DR4 positive suggests that certain genes in the HLA-D/DR region may carry a particular disease risk which the usual immunological typing techniques cannot at present demonstrate. These differences between diabetic and non-diabetic HLA-DR4 may yet enable us to explain the association with complement and Bf alleles through linkage disequilibrium.

Non-HLA genes

Approximately 50% of non-diabetics are HLA-DR3 or DR4 and yet only about 0.1% of the population develops IDDM. How can so many people carry the susceptibility gene when only a few develop the disease? Non-genetic factors must in part explain this discrepancy. Further studies of HLA-DR subtypes, complement and Bf alleles should enable us to define further the difference between HLA-DR3 and 4 subjects with and without IDDM. Since a large number of autoimmune disorders are associated with HLA-DR3 the question arises as to which factor, be it genetic or non-genetic, confers that specificity which produces IDDM rather than, for example, chronic active hepatitis. There is evidence for a second non-HLA-linked gene which predisposes to IDDM. The insulin gene on the short arm of chromosome 11 is flanked by a polymorphic region with three major alleles: a common small Class 1 allele averaging 570 base pairs, a rare intermediate Class 2 allele of 1320 base pairs and a large Class 3 allele which averages 2470 base pairs. In a study of 113 unrelated IDDMs and 83 non-diabetic subjects there was a significantly higher frequency of both Class 1 alleles and genotypes containing two Class 1 alleles in the diabetics (14). This important observation needs to be confirmed but preliminary studies from other groups give reason to believe it will be. Confirmation of linkage between IDDM and the Class 1 allele must await family studies.

The search for other non-HLA markers has been less fruitful. A preliminary observation indicated an association between the Kidd (Jk) red blood cell marker located on Chromosome 2 and IDDM (15). This observation has not been confirmed by the same authors in an extended study of 103 patients with IDDM (16). In another study of 133 families with IDDM there was strong evidence that Kidd and IDDM were not linked (17). Assuming three genetic models (autosomal recessive, additive and dominant) the lod scores at zero recombination were −18.51, −11.62 and −6.03 for each model respectively (a positive lod score would suggest linkage). An interesting but very preliminary observation has suggested linkage between IDDM and an immunoglobulin gene allotype on Chromosome 2, which codes for the constant region of kappa light chain antibodies (18). Since constant region genes are closely linked to variable region genes the suggestion is that the linkage is between IDDM and variable region genes. A study of 4 patients with Graves' disease and 6 with IDDM and Graves' disease showed that all ten patients shared the same kappa light chain allotype with a similarly affected sib. This observation indicates linkage between Graves' disease and this light chain allotype. Two further families were studied in whom the proband had IDDM and a similarly affected sib. In both the diabetics shared the same kappa light chain allotype. The result from these two families were pooled with those from the six families with IDDM and Graves' disease and the authors concluded that IDDM also showed linkage with certain light chain allotypes. This conclusion is not valid since it ignores the established linkage between Graves' disease and these allotypes and is based on only two observations.

Acetylator status is another possible genetic marker for IDDM. However, all the recently reported studies have been designed to assess a relationship between acetylator status and diabetic neuropathy. Fast acetylators were found in 74% of 116 IDDM patients, 54% of non-insulin-dependent diabetics and 48% of non-diabetics in one study (19) and in 49% of IDDMs and 37% of non-diabetics in another (20). It remains to be determined whether acetylator status is influenced by metabolic changes and whether this association is found in an unbiased population study.

Non-insulin-dependent diabetes (NIDDM)

The genetics of NIDDM is distinct from that of IDDM. The two types breed true. NIDDM, being much the commoner type in all communities, is often found in relatives of IDDM subjects but no more often than in the general population (21). There is a strong inherited component in the etiology of NIDDM which is unassociated with HLA types. This is proved by twin studies.

Twin Studies in NIDDM

Concordance in identical (monozygotic) twins with respect to diabetes (or any other disease) does not prove that it is genetically determined; co-twins usually share the same environment, at least in early life, and will therefore be concordant (both twins affected) for diseases such as measles or tuberculosis, because they are both exposed to the infecting organism. However, if twin pairs are concordant for a disease with onset in later life, when co-twins are living apart and thus exposed to different environments, the evidence becomes more persuasive.

In the case of NIDDM concordance among identical twins is high; more so than for IDDM (1). Among 53 pairs of identical twins 48 were concordant for NIDDM, only 5 discordant. Furthermore in the 5 discordant pairs the affected twins had been discovered to be diabetic only within the previous 5 years and the unaffected twins might therefore be expected to become diabetic themselves.

When the 5 unaffected twins were tested by glucose challenge mean glucose values were raised, insulin secretion was diminished and metabolite values were also abnormal (22). It might be concluded from this that most or all of these 'unaffected' twins are destined to become diabetic but it remains to be established whether this will be so.

Later results on this series of twins (unpublished) have shown a larger number of discordant pairs, highlighting the risks of biased ascertainment in studies of this kind in which diabetic twins are reported, not through population surveys, but by their physicians because they happen to have been diagnosed as such. Nevertheless it remains true that of 37 pairs in which NIDDM was diagnosed in one twin before 1970 the other has become diabetic in every case, 75% of them within 6 years.

This high degree of concordance for NIDDM is seen despite the fact that co-twins are almost always living apart when diabetes is diagnosed in the index twin and, perhaps more important and surprising, when neither twin is obese and when their weights are widely different. Co-twins differed from each other at the time of diagnosis by 5 kg or more in 75% of cases and by more than 15 kg in about 30% and it was as often that the diagnosis was made first in the lighter twin as it was in the heavier.

These results, whilst not refuting the well-known association of NIDDM with obesity, cast doubt upon its etiological significance. Furthermore, they suggest that other environmental, or non-genetic factors, such as diet or occupation are also unlikely to play important roles in the production of NIDDM, at least in these twin pairs.

Is NIDDM a single entity?

We have spoken as if NIDDM were a single disease but there is little direct evidence for this belief and considerable reason to doubt it.

NIDDM usually appears in late life but it has been recognized for many years that it may be diagnosed in childhood. It may then be referred to as maturity-onset diabetes (a term now no longer used) of youth, or MODY. This is a useful but purely descriptive term. It is probable that MODY itself is not a single disorder; indeed some cases of MODY turn out, on follow-up, to be insulin-dependent diabetes of unusually slow development.

However, the majority of cases are probably due to the apparently discrete disorder which we prefer to call by the neutral term Mason-type diabetes – after the proposita (23). The features of this type of diabetes are that it is often, although by no means always, diagnosed in childhood or early adult life, it is and remains non-insulin-requiring, and it is inherited as an autosomal dominant – as shown by inheritance through three or more consecutive generations, a ratio of affected to unaffected among the offspring of cases of about 1:1 and the presence of non-insulin-requiring diabetes in one parent of affected cases. This type of diabetes was described over half a century ago (24) but its frequency and importance have only recently come to be appreciated (25). It is not a rare condition, as has often been suggested; if all young diabetics are at once put on insulin treatment, even in the absence of ketonuria, cases of Mason-type diabetes are likely to be missed and the syndrome may therefore be thought to be rare.

This type of diabetes is not linked with HLA (26) nor to variations of the flanking region of the insulin gene (27) (see next section).

Insulin and insulin receptor variants

Proinsulin is the precursor of insulin and C-peptide. Proinsulin has a low insulin-like biological activity but it cross-reacts with the insulin antibody used in the radioimmunoassay of serum insulin. Normally less than 10% of insulin immunoreactivity is due to proinsulin. A rare syndrome of familial hyperproinsulinemia has been described, in which affected patients have very high levels of proinsulin, presumably due to deficient breakdown of the parent molecule to insulin and C-peptide (28). The defect is transmitted through families as an autosomal dominant trait. Affected individuals have in addition normal circulating insulin, which probably accounts for their normal glucose tolerance. However, in a few subjects the level of normal insulin may be inadequate and patients with NIDDM and hyperproinsulinemia have been described (28). When a hormone with reduced biological activity is produced it may be secreted to excess. Therefore the search for other insulin variants has centered on those patients with hyperglycemia and hyperinsulinemia typical of insulin resistance but in whom the response to exogenous insulin is normal. Three mutant insulines from such individuals have been described (29). One, designated insulin Chicago, has been identified as normal insulin except for the 25 position on the β-chain where leucine has been substituted for phenylalanine. In two of these three patients it has been possible to demonstrate mutation at a site corresponding to B24 or 25 in one insulin gene allele. Insulin extracted from pancreatic tissue of the patient with a B25 substitution contained both normal insulin and the variant insulin, suggesting co-dominant expression of both insulin alleles. The importance of these observations and their relevance, if any, to the etiology of NIDDM in general remains to be determined.

A further patient with mild diabetes, fasting hyperinsulinemia and normal sensitivity to exogenous insulin had a serine for phenylalanine substitution at Position 24 on the insulin β-chain (30). Restriction-endonuclease cleavage of DNA showed loss of the Mbo11 recognition site in one allele of the insulin gene consistent with a point mutation at this site. A study of her family revealed five additional affected relatives in three generations with variable degrees of glucose tolerance, ranging from normal to diabetic.

A genetic deficiency of insulin receptors causing insulin resistance and severe diabetes has been described in a 14-year-old girl (31). The patient had normal circulating insulin and no detectable insulin receptor antibodies. However, insulin binding to erythrocytes, monocytes, adipocytes and cultured fibroblasts was markedly reduced. Insulin-stimulated glucose transport both in vivo, using a euglycemic clamp, and in isolated adipocytes was decreased. The patient's mother and two sisters were also insulin-resistant with hyperinsulinemia.

Insulin gene

A polymorphic region flanking the human insulin gene on the short arm of Chromosome 11 can be described as a locus with at least three classes of alleles. We have already mentioned the recent report suggesting an association between two Class 1 alleles and IDDM (RR = 3.9) (14). The same study reported a more modest association in Caucasians with NIDDM and possession of two Class 1 alleles (RR = 2.1) (14). Other studies in Caucasians have shown no difference (32) or an increase in genotypes containing two Class 3 alleles in NIDDMs (33). The picture therefore is far from clear. In one study (32) the population was racially mixed. Selection of an appropriate non-diabetic control population is difficult as the incidence of

NIDDM increases with age. Therefore old people (mean age 67) with normal glucose tolerance have been selected, though they might represent a biased group of survivors (34). This possible bias is all the more pertinent since a higher frequency of Class 3 alleles has been described in diabetic and non-diabetic groups with atherosclerosis (34). Thus the association between Class 3 alleles and NIDDM may be due to the high frequency of atherosclerosis in NIDDM. An increased frequency of Class 3 alleles in patients with hypertriglyceridemia has been reported but needs to be confirmed (35).

Confirmation of the putative link between NIDDM and a polymorphic locus near the insulin gene must await family studies. Studies have been performed in families with maturity-onset diabetes of the young (Mason-type diabetes) in whom diabetes is not linked to the insulin gene (27, 36).

If the association between the polymorphic locus and diabetes is confirmed, it remains unclear what role it might play in the etiology of the disease. There is no evidence to suggest that these alleles influence insulin gene expression. It is unlikely that this region is required for expression of the insulin gene since a similar region is absent around the rat insulin gene. It is unlikely that it codes for a protein since every third amino acid would be glycine or proline. Finally, it is difficult to reconcile the proposed association of Class 1 alleles with both IDDM and NIDDM in the light of all we know about the genetic and pathogenetic differences between these diseases.

Chlorpropamide alcohol flushing (CPAF)

Facial flushing after alcohol in diabetics taking chlorpropamide was first reported soon after chlorpropamide was introduced more than 25 years ago. The suggestion that this harmless drug side effect might be inherited and linked to some cases of NIDDM came from the observation of CPAF in two cases of Mason-type diabetes (37), Mrs. Mason and her daughter. It soon became apparent that CPAF commonly occurred in other, more common types of NIDDM (38); indeed about one-third of all NIDDMs, perhaps more, show the reaction. It also occurs in IDDMs and in non-diabetics.

The significance of CPAF is confused largely because of difficulty in its assessment – the reaction is subjective (although associated with objective evidence of facial temperature rise) and is to some extent dependent upon chlorpropamide dosage. There is still no generally accepted technique for testing for CPAF although a dose which leads to a blood level of over 40 mg/l and an assessment which combines subjective sensation of flushing with a rise of facial temperature, from a resting temperature of no more than 32 °C, of 1.5° or more provide a good separation of 'flushers' from 'non-flushers', with only a few 'intermediates'.

The original suggestion was that CPAF is inherited as a simple autosomal dominant (37). Evidence of its genetic character comes from studies in identical twins who are in all, or nearly all, cases concordant for CPAF even when discordant for diabetes; and from the fact that in those 'flushers' whose parents have been tested one has been found to be positive, as have half of their siblings.

In view of the technical difficulties of CPAF testing and doubts about its frequency and association with diabetes these observations should be treated with caution but it still remains probable that CPAF is, in some families at least, an inherited phenomenon (39–43).

Does this tell us anything about non-insulin-dependent diabetes? The suggestion of a peculiar association of CPAF with NIDDM did not take account of the fact that CPAF is seen in IDDMs and in non-diabetics, if with lesser frequency.

In some families with Mason-type diabetes, CPAF is strongly associated with diabetes and may even be a marker for the future appearance of diabetes in unaffected offspring. In other families, however, there seems to be no association (44). These conflicting results may be due to differences in techniques of testing or to Mason-type diabetes being itself a heterogeneous grouping – or both.

With improved techniques of CPAF assessment, measurements of serum levels of acetaldehyde (higher in 'flushers' than in 'non-flushers') and perhaps of liver aldehyde dehydrogenase and of serum levels of metenkephalin (increased by chlorpropamide and alcohol in both flushers and non-flushers), we may learn more about the pathogenesis of the reaction, its mode of inheritance and its association and relevance, if any, to non-insulin-dependent diabetes.

Microvascular complications of diabetes

Complications affecting especially the retina and glomerulus are common in diabetes. Great efforts have been made to establish that they are related to the degree of diabetic control, or rather lack of it. The prevailing view is that the better the control the less the frequency and severity of the complications.

There is certainly much clinical evidence to support this view, but is it the whole truth? Could other, perhaps genetic, factors play a role? An immediate objection to accepting the view that complications result exclusively from poor control is the frequent case of the badly controlled diabetic who escapes all complications. Extensive background retinopathy may be seen at the time of diagnosis, especially in subjects with NIDDM. On the other hand series of diabetics studied after 40 years or more include a high proportion, as much as one third, who are free of all detectable complications (45). These incongruities have raised the suspicion that constitutional factors are involved in the appearance and non-appearance of diabetic complications.

Some support for this comes from identical twin studies. In a series of 85 pairs, 48 IDDM and 37 NIDDM, the co-twins resembled each other in respect of the presence and severity of retinopathy, especially in the NIDDM pairs (46). Classifying retinopathy as nil, background or severe co-twins in 35 of the 37 NIDDM pairs, all of whom had been diabetic for at least 9 years, were in the same category. Among the IDDM pairs, however, the similarity was much less marked; of 10 pairs in which the co-twins had been diabetic for the same time, 5 showed striking differences between co-twins. It seems from this study, therefore, that a genetic element in the pathogenesis of diabetic microvascular disease may be strong in NIDDM but less so in IDDM. Nevertheless, whatever the genetic background, the presence of diabetes seems to be necessary before microvascular disease appears; none of the unaffected co-twins showed any retinopathy. When studies were performed of the basement membrane thickness of muscle capillaries, thickening was found in some of the diabetic twins but in none of the unaffected co-twins (47, 48).

Microvascular complications are rare in Mason-type diabetes and, when present, nearly always mild (49). This might be due to the mildness of the diabetes itself but that does not seem to protect against complications in other forms of non-insulin-dependent diabetes and the relative freedom from complications may be part of the inherited picture.

The strong association of Mason-type diabetes with CPAF, at least in some families, raised the question of a link between CPAF and relative freedom from complications. For the reasons already discussed, the evidence on this point should be viewed with reserve but the possibility of a connection has not yet been disproved and the potential importance of an association is so great that the matter is still worth pursuing.

Finally, there have been suggestions that another diabetic complication, neuropathy, may be linked to an inherited feature, acetylator status, fast acetylators being less prone to develop peripheral neuropathy. However, the association was weak and was confirmed in a study of 116 diabetics, both IDDM and NIDDM, from one center (50) in which, however, the question was raised of whether acetylator status might be a genetic marker of diabetes itself. Since fast acetylation was found in both IDDMs and NIDDMs, whose genetic predisposition to diabetes is so different, this prospect seems unlikely.

Evidence linking HLA types and diabetic complications in IDDMs is conflicting. The best present evidence is that there is no association.

References

1. Barnett AH, Eff C, Leslie RDG, Pyke DA (1981): Diabetes in identical twins: a study of 200 pairs. *Diabetologia*, *20*, 87.
2. Johnston C, Pyke DA, Cudworth AG, Wolf E (1983): HLA-DR typing in identical twins with insulin-dependent diabetes: a difference between concordant and discordant pairs. *Br. Med. J.*, *286*, 253.
3. Platz P, Jakobsen BK, Morling N et al (1981): HLA-D and -DR antigens in genetic analysis of insulin dependent diabetes mellitus. *Diabetologia*, *21*, 108.
4. Wolf E, Spencer KM, Cudworth AG (1983): The genetic susceptibility to Type 1 (insulin-dependent) diabetes, analysis of the HLA-DR association. *Diabetologia*, *24*, 224.
5. Rotter JI, Anderson CE, Rubin R, Congleton JE, Terasakipi, Rimoin DL (1983): HLA genotype study of insulin-dependent diabetes, the excess of DR3/DR4 heterozygotes allows rejection of the recessive hypothesis. *Diabetes*, *32*, 169.
6. Cudworth AG (1983): Type I diabetes mellitus. *Diabetologia*, *14*, 281.
7. Irvine WJ (1977): Classification of idiopathic diabetes. *Lancet*, *1*, 638.
8. Bottazzo G, Cudworth AG, Moul D, Doniach D, Festenstein H (1978): Evidence for a primary autoimmune type of diabetes mellitus. *Br. Med. J.*, *2*, 1253.
9. Spencer KM, Tarn A, Dean BM, Lister J, Bottazzo GF (1984): Fluctuating islet cell autoimmunity in unaffected relatives of patients with insulin dependent diabetes. *Lancet*, *1*, 764.
10. Pittman WB, Acton RT, Berger BD et al (1982): HLA-A, -B, and -DR associations in type I diabetes mellitus with onset after age forty. *Diabetes*, *31*, 122.
11. Wolf E, Cudworth AG, Markwick JR et al (1982): The Bf system in diabetes – gene interaction or linkage disequilibrium. *Diabetologia*, *22*, 85.
12. McCluskey J, McCann WJ, Kay PH et al (1983): HLA and complement allotypes in type I (insulin-dependent) diabetes. *Diabetologia*, *24*, 162.
13. Owerbach D, Lernmark A, Platz P et al (1983): HLA-D region B chain DNA endonuclease fragments differ between HLA-DR identical healthy and insulin-dependent diabetic individuals. *Nature (London)*, *303*, 815.
14. Bell GI, Horita S, Karam JH (1984): A polymorphic locus near the human insulin gene in association with insulin-dependent diabetes mellitus. *Diabetes*, *33*, 176.
15. Hodge SE, Anderson CE, Weiswanger K et al (1981): A second genetic locus for insulin-dependent diabetes mellitus (IDDM), evidence for close linkage between IDDM and Kidd blood group. *Lancet*, *2*, 893.
16. Hodge SE, Anderson CE, Weiswanger K et al (1983): Association studies between type I (insulin-dependent) diabetes and 27 genetic markers: lack of association between type 1 diabetes and Kidd blood group. *Diabetologia*, *25*, 343.
17. Dunsworth TS, Rich SS, Swenson J, Barbosa J (1982): No evidence for linkage between diabetes and the Kidd marker. *Diabetes*, *31*, 991.
18. Adams DD, Adams YJ, Knight TG et al (1984): A solution to the genetic

and environmental puzzles of insulin-dependent diabetes mellitus. *Lancet*, *1*, 420.
19. Shenfield GM, McCann VJ, Tjokresctio R et al (1982): Acetylator status and diabetic neuropathy. *Diabetologia*, *22*, 441.
20. Bodansky HJ, Wolf E, Cudworth AG et al (1982): Genetic and immunologic factors in microvascular disease in type I insulin-dependent diabetes. *Diabetes*, *31*, 70.
21. Irvine WJ, Toft AD, Holton DE et al (1977): Familial studies of type I and type II idiopathic diabetes mellitus. *Lancet*, *2*, 325.
22. Barnett AH, Spiliopoulos AJ, Pyke DA et al (1981): Metabolic studies in unaffected co-twins of non-insulin dependent diabetics. *Br. Med. J.*, *1*, 1656.
23. Tattersall RB (1974): Mild familial diabetes with dominant inheritance. *Q. J. Med.*, *43*, 339.
24. Cammidge PJ (1928): Diabetes mellitus and heredity. *Br. Med. J.*, *2*, 738.
25. Tattersall RB, Fajans SS (1975): A difference between the inheritance of classical juvenile onset and maturity onset type diabetes of young people. *Diabetes*, *24*, 44.
26. Nelson PG, Pyke DA (1976): Genetic diabetes not linked to the HLA locus. *Br. Med. J.*, *1*, 196.
27. Bell JI, Wainscoat JS, Old JM et al (1983): Maturity onset diabetes of the young is not linked to the insulin gene. *Br. Med. J.*, *1*, 590.
28. Robbins DC, Shoelson SE, Rubenstein AH, Tager HS (1984): Familial hyperproinsulinaemia: two cohorts secreting indistinguishable Type II intermediates of proinsulin conversion. *J. Clin. Invest.*, *73*, 714.
29. Shoelson S, Haneda M, Blix P et al (1983): Three mutant insulins in man. *Nature (London)*, *302*, 540.
30. Haneda M, Polansky KS, Berganstal RM et al (1984): Familial hyperinsulinaemia due to a structurally abnormal insulin: definition of an emerging new clinical syndrome. *N. Engl. J. Med.*, *310*, 1288.
31. Scarlett JA, Kolterman OG, Moore P et al (1982): Insulin resistance and diabetes due to a genetic defect in insulin receptors. *J. Clin. Endocrinol. Metab.*, *55*, 123.
32. Rotwein P, Chergwin J, Province M et al (1983): Polymorphism in the 5′-flanking region of the human insulin gene: a genetic marker for non-insulin dependent diabetes. *N. Engl. J. Med.*, *308*, 65.
33. Owerbach D, Nerup J (1982): Restriction fragment length polymorphism of the insulin gene in diabetes mellitus. *Diabetes*, *31*, 275.
34. Owerbach D, Billesbolle P, Schroll M et al (1982): Possible association between DNA sequences flanking the insulin gene and atherosclerosis. *Lancet*, *2*, 1291.
35. Jowett NI, Williams LG, Hitman GA, Galton DJ (1983): An insulin gene polymorphism that relates to diabetic hypertriglyceridaemia. *Diabetes*, *25*, 168.
36. Owerbach D, Thomsen B, Johansen K et al (1983): DNA insertion sequences near the insulin gene are not associated with maturity-onset diabetes of young people. *Diabetologia*, *25*, 18.
37. Leslie RDG, Pyke DA (1978): Chlorpropamide alcohol flushing: a dominantly inherited trait associated with diabetes. *Br. Med. J.*, *2*, 1519.

38. Wiles PG, Pyke DA (1984): The chlorpropamide alcohol flush. *Clin. Sci.* (in press).
39. Ng Tang-Fui S, Keen H, Jarrett RJ et al (1983): Epidemiological study of prevalence of chlorpropamide alcohol flushing in insulin dependent diabetics, non-insulin dependent diabetics and non-diabetics. *Br. Med. J.*, *2*, 1509.
40. Johnston C, Wiles PG, Pyke DA (1984): Chlorpropamide-alcohol flush: the case in favour. *Diabetologia*, *26*, 1.
41. Hillson RM, Hockaday TDR (1984): Chlorpropamide alcohol flush: a critical re-appraisal. *Diabetologia*, *26*, 6.
42. Ng Tang-Fui S, Keen H, Jarrett J, Gossain V, Marsden P (1983): Test for chlorpropamide alcohol flush becomes positive after prolonged chlorpropamide treatment in insulin-dependent and non-insulin dependent diabetics. *N. Engl. J. Med.*, *309*, 93.
43. Kobberling J, Bengsch N, Bruggesboer B et al (1980): The chlorpropamide alcohol flush – lack of specificity for non-insulin-dependent diabetes. *Diabetologia*, *19*, 359.
44. Panzram G, Adolph W (1982): Chlorpropamide alcohol flush test (CPAF) in young MODY diabetics. *Endokrinologie*, *79/2*, 221.
45. Oakley WG, Pyke DA, Tattersall RB, Watkins PJ (1974): Long-term diabetes: a clinical study of 92 patients after 40 years. *Q. J. Med.*, *43*, 145.
46. Leslie RDG, Pyke DA (1982): Diabetic retinopathy in identical twins. *Diabetes*, *31*, 19.
47. Ganda OM, Williamson JR, Soeldner JS et al (1983): Muscle capillary basement membrane width and its relationship to diabetes mellitus in monozygotic twins. *Diabetes*, *32*, 549.
48. Barnett AH, Spiliopoulos AJ, Pyke DA et al (1983): Muscle capillary basement membrane in identical twins discordant for insulin-dependent diabetes. *Diabetes*, *32*, 557.
49. Fajans SS, Cloutier MC, Crowther RL (1978): Clinical and aetiological heterogeneity of idiopathic diabetes mellitus. *Diabetes*, *27*, 1112.
50. Bodansky HJ, Drury PL, Cudworth AG et al (1981): Acetylator phenotypes and type 1 (insulin-dependent) diabetics with microvascular disease. *Diabetes*, *30*, 907.

The Diabetes Annual/1
K.G.M.M. Alberti and L.P. Krall, editors

ISBN 0444 90 343 7
$0.85 per article per page (transactional system)
$0.20 per article per page (licensing system)

4 Immunological aspects of therapy

W.G. REEVES

Interest in the immunological properties of insulin continues to increase. This is largely due to the fact that its primary and tertiary structures are well documented; a number of synthetic analogues have been prepared, species variants are available and it can be obtained in high purity. Furthermore, insulin is the only protein antigen with these characteristics that is frequently injected into man (1). This has enabled important observations to be made concerning the genetic control of insulin antibody production; the nature of which may have implications for the pathogenesis of diabetes itself (2, 3). Recently there has been renewed interest in antibodies with specificity for the insulin receptor and in the possibility that such antibodies may arise as part of the normal anti-idiotype response to the production of insulin antibody: the term 'idiotype' referring to the specific chemical configuration of the antigen-combining site of an antibody – in this case specific for insulin. Another important development is the finding that immunological abnormalities are present for some considerable time before the seemingly 'acute onset' of Type 1 diabetes in man and that similar changes are seen in the BB rat. A dramatic response to the administration of cyclosporin A in pre-diabetic rats has led to trials of cyclosporin in man and this, and other work, has increased the likelihood of successful immunological manipulation in the future (4, 5).

The immune response to injected insulin

Insulin antibodies

The majority of human subjects given subcutaneous injections of bovine, porcine or human insulin develop insulin antibodies gradually during the first 12 months of treatment. These are predominantly of IgG class but are non-precipitating and it is for this reason that most assays for their determination involve the use of radio-labelled insulin in conjunction with a means of separating labelled insulin 'bound' to its antibody from that which remains 'free' in the supernatant. The more important sources of variation

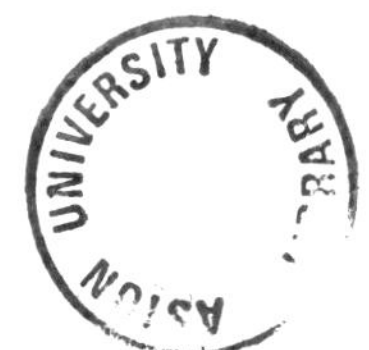

in assay technique and the results derived therefrom have been reviewed recently (6) and information from an international insulin antibody workshop (7) has highlighted the need for standardization of assay conditions and the manner in which results are expressed. A great deal has been published about insulin antibodies but, unfortunately, a significant proportion records the use of indifferent, and sometimes spurious, methodology which can prove a nightmare to the naive investigator.

Various factors affect the magnitude of the immune response to injected insulin (Table 1). Proinsulin contamination greatly enhances the immunogenicity of insulin preparations, and mice genetically unresponsive to purified insulin can produce insulin antibodies following immunization with the more elaborate proinsulin molecule (8). Thus, it was not too surprising that a comparison between conventional bovine insulin (containing > 10,000 p.p.m. proinsulin) and a purified bovine insulin preparation (containing 20–40 p.p.m. proinsulin) did not show a significant difference in insulin antibody level (9). A more recent study using bovine insulin purified to less than 1 p.p.m. does show a significant reduction in the ability to induce insulin antibody although bovine insulin purified to this degree remains more immunogenic than highly purified preparations of porcine or human sequence (10) and the greater immunogenicity of the bovine molecule has been demonstrated in other studies using proinsulin-free material (11).

Many studies have demonstrated the reduced immunogenicity of highly purified porcine insulin preparations (e.g. 12, 13) and it had been suggested that insulin antibodies would become a thing of the past following the introduction of preparations containing insulins of human sequence. However, the single amino acid substitution at the B30 position (threonine in human to alanine in porcine insulin) was never sufficient explanation for the residual immunogenicity of porcine preparations and it was not too

TABLE 1 *Factors affecting the immunogenicity of insulin*

Preparation
Proinsulin contamination
Native molecule, i.e. species
Physico-chemical changes,
e.g. deamidation, dimerisation
Formulation
Site and mode of injection
Recipient
Metabolic status
Genetic background

surprising to find that, when the appropriate comparisons were made, human insulin turned out to be of comparable immunogenicity to that of porcine insulin of similar purity. Many studies have looked at these differences and some are still in progress but it does look as if there is no detectable difference between the two when cross-over studies are performed in patients already established on insulin treatment (14, 15), whereas comparisons made between two matched cohorts receiving either human or porcine insulin from their first insulin exposure can show a minor difference (in favor of human insulin) particularly when the follow-up period is extended for 12 months or more (16, 18).

The physico-chemical reasons why formulations of human insulin administered subcutaneously induce antibody production in contrast to the natural state in vivo are poorly understood but the insulin molecule is prone to aggregation and deamidation and the rate at which these processes take place is affected by the temperature, pH, insulin and zinc concentrations at which insulin preparations are stored. The avoidance of a crystallization step during preparation has also been shown to reduce the immunogenicity of bovine isophane insulin (19). Acid soluble preparations of conventional bovine insulin induce rather higher levels of antibodies reactive with contaminating molecules e.g. pancreatic polypeptide and proinsulin, as well as insulin itself (20) but there is probably little difference in overall immunogenicity between neutral soluble and insoluble preparations whether the latter are produced as insulin zinc suspensions or by complexing with protamine as in the isophane or NPH preparation.

There are few data as yet concerning the difference in immunizing potential of insulins administered by intermittent subcutaneous injection vs. continuous subcutaneous infusion or administration by subcutaneous vs. intravenous routes. Initial reports of amyloidosis developing following continuous insulin infusions have not been confirmed (21, 22). Further reports and comparisons in man are awaited.

A remarkably large variation in antibody response is seen within a group of individuals treated with a standard insulin preparation. The metabolic status of the individual may play a part either in terms of impairment of the immune system in the more severely ill diabetic patient at presentation or in relation to the level of residual B-cell function when exogenous insulin therapy is started. However, in a prospective study conducted in Nottingham we did not find any evidence of a relationship between B-cell function at the time of starting insulin and the levels of insulin antibody produced 6 months later, although there was a suggestion that patients who had had symptoms of diabetes for more than 5 weeks prior to insulin therapy produced lower levels of antibody (20).

Several studies – mostly retrospective – point to an important genetic contribution and we have recently been able to confirm the original observation by Bertrams et al. (23) that patients possessing the HLA-B8 histocompatibility antigen are generally very unresponsive even to the more immunogenic bovine insulins (20). The B8/DR3 haplotype often contains a null gene at the C4A locus and this, in conjunction with evidence that individuals bearing this haplotype are less able to clear immune complexes, may indicate a non antigen-specific abnormality of immunity. Patients bearing the HLA-DR4 haplotype do not show a bias toward high or low responsiveness (3, 24) whereas those that possess HLA-DR7 show much higher levels of insulin antibody (20). This appears to be an antigen-specific phenomenon and may indicate the presence of an immune response gene for insulin (3). Little weight can be given to a report suggesting that DR4-positive individuals are hyper-responsive to insulin (25) as the method of antibody characterization used raises considerable difficulties of analysis and interpretation (see ref 6).

A study by Nakao et al. indicated that variation in the IgG heavy chain allotypes (the Gm system) correlates with the magnitude of the immune response to insulin (26) and our data is in keeping with this observation (20). The dual contribution of genes lying within both HLA and Gm systems has been described for other specific immune responses and emphazises the need for patient groups of adequate size matched with control groups of a similar genetic background in any comparison of insulin immunogenicity in man.

Anti-idiotype and anti-receptor antibodies

There is abundant evidence that if antibody of a particular specificity is purified and injected into another animal, some antibody will be produced having specificity for the individual chemical configuration of the antigen combining site or *idiotype* of the first antibody. Anti-idiotype antibodies can be detected in the same individual that produced the first, idiotype-bearing, antibody and there may be even further recognition phases of the immune response forming an immunological network by which the initial response is regulated (27). Studies in experimental animals have demonstrated that antibodies reactive with insulin receptor-bearing cells can be induced by immunization with insulin and that these antibodies can be blocked or bound by insulin antibodies themselves (28). These antibodies have been interpreted as having anti-idiotype specificity, although they were characterized by virtue of their insulin-like effects on adipocytes. Others have found that normal human IgG can stimulate adipocyte lipogenesis; that this is mediated by the Fc fragment of the IgG molecule and can be neutralized by anti-Fc antisera (29). Whether these, or other serum proteins, can function as non-specific carrier proteins for insulin is still a matter for conjecture.

Naturally occurring anti-insulin receptor antibodies may either stimulate or block the insulin receptor and an individual serum may contain a variety

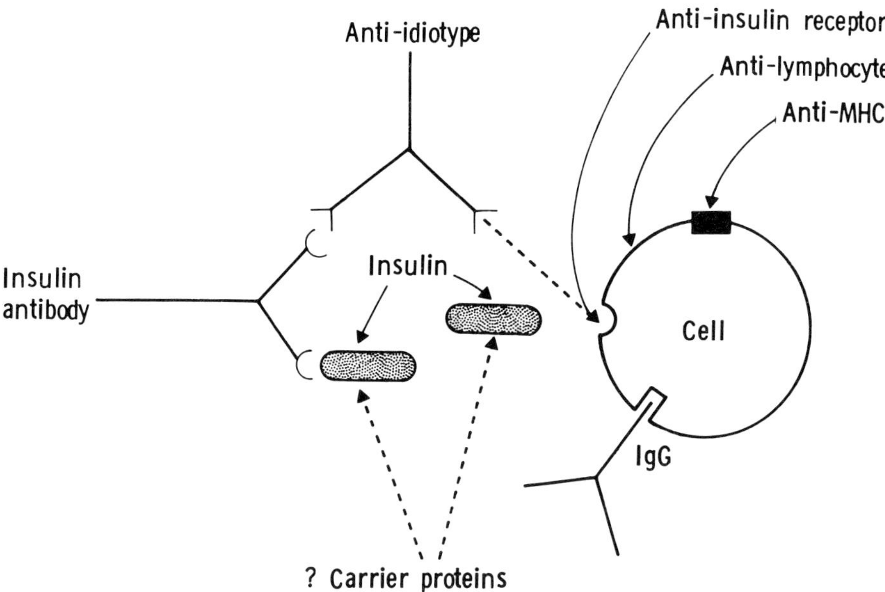

FIG. 1. *Antibodies (and other proteins) that may bind to insulin or insulin-receptor bearing cells.*

of receptor binding specificities (30). Figure 1 indicates diagrammatically how an anti-idiotype antibody induced by the idiotype of an insulin specific antibody might be able to react with at least part of the insulin receptor and compete for insulin binding to it. The insulin receptor-bearing cell is shown bearing, in addition, a receptor for the Fc portion of IgG and glycoproteins forming part of the major histocompatibility complex (MHC). The insulin-receptor bearing cells most often used in in-vitro work are IM-9 cells derived from a lymphoblastoid cell line, monocytes, erythrocytes or adipocytes (31) and a further complexity for much of this work is that anti-lymphocyte antibodies (of both IgM and IgG classes) are present in a variety of diseases including Type 1 diabetes and are found in higher frequency in the first 12 months after presentation and in those patients bearing the HLA-B8/DR3 haplotype (32). Thus, the report of anti-insulin receptor antibodies of IgM class in the sera of 10/22 children with Type 1 diabetes prior to insulin treatment has to be interpreted with care (33). The equation of anti-idiotype antibodies with anti-receptor antibodies has yet to be proved and this will require adequate definition of both 'idiotype' and 'receptor' and the use of rigorous controls. Recent work also demonstrates that insulin receptors are structurally and functionally associated with MHC glycoproteins (34, 35) and therefore antibodies with specificity for HLA may also be active in these systems.

Clinical sequelae

Some of the possible sequelae of the formation of insulin antibodies are listed in Table 2. Insulin allergy, insulin resistance and injection site lipo-atrophy have each become relative rarities following the introduction of highly purified insulins (36). Severe, and occasionally life-threatening, insulin allergy still occurs although there is usually a history of treatment with bovine insulin preparations in the past and skin-testing with these preparations can exacerbate the condition. Effects of insulin antibodies on diabetic control are more subtle and have proved difficult to analyse in view of the marked heterogeneity of insulin antibody production among groups of insulin-treated patients. If diabetic control is optimized and maintained, a relationship is seen in antibody-producing patients between the changes in their antibody levels and their insulin dose requirement on transfer from a more to a less immunogenic insulin regimen and vice versa (13). Although insulin antibodies have often been considered the villain of the piece there is evidence that, in the absence of endogenous insulin secretion, diabetic control may be better in patients with higher levels of antibody (37) and that hyperglycemia develops more slowly following insulin withdrawal in patients possessing plentiful insulin antibody (38). These, and other studies, support the view that insulin antibody acts as a 'sponge' or 'buffer' to damp oscillations in free insulin. Sodoyez et al. (39) have recently demonstrated that ^{125}I-insulin localizes to hepatocytes in control animals but to Kupffer cells in insulin antibody treated animals. It is still possible, however, that the Kupffer cell bound insulin is slowly released and acts on insulin receptors on the hepatocyte.

The ability of insulin to dissociate from its antibody as the free insulin level falls means that hypoglycemia can occur long after the last injection of insulin has been given and will be more readily seen at times of carbohydrate restriction or increased utilization. It should be easier to plan an insulin regimen to suit the C-peptide negative patient who relies entirely on the subcutaneous route but regimens may need to match the degree of antibody buffering present (37, 40).

TABLE 2 *Clinical sequelae of insulin antibody production*

Insulin allergy
Injection site lipo-atrophy
Insulin resistance
Effects on diabetic control
Hypoglycemia
Duration of remission period
Placental transfer
Effects on micro- or macrovasculature

Much has been written about 'spontaneous' hypoglycemia in association with the seemingly spontaneous development of insulin antibodies. The largest body of evidence comes from Japan (41) and in many of the cases described the phenomenon is linked with the administration of antithyroid drugs. Virtually all the cases of spontaneous hypoglycemia with insulin antibodies in which we have been involved have been factitious in nature; due to the self-administration of insulin (42) and it has not been our experience to find insulin antibodies in the absence of exogenous insulin administration. The report by Palmer et al. (43) sets a relatively low and arbitrary binding level above which patients are deemed to have 'insulin antibodies' and records their presence in 16% of patients with juvenile-onset diabetes prior to insulin treatment. They suggest that low levels of insulin antibody may be a marker of B-cell damage but this has yet to be confirmed by others.

It has been suggested that there is a negative correlation between the length of partial remission in Type 1 diabetes and the degree of insulin antibody production. Patients bearing the B8/DR3 haplotype have, generally, much better residual B-cell function at presentation than those with the DR4 haplotype. DR3 associates with hyporesponsiveness to insulin (see above) and it is possible that these two facts are not causally related. A recent study by Ludvigsson supports their coexistence (44) but provides no evidence in favor of the view that insulin antibodies have negative effects on B-cell function. A recent study conducted in the UK provides evidence to suggest that the remission period is due partly to an improvement in B-cell function and partly to a decrease in peripheral insulin resistance but found no correlation between remission and the level of insulin antibody (45).

Babies born to diabetic mothers show increased secretion of insulin and proinsulin and may develop hypoglycemia. Although the babies of mothers with insulin antibodies show concentrations of antibodies similar to those of their mothers, the total levels of immuno-reactive insulin are higher in these babies due in part to increased proinsulin binding (46). Insulin and proinsulin can be transferred across the placenta complexed to insulin or proinsulin-specific antibody (47) and this may explain the increased frequency of hypoglycemia in babies with insulin antibodies.

The possibility that insulin antibodies, and the complexes they may form with injected insulin, may have adverse effects on the vascular complications of diabetes has been a source of anxiety for many years (48). It is fairly easy to detect immune complex-like material in the sera of diabetic patients, whether they have been treated with exogenous insulin or not, but abnormalities on complement testing are rarely found (49) and thus their inflammatory potential is in doubt. A multitude of methods have been used for the detection of immune complexes (IC) but even when similar methods are used e.g. the solid-phase C1q binding assay, reports disagree concerning the existence of a correlation with the levels of IC and the presence of micro-angiopathy (50, 51). I am not aware of any evidence that supports a link between the presence of insulin:anti-insulin IC and micro-angiopathy although this might be obtained by using more sophisticated methods for the immunochemical characterization of soluble IC (52). A study from Oxford demonstrated that higher glucose levels and the possession of HLA-DR4 contributed as independent variables toward the risk of developing diabetic retinopathy (53). As HLA-DR4 does not correlate with higher levels of insulin antibody, this effect is probably mediated by a non antibody-dependent mechanism.

A closely argued case has been made for the role of insulin in the pathogenesis of atherosclerosis, with special reference to the insulin-treated diabetic (54). The production of insulin antibodies in response to insulin therapy is associated with a very considerable rise in levels of immunoreactive insulin (IRI) in the circulation (55) and it seems more likely that any adverse effect of the formation of insulin:insulin antibody complexes in the circulation is likely to be due to the sequestration of considerable amounts of metabolically active insulin within the vascular compartment where it can stimulate smooth muscle cell proliferation and lipid synthesis within the arterial wall (54). Experimentally, elevated levels of insulin antibodies and IRI have been shown to induce increased triglyceride synthesis (56) and more attention probably needs to be paid to macroangiopathic complications when considering the adverse effects of insulin antibody production.

Immunotherapy of Type 1 diabetes

The case for an important contribution by the immune system to the pathogenesis of Type 1 diabetes has been considerably strengthened during the last few years (57, 58). Work from the Barts/Windsor study has clearly demonstrated the existence of a long prodromal period – in which a number of immunological abnormalities can be detected – prior to the development of the acute symptoms of diabetes and a requirement for insulin replacement therapy (59). Several animal models of spontaneous Type 1-like diabetes are available; two of which, the bio-breeding (BB) rat and the non-obese diabetic (NOD) mouse, show immunological abnormalities similar to those found in man, including the presence of islet cell surface antibodies (ICSA) (60). Although viruses are very likely to be the triggering agency in genetically susceptible individuals (57) it is still far from clear whether the resulting mayhem develops as a consequence of a relative incapacity or over-exuberance of the immune system of the susceptible subject. Patients bearing the HLA-B8/DR3 haplotype show an increased incidence of various abnormalities of the immune system, e.g. the presence of null genes at the

C4 loci and IgA deficiency (57), and abnormalities of lymphocyte subpopulations are present from an early stage in many patients with Type 1 diabetes (61). Recent work in the BB rat has shown that the presence of two independent genes is required for the development of diabetes: one causes the T-cell lymphopenia, whereas the other is linked to the major histocompatibility RT1 locus analogous to the HLA system in man (62).

Thus, it is of paramount importance to discover more about the site of action of the susceptibility genes for Type 1 diabetes in man in order to design appropriate therapeutic strategies to prevent or ameliorate this otherwise life-long condition. We know remarkably little about the ability of human B-cells to regenerate after injury and it is possible that promotion of this process could yield a very significant therapeutic gain.

Most forms of immunological intervention tried thus far have been based on the premise that general (i.e. 'broad-spectrum') immunosuppression will offer overall benefit to the recently diagnosed or prodromal diabetic (63–65). Experience of the use of non-specific immunosuppression in other situations e.g. for the control of graft rejection and in the treatment of other autoimmune diseases, has emphasized the hazards of blotting out immune responsiveness nonspecifically – the chief consequence being a serious risk of developing opportunistic infection and virally induced lymphoproliferative disease (66). One could argue that patients submitted to the combined regimen of anti-lymphocyte globulin (15 infusions during a 3-week period), prednisone (150 mg/day decreasing to 20 mg/day with further reduction), azathioprine (3 mg/kg for one month prior to reduction) and intensive plasmapheresis have survived in spite of their treatment (67), although in 1 of 4 patients treated in this way a complete remission has been observed for 15 months.

There is no lack of measures by which nonspecific immunosuppression may be achieved (66) and individual approaches such as plasmapheresis (68), total lymphoid irradiation (63) and the use of monoclonal antibodies against T-cells and their subsets (65) have been promoted.

The observation that the administration of cyclosporin A prevents the development of diabetes in a very large majority of susceptible BB rats (69) has encouraged the view that timely intervention with immunosuppressive drugs of this kind may have a future in preventing the development of diabetes in man, and pilot studies have documented some benefit from the use of cyclosporin in diabetes of recent onset (70,71). Side-effects include hirsutism, paresthesiae, gingival hyperplasia, nephrotoxicity, reduction in blood hemoglobin levels and a risk of lymphoma. In view of this drug's variable absorption, Stiller's group have adjusted dosage by measurement of serum levels (70). Further, and more elaborate, studies are planned but it is clear that these should only be attempted in a clinical research setting (65) with great attention being paid to the selection of cases, matching of controls and determination of what constitutes 'successful intervention'.

The introduction of cyclosporin has produced significant benefits in organ transplantation and the control of graft-versus-host disease in bone marrow transplantation. It is not yet clear whether the same risks are justified in the management of diabetes.

Pancreatic transplantation continues to be pursued with vigor as a means of correcting B-cell failure but a recent and illuminating finding is that successful grafts show a fairly rapid and selective loss of B-cells (72) which makes an interesting parallel with recurrence of the original immunologically mediated disease when certain kinds of glomerulonephritis are treated by renal transplantation.

Conclusions

1. Many factors affect the immunogenicity of injected insulin including: (a) characteristics of the *preparation* used, e.g. proinsulin contamination, its species, its physico-chemical state and formulation, the site and mode of injection, and (b) characteristics of the individual *recipient* e.g. metabolic status and genetic background.
2. Greater attention needs to be given to the validation and standardization of insulin antibody methods and the ways in which data are analysed and reported.
3. Human sequence insulin is of comparable immunogenicity to highly purified porcine preparations, although a modest reduction in antibody production has been observed when human and porcine insulins are compared over a period of 12 months or more, in patients receiving insulin for the first time.
4. Patients bearing the HLA-B8/DR3 haplotype are remarkably unresponsive to insulin (as an antigen); whereas those positive for HLA-DR7 show much greater levels of insulin antibody. The possession or lack of HLA-DR4 appears to have no effect on insulin production. The IgG Gm allotype markers also contribute to the genetic effect, emphasizing the need for patient groups of adequate size matched with control groups of a similar genetic background in any comparison of insulin immunogenicity in man.
5. Recent work has suggested that insulin receptor antibodies may commonly occur in Type 1 diabetes and can arise as part of the anti-idiotype response to insulin. However the equation of anti-idiotype and antireceptor antibodies has yet to be proved and this will require adequate definition of both ‘idiotype’ and ‘receptor’ and the use of rigorous controls.
6. Insulin antibodies cause problems in some patients but may be beneficial in others by virtue of their buffering effect on free insulin levels. It is unlikely that they have a significant role in exacerbating diabetic microangiopathy although their ability to sequester large amounts of metabolically active insulin within the vascular compartment may accelerate the atherosclerotic process.

7. The immune system is intimately involved in the pathogenesis of Type 1 diabetes although whether susceptibility to develop the disease results from a relative incapacity or over-exuberance of the immune system is unclear. Most forms of immunological intervention tried thus far have been based on the latter premise and preliminary results with cyclosporin A have encouraged the setting up of formal trials of this immunosuppressive agent. It does, however, have various important side effects and it is not yet clear whether these risks are justified in the management of diabetes.

References

1. Keck K, Erb P (Eds) (1981): *Basic and Clinical Aspects of Immunity to Insulin*. Walter de Gruyter, Berlin.
2. Reeves WG (1983): The immunology of β cell failure: a case for immune response genes? *Immunol. Today*, *4*, 207.
3. Reeves WG, Gelsthorpe K, Van der Minne P, Torensma R, Tattersall RB (1984): HLA phenotype and insulin antibody production. *Clin. Exp. Immunol.*, *57*, 443.
4. Kolb H, Schernthaner G, Gries FA (Eds) (1983): *Diabetes and Immunology: Pathogenesis and Immunotherapy*. Hans Huber, Bern.
5. Andreani D, Di Mario U, Federlin KF, Heding LG (Eds) (1984): *Immunology in Diabetes*. Kimpton, London.
6. Reeves WG (1983): Insulin antibody determination: theoretical and practical considerations. *Diabetologia*, *24*, 399.
7. Kurtz AB, Reeves WG, Smith WC, Spradlin CT (1984): Inter-laboratory insulin antibody workshop: a report of a collaborative study in Europe and the United States. *Diabetologia*, *27*, 300A.
8. Kapp JA, Strayer DS (1978): H-2 linked Ir gene control of antibody responses to porcine insulin. *J. Immunol.*, *121*, 978.
9. Peacock I, Taylor A, Tattersall RB, Douglas CA, Reeves WG (1983): Effects of new insulins on insulin and C-peptide antibodies, insulin dose and diabetic control. *Lancet*, *1*, 149.
10. Wilson RM, Douglas CA, Tattersall RB, Reeves WG (1984): Immunogenicity of highly purified bovine insulin: a comparison with conventional bovine and highly purified human insulins. Submitted for publication.
11. Holman RR, Steemson J, Darling P, Reeves WG, Turner RC (1984): Human ultralente insulin. *Br. Med. J.*, *288*, 665.
12. Heding LG, Larsson Y, Ludvigsson J (1980): The immunogenicity of insulin preparation. Antibody levels before and after transfer to highly purified porcine insulin. *Diabetologia*, *19*, 511.
13. Walford S, Allison SP, Reeves WG (1982): The effect of insulin antibodies on insulin dose and diabetic control. *Diabetologia*, *22*, 106.
14. Mann NP, Johnston DI, Reeves WG, Murphy MA (1983): Human insulin and porcine insulin in the treatment of diabetic children: comparison of metabolic control and insulin antibody production. *Br. Med. J.*, *287*, 1580.

15. Home PD, Mann NP, Hutchison AS, Park R, Walford S, Murphy M, Reeves WG (1984): A fifteen month double-blind crossover study of the efficacy and antigenicity of human and pork insulins. *Diabetic Med.*, *1*, 93.
16. Fineberg SE, Galloway JA, Fineberg NS, Rathbun MJ, Hufferd S (1983): Immunogenicity of recombinant DNA human insulin. *Diabetologia*, *25*, 465.
17. Schernthaner G, Borkenstein M, Fink M, Mayr WR, Menzel J, Schober E (1983): Immunogenicity of human insulin (Novo) or pork monocomponent insulin in HLA-DR-typed insulin-dependent diabetic individuals. *Diabetes Care*, *6*, 43.
18. Iavicoli M, Di Mario U, Coronel GA, Dawud AM, Arduini P, Leonardi M (1984): Semisynthetic human insulin: biologic and immunologic activity in newly treated diabetic subjects during a six-month follow-up. *Diabetes Care*, *7*, 128.
19. Hansen B, Lernmark A, Nielsen JH, Owerbach D, Welinder B (1982): New approaches to therapy and diagnosis of diabetes. *Diabetologia*, *22*, 61.
20. Reeves WG, Barr D, Douglas CA, Gelsthorpe K, Hanning I, Skene A, Wells L, Wilson RM, Tattersall RB (1984): Factors governing the human immune response to injected insulin. *Diabetologia*, *26*, 266.
21. Mauer SM, Buchwald H, Groppoli TJ, Rohde TD, Wigness BD, Rupp WM, Steffes MW (1983): Failure to find amyloidosis in dogs treated with long-term intravenous insulin delivered by a totally implantable pump. *Diabetologia*, *25*, 448.
22. Pickup JC, Bending JJ, Keen H (1984): Insulin pump therapy and serum amyloid A. *Lancet*, *1*, 853.
23. Bertrams J, Jansen FK, Gruneklee D, Reis HE, Drost H, Beyer J, Gries FA, Kuwert A (1976): HLA antigens and immunoresponsiveness to insulin in insulin-dependent diabetes mellitus. *Tissue Antigens*, *8*, 13.
24. Bodansky HJ, Wolf E, Cudworth AG, Dean BM, Nineham LJ, Bottazzo GF, Matthews JA, Kurtz AB, Kohner EM (1982): Genetic and immunologic factors in microvascular disease in Type 1 insulin-dependent diabetes. *Diabetes*, *31*, 70.
25. Sklenar I, Neri TM, Berger W, Erb P (1982): Association of specific immune response to pork and beef insulin with certain HLA-DR antigens in Type I diabetes. *Br. Med. J.*, *285*, 1451.
26. Nakao Y, Matsumoto H, Miyazaki T, Mizuno N, Arima N, Wakisaka A, Okimoto K, Akazawa Y, Tsuji K, Fujita T (1981): IgG heavychain (Gm) allotypes and immune response to insulin in insulin-requiring diabetes mellitus. *N. Engl. J. Med.*, *304*, 407.
27. Bona CA, Pernis B (1984): Idiotypic networks. In: *Fundamental Immunology*, Chapter 22, p 577. Editor: W.E. Paul. Raven Press, New York.
28. Shechter Y, Maron R, Elias D, Cohen IR (1982): Autoantibodies to insulin receptor spontaneously develop as anti-idiotypes in mice immunized with insulin. *Science*, *216*, 542.
29. Khokher MA, Janah S, Dandona P (1983): Human immunoglobulin G stimulates human adipocyte lipogenesis. *Diabetologia*, *25*, 264.
30. Kahn CR, Kasuga M, King GL, Grunfeld C (1982): Autoantibodies to insulin *Ciba Symposium (No. 90) on Receptors, Antibodies and Disease*, p 91. Pittman, London.

31. Pedersen, O (1983): Insulin receptor assays used in human studies: merits and limitations. *Diabetes Care*, *6*, 301.
32. Herold KC, Huen AH-J, Rubenstein AH, Lernmark A (1984): Humoral abnormalities in Type 1 (insulin-dependent) diabetes mellitus. In: *Immunology in Diabetes*, Chapter 8, p 105. Editors: D. Andreani, K.F. Federlin, U. DiMario and L.G. Heding. Kimpton, London.
33. Maron R, Elias D, de Jongh RM, Bruining GJ, Van Rood JJ, Shechter Y, Cohen IR (1983): Autoantibodies to the insulin receptor in juvenile onset insulin-dependent diabetes. *Nature (London)*, *303*, 817.
34. Simonsen M, Olsson L (1983): Possible roles of compound membrane receptors in the immune system. *Ann. Immunol. (Inst. Pasteur)*, *134D*, 85.
35. Fehlmann M, Brossette N, Van Obberghen E (1984): Interaction between insulin receptors and major histocompatibility complex antigens. *Diabetologia*, *27*, 273A.
36. Reeves WG, Allen BR, Tattersall RB (1980): Insulin-induced lipoatrophy: evidence for an immune pathogenesis. *Br. Med. J.*, *280*, 1500.
37. Gray RS, Borsey DQ, Kurtz A, Rainbow S, Smith AF, Elton RA, Duncan LJP, Clarke BF (1981): Relationship of glycosylated haemoglobin to C-peptide secretory status and antibody binding of insulin in insulin-dependent diabetes. *Horm. Metab. Res.*, *13*, 599.
38. Vaughan NJA, Matthews JA, Kurtz AB, Nabarro JDN (1983): The bioavailability of circulating antibody-bound insulin following insulin withdrawal in Type 1 (insulin-dependent) diabetes. *Diabetologia*, *24*, 355.
39. Sodoyez-Goffaux F, Sodoyez JC, De Vos CJ (1984): Effect of guinea pig insulin serum on insulin metabolism: autoradiographic and scintigraphic studies. *Diabetologia*, *25*, 195.
40. Bolinger RE, Morris JH, McKnight FG, Diederich DA (1964): Disappearance of I^{131}-labelled insulin from plasma as a guide to management of diabetes. *N. Engl. J. Med.*, *270*, 767.
41. Hirata Y (1983): Methimazole and insulin autoimmune syndrome with hypoglycaemia. *Lancet*, *2*, 1037.
42. Kurtz AB, Harrington MG, Matthews JA, Nabarro JDN (1979): Factitious diabetes and antibody mediated resistance to beef insulin. *Diabetologia*, *16*, 65.
43. Palmer JP, Asplin CM, Clemons P, Lyen K, Tatpati O, Raghu PK, Paquette TL (1983): Insulin antibodies in insulin-dependent diabetics before insulin treatment. *Science*, *222*, 1337.
44. Ludvigsson J (1984): Insulin antibodies in diabetic children treated with monocomponent porcine insulin from the onset: relationship to B-cell function and partial remission. *Diabetologia*, *26*, 138.
45. Cartwright BJ, Gerlis LS, Owens DR, Pennock CA, Owens C, Waterfield M, Bloom SR (1984): Remission in Type I (insulin-dependent) diabetes is related to increased insulin sensitivity. Submitted for publication.
46. Heding LG, Persson B, Stangenberg M (1980): B-cell function in newborn infants of diabetic mothers. *Diabetologia*, *19*, 427.
47. Bauman WA, Yalow RS (1981): Transplacental passage of insulin complexed to antibody. *Proc. Natl Acad. Sci. USA*, *78*, 4588.
48. Reeves WG (1980): Immunology of diabetes and insulin therapy. In: *Recent*

Advances in Clinical Immunology, 2nd ed, Chapter 7, p 183. Editor: R.A. Thompson. Churchill/ Livingstone, Edinburgh.
49. Charlesworth JA, Campbell LV, Catanzaro R, Pussell BA, Pasterfield GV, Peake P (1982): Immune complexes in diabetes mellitus: studies of complement utilisation and tissue deposition. *J. Clin. Lab. Immunol.*, *8*, 163.
50. Abrass CK, Heber D, Lieberman J (1983): Circulating immune complexes in patients with diabetes mellitus. *Clin. Exp. Immunol.*, *52*, 164.
51. Dimario U, Ventriglia I, Iavicoli M, Guy K, Andreani D (1983): The correlation between insulin antibodies and circulating immune complexes in diabetics with and without microangiopathy. *Clin. Exp. Immunol.*, *52*, 575.
52. Svehag S-E, Baatrup G, Petersen I (1984): Characterisation of circulating immune complexes and their solubilization by complement. In: *Recent Developments in Clinical Immunology*, Chapter 5, p 111, Editor: W.G. Reeves. Elsevier, Amsterdam.
53. Dornan TL, Ting A, McPherson CK, Peckar CO, Mann JI, Turner RC, Morris PJ (1982): Genetic susceptibility in the development of retinopathy in insulin-dependent diabetics. *Diabetes*, *31*, 226.
54. Stout TW (1979): Diabetes and atherosclerosis – the role of insulin. *Diabetologia*, *16*, 141.
55. Kurtz AB, Nabarro JDN (1980): Circulating insulin-binding antibodies. *Diabetologia*, *19*, 329.
56. Falholt K, Heding LG (1982): Intracellular muscle enzymes in pigs with high levels of insulin antibodies. *Diabetologia*, *22*, 386.
57. Reeves WG (1983): Immunological aspects of diabetes. In: *Immunology in Medicine: a Comprehensive Guide to Clinical Immunology, 2nd ed*, Chapter 20, p 365. Editors: E.J. Holborow and W.G. Reeves. Grune and Stratton, London.
58. Bottazzo GF (1984): β cell damage in diabetic insulitis: are we approaching a solution? *Diabetologia*, *26*, 241.
59. Gorsuch AN, Spencer KM, Lister J, McNally JM, Dean BM, Bottazzo GF, Cudworth AG (1981): Evidence for a long prediabetic period in type 1 (insulin-dependent) diabetes mellitus. *Lancet*, *2*, 1363.
60. Rossini A, Mordes JP, Like AA (1984): Animal models of insulin-dependent diabetes mellitus. In: *Immunology in Diabetes*, Chapter 3, p 35. Editors: D. Andreani, K.F. Federlin, U. DiMario and L.G. Heding. Kimpton, London.
61. Pozzilli P, DiMario U (1984): Lymphocyte subpopulations and circulating immune complexes: their relationship in the pathogenesis of Type 1 (insulin-dependent) diabetes. In: *Immunology in Diabetes*, Chapter 10, p 133. Editors: D. Andreani, K.F. Federlin, U. DiMario and L.G. Heding. Kimpton, London.
62. Buse J, Ben-Nun A, Klein KA, Eisenbarth GS, Seidman JG, Jackson RA (1984): Specific Class II histocompatibility gene polymorphism in BB rats. *Diabetes*, *33*, 700.
63. Cahill GF (1983): Early intervention in insulin-dependent diabetes mellitus. In: *Diabetes and Immunology: Pathogenesis and Immunotherapy*, p 108. Editors: H. Kolb, G. Schernthaner and F.A. Gries. Hans Huber, Bern.
64. Gries FA (1983): Immunotherapy of type 1 diabetes. In: *Diabetes and Immunology: Pathogenesis and Immunotherapy*, p 134. Editors: H. Kolb, G. Schernthaner and F.A. Gries. Hans Huber, Bern.

65. Rabinowe SL, Eisenbarth GS (1984): Immunotherapy of type I (insulin-dependent) diabetes mellitus. In: *Immunology in Diabetes*, Chapter 13, p 171. Editors: D. Andreani, K.F. Federlin, U. DiMario and L.G. Heding. Kimpton, London.
66. Reeves WG (1983): Therapeutic manipulation of the immune response. In: *Immunology in Medicine: a Comprehensive Guide to Clinical Immunology, 2nd ed.*, Chapter 32, p. 613. Editors: E.J. Holborow and W.G. Reeves. Grune and Stratton, London.
67. Leslie RDG, Pyke DA (1980). Immunosuppression of acute insulin-dependent diabetes. In: *Immunology of Diabetes*, Chapter 25, p 345. Editor: W.J. Irvine. Teviot, Edinburgh.
68. Ludvigsson J, Heding L, Lieden G, Marner B, Lernmark A (1983): Plasmapheresis in the initial treatment of insulin-dependent diabetes mellitus in children. *Br. Med. J.*, *286*, 176.
69. Laupacis A, Stiller CR, Gardell C et al (1983): Cyclosporin prevents diabetes in BB Wistar rats. *Lancet*, *1*, 10.
70. Stiller CR, Laupacis A, Dupre J, Jenner MR, Keown PA, Rodger W, Wolfe BMJ (1983): Cyclosporin for treatment of early type I diabetes: preliminary results. *N. Engl. J. Med.*, *308*, 1226.
71. Assan R, Feutren G, Debray-Sachs M, Quiniou-Debrie MC, Chatenoud L, Hors J, Bach JF (1984): Administration of cyclosporin A to recently-diagnosed Type I (insulin dependent) diabetic patients. *Diabetologia*, *27*, 253A.
72. Sutherland DER (1984): Pancreas transplantation: an overview and current status of cases reported to the registry by mid-1983. In: *Immunology of Diabetes*, Chapter 16, p 195. Editors: D. Andreani, K.F. Federlin, U. DiMario and L.G. Heding. Kimpton, London.

The Diabetes Annual/1
K.G.M.M. Alberti and L.P. Krall, editors

ISBN 0444 90 343 7
$0.85 per article per page (transactional system)
$0.20 per article per page (licensing system)

5 Tropical diabetes

V. MOHAN, A. RAMACHANDRAN AND M. VISWANATHAN

Most of the developing countries of the world are situated in tropical regions. During the past few years it has been observed that the profile of diabetes in the tropics shows certain basic differences from that seen in western countries. In tropical countries, several factors influence the profile of diabetes and Skrabalo and Katona (1) have summarized these in a recent review. They include 'varying climatic conditions, nomadic ways of life, various customs, traditions, cultures, religions, caste systems, widespread poverty etc.' In a disease with a genetic predisposition, but whose clinical profile is greatly influenced by environmental forces, the effect of these multiple factors can well be imagined.

The late Kelly West strongly believed that the study of diabetes in the tropics was worthwhile and, in his own words, diabetes in the tropics provided 'some lessons for western diabetology' (2). He justifies the use of the term 'tropical diabetes' to describe the variety of diabetes seen in tropical regions. In a recent book, '*Secondary Diabetes*', many aspects of diabetes in the tropics have been brought to light (3). The peculiarities in the diabetes syndrome in the tropics with respect to the frequency, types and manifestations of diabetes include the following: (a) difference in genetic pattern of diabetes in tropical regions; (b) a low prevalence rate of classic insulin-dependent (juvenile-onset) diabetes mellitus; (c) younger age at onset of non-insulin-dependent diabetes (NIDDM); (d) reversal of sex ratio, with male preponderance; (e) peculiar types of malnutrition diabetes such as 'J' type and tropical pancreatic diabetes; and (f) large-scale use of high-carbohydrate high-fiber diets, in the treatment of diabetes mellitus. We shall consider some of these factors, highlighting the 'new' as well as the 'old' information.

Genetic factors in tropical diabetes

Information is relatively sparse on the genetics of diabetes in tropical countries. Recent studies on the HLA profile and the properdin (BF) system have shown some interesting results.

HLA studies

Srikantia and co-workers (4) have reported on the HLA antigens in Type 1 diabetes mellitus (IDDM) in North India. The frequency of HLA-Bw21 was significantly increased and that of B7 significantly reduced. HLA-B8, B15 and B18, which are associated with insulin-dependent diabetes (IDDM) in Caucasians, did not have any significant association with IDDM in this series of patients. The Japanese found an association with HLA-Bw22 J1 (Bw54), which is different from that noted in the above study.

A recent study from South India by Kirk et al. (5) has shown still more interesting findings. The HLA profile in IDDM in South India is quite different from that reported from North India. In the South, HLA-B8 is associated with IDDM, which is similar to the findings in the Caucasian IDDM. However, unlike the latter findings, there was no association with B15. These studies appear to provide evidence for genetic differences in susceptibility to IDDM between Indians and Caucasians and even between the North- and South-Indian populations. They also corroborate the earlier studies of Hammond and Asmal (6), who reported the HLA profile in Indian IDDM patients in South Africa. It was noted that while the Dravidian (South-Indian) IDDM population in S. Africa showed an increased prevalence of HLA-B8, this was not seen in the Aryan (North-Indian) population.

Even within the tropical belt, there are likely to be differences in the HLA associations with IDDM. Lee et al. (7) reported that the HLA association with IDDM in the Chinese population was with DR3 and HLA-A9 but not with B8. Thus the HLA-linked susceptibility to IDDM seems to be fairly specific to the population studied and there are definite differences in the HLA association in different races.

Serjeantson et al. (8) reported an interesting study of HLA and NIDDM in Fiji Indians. There was a significant increase in Bw61 in NIDDM Fiji patients of Indian origin. This study is interesting because it is one of the few reports of an HLA association with NIDDM type of diabetes. The only other report of an HLA association with NIDDM has been in a study of South African Blacks of the Xhosa tribe in whom an association between HLA-A2 and NIDDM was noted (9).

Studies on properdin (BF) system

The properdin (BF) system which is associated with the alternate complement pathway, is situated close to the HLA region on Chromosome 6. There have been reports of associations between the BF system and IDDM in Caucasian races. Recent studies have shown an association between the BF system and IDDM in Indian populations.

The BF haplotype associated with IDDM in Caucasian populations is the

TABLE 1. *HLA and properdin (BF) haplotypes associated with IDDM in Caucasians and Indians*

Race	HLA	BF system
Caucasian	B8 B15 DR3 DR4	BFS
N. Indian	Bw21	BFS1
S. Indian	B8	BFF

BFS. An association between the properdin system and insulin-dependent diabetes in South India has been reported by Kirk et al. (10). There was a significant increase among IDDM patients, as compared with controls, in the BFF phenotype and a corresponding fall in the BFS phenotype. This increase in the BFF phenotype was reflected also in a significant difference in the BFF gene frequency between IDDM patients and controls. There were no significant differences between controls and NIDDM. The relative risk for the BFF phenotype in IDDM was 4.1.

In contrast to the previous reported results for North Indian IDDM patients (11) there was no significant association of the BFS1 haplotype with either IDDM or NIDDM patients in the South Indian population studied. This suggests that the susceptibility allele(s) for IDDM in South India arose independently from the susceptibility allele(s) in North India. Alternatively, it is possible that a different etiological factor with a distinctive genetic susceptibility is present in the South Indians.

In summary, the above studies on HLA and BF system do seem to indicate that (a) differences exist between the Indian and Caucasian races with respect to susceptibility to IDDM; and more interestingly, (b) there are differences between the North and South Indians. These findings are summarized in Table 1. Studies are urgently required in other populations in tropical regions to see whether any definite pattern of susceptibility to IDDM emerges for countries within the tropical belt.

Studies on genetics of NIDDM patients

Few studies have been reported on the genetics of NIDDM patients in tropical countries. Viswanathan (12) published the results of a 20-year follow-up study on relatives of diabetic patients. Preliminary observations suggest that the genetic factor appears to be stronger in Indian diabetics compared with other races. When one parent had diabetes 11.3% of all offspring had diabetes and when both parents were diabetic, 25.1% of all offspring had diabetes. When those above 40 years of age were analysed, as many as 55.6% of the offspring of two diabetic parents had overt diabetes. This study was based on a questionnaire method. Obviously, if all offspring were tested, the figure would be much higher. These prevalence rates for diabetes in the offspring of conjugal diabetics are the highest reported for any population studied, suggesting that in Indian diabetics, the genetic factor is stronger than in Caucasian races.

Mohan et al. (13) reported the preliminary observations on a unique long-term project on primary prevention of diabetes. Detailed pedigree charts of offspring of over 2000 'conjugal' diabetic couples and equal number of offspring of 'one-parent diabetic' and 'no-parent diabetic' couples have been collected at the Diabetes Research Centre in Madras. The study includes glucose tolerance tests, insulin and C-peptide assay in the offspring with a view to detect early biochemical markers. In the next phase of the project which is now underway at the center, steps are being taken to prevent the influence of environmental diabetogenic factors.

Malnutrition diabetes

One of the types of diabetes peculiar to tropical regions is that associated with malnutrition. The two major forms of malnutrition diabetes are 'J-type diabetes' and 'tropical pancreatic diabetes'.

The 'J-type' diabetes was described by Hugh Jones in 1955 (14) and was thus named because it was first observed in Jamaica. It has several distinctive characteristics: (1) Despite severe hyperglycemia, ketosis is uncommon. (2) There is often resistance to insulin. (3) Patients are lean and often grossly emaciated. (4) There is usually a history of extreme poverty and childhood malnutrition. (5) Onset of diabetes occurs usually between 15 and 40 years.

The second form of malnutrition-associated diabetes is tropical pancreatic diabetes (TPD). In this form of diabetes, in addition to the features seen in the J-type diabetes, patients have evidence of chronic pancreatitis with pancreatic calcification and fibrosis. For this reason, it has also been referred to as the pancreatic fibrosis-calcification syndrome or the Zuidema syndrome (15).

The clinical features of TPD have been recently reviewed in detail (16). They include the following: (a) young age at onset with male preponderance; (b) history of recurrent pain in the abdomen from childhood; (c) evidence of pancreatic fibrosis and/or calcification; (d) steatorrhea; (e) evidence of protein/calorie malnutrition.

Patients with both forms of malnutrition diabetes are usually insulin-dependent in so far as they need insulin for maintaining health and life. However, they do not develop ketoacidosis, even if the insulin injections are withdrawn for long periods of time. The ketosis-resistant nature of malnutrition diabetes has long remained a matter of debate. Recent work has thrown some light on the probable explanation for this. Mohan et al. (17) reported on the pancreatic B-cell function by estimating C-peptide levels in patients with TPD in comparison with classic IDDM and NIDDM patients (Fig. 1).

It was seen that in general, all diabetics showed lower post-glucose stimulated C-peptide levels in comparison with non-diabetic controls. The NIDDM patients had the highest C-peptide values among the diabetic groups. IDDM patients had very low C-peptide levels. Patients with TPD had higher post-glucose C-peptide levels than the IDDM patients, the difference being statistically significant ($P < 0.001$). It was concluded that the higher B-cell reserve in patients with TPD was probably responsible for the ketosis-resistant nature of the diabetes seen in TPD. It is known that even partial preservation of B-cell reserve can protect against ketoacidosis. Another report from India (18) on C-peptide levels in young ketosis-resistant diabetes (J-type) presented similar results.

Another explanation for the ketosis-resistant nature of J-type diabetes

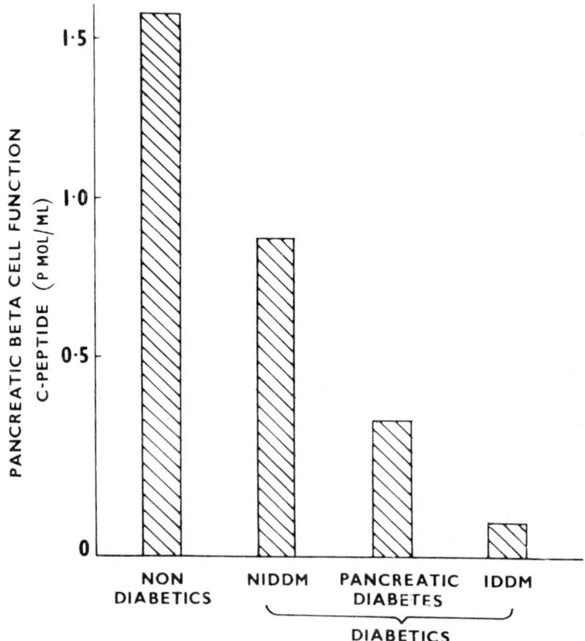

FIG. 1. *Post-glucose stimulated C-peptide levels in tropical pancreatic diabetics compared with NIDDM, IDDM and non-diabetic controls.*

was provided by Rao et al. (19), who reported on the suppressible glucagon secretion in this type of diabetes. They found that fasting glucagon levels were similarly elevated in both classic Type 1 diabetic subjects and the J-type diabetics compared with non-obese non-diabetic controls. After oral glucose administration however, glucagon responses were strikingly dissimilar in the two groups. In Type 1 diabetic individuals, glucagon levels rose paradoxically during OGTT, while in the J-type diabetics levels fell after glucose. The authors concluded that postprandial glucagon suppressibility may be responsible for the ketosis resistance that is characteristic of J-type diabetes.

It is possible that the ketosis-resistant nature of the malnutrition associated diabetes is due to a combination of many factors. These factors include higher C-peptide levels and postprandial glucagon suppressibility.

Very recently Mohan et al. (20), in a more detailed study of TPD, have reported that the clinical spectrum of TPD patients is heterogeneous. The majority of patients do belong to the ketosis-resistant insulin-requiring group described above. However, a small subgroup exhibited ketosis, although ketoacidosis and coma were very infrequent. In the latter the C-peptide levels were indistinguishable from classic IDDM. Another small subgroup showed a positive response to oral drugs, and in this group the C-peptide levels were much higher than in the insulin-requiring cases. Another new feature of TPD noted in this series from Madras is that malnutrition, which was previously considered as an important feature of TPD, was seen only in a minority of the cases. This suggests that factors apart from malnutrition could also be important in the pathogenesis of TPD seen at Madras.

McMillan and Geevarghese (21) have put forward an interesting hypothesis to explain the pathogenesis of malnutrition diabetes. The geographic distribution of malnutrition diabetes coincides with that of cassava ingestion. Cassava is known to contain cyanide-containing glycosides. Ingested cyanide is normally detoxified by conversion of thiocyanate. This detoxification requires sulphur, which is usually derived from aminoacid sources. McMillan and Geevarghese conducted animal experiments to see whether cyanide was capable of producing pancreatic damage and diabetes. Studies in the rat showed the following results: (a) a remarkable ability to detoxify ingested cyanide; (b) a reduction in urinary thiocyanate excretion when protein intake is lowered (especially during growth); (c) production of marked hyperglycemia by either oral or parenteral cyanide; and (d) the development of cyanosis and epidermal changes when there was prolonged exposure to cyanide. McMillan and Geevarghese concluded that their work supported a role for cyanide in the pathogenesis of malnutrition diabetes.

The cassava-cyanide hypothesis might explain the occurrence of malnutrition diabetes in the state of Kerala in India and other parts where cassava is regularly consumed. However, in Madras and several other parts of

India, virtually no cassava is eaten. Yet malnutrition diabetes is seen also in these parts. This suggests that factors apart from cassava ingestion seem to play a role in the causation of malnutrition diabetes. Therefore, its etiology still remains an enigma and more studies are certainly needed on this subject.

Mngola (22), in a review of the African pancreatic diabetes, described yet another form of tropical diabetes, which he calls the Kenyan type or 'K-type' of pancreatic diabetes to distinguish this from the 'Madras type'. Its main features are: (1) Patients with the 'K-type' of diabetes consume a local alcoholic brew called Changaa. (2) They do not have evidence of malnutrition. (3) Ketoacidosis is common. (4) There is usually no insulin resistance.

In summary, while the occurrence of malnutrition-associated diabetes in tropical regions is quite common, the clinical picture is far from uniform. There is heterogeneity with respect to occurrence of malnutrition itself, the biochemical profile, the pancreatic B-cell responses, the presence or absence of pancreatic calcification and the response to therapy.

Use of high-carbohydrate high-fiber diet on a large scale in treatment of diabetes

In most tropical regions, carbohydrate constitutes 70–80% of the total calories of the diet of the general population. As early as 1958, Viswanathan and colleagues at Madras started trying diets with a higher carbohydrate content. Initial studies at the Diabetes Research Centre. Madras, with the use of the high carbohydrate diet over a period of 10 years (23) showed that the diet was effective in the control of diabetes. Later, the protein content of the diet was raised by adding vegetable proteins in

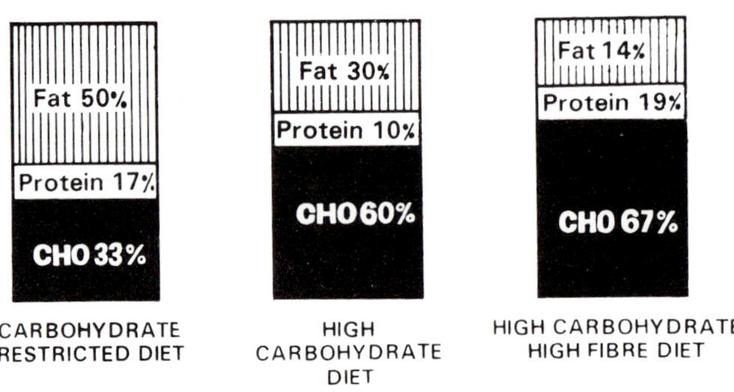

FIG. 2. *Evolution of the use of the high-carbohydrate high-fiber (HCHF) diet at the Diabetes Research Centre (DRC), Madras, India.*

the form of pulses and legumes. This increased not only the protein but also the fiber content of the diet. A study of the fiber content of the diet used at the Diabetes Research Centre, Madras, was done at the University of Kentucky, Lexington, USA, which showed that it contained 52 grams of dietary fiber. This was approximately double the fiber content of the standard American Diabetic Association diet used at that time. Hence the diet was called the high-carbohydrate high-fiber (HCHF) diet. Figure 2 shows the evolution of our HCHF diet.

Overall, the high-carbohydrate diet was used in over 18,000 diabetics at the Diabetes Research Centre over a period of 22 years (24). A series of studies on the efficacy of the diet in the control of diabetes, the effect on serum lipids and on the insulin responses to glucose load have been published by Viswanathan and his colleagues. In a recent review they have summarized the long-term benefits of the HCHF diet in Indian diabetics (25):

1. The patients' acceptance and adherence to the diet has been very satisfactory because it is similar to the diet of the general population.
2. The diet is very useful in achieving rapid and effective control of diabetes which can be sustained for years.
3. The dose of hypoglycemic agents is small.
4. In many cases, the hypoglycemic drugs could later be withdrawn.
5. The concentrations of both serum cholesterol and triglycerides show an impressive fall which is sustained for many years.
6. The fall in serum cholesterol levels was mainly due to decreased LDL cholesterol levels. This resulted in a decrease in the ratios of total cholesterol/HDL cholesterol and LDL/HDL cholesterol (26).
7. The HCHF diet improves many aspects of metabolism. Evidence of this

TABLE 2. *Composition of high-carbohydrate high-fiber (HCHF) diet of the Diabetes Research Centre, Madras, India*

	Grams	Calories	% of total calories
Carbohydrate	301	1204	67
Protein	86	344	19
Fats	28	252	14
Total calories		1800	
Dietary fiber content		52 g	
Source of fiber	Whole cereals, pulses and legumes and green leafy vegetables		

was seen in a recent study where nerve conduction velocity was found to improve even within a period of one week of treatment (27).

8. The IRI responses to glucose load showed lowered insulin levels after long-term treatment with the HCHF diet. This suggested improved peripheral sensitivity to insulin in patients on HCHF diets (28).

Table 2 shows the composition of the HCHF diet used at the Madras Centre.

Conclusions

'Tropical diabetes', although not a homogeneous entity does have distinctive characteristics of its own. Genetic, nutritional, dietary and other factors seem to be responsible for at least some of the differences noted in 'tropical diabetes' compared with diabetes in the West.

Studies on the HLA and properdin (BF) factors have brought out definite differences in the genetic susceptibility to IDDM between the tropical and Caucasian races. The role of genetic factors in causation of NIDDM appears to be very high in the Indian races. These studies should now be extended to other countries in the Afro-Asian region.

The successful use of the HCHF diet on a long-term basis at the Madras Centre provide ample evidence that, at least for tropical regions, this is probably the best form of dietary therapy.

Finally, malnutrition diabetes continues to provide a fascinating area for research. Recent studies have shown the possible etiological link between cassava ingestion and pancreatic diabetes. However, this hypothesis will not explain the etiology of the 'Madras type' of tropical pancreatic diabetes since cassava is not consumed in Madras. At least two explanations for the ketosis-resistant nature of malnutrition diabetes have been put forward. More studies are required on malnutrition diabetes since this could throw significant light on the understanding of other types of diabetes as well.

References

1. Skrabalo Z, Katona G (1982): Problems of the developing nations. In: *World Book of Diabetes in Practice, 1982*, p 157. Editors: L.P. Krall and K.G.M.M. Alberti. Excerpta Medica, Amsterdam.
2. West KM (1980): Diabetes in the tropics: some lessons for western diabetology. In: *Secondary Diabetes: The Spectrum of the Diabetic Syndromes*. p 249. Editors: S. Podolsky and M. Viswanathan. Raven Press, New York.
3. Podolsky S, Viswanathan M (Eds) (1980): *Secondary Diabetes: The Spectrum of the Diabetic Syndromes*. Raven Press, New York.
4. Srikantia S, Mehra NK, Vaidya MC, Malaviya AN, Ahuja MMS (1981):

HLA antigens in Type I (insulin dependent) diabetes mellitus in North India. *Metabolism*, *20*, 992.
5. Kirk RL, Ranford PR, Serjeantson SW, Thompson AR, Chetty SMM, Lily J, Mohan V, Ramachandran A, Snehalatha C, Viswanathan M (1984): HLA, complement C2, C4, properdin factor B and glyoxalase types in South Indian diabetics. In press.
6. Hammond MG, Asmal AC (1980): HLA and insulin dependent diabetes in South African Indians. *Tissue Antigens*, *15*, 244.
7. Lee TD, Zhaio T, Chi Z, Wong H, Shen M, Rochey G (1984): HLA-A and B and HLA-DR phenotypes in mainland Chinese patients with diabetes mellitus. *Tissue Antigens*, *22*, 92.
8. Serjeantson SW, Ryan DP, Ram P, Zimmet P (1981): HLA and non-insulin dependent diabetes in Fiji Indians. *Med. J. Aust.*, *1*, 462.
9. Briggs BR, Jackson WPU, Du Toit ED, Botha MC (1980): The histocompatability antigens distribution in Southern African Blacks (Xhosa) *Diabetes*, *29*, 68.
10. Kirk RL, Ranford PR, Viswanathan M, Mohan V, Ramachandran A, Snehalatha C, Chetty SMM, John L (1983): Another association between properdin system (BF) and insulin dependent diabetes in S. India. *Tissue Antigens*, *22*, 170.
11. Kirk RL, Ranford PR, Theophilus J, Ahuja MMS, Mehra NK, Vaidiya MC (1982): The rare factor BFS_1 of the properdin system strongly associated with insulin dependent diabetes in N. India. *Tissue Antigens*, *20*, 303.
12. Viswanathan M (1981): Prevention in diabetes. *J. Assoc. Physicians India*, *29*, 251.
13. Mohan V, Ramachandran A, Viswanathan M (1983): Primary prevention of diabetes. A project of the Diabetes Research Centre, Madras, India. *Bull. Delivery Health Care Diabetics Developing Countries*, *4*, 9.
14. Hugh-Jones P (1955): Diabetes in Jamaica. *Lancet*, *2*, 891.
15. Zuidema PJ (1955): Calcification and cirrhoses of the pancreas in patients with malnutrition. *Trop. Geogr. Med.*, *7*, 229.
16. Viswanathan M (1980): Pancreatic diabetes in India. An overview. In: *Secondary Diabetes*, p 105. Editors: S. Podolsky and M. Viswanathan. Raven Press, New York.
17. Mohan V, Snehalatha C, Ramachandran A, Jayashree R, Viswanathan M (1983): Pancreatic beta cell function in tropical pancreatic diabetes. *Metabolism*, *32*, 1091.
18. Sood R, Ahuja MMS, Kamarkar MG (1983): Serum c-peptide levels in young ketosis resistant diabetics. *Indian J. Med. Res.*, *78*, 661.
19. Rao RH, Vigg BL, Rao KS (1983): Suppressible glucagon secretion in young, ketosis resistant type J diabetic patients in India. *Diabetes*, *32*, 1168.
20. Mohan V, Mohan R, Aruna AC, Susheela L, Snehalatha C, Ramachandran A, Viswanathan M, Bharani G, Mahajan VK, Kohner EM (1984): Tropical pancreatic diabetes in S. India. Heterogeneity in clinical and biochemical profile. *Diabetologia*, *27*, 311A.
21. McMillan DE, Geevarghese PJ (1979): Dietary cyanide and tropical malnutrition diabetes. *Diabetes Care*, *2*, 202.

22. Mngola EN (1982): African pancreatic diabetes. In: *World Book of Diabetes in Practice 1982*, p 176. Editors: L.P. Krall and K.G.M.M. Alberti. Excerpta Medica, Amsterdam.
23. Viswanathan M (1968): High carbohydrate diet in diabetes. *J. Diabetic Assoc. India*, *8*, 853.
24. Viswanathan M, Ramachandran A, Mohan V, Snehalatha C (1981): High carbohydrate high fibre diet in diabetes. *J. Diabetic Assoc. India*, *30*, 90.
25. Viswanathan M, Snehalatha C, Ramachandran A, Mohan V (1979): High carbohydrate diet in diabetes. Long term experience. In: *Proceedings of the Tenth International Diabetes Federation Congress, Vienna*, p 84. Editor: W. Waldhäusl. Excerpta Medica, Amsterdam.
26. Susheela L, Shyamsundar R, Ramachandran A, Mohan V, Viswanathan M (1983): Favourable alterations in serum Total/HDL and LDL/HDL cholesterol ratios after gluco-regulation in newly diagnosed NIDDM. *Diabetologia Croat.*, *12*, 17.
27. Shyamsundar R, Mohan V, Ramachandran A, Viswanathan M, Velmurugendran CU, Murugesan A (1983): Rapid improvement in motor nerve conduction velocity after antidiabetic therapy. *Diabetologica Croat.*, *12*, 117.
28. Viswanathan M, Snehalatha C, Ramachandran A, Mohan V (1983): Effect of the high carbohydrate high fibre diet on immunoreactive insulin level in diabetics. *J. Diabetic Assoc. India*, *23*, 45.

The Diabetes Annual/1
K.G.M.M. Alberti and L.P. Krall, editors

ISBN 0444 90 343 7
$0.85 per article per page (transactional system)
$0.20 per article per page (licensing system)

7 Insulin therapy: conventional

MICHAEL BERGER

Since 1922, insulin substitution therapy has been based upon daily subcutaneous injections of the hormone carried out by the patient. With the development of new methods and technologies of insulin replacement by continuous infusion of the hormone or by transplantation of insulin-producing cells (as described in Chapters 8, 9, and 12) the treatment with subcutaneous insulin injections has been termed 'conventional insulin therapy'.

As the concept of a causal relationship between the quality of metabolic control and the development of diabetic microangiopathy has become widely accepted during the past ten years, more and more diabetologists and their patients tend to strive for (near-) normoglycemia, or at least for substantial improvements of glucose homeostasis. As a consequence, a number of attempts have been made in order to increase the efficacy of the conventional insulin therapy, in that it has become obvious that the new 'un-conventional' modes of insulin replacement therapy will only be available on an experimental basis or for a restricted number of patients, at least for quite some time.

Recent attempts to improve conventional insulin therapy have been based largely on the new technologies for metabolic self-control and, to a lesser extent, on the development of new insulin preparations and injection materials. A considerable amount of clinical investigation has been devoted to the riddles and apparent vagaries of the absorption process of insulin from its subcutaneous depot into the circulation. Thus, systematic attempts have been made to study, and, if possible, to standardize the bioavailability of subcutaneously injected insulin preparations. New insight into the pharmacokinetics and clinical pharmacology of conventional insulin therapy has become possible due to advances in the assessment of serum free insulin concentrations in diabetic patients. It has become evident that the preferential use of long-acting insulin preparations, which have been widely advocated during the past 30 years, results in a most unphysiological, persisting hyperinsulinemia. Thus, various strategies have been developed recently to adapt conventional insulin therapy more closely to the physiological pattern of insulin secretion. As a consequence, different concepts of intensified (conventional) insulin therapy have been proposed (1), all of which include the preferential use of short-acting (regular) insulin before the main meals in addition to a 'basal' component of insulin substitution, which is delivered by one or two daily injections of intermediate- or long-acting insulin preparations. In particular, the pre-meal bolus injections of regular insulin are variable, and are adjusted by the patient, on the basis of the actual results of self-monitoring of glycemia or glucosuria and of the amount of carbohydrate to be consumed. These new concepts of intensified conventional insulin therapy (ICT) require an increasing level of understanding, cooperation and compliance. They have gained in popularity with patients and physicians since they should eventually lead to better metabolic control and to more independence from the earlier rigid dietary regimens.

In essence, these apparently 'new' concepts of conventional insulin therapy represent a return to the original philosophy of diabetes treatment proposed by Joslin and other pioneers of modern diabetes some sixty years ago (2); systematic education of the patient in order to have him/her give insulin as independently as possible on the basis of regular metabolic self-monitoring and frequent adaptations of the dosage of premeal regular insulin injections.

Absorption of subcutaneously injected insulin – bioavailability of exogenous insulin

Many of the difficulties and unexplained variations in subcutaneous insulin replacement therapy have been attributed to the absorption process of the exogenous insulin from its subcutaneous depot into the circulation. The inter- and intra-individual differences in the anatomical structure of subcutaneous tissues as well as the potential enzymatic and physicochemical reactions facing the insulin molecule on its way from the injection needle into the circulation would be expected to make the bioavailability of subcutaneously administered insulin variable and sometimes even unpredictable. With the increasing interest in an improvement of metabolic control in insulin-treated diabetic patients, intensive efforts have been made to investigate the molecular biology and the pharmacokinetics of the absorption process for various insulin preparations in recent years. The interpretation of these investigations has been clouded by methodological problems. Formerly, studies on the insulin absorption process depended on indirect assessment techniques based upon the disappearance of radioactivity measured by external counting above the injection site of iodinated insulin preparations (3). For a number of reasons these methods have been criticized (4), especially when applied in studies on regular (soluble) insulin preparations since it has been repeatedly documented that a substantial amount of insulin is (enzymatically) degraded at the subcutaneous site of injection (4–6). However, the exact percentage of insulin degraded *in situ* is as yet uncertain and may vary at different injection sites, from patient to patient, and from one insulin preparation to another. More recent investigations of insulin pharmacokinetics and bioavailability have therefore con-

TABLE 1. *Factors influencing the absorption of subcutaneously injected regular insulin*

Acceleration	Delaying effect
Abdominal injection	Thigh injection
High temperatures (e.g. hot bath)*	Low temperatures*
Muscular exercise*	Injection into lipodystrophic areas
Aprotinin, lidocain, etc.	Galenic procedures in order to prolong insulin action (protamine-insulin crystallization etc.)
	Interaction of regular insulin with long-acting insulin preparations in insulin mixtures
Low insulin strength (e.g. U-20)	High insulin strength (e.g. U-100)
Human insulin	

* When applied up to 30 min after the subcutaneous injection of insulin.

centrated on direct measurement of circulating levels of exogenous insulin. The molecular processes underlying the absorption of insulin from the subcutaneous extracellular space into the capillaries and (to a much lesser extent), into the lymph vessels remain to be elucidated. Nevertheless, a number of factors which influence the absorption rates have been consistently identified in various investigations (4, 9–12). Some of these factors are summarized in Table 1.

As a result of differences in the anatomical structures, regular insulin is more rapidly absorbed when injected into the abdomen compared to injections into the thigh or the arm. Similarly, the absorption rate and the bioavailability of regular insulin can be augmented by increasing the temperature at and around the injection site. Differences in the bioavailability of insulin related to the subcutaneous injection technique have also been described (8). Substantial increases in the rate of insulin absorption and its hypoglycemic effect are documented for physical exercise and massage of the injection site. Both physical activity involving parts of the body where insulin had been injected before and the massage of the injection site result in an acceleration of the absorption process of regular insulin and in a potentiation of its blood glucose lowering action, demonstrable both in clinical investigations with normal subjects and in insulin-treated diabetic patients (4, 13). However, it should be noted that most of these studies have been restricted to the use of regular (soluble) insulin preparations, and, more importantly, consistent with the kinetics of the insulin absorption process (4, 14), all of these effects are only demonstrable if applied immediately after or at the most within 30 minutes of the subcutaneous administration of insulin.

Some other phenomena, such as accelerated insulin absorption associated with smoking or with a sauna bath have not been confirmed in subsequent studies using a direct method to follow insulin pharmacokinetics (15).

Comparatively limited information is available with regard to the absorption process and the bioavailability of (medium-) long-acting insulin preparations (4, 8, 16–19). Again, methodological problems render the interpretation of most of the published data difficult. It seems, however, fair to conclude that very large differences exist with regard to the timing of peak hypoglycemic action and duration of action from one patient to another, as well as between injection sites. On the other hand, the bioavailability of long-acting insulin preparations seems to be somewhat more resistant to the various factors which are known to alter the absorption kinetics of regular insulin preparations (see Table 1).

Controversial data have been published recently with respect to the miscibility of long-acting and regular insulin preparations, an area which has become more important as ICT has gained in popularity. From a number of studies, it can be concluded that no problems arise when NPH insulin preparations and regular insulins are mixed in one syringe before injection (4, 7, 8, 20). By contrast, substantial amounts of regular insulin (Actrapid®) seem to become attached to the insulin-zinc crystals when mixed with lente-type preparations (Monotard® or Human Ultratard®) in one syringe. This results in the diminution of the short-acting component of the insulin mixture (4, 21, 22). In keeping with clinical experience, such a loss of regular insulin can be avoided when the regular-lente (porcine Actrapid®–Monotard®) mixture is injected immediately after preparation of the mixture (4, 20). In one recent study, however, the loss of the fast action of the human regular-type insulin (Human Actrapid®–Monotard® was independent of the time interval between the preparation of the mixture and its administration (23). Whether differences in the ratio between the insulin preparations mixed in these studies, species differences, and/or other methodological differences were responsible for the contrasting results from these investigations remains to be elucidated. Further systematic studies of the clinically important area of insulin miscibility are urgently needed.

Since the acceleration of insulin absorption from its subcutaneous injection site would obviously represent a chance for a more physiological insulin substitution therapy, various pharmacological attempts (4, 8, 24, 25) have been made to accelerate the pharmacokinetics of insulin either via a stimulation of local blood flow (e.g. by aprotinin or local anesthetics) or by inhibiting local degradation of insulin (e.g. by aprotinin, ophthalmic aid or other substances). These attempts have, however, as yet not resulted in practically relevant suggestions.

In this context, it might be of note that the change of insulin strength from U-40 to U-100 which is currently being carried out in a number of countries might well be associated with a slight decrease in the absorption rate of regular insulin (8, 12, 26–28). Whether or not these differences are of clinical significance remains to be clarified.

Particular problems with the absorption and bioavailability of subcutaneously injected insulin

Over and above the described variations of insulin pharmacokinetics, a number of conditions have been described in which specific problems with the absorption of insulin from its subcutaneous depot resulting in major difficulties to achieve stable metabolic control have been identified or suggested. Thus, a number of case reports have been published describing a particular resistance against exogenous insulin when administered subcutaneously (1, 8). These patients respond adequately to intravenously administered insulin, have low insulin-binding antibody titers and unaltered insulin receptors, but they seem to require very large insulin dosages when treated subcutaneously. Clinically these patients seem to represent a rather heterogenous group and any complete description of the 'syndrome' is hampered by the fact that the 'resistance against subcutaneous insulin' does not appear to be a constant feature of these patients. In some studies, excessive degradation of insulin by tissue extracts and/or the patients' sera has been found, or local sequestration at the injection site has been suggested (29–31). As a consequence, attempts have been made to inhibit such excessive local insulin degradation and/or increase the local blood flow by injecting aprotinin (or lidocain) together with the insulin solution (1, 29, 30, 32). The long-term results of such therapeutic trials have been largely disappointing, however, and the therapeutic use of subcutaneous aprotinin injections must be discouraged because of the hazard of anaphylactic reactions (1, 33, 34). More recently, Misbin et al. (35) have described an interesting case of resistance against subcutaneously injected insulin due to excessive insulin degradation *in situ* causally related to a lack of the insulin-like growth factor IGF_2.

Just as heterogeneous is the group of patients often referred to as 'brittle diabetics'. These patients present with erratic variations of insulin requirements precipitating frequent episodes of diabetic ketoacidosis or severe hypoglycemia necessitating hospitalization. The majority of these patients have been shown to have serious psycho-social and behavioral problems causing the mismanagement of their diabetes. Some true cases of 'brittle diabetes' may, however, exist. Controversial reports have been published as to the possible involvement of bizarre patterns of insulin absorption in the etiology of these cases (1, 36, 37). A recent report by Williams et al.

(38) points to abnormal patterns of local blood flow in response to the subcutaneous insulin injection as a hypothetical mechanism of the brittleness of metabolism in these patients.

A factor well known to interfere with the bioavailability of subcutaneously injected insulin is the binding of insulin to circulating insulin antibodies. In the presence of high titers of circulating insulin-binding antibodies (IBA), clinical insulin resistance may occur, in rare cases requiring the administration of extremely large doses of insulin independent of the route of its administration (see Chapter 4). These cases of immunological insulin resistance have, however, become extremely rare since the introduction of highly purified insulin preparations more than ten years ago. The disappearance of acid-pH insulin preparations from the market and the gradual replacement of bovine insulins by porcine or human insulin preparations is expected to further reduce the incidence of immunologic resistance. Circulating insulin antibodies in smaller quantities can, however, be detected in almost all insulin-treated diabetic patients if appropriate assay methodologies are used (39). In fact, the presence of small to moderate quantities of IBA has often been considered as clinically beneficial since the pool of bound insulin would tend to stabilize metabolic homeostasis by preventing rapid changes of the biologically active 'free insulin' in the serum.

As the presence of small to moderate quantities of circulating IBA may have been a stabilizing factor (40) in the framework of an insulin therapy preferentially based upon long-acting insulin and a rigid diet distributed over 6–8 meals per day, the binding of exogenous insulin will prevent the more rapid oscillations of serum-free insulin intended by the preferential use of regular insulin during ICT. Thus, in patients with moderate titers of IBA the use of regular insulin before a meal may fail to elicit an adequate rise of circulating free insulin to cover the intake of carbohydrates and to prevent postprandial hyperglycemia. Several hours later, however, the prolonged release of biologically active insulin from the insulin–antibody-complexes may lead to unexpected hypoglycemia. Figure 1 illustrates the disturbance of the bioavailability of regular insulin given as a pre-meal bolus by circulating IBA. After one year of continuous subcutaneous insulin infusion (CSII) with a highly purified regular porcine insulin preparation, IBA titers had been substantially reduced: in response to an identical bolus injection of regular insulin a rapid increase of free insulin was elicited – adequate to result in normoglycemia following the standardized meal.

On the other hand, a recent series of investigations reported by Bolli et al. (41) have indicated that the presence of IBA, even in rather small quantities, is a leading cause of prolonged hypoglycemia in insulin-treated diabetic patients. In these studies, changes of the bioavailability of exogenous regular insulin due to the presence of IBA were causally related to the prolongation of hyperinsulinemia and hypoglycemia. In conclusion, the

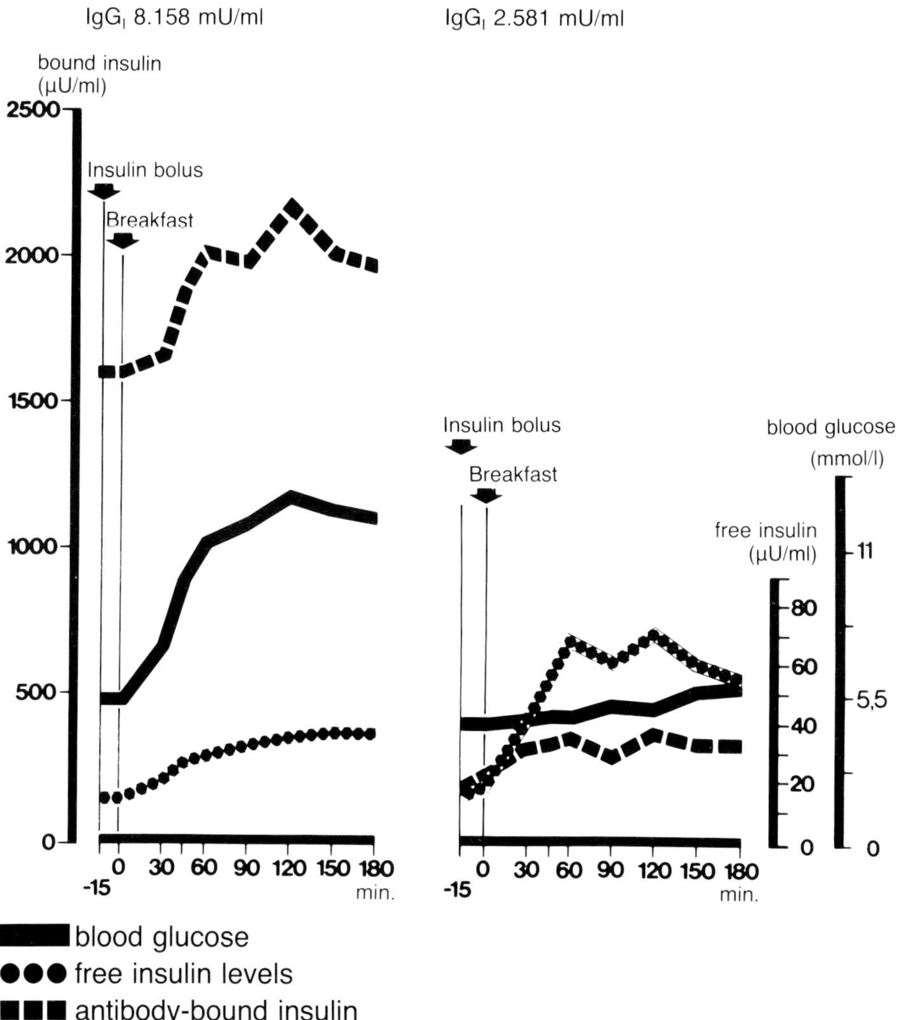

FIG. 1. *Effect of circulating insulin-binding antibodies IgG_I on the pharmacokinetics and bioavailability of subcutaneously injected regular insulin. An insulin bolus of regular subcutaneously injected insulin was given to a 24-year-old Type 1 (insulin-dependent) diabetic woman on two occasions one year apart. At the time of the first test, the patient had substantially elevated titers of circulating insulin antibodies IgG_I due to previous treatment with Surfen® bovine insulin preparations. Thereafter, the patient was treated with continuous subcutaneous insulin infusion using porcine Actrapid® insulin diluted in 0.9% saline, as a result of which IgG_I levels fell considerably over the period of one year. Test conditions, insulin dose and preparation, and the test meal were identical on both occasions.*
(From Goldgewicht et al. (80), by courtesy of the Editors of Diabetologia.)

more recent data suggest that circulating IBA may upset the bioavailability of subcutaneously injected regular insulin by prolongation of the half-life of exogenous insulin in the serum. At least for insulin treatment strategies preferentially based upon the use of regular insulin, such as ICT (or continuous subcutaneous insulin infusion), the presence of IBA should thus be disadvantageous and attempts should be made to lower IBA titers or prevent their development.

Human insulin

During the past three years, considerable attention has been devoted to the introduction, pharmacological and clinical evaluation of human insulin preparations (42, 43). Although the absorption of regular human insulin appears to be slightly, but significantly faster when compared to the respective porcine insulin preparations, according to the majority of the published reports, it remains doubtful whether this difference is substantial enough to present a definite advantage in clinical practice. Indeed, such a clinical benefit seems rather unlikely (44). On the other hand, at least some of the (medium-) long-acting human insulins have a considerably shorter duration of action than the respective bovine and porcine preparations (45, 46). The reasons for those differences are at present poorly understood and it remains to be determined whether as yet unidentified steps in the manufacture of some long-acting human insulins are responsible for this phenomenon.

Also unexpected and as yet unexplained is the observation that miscibility with regular insulin differs between human and bovine ultralente preparations. Thus, it appears that the mixture of regular and human-ultralente insulins removes the short-acting component of the regular insulin instantaneously, whereas this phenomenon may be avoided when mixtures of regular insulin and bovine ultralente insulin are injected immediately after the mixing procedure (21). Likewise, it appears that the miscibility of lente-type insulins differs quite markedly between human and porcine insulin preparations.

Much attention has been paid to the consequence of the introduction of human insulin preparations with regard to the formation of IBA. In patients previously treated with bovine insulin, IBA titers have been repeatedly demonstrated to fall when therapy is changed to human insulin (47, 48). In patients previously treated with highly purified porcine insulin preparations, IBA titers are already rather low or at the lower limit of detectability, and thus an effect of changing over to human insulin, if any, has been difficult to document (48).

The hope that the exclusive use of human insulin preparations would not induce any IBA formation at all has not been fulfilled. However, from the available data of a number of studies in process it can be concluded that the development of IBA is less marked when insulin therapy is initiated with human insulin preparations as compared to porcine insulins (49–51). Whether the *statistical* difference in these studies is of any clinical significance remains to be seen. If one assumes, however, that any potential disturbance of the bioavailability of subcutaneously injected insulin by circulating IBA should be prevented, it seems reasonable to advocate the use of human insulin in all newly discovered Type 1 diabetic patients, a policy which is presently followed by many diabetologists.

In cases of immunologically induced complications of bovine or porcine insulin therapy, it is advisable to change to the use of human insulins. This has been successful in many, but not all patients with insulin allergies and immunologic insulin resistance (see also Chapter 4).

It is of note that no differences have been reported between biosynthetic and semisynthetic regular insulins in all aspects studied. Isolated observations on differences between human and porcine insulin preparations with regard to the hormonal counterregulation and the subjective symptoms following insulin-induced hypoglycemia have not been substantiated (43).

In conclusion, the introduction of human insulin preparations into clinical practice marks an impressive technological advance in the area of mass production of therapeutically used polypeptide hormones. Its practical benefit for the achievement of satisfactory metabolic control in diabetic patients seems, however, quite limited.

Injection materials

Considerable technical advances have been made concerning the mass production of disposable plastic syringes. These syringes can be used repeatedly without any increased risk of local or systemic infections (52). Their precision represents a substantial advance over the glass syringes formerly in use and has made not only the introduction of U-100 insulins possible, but it has also increased the reliability in the practice of even minor adaptations of the insulin dosage as carried out by patients. Problems with dead space (53) and differences in the accuracy of the new plastic syringes (54) need, however, to be taken into account.

Administration of insulin through intestinal or nasal mucosa

As long as insulin has been available for the treatment of diabetic patients, trials have been conducted in order to avoid the necessity of insulin injections (2). During the past few years, attempts to elucidate the possibility for rectal administration of the hormone (55, 56, 57, 58) or for a peroral (59, 60) use have been made, mainly using animal models. A lot of publicity has been focused upon recent trials to investigate the nasal administration of insulin (61, 62). The practicability of such attempts awaits further evaluation, especially since only minute percentages of the administered insulin are absorbed and the bioavailability of nasally given insulin appears to be subject to a rather large number of modulating factors.

Intensified conventional insulin treatment (ICT)

Under the heading of ICT, a number of more recently proposed strategies of insulin treatment can be summarized (1, 63). Common to all of them is a physiology-oriented insulin injection regime which differentiates between a basal insulin component delivered by (medium-) long-acting insulins and the prandial insulin requirements preferentially covered by two or more daily injections of regular insulin before the main meals. The term ICT describes the strategy of diabetes care as such, rather than merely suggesting a certain type of insulin treatment. Thus for all subtypes of ICT, the education of the diabetic patient to conduct the treatment as independently as possible represents the *conditio sine qua non*. The treatment is based upon systematic self-monitoring of glycemia or glycosuria and the patient's ability to modify the insulin dose according to the degree of glycemic control and to his/her immediate plans to eat or to engage in physical activity. Thus, the success of ICT relies essentially on the understanding and cooperation of the patient; hence diabetes education becomes *the* cornerstone of any attempt to carry out ICT. In addition to the influence of the renewed understanding of physiology, the development of ICT strategies has greatly profited from the experience of patients and their physicians with metabolic self-monitoring, from the recent advances in diabetes education techniques (64), and from the experiences gained with continuous subcutaneous insulin therapy (CSII). It is worth noting that many recent developments in the clinical care of Type 1 diabetic patients, such as the successful attempts to liberalize the hitherto rigid dietary regimen (65) and the use of algorithms for pre-meal or pre-exercise insulin dose adjustments were first studied in patients on CSII before they were introduced to patients on ICT.

Recently, Schade et al. (1) have reviewed the various theoretical and practical aspects of ICT in detail: in essence, four different strategies for insulin replacement therapy by subcutaneous injections can be differentiated (Table 2). Patient and physician should review the possibilities, advantages and disadvantages of these strategies for each individual case before a particular insulin regimen is initiated. Very often, a stepwise advance takes place with increasing knowledge and experience on the part of the patient. Thus, it might be advisable to begin with *ICT-Type A* on a routine basis. For many patients this type of insulin therapy will turn out to be satisfactory, if insulin dosages are frequently adjusted by the patient in order to achieve acceptable degrees of metabolic control. A certain percen-

TABLE 2. *Strategies of intensified conventional insulin therapy (ICT)*

Strategy	Insulin injections			
	Before breakfast	Before lunch	Before supper	At bed-time
ICT-Type A	*Mixture of:* lente or NPH + regular	–	*Mixture of:* lente or NPH + regular	–
ICT-Type B	*Mixture of:* lente or NPH + regular	–	regular	lente or NPH
ICT-Type C	*Mixture of:* lente or NPH + regular	regular	regular	lente or NPH
ICT-Type D	Regular	regular	regular	ultralente*

* Depending on the ultralente preparation used and the life-style (nutrition, physical activity etc.) of the patient, the ultralente injection in strategy ICT-Type D might be given at any other time of the day.

tage of patients, however, will find it difficult to achieve (near-) normal fasting glycemia using *ICT-Type A*. In many of these cases, it has turned out to be beneficial to give the second daily injection of medium long-acting insulin as a bed-time injection (66), in order to increase the serum free insulin levels in the early morning hours. Very often, the actual dose of the medium-long-acting insulin can be reduced when giving it at bed-time, thus decreasing the risk of nocturnal hypoglycemia (*ICT-Type B*).

With increasing education and experience, an increasing number of patients prefer to take an additional injection of regular insulin at lunch-time (*ICT-Type C*), in order to be able to vary the time and the content their lunch more freely. The morning medium-long-acting insulin dose is reduced with this type of insulin therapy, and the patient may adapt the pre-lunch regular insulin dose according to the actual glycemia and the amount of carbohydrate to be ingested. The relative freedom of choice with regard to the timing of the lunch might be lost if the morning injection of medium long-acting insulin is omitted.

Finally, it has been advocated that the administration of long-acting insulin should be decreased to one injection per day (*ICT-Type D*) in an attempt to lower the constant 'basal' insulinemia to as low (and physiological) levels as possible. Such an insulin regimen can be constructed by injecting long-acting insulin preparations (of the ultra-lente type) once daily (67,68). Thus, it has been suggested to use once daily injections of bovine Ultralente® insulin either in the morning or pre-supper or at bed-time. The aim of such insulin therapy would be to mimic the basal component of CSII by ultralente type insulin preparations. In keeping with the experience from CSII, the long-acting insulin dose should not exceed 40 to 50% of the total daily insulin requirement. Obviously, numerous variations of these basic schemes are possible. Thus, adjustments have to be made for instance for shift-workers, patients who dislike eating large English-type breakfast, and other alterations to 'normal' life-styles.

A number of studies have attempted to compare the efficacy of the various ICT strategies (and CSII) in achieving (near-) normoglycemia (1, 63, 69–76). In general, any ICT can result in satisfactory degrees of metabolic control in most patients. The long-term success will depend in the most part on the cooperation of the patient. Thus, it appears most important to find out together with the patient which one of the ICT strategies suits his personal life-style and his individual preferences best. Since patients vary quite substantially in their individual preferences and acceptance of different treatment strategies, it seems of limited interest to conduct 'controlled' trials in order to compare various ICTs against each other or with CSII in order to find out whether any one of them is most effective. In the short-term, any one of the intensive types of diabetes treatment regimens will turn out to be better than the previous insulin therapy with one or two daily injections of (medium-) long-acting insulins without metabolic self-control. In the long-term, however, it is the patient who has to decide which one of the ICTs (or CSII) he or she believes to be most acceptable – if stable metabolic control is to be achieved.

Many patients manage to work out individual algorithms for the insulin dosage based upon their own experience with self-monitoring of glycemia (or glucosuria). A number of basic rules for such algorithms have been suggested (1, 77). In pregnant diabetic patients such algorithms for ICT including 6 or more daily injections of regular insulin have been used most successfully by Jovanovic et al. (78) and others to achieve normoglycemia throughout pregnancy.

In unselected groups of Type 1 (insulin-dependent) diabetic patients referred to a specialized diabetes unit substantial improvements of metabolic control and other parameters of diabetes care have been documented as a result of an integrated approach of intensive diabetes education and ICT (79).

Any attempt to improve the overall degree of metabolic control and to lower glycemia to (near-) normal values is expected to raise the risk of severe hypoglycemia. With the exception of one recent report from the Hôtel-Dieu (80), unfortunately, almost no valid data are available as to the incidence of severe hypoglycemia in insulin-treated diabetic patients which might serve as a reference for further studies on the risk of hypoglycemia during ICT or CSII. Preliminary data from our own studies seem to indicate, however, that the risk of severe hypoglycemia is not unduly increased in well educated patients on ICT (nor on CSII) when compared to the – admittedly limited – data from other series (81). A number of recent investigations have been carried out in order to describe particular risk factors for the development of severe hypoglycemia in Type 1 (insulin-dependent) diabetic patients. These studies have initially concentrated on potential abnormalities of hormonal counterregulation following insulin-induced hypoglycemia (82–89). Some defects seem to have been discovered, although it remains to be established to which extent such defects of catecholamine and/or glucagon counterregulation are reversible with increased degrees of metabolic control. Eventually, these studies should be instrumental in selecting a subgroup of diabetic patients at particularly high risk of developing severe hypoglycemia (83, 86, 87); it might be advisable then to exclude such patients from intensive efforts to strive for (near-) normoglycemia by ICT or CSII. The most recent studies of Bolli et al. (41) seem to point to the circulating levels of IBA as a major risk for developing hypoglycemia; it is expected that this particular risk factor can be eliminated by the use of highly purified porcine or human insulin preparations.

Whether the undisputed efficacy of ICT in achieving improvements of metabolic control and in freeing patients from rigid regimens of diet and life-style, as shown in some diabetes centers, can be made available to larger populations of diabetic patients will depend mainly on a marked increase in the quality and quantity of diabetes education facilities worldwide.

References

1. Schade DS, Santiago JV, Skyler JS, Rizza RA (1983): *Intensive Insulin Therapy*. Excerptà Medica, Amsterdam.
2. Rinke S, Berger M (1983): *Die ersten Jahre der Insulin-Therapie*. Zuckschwerdt, München.
3. Binder C (1969): *Absorption of Injected Insulin*. Munksgaard, Copenhagen.
4. Berger N, Cüppers HJ, Hegner H et al (1982): Absorption kinetics and biological effects of subcutaneously injected insulin preparations. *Diabetes Care*, *5*, 77.
5. Kobayashi T, Sawano S, Itoh T et al (1983): The pharmacokinetics of insulin after subcutaneous infusion or bolus subcutaneous injection in diabetic patients. *Diabetes*, *32*, 331.
6. Fischer U, Freyse EJ, Jutzi E et al (1983): Absorption rates of subcutaneously injected insulin in the dog as calculated from the plasma insulin levels by means of a simple mathematical model. *Diabetologia*, *24*, 196.
7. Galloway JA, Spradlin CT, Nelson RL et al (1981): Factors influencing the absorption, serum insulin concentration, and blood glucose responses after injections of regular insulin and various insulin mixtures. *Diabetes Care*, *4*, 366.

8. Binder C, Lauritzen T, Faber O, Pramming S (1984): Insulin pharmacokinetics. *Diabetes Care*, *7*, 188.
9. Binder C (1983): A theoretical model for the absorption of soluble insulin. In: *Artificial Systems for Insulin Delivery*, p 53. Editors: P. Brunetti, K.G.M.M. Alberti, A.M. Albisser, K.D. Hepp and M. Massi-Benedetti. Raven Press, New York.
10. Berger M, Jörgens V (1983): *Praxis der Insulin Therapie*. Springer, Berlin-Heidelberg-New York.
11. Kolendorf K, Bojsen J, Deckert T (1983): Clinical factors influencing the absorption of ^{125}I-NPH-insulin. *Horm. Metab. Res.*, *15*, 274.
12. Hildebrandt P, Sestoft L, Nielsen SL (1983): The absorption of subcutaneously injected short-acting soluble insulin: Influence of injection technique and concentration. *Diabetes Care*, *6*, 459.
13. Dillon RS (1983): Improved serum insulin profiles in diabetic individuals who massaged their insulin injection sites. *Diabetes Care*, *6*, 399.
14. Berger M, Halban PA, Offord RE et al (1979): Absorption kinetics of subcutaneously injected insulin: Evidence for degradation at the injection site. *Diabetologia*, *17*, 97.
15. Mühlhauser I, Cüppers HJ, Berger M (1984): Smoking and insulin absorption from subcutaneous tissue. *Br. Med. J.*, *288*, 1875.
16. Kolendorf K, Bojsen J (1983): Kinetics of subcutaneous NPH insulin in diabetics. *Clin. Pharmacol. Ther.*, *31*, 494.
17. Kolendorf K, Bojsen J (1982): Biotelemetric detection of the disappearance rate of subcutaneously injected ^{125}I-NPH-insulin in diabetic patients. *Clin. Physiol. (Stockholm)*, *2*, 13.
18. Lauritzen T, Pramming S, Gale EAM et al (1982): Absorption of isophane (NPH) insulin and its clinical implications. *Br. Med. J.*, *285*, 159.
19. Deckert T, Hansen B, Kolendorf K et al (1982): Absorption of NPH-insulin from subcutaneous tissue: a methodological study in pigs. *Acta Pharmacol. Toxicol.*, *51*, 30.
20. Kolendorf K, Bojsen J, Deckert T (1983): Absorption and miscibility of regular porcine insulin after subcutaneous injection in insulin-treated diabetic patients. *Dabetes Care*, *6*, 6.
21. Mühlhauser I, Broermann C, Tsotsalas M, Berger M (1984): Miscibility of human and bovine ultralente insulin with soluble insulin. *Br. Med. J.*, in press.
22. Nolte MS, Poon V, Grodsky GM et al (1983): Reduced solubility of short-acting soluble insulins when mixed with longer-acting insulins. *Diabetes*, *32*, 1177.
23. Heine RJ, Bilo HJG, Fonk T (1984): Absorption kinetics and action profiles of mixtures of regular and intermediate acting insulins. *Diabetologia*, *27*, in press.
24. Offord RE, Philippe J, Davies et al (1979): The inhibition of degradation of insulin by ophthalmic acid and a bovine pancreatic protease inhibitor. *Biochem. J.*, *182*, 249.
25. Williams G, Pickup JC, Bowcock S et al (1983): Subcutaneous aprotinin causes local hyperaemia. A possible mechanism by which aprotinin improves control in some diabetic patients. *Diabetologia*, *24*, 91.

26. Swift PGF, Kennedy JD, Gerlis LS (1983): Change to U-100 insulin does not appear to affect insulin absorption. *Br. Med. J.*, *286*, 1015.
27. Chantelau EA, Sonnenberg GE, Rajab A, Broermann C, Best F, Berger M (1984): Absorption of subcutaneously administered regular human and porcine insulin in different concentrations. *Diabète Métab.*, in press.
28. Williams G, Pickup JC, Keen H (1983): U-100 Insulin and insulin absorption. *Br. Med. J.*, *286*, 1437.
29. Freidenberg GR, White N, Cataland S et al (1981): Diabetes responsive to intravenous but not subcutaneous insulin: effectiveness of aprotinin. *N. Engl. J. Med.*, *305*, 363.
30. Maberly GF, Wait GA, Kilpatrick JA et al (1982): Evidence for insulin degradation by muscle and fat tissue in an insulin resistant diabetic patient. *Diabetologia*, *23*, 333.
31. Calle-Pascual AL, Maranes-Pallardo JP, Charro-Salgado AL (1983): Resistencia a la insulina por aumento de la actividad de las enzimas proteoliticas en el lugar de la inyeccion de la insulina. Su estudio en sujetos diabeticos insulino-dependientes (DID). *Med. Clin. (Barcelona)*, *80*, 524.
32. Müller WA, Taillens C, Léreret S et al (1980): Resistance against subcutaneous insulin successfully managed with aprotinin. *Lancet*, *1*, 1245.
33. Berger M, Misbin RI, Duckworth WB et al (1981) Diabetes resistant to subcutaneous insulin: effect of aprotinin. (Letter to the Editor) *N. Engl. J. Med.*, *305*, 1413.
34. Pickup JC, Williams G, Bilous R, Keen H (1981): Resistance against subcutaneous insulin: effect of aprotinin (Letter). *N. Engl. J. Med.*, *305*, 1413.
35. Misbin RI, Almira EC, Froesch ER et al (1983): Resistance to subcutaneous and intramuscular insulin associated with deficiency of insulin-like growth factor (IGF) 2. *Metab. Clin. Exp.*, *32*, 537.
36. Home PD, Massi-Benedetti M, Gill GV et al (1982): Impaired subcutaneous absorption of insulin in 'brittle' diabetics. *Acta Endocrinol.* (*Copenhagen*), *101*, 414.
37. Pickup JC, Williams G, Jones P, Keen H (1983): Clinical features of brittle diabetic patients unresponsive to optimized subcutaneous insulin therapy. *Diabetes Care*, *6*, 279.
38. Williams G, Pickup JC, Clark A et al (1983): Changes in blood flow close to subcutaneous insulin injection sites in stable and brittle diabetics. *Diabetes*, *32*, 466.
39. Reeves WG (1983): Insulin antibody determination: theoretical and practical considerations. *Diabetologia*, *24*, 399.
40. Vaughan NJA, Matthews JA, Kurtz AB, Nabarro JDN (1983): The bioavailability of circulating antibody-bound insulin following insulin withdrawal in type 1 (insulin-dependent) diabetes. *Diabetologia*, *24*, 355.
41. Bolli GB, Dimitriadis GD, Pehling GB, Baker BA, Haymond MW, Cryer PE, Gerich JE (1984): Abnormal glucose counterregulation after subcutaneous insulin in insulin-dependent diabetes mellitus. *N. Engl. J. Med.*, *310*, 1706.
42. Sonnenberg GE, Berger M (1983): Human insulin – much ado about one amino acid? *Diabetologia*, *25*, 457.

43. Johansen K (1983): Human insulin – medical progress? *Metab. Clin. Exp.*, *32*, 528.
44. Sonnenberg GE, Chantelau EA, Sunderman S et al (1982): Human and porcine insulins are equally effective in subcutaneous replacement therapy. *Diabetes*, *31*, 600.
45. Galloway JA, Peck FB, Fineberg SE et al (1982): The US 'New Patient and Transfer' studies. *Diabetes Care*, *5*, *Suppl. 2*, 135.
46. Massi-Benedetti M, Bueti A, Mannino D et al (1984): Kinetics and metabolic activity of biosynthetic NPH insulin evaluated by the glucose clamp technique. *Diabetes Care*, *7*, 132.
47. Peacock I, Tattersall RB, Taylor A et al (1983): Effects of new insulins on insulin and c-peptide antibodies, insulin dose, and diabetic control. *Lancet*, *1*, 149.
48. Skyler JS (Ed.) (1982): Symposium on Human Insulin of Recombinant DNA Origin. *Diabetes Care*, *5*, *Suppl. 2*.
49. Iavicoli M, Di Mario U, Coronel GA et al (1984): Semisynthetic human insulin: biologic and immunologic activity in newly treated diabetic subjects during a six-month follow-up. *Diabetes Care*, *7*, 128.
50. Fineberg SE, Galloway JA, Fineberg NS et al (1983): Immunogenicity of recombinant DNA human insulin. *Diabetologia*, *25*, 465.
51. Heding LG, Marshall MO, Persson B et al (1984): Immunogenicity of monocomponent human and porcine insulin in newly diagnosed type 1 (insulin-dependent) diabetic children. *Diabetologia*, *27*, 96.
52. Oli JM, Gugnani HC, Ojiegbe GC (1982): Multiple use of ordinary disposable syringes for insulin injections. *Br. Med. J.*, *284*, 6311.
53. Hall GH, Thompson CJ, Palmer A (1984): Danger of dead space in U-100 insulin syringes. *Br. Med. J.*, *288*, 284.
54. Skodda H, Warzecha P, Mühlhauser I et al (1983): The quality of different insulin syringes. *Diabetologia*, *25*, 194A.
55. Yagi T, Hakui N, Yamasaki Y et al (1983): Insulin suppository: enhanced rectal absorption of insulin using an enamine derivative as a new promotor. *J. Pharm. Pharmacol.*, *35*, 177.
56. Kim S, Kamada A, Higuchi T, Nishihata T (1983): Effect of enamine derivatives on the rectal absorption of insulin in dogs and rabbits. *J. Pharm. Pharmacol.*, *35*, 100.
57. Nishihata T, Rytting JH, Kamada A et al (1983): Enhancement of rectal absorption of insulin using salicylates in dogs. *J. Pharm. Pharmacol.*, *35*, 148.
58. Fujita S, Kamado K, Takimoto T et al (1983): Insulin suppositories to stabilize brittle diabetes. In: *Current and Future Therapies with Insulin*. p 268. Editors: N. Sakamoto and K.G.M.M. Alberti. Excerpta Medica, Amsterdam-Oxford-Princeton.
59. Dobre V, Georgescu D, Simionescu L et al (1983): The entrapment of biologically active substances in liposomes. I. Effects of the oral administration of liposomally entrapped insulin in normal rats. *Rev. Roum. Biochim.*, *20*, 15.
60. Rossels AN, Bukhman AA, Vakhrusheva LL et al (1983): The possibility to use liposomes for oral insulin introduction in diabetes mellitus. *Khim. Farm. Zh.*, *17*, 52.

61. Pontiroli AE, Alberetto M, Secchi A et al (1982): Insulin given intranasally induces hypoglycaemia in normal and diabetic subjects. *Br. Med. J.*, *284*, 303.
62. Moses AC, Gordon GS, Carey MC, Flier JS (1983): Insulin administered intranasally as an insulin-bile salt aerosol. Effectiveness and reproducibility in normal and diabetic subjects. *Diabetes*, *32*, 1040.
63. Schiffrin A (1982): Treatment of insulin-dependent diabetes with multiple subcutaneous insulin injections. *Med. Clin. N. Am.*, *66*, 1251.
64. Assal JP, Berger M, Canivet J, Gay N (Eds) (1983): *Diabetes Education. How to Improve Patient Education.* Excerpta Medica, Amsterdam-Oxford-Princeton.
65. Chantelau EA, Bockholt M, Lie KT et al (1984): Diet and pump-treated diabetes: a long-term follow-up. *Diabète Métab.*, *9*, 277.
66. Francis AJ, Home PD, Hanning I et al (1983): Intermediate acting insulin given at bedtime: effect on blood glucose concentrations before and after breakfast. *Br. Med. J.*, *286*, 1173.
67. Turner RC, Phillips MA, Ward EA et al (1983): Ultralente based insulin regimens – clinical applications, advantages and disadvantages. *Acta Med. Scand.*, *213*, *Suppl. 671*, 75.
68. Turner RC, Phillips M, Jones R et al (1982): Ultralente-based insulin regimens in insulin-dependent diabetics. In: *Insulin Update 1982*, p 157. Editor: J.S. Skyler. Excerpta Medica, New York.
69. Schiffrin A, Belmonte M (1981): Combined continuous subcutaneous insulin infusion and multiple subcutaneous injections in type I diabetic patients. *Diabetes Care*, *4*, 595.
70. Schiffrin A, Belmonte M (1982): Comparison between continuous subcutaneous insulin infusion and multiple insulin injections of insulin. *Diabetes*, *31*, 255.
71. Schiffrin A, Desrosiers M, Aleyassine H, Belmonte M (1984): Intensified insulin therapy in the type I diabetic adolescent: a controlled trial. *Diabetes Care*, *7*, 107.
72. Home PD, Capaldo B, Burrin JM et al (1982): A crossover comparison of continuous subcutaneous insulin infusion (CSII) against multiple insulin injections in insulin-dependent diabetic subjects: improved control with CSII. *Diabetes Care*, *5*, 466.
73. Nathan D, Lou P, Avruch J (1982): Intensive conventional and insulin pump therapy in adult Type 1 diabetes: a crossover study. *Ann. Intern. Med.*, *97*, 31.
74. Reeves ML, Seigler DE, Ryan EA, Skyler JS (1982): Glycaemic control in insulin-dependent diabetes mellitus. Comparison of outpatient intensified conventional therapy with continuous subcutaneous insulin infusion. *Am. J. Med.*, *72*, 673.
75. Skyler JS, Seigler DE, Reeves ML (1982): A comparison of insulin regimens in insulin-dependent diabetes mellitus. *Diabetes Care*, *5*, *Suppl. 1*, 11.
76. Dupré J, Champion M, Rodger NW (1982): Advances in insulin delivery in the management of diabetes mellitus. *Clin. Endocrinol. Metab.*, *11*, 525.
77. Skyler JS, Miller NE, O'Sullivan MJ et al (1982): Use of insulin in insulin-dependent diabetes mellitus. In: *Insulin Update 1982*, p 125. Editor: J.S. Skyler. Excerpta Medica, New York.

78. Jovanovic L, Peterson CM, Saxena BB et al (1980): Feasibility of maintaining normal glucose profiles in insulin-dependent diabetic women. *Am. J. Med.*, *68*, 105.
79. Mühlhauser I, Jörgens V, Berger M et al (1983): Bicentric evaluation of a teaching and treatment programme for type 1 (insulin-dependent) diabetic patients: improvement of metabolic control and other measures of diabetes care for up to 22 months. *Diabetologia*, *25*, 470.
80. Goldgewicht C, Slama G, Papoz L, Tchobroutsky G (1983): Hypoglycaemic reactions in 172 type 1 (insulin-dependent) diabetic patients. *Diabetologia*, *24*, 95.
81. Koch J, Mühlhauser I, Jörgens V et al (1983): Incidence and management of severe hypoglycaemia in 402 type 1 diabetic patients (Abstract). *Diabetologia*, *25*, 171.
82. Kleinbaum J, Shamoon H (1983): Impaired counterregulation of hypoglycaemia in insulin-dependent diabetes mellitus. *Diabetes*, *32*, 493.
83. Unger RH (1983): Insulin-glucagon relationships in the defense against hypoglycaemia. *Diabetes*, *32*, 575.
84. Bergenstal RM, Polonsky KS, Pons G et al (1983): Lack of glucagon response to hypoglycaemia in type 1 diabetics after long-term optimal therapy with continuous subcutaneous insulin infusion pump. *Diabetes*, *32*, 398.
85. Cryer PE, Gerich JE (1983): Relevance of glucose counterregulatory systems to patients with diabetes: critical rôles of glucagon and epinephrine. *Diabetes Care*, *6*, 95.
86. White NH, Skor DA, Cryer PE et al (1983): Identification of type 1 diabetic patients at increased risk for hypoglycaemia during intensive therapy. *N. Engl. J. Med.*, *308*, 485.
87. Boden G, Hoeldtke RD (1983): Making intensified insulin treatment safer. *Ann. Intern. Med.*, *99*, 268.
88. Bolli G, De-Feo P, Compagnucci P et al (1983): Abnormal glucose counterregulation in insulin-dependent diabetes mellitus. Interaction of anti-insulin antibodies and impaired glucagon and epinephrine secretion. *Diabetes*, *32*, 134.
89. Bolli G, De-Feo P, Periello G et al (1984): Mechanisms of glucagon secretion during insulin-induced hypoglycaemia in man. The rôle of the beta cell and arterial hyperinsulinaemia. *J. Clin. Invest.*, *73*, 917.
90. Chantelau EA, Sonnenberg GE, Heding LG, Berger M (1984): Impaired metabolic response to regular insulin in the presence of a high level of circulating insulin-binding immunoglobulin G. *Diabetes Care*, *7*, 403.

The Diabetes Annual/1
K.G.M.M. Alberti and L.P. Krall, editors

ISBN 0444 90 343 7
$0.85 per article per page (transactional system)
$0.20 per article per page (licensing system)

8 Open-loop continuous insulin infusion in management of insulin requiring diabetes mellitus

J. DUPRÉ

So-called open-loop continuous infusion of insulin has long been used in the acute management of metabolic disorders in diabetes. The development of this technique for long-term management of the disease depended in part on knowledge of the physiology of insulin secretion, and on experience with closed-loop delivery of insulin by means of the artificial endocrine pancreas (AEP), but has nevertheless been largely empirical. Early experience with portable pumps, with effectively continuous intravenous (CIVII) or subcutaneous (CSII) delivery of insulin and dispensing with on-line feedback control in response to the concentration of glucose in the blood, suggested that programs using fixed rate background ('basal') infusions, with empirically determined pre-meal supplements, could result in control of glycemia superior to that expected with conventional (once-or-twice daily) injections of mixed insulins in IDDM (1, 2). In these preliminary studies controlled comparisons with the conventional therapies were not carried out, and since the improvement in glycemic control in some subjects was associated with increased daily dosage of insulin, as well as with intensified monitoring of the blood glucose concentrations, it could be questioned how far the response was dependent on the infusion technique itself. However, paired comparisons with conventional and CSII techniques in subjects with IDDM studied under similar conditions of management showed that CSII resulted in superior control of blood glucose levels (3). This was followed by use of the method in more standard clinical situations (4), and more recently by controlled trials in which the results of conventional therapy and of subcutaneous infusion therapy were subjected to the more rigorous comparisons described below (5, 6). Thus the results obtained with delivery of insulin by the subcutaneous route at present provide the benchmark experience with open-loop systems for comparison with the effects of administration of insulin by other routes or by conventional depot injection therapy. It is important to note that application of these methods and assessment of their results have depended heavily not only on the availability of techniques for rapid approximate measurement of capillary blood glucose concentrations, but also on the determination of glycosylated hemoglobin levels as an independent means of assessing the concentrations of glucose prevailing in the blood.

EVOLUTION OF PROGRAMS FOR OPEN-LOOP CONTINUOUS INSULIN INFUSION IN IDDM

Empirical selection of programs and targets for control of glycemia with CSII

With use of CSII and programs employing fixed-rate basal infusions, together with pre-meal supplements given as boluses, attempts to maintain strict normoglycemia are associated with an undesirable risk of hypoglycemia overnight or at intervals of more than 3 hours after meals, so that compromise targets for control of plasma concentrations have generally been adopted. These are commonly in a range leading to average blood glucose levels of approximately 100 mg/dl (5.6 mmoles/l) before the main meals (7). When such targets are accepted the postprandrial rise of plasma glucose concentration frequently exceeds the normal range, with concentrations rising to 160–180 mg/dl (8.9–10 mmoles/l). Substantial experience with this type of program has now accumulated, and the diurnal profiles of glycemic control attainable with long-term use under everyday conditions have been reported (8) (Fig. 1). The resulting mean blood glucose and glycohemoglobin levels in studies with groups of subjects with IDDM during CSII have generally fallen close to the upper limits defined in normal subjects (5, 6, 8).

Optimization of basal rates of delivery of insulin in management of IDDM by CSII

Theoretical and practical considerations suggest that diurnal variation of the basal rate of delivery of insulin, particularly with an increase in the rate during the dawn hours before breakfast, may improve control of glycemia without increasing the risk of hypoglycemia (9). Experience with fixed basal-rate programs suggests that some subjects are at risk for development of hypoglycemia in the small hours of the night when the program delivers sufficient insulin to produce target control of glycemia before breakfast. This phenomenon has been related to findings with closed-loop insulin delivery systems, which have shown that an increased rate of delivery occurs when the AEP is used to ‘clamp’ the blood glucose concentration at normal fasting levels during the dawn hours (10). The physiology of the

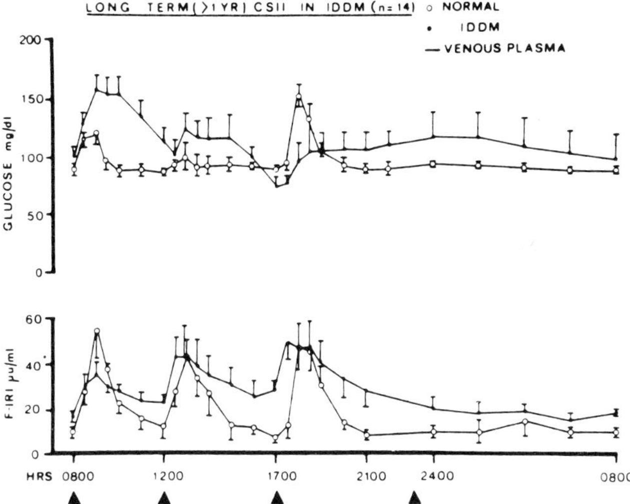

FIG. 1. *Mean diurnal plasma concentrations of glucose and free immunoreactive insulin in normal volunteers and in volunteers with IDDM during long-term CSII. CSII continued for more than 1 year in every subject. Subjects attended the unit either for breakfast, lunch, supper, or for an overnight study, on different occasions. The periods of study were selected so that a composite 24-hour profile could be assembled from the results. Serum free-immunoreactive insulin was determined after extraction of serum, equilibrated at 37 °C, with PEG. The meals were in accordance with the current diets of all subjects. Reproduced from Dupré et al. (8), by courtesy of the Editors of Clinical and Investigative Medicine.*

so-called dawn phenomenon remains to be clarified. It has been shown that it cannot be attributed simply to the effects of identified counter-regulatory hormones (11), and evidence has been obtained suggesting that the clearance of insulin from the blood may increase during this period of greater apparent demand for the hormone (12, 13). Experience with programmable portable pumps used for CSII shows that the use of a lower basal rate of delivery of insulin in the interval between (approximately) midnight and 3:00 or 4:00 a.m., with an increase in the subsequent hours before breakfast, can improve glycemic control in some subjects. However, it should be noted that the use of variable basal rates of infusion of insulin overnight with CSII is not necessary for maintenance of target control of glycemia in all patients, and probably is essential only in a minority, when optimal basal infusion rates are combined with appropriate meals and insulin supplements in the evening. Nevertheless, rigorous assessment of the capacity of more complex insulin infusion programs to improve mean glucose levels without increasing the risk of hypoglycemia has not yet been undertaken. The wide range of adaptability of a variety of insulin delivery programs for

CSII in combination with appropriate diet and exercise is illustrated by demonstration of the efficacy of a program which did not incorporate premeal supplementary doses of insulin, but relied on two-step diurnal variation of the basal rate (14).

Pulsatile delivery of insulin: advantages and limitations

In the interests of simplicity of design, reduction of size, and economy of operation, pulsatile delivery of infusate is provided by most of the instruments. It is convenient to vary the rate of delivery by varying the pulse intervals. The degree to which these intervals can be prolonged during basal infusion of insulin has recently been examined (15). It was found that the control of glycemia varied little when the intervals between pulses were increased to as much as two hours, presumably due to the depot effect associated with delivery into the subcutaneous tissue. It should be noted that care must be taken with wide pulse-interval programs of basal infusion to take account of the total interval between doses that may result from random interruptions, since on temporary removal of the pump the time elapsing between the pulses that precede and follow the interruption may be much greater than the period of removal.

Adaptability of open-loop insulin therapy to performance of exercise

The liability to symptomatic hypoglycemia during or after exercise is a well-recognized hazard in the course of conventional treatment of IDDM. This risk may result from effects of exercise on clearance of glucose from the blood, but appears also to depend on hyperinsulinemia, and on increases in the blood levels of insulin consequent on its mobilization from injection sites. As a result the physiologic increase in the rate of appearance of glucose that occurs in non-diabetic subjects during exercise is inhibited, so that glucose removal exceeds glucose production, and hypoglycemia ensues (16). Experience with CSII in management of patients with IDDM in the course of exercise in the postabsorptive state suggests that the risk of hypoglycemia is small in subjects with competent counter-regulatory mechanisms. Under these conditions, with continued infusion of insulin at the empirically determined basal rate, vigorous exercise is accompanied by approximately-matching increases of glucose disposal and glucose production, so that hypoglycemia is prevented (17). It is notable that glucose turnover was normal in the normoglycemic postabsorptive state in these subjects with IDDM during CSII. In regard to the response to exercise under these conditions there appears to be little difference between open-loop systems employing subcutaneous delivery and open-loop systems making use of intravenous delivery of insulin (17, 18). This is presumably because the depot effect in the subcutaneous delivery site (at time intervals sufficiently long after the preceding meal supplement) is not great enough to allow significant mobilization of insulin from the infusion site. However, experience during CSII when exercise is undertaken after a meal, and the blood glucose concentration is falling towards the postabsorptive level, shows that the subjects may be at risk for symptomatic hypoglycemia (19). Studies of the effects of exercise after a meal with closed-loop systems (AEP) shed light on the problem of postprandial exertion during CSII (20). With continuous intravenous administration of insulin it is found that sharp curtailment of the delivery of insulin is necessary when exercise is taken after a meal (21). This could be due to the effects of exercise on intestinal absorption of nutrients, as well as on the clearance of glucose from the systemic pool. Programs of delivery of insulin by the subcutaneous route cannot be adjusted acutely and effectively in response to exercise. Thus, appropriate precautions similar to those familiar to conventionally treated subjects with IDDM must be employed with CSII when exercise is undertaken after a meal during CSII.

LONG-TERM EFFECTS OF CSII IN IDDM

Control of metabolism with CSII

Experience of the use of CSII in management of IDDM now extends to more than five years' duration, and a number of subjects have maintained this treatment under everyday conditions for such periods, with metabolic control superior to that obtained in historical experience with conventional therapy. This experience prompted consideration of the feasibility and propriety of controlled studies of the effects of intensive therapies on the complications of diabetes.

Controlled comparisons of glycemia during conventional therapy and open-loop infusion therapy

The past two years have witnessed reports of controlled (randomized) comparisons of conventional (once-or-twice daily) injection therapy and of CSII in IDDM, in studies of up to two years' duration, in single-center and collaborative multi-center trials, in which attempts were also made to assess the effects of these treatments on the complications of the disease. In design the studies carried out at the Steno Hospital in Denmark (5), and by the KROC Collaborative Study Group in six centers in North America and the United Kingdom (6), were broadly similar. Groups of volunteers with long-term IDDM (with absent or negligible endogenous secretion of insulin as tested by the concentration of immunoreactive C-peptide in the blood) were randomly assigned to continued conventional therapy or to management by means of CSII. In both studies the subjects exhibited background retinopathy at entry. Variable but not severe degrees of renal impairment were present in some subjects, and hypertensive subjects were excluded. It is important to note that conventional therapy was not intensified in either study, since it was not intended to determine the relative optimal capabilities of CSII and depot injection therapy in control of glycemia. Under these conditions both groups of investigators succeeded in recruiting and randomizing sets of volunteers with similar characteristics at entry. Both studies resulted in clear separation of glycemic control in the two treatment groups in terms of the mean profiles of plasma glucose concentration, and of the mean proportions of glycosylated hemoglobin attained after equilibration, throughout the study periods. The mean indices of glycemic control reported at 1 year of study by the Steno Hospital Group (Fig. 2) and at 8 months of study by the KROC Collaborative Study Group (Fig. 3), were remarkably similar in both conventional and infusion-treated groups of subjects. The metabolic control achieved in the CSII groups in these studies was very similar to that reported in uncontrolled studies using this technique, while no major change in the glycemic control of the conventionally-treated patients occurred after entry. At the same time it is

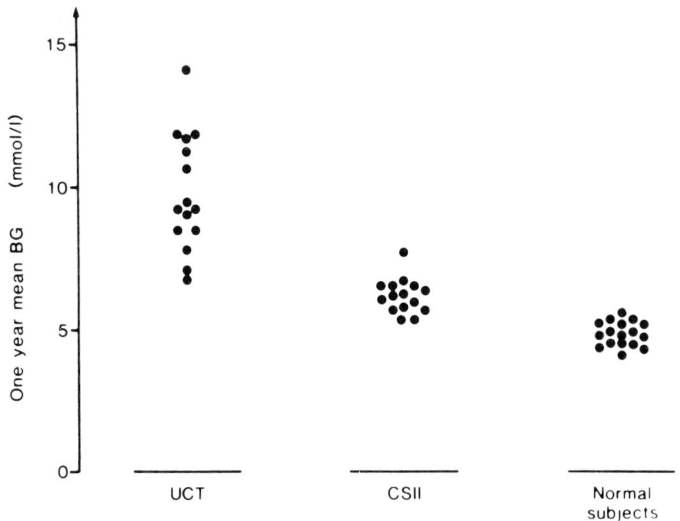

FIG. 2. *Mean glycemia during one year of conventional and CSII therapy in IDDM, compared with normal subjects. For patients each spot represents a mean of approximately 170 measurements (seven samples per day every second week for a year). For normal subjects each spot represents seven measurements a day during 3 consecutive days. Reproduced from Lauritzen et al. (5), by courtesy of the Editors of the Lancet.*

clear from the variability of control among subjects in the two treatment groups in both studies that 'overlap' of the results in the treatment groups occurred. The Steno Hospital group have indicated continued maintenance of similar and well-separated mean levels of glycemic control in the two groups through a second year of study (22). Whether such separation of the mean levels of glycemia can be maintained through longer periods of time remains to be determined.

Biochemical effects of open-loop insulin infusion therapy other than alteration of blood glucose levels

The effects of CSII on metabolites other than glucose were examined in uncontrolled studies in which the effects of this mode of therapy in control

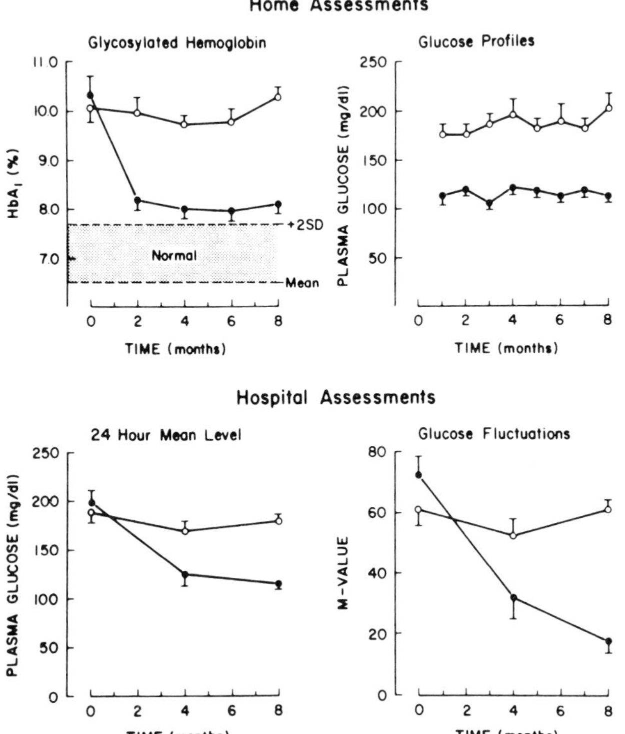

FIG. 3. *Glycemic control during conventional and CSII therapy of eight months' duration in the KROC Study Group Trial. Home and hospital assessments of glycemic control in patients randomly assigned to continuous subcutaneous insulin infusion (solid circles) or unchanged conventional injection treatment (open circles). HbA$_I$ denotes glycosylated hemoglobin. Reproduced from KROC Study Group (6), by courtesy of the Editors of the New England Journal of Medicine.*

of glycemia were explored. By comparison with historical control observations, early experience with CSII in IDDM showed that improvement of glycemic control was also associated with superior control of the concentrations of lactate, pyruvate, 3-hydroxybutyrate and alanine (23), and of cholesterol, triglyceride and free fatty acids (24), in the blood, through periods of one or two weeks. While controlled comparisons of the effects of these two modes of therapy and longer-term studies of these effects have yet to be reported, it has been shown that improvement of lipidemia persists, and that the fall of total triglyceride concentration in the blood is associated with increased levels of high density lipoprotein (25).

CSII in management of IDDM under standard clinical conditions

Since the development of effective programs for management of IDDM by CSII, a growing number of patients have been managed by means of this technique under standard clinical conditions, with quite similar results (4). Nevertheless in clinical practice the use of the technique has extended to a wider variety of patients, including some with Type 2 diabetes, and some with advanced complications of the disease.

Open-loop insulin infusion in non-insulin-dependent diabetes mellitus

Preliminary studies of CSII in patients with NIDDM have shown that the control of glycemia attainable is at least as good as that recorded in subjects with IDDM, as might be expected (26, 27). The question whether this technique has a place in management of NIDDM remains to be resolved by means of further assessments of the efficacy, safety, acceptability and benefits of open-loop CSII treatment programs in insulin-requiring NIDDM.

Comparisons of open-loop continuous insulin infusion therapy and intensified multiple subcutaneous depot injection therapies in IDDM

The possible effects of self-monitoring of capillary blood glucose concentrations in subjects with IDDM, and improvements in the use of mixed insulins delivered by injection, have raised the question whether intensified conventional depot injection therapy (once or twice a day) can match continuous open-loop infusion therapies in control of glycemia in IDDM. It has been claimed that optimization of therapy with twice-daily injection of rapid- and longer-acting insulins, adjusted in relation to the effects determined by monitoring of capillary blood glucose concentrations, can match the glycemic control attainable with CSII (28). Comparisons with further intensified injection therapy using three or more injections a day, have suggested that the attainable control of glycemia can approach or match that with

CSII (29). While group studies have demonstrated superior mean control of glycemia with the infusion technique, individual subjects may match the effects of CSII with multiple (> 2/day) injection regimens. The issue of the acceptability of these intensified regimens by comparison with conventional therapy has not been addressed in a systematic way, and must in any case be highly dependent on the outcome of technical developments, and on assessment of the risks and benefits of open-loop and other insulin treatment regimens.

Delivery of insulin by non-subcutaneous routes in open-loop programs for management of IDDM, and comparisons of these techniques with intensified depot injection therapy

Continuous insulin infusion by the intravenous route

Continuous intravenous insulin infusion, like CSII, has yielded metabolic control superior to that attained historically with conventional depot injection therapy (30). Controlled comparisons of open loop intravenous insulin therapy with open loop subcutaneous infusion therapy in IDDM have not been carried out. Nevertheless the results with intravenous infusion therapy appear to be comparable, in terms of glycemic control, with those of CSII. The technique of intravenous infusion is more adaptable to acute changes of the program in response to exercise and variation of meals (20). However, the continuing risk of infection associated with vascular access with portable external infusion devices has limited the use of this method to experimental studies of relatively short duration.

The risks of infection contingent upon vascular access with use of external infusion devices is potentially eliminated by implantation of the infusion systems. Provided the problems of long-term intravascular infusion devices can be solved, and given the necessary reliability of the infusion system and availability of suitable insulin formulations, this route of delivery of insulin remains the most attractive approach to physiologic replacement treatment with insulin. This route furthermore offers potential access to the hepatic portal system, with simulation of the physiologic route of delivery. Although problems associated with the instrumentation and the formulation of insulin for use in the reservoirs have not yet been solved, this approach may be best suited in the long-run to development of open-loop treatment with implantable devices (31).

Continuous insulin infusion by the peritoneal route

Delivery of insulin into the peritoneal cavity has practical and theoretical attractions (32). The peritoneal space is easily accessible, while the risks of infection can be minimized by use of available techniques with external infusion devices, and can be largely eliminated by implantation of the devices. Nevertheless, clear evidence of the advantages of delivery of insulin into the peritoneal cavity that have been postulated as results of partial hepatic portal delivery of the hormone is lacking, and practical problems associated with implantation and delivery of insulin from the devices have suggested that this technique is not yet capable of general application (33).

Continuous insulin infusion by the intramuscular route

In attempts to develop a practical technique for management of IDDM in those subjects who cannot be controlled with subcutaneous insulin injections, and in whom better responses to continuous intravenous infusion of insulin have suggested that degradation of insulin may occur at the subcutaneous delivery site, continuous intramuscular infusion of insulin (34) has been employed. The results suggest that this may be a useful option in management of this rare and hazardous condition (35).

Concentrations of insulin in the blood during open-loop insulin therapy in IDDM

During CSII in IDDM the mean levels of free immunoreactive insulin (FIRI) in the blood are significantly higher than normal (8). Continuous open-loop insulin infusion by this route in IDDM makes use of daily dosage generally not exceeding and frequently less than that employed with conventional therapy, in spite of improvement of glycemic control. The resulting diurnal concentrations of FIRI in the blood have been similar to those associated with conventional depot injection therapy in terms of the mean values (36). Thus in spite of difficulties in interpretation of the results of assays for free insulin in the blood in subjects who may have developed insulin antibodies, there is no evidence of an increased hazard dependent on relative hyperinsulinemia with CSII by comparison with conventional insulin therapy. Open-loop intravenous insulin therapy was developed largely on the basis of experience with the artificial endocrine pancreas (AEP), with which virtual normalization of blood glucose was achieved in association with evidence of marked hyperinsulinemia, and this feature has been reproduced in some studies with open-loop intravenous infusion programs (37). With continuous intraperitoneal insulin infusion the postulated benefit of relative lowering of systemic blood levels of insulin dependent on partial portal delivery of insulin and increased hepatic action and extraction of the hormone has not yet been clearly substantiated. The conclusion that CSII does not cause significant hyperinsulinemia relative to conventional therapy is supported by the results of studies of erythrocyte insulin receptor function in comparisons among normal subjects and subjects with

IDDM treated by conventional therapy or CSII. The findings were consistent with very slight down regulation of receptor function in the diabetics, with no detectable difference between the treatment groups (38).

CLINICAL RISKS AND BENEFITS OF MANAGEMENT OF IDDM BY MEANS OF CSII

While the long-term risks and possible benefits of CSII remain uncertain in the absence of controlled comparisons, accumulating experience with the technique permits documentation of some of the hazards. Furthermore, relatively short-term controlled comparisons of the effects of CSII and conventional therapy on the complications of diabetes and on some of the recognized hazards have now been reported.

Risks of instrument failure

While it may be expected that the hazards of instrument failure other than those leading to interruption of delivery of insulin will be largely eliminated by technical improvements, such interruption is bound to occur inadvertently at an irreducible rate with portable battery-powered instruments. The effects of deliberate interruption of CSII treatment on the development of hyperglycemia and ketosis, and some of the underlying pathophysiological mechanisms, have been examined experimentally (3, 17, 39, 40). The rate of development of hyperglycemia varies with the timing of interruption of insulin infusion in relation to preceding meals, and their associated supplementary doses of insulin. It appears that a rise in the concentration of glucose in the blood begins within an hour or two of the descent of FIRI levels below those associated with maintenance of target control of glycemia in the postabsorptive state. Within 5–6 hours the concentration of glucose in the blood approaches the renal threshold. Within these few hours the expected rises of plasma concentrations of ketone bodies and of non-esterified fatty acids also begin. The rise in the concentration of glucose in the blood may precede detectable increases of the concentrations of the 'counter-regulatory' hormones, and the early developmenty of hyperglycemia appeals to be largely due to a fall in the clearance of glucose without an accompanying increase in endogenous glucose production. This finding is in contrast to the results of studies with interruption of continuous intravenous infusion of insulin after short-term maintenance of normoglycemia in IDDM. It remains to be determined whether the longer-term effects of CSII render the subject less liable to rapid increases of endogenous production of glucose when insulin delivery is interrupted. It is apparent from clinical experience that there is substantial individual variation among subjects with IDDM with respect to the rate of metabolic deterioration under these conditions. The degree to which this variation is related to the buffering effect of antibody-bound insulin in the blood has yet to be determined. Thus it appears that accidental interruption of delivery of insulin during these programs is not a major hazard when careful routines are employed to detect escape from control within periods not exceeding the overnight interval.

Risks of intercurrent stress and its impact on metabolic control during CSII

Clinical experience with CSII in IDDM suggests that the rate of occurrence of episodes of diabetic ketoacidosis may be higher than that associated with conventional depot injection therapy (41). This impression is supported in the results of the multi-center controlled comparison of conventional and CSII techniques (6). It has become apparent that these episodes cannot be attributed simply to instrument failure, and that they can sometimes occur in association with minor identifiable intercurrent stresses, such as infections or emotional upsets, and occasionally without identifiable cause. It is thus of the greatest importance to recognize this phenomenon, and to recommend appropriate responses on the part of the subjects. Continued monitoring of capillary blood glucose levels is essential for detection of hyperglycemic 'escape', and under conditions that may have to be defined for each individual it is necessary to monitor for the development of ketosis. It is also necessary for some subjects to resort to intramuscular injection of insulin, and to seek emergency medical advice and assistance when episodes of hyperglycemia with ketonuria develop. The apparently increased liability to ketoacidosis during CSII by comparison with conventional therapy may be due to the low levels of FIRI prevailing in the blood during the basal infusion of insulin, after clearance of premeal supplementary doses of the hormone.

Adverse effects related to the subcutaneous catheter and the delivery system

While local infection as a result of injections in the course of conventional therapy is exceedingly rare, it has become apparent that reactions at the infusion site are relatively common during CSII (42). The frequency of localized infections is greater than with depot injection therapy. It may be related to a more obvious degree to the hygienic and antiseptic precautions taken by the patient, to the frequency of changing of infusion sites, and to the speed of response of the patient to such adverse reactions.

The hazards and adverse reactions discussed above are predictable risks of CSII. Although this technique makes use of a well-proven therapeutic agent delivered in conventional vehicles by standard dosage and route, it is clear that the possibility exists of unexpected and specific hazards. These may be related to the properties of insulin under the conditions of its use in CSII (43), to chemical contamination of the infusate as result of prolonged exposure to the materials of the system (44), or to unknown causes.

Risk of amyloidosis during long-term continuous insulin infusion therapy

It has been suggested as a result of observations in animals (45) and in patients with diabetes mellitus that long-term parenteral delivery of insulin, particularly by continuous subcutaneous infusion, is associated with a risk of development of systemic amyloidosis (46). However, the suggestion that increased levels of amyloid-related proteins are present in the blood of patients receiving long-term infusion therapy with insulin has not been confirmed (47), and it remains to be established whether there is a significant difference in this respect between conventional and open-loop infusion treatments.

Incidence of hypoglycemia during open-loop insulin therapy

Uncontrolled clinical experience with CSII suggested that the risk of hypoglycemia, in spite of near-normalization of the blood glucose in many subjects, is not greater than with subcutaneous depot therapy (1, 2, 8). The controlled multi-center comparisons have demonstrated that the rate of occurrence of chemical hypoglycemia (blood glucose < 50 mg/dl, 2.8 mmol/l) is probably greater during CSII than during conventional therapy, but that episodes of severe symptomatic hypoglycemia are not more frequent during CSII (6).

Mortality associated with CSII

Documentation of the mortality of subjects undergoing CSII in management of diabetes mellitus has recently been attempted (48). Ascertainment of the use of the technique in subjects with diabetes at large in the United States was attempted by the Center for Disease Control, with analysis of the circumstances of deaths occurring among patients using insulin pumps. The denominator was arrived at by collecting information concerning the number of insulin pumps supplied to the community with diabetes, with attempts to verify the use of the instruments. This material documents the use of CSII by several thousand subjects with diabetes, through experience representing many thousand patient-years of treatment. Analysis suggested that there is no excess of deaths among these subjects above that to be expected when account is taken of the demography and clinical histories of the group. At the same time this study led to documentation of a number of instances of treatment-related deaths. These include death attributable to septicemia consequent on infection at the infusion site, death due to the development of ketoacidosis, and death probably due to hypoglycemia with or without disordered function of the instrument. It is evident that controlled comparisons of the rates of occurrence of major adverse effects and the mortality associated with conventional therapy and CSII are virtually impossible, but it may be said that this cumulative experience has revealed no important deterrent to the application of the technique of CSII in management of diabetes under appropriate experimental or clinical conditions.

EFFECTS OF IMPROVED GLYCEMIC CONTROL ON COMPLICATIONS OF DIABETES MELLITUS

Uncontrolled studies of the complications of diabetes during open-loop insulin therapy

In the course of studies of the feasibility, safety and effectiveness of CSII in control of glycemia in IDDM, initial experience in subjects who exhibited the complications of diabetes mellitus encouraged the hope that these treatment regimens might reverse the complications. However, subsequently more substantial though uncontrolled observations have shown that the degree of metabolic control attainable with CSII is clearly not associated with systematic reversal or arrest of the established microvascular complications of diabetes (40, 50). The question whether these complications can be prevented or their progression inhibited can therefore be addressed only in controlled studies.

Controlled studies of the complications of diabetes during open-loop insulin therapy

Experience with CSII as the most widely tested of the open-loop techniques has led the proponents to suggest that this method is capable of application in large-scale trials of the effects of metabolic control on the complications of diabetes. The controlled trials carried out by the Steno Hospital group (5) and the KROC Collaborative Study Group (6) were expressly developed to test the feasibility of this approach and have yielded valuable preliminary findings.

Effects of CSII on diabetic retinopathy

The subjects recruited to the Steno Hospital Study (5) and the KROC Collaborative Study (6) exhibited background retinopathy, with a range of severity from very mild to less-than that defined as 'high-risk' or preproliferative retinopathy. In the Steno Hospital Study the assessment of retinopathy was based on serial fundus photographs, which were assessed in a blinded fashion by expert participants in the study. The overall conclusion from comparisons of the two treatment groups at one year into the study showed that there was a slight but significantly greater progression of retinopathy in the CSII-treated group. The difference between the two treatment groups was largely attributable to a greater rate of development of nerve fiber layer infarcts (cotton-wool spots) in the CSII-treated group. The preliminary report from the Steno Hospital Group describing analysis of fundus photographs at two years, with continuation of the patients in their original treatment groups, suggests that the difference between the two groups is not maintained, though overall the progression of retinopathy continued (22). In the study of the KROC Collaborative Group, the assessment of retinopathy was based on stereo-color fundus photographs taken at entry and after eight months of treatment, with 'blinded' assessment conducted independently at the Wisconsin Center. The techniques used were established through experience with the photographs obtained in the diabetic retinopathy studies carried out in the United States (51, 52). These assessments again documented objective evidence of systematic progression of retinopathy through the eight month study period in both treatment groups (Fig. 4). As in the Steno Hospital Study, the progression of retinopathy was marginally greater in the CSII treatment group, and this difference was again largely attributable to increased numbers of nerve-fiber-layer infarcts.

It is important to point out that the differences between the treatment groups in both studies were not great and were not associated with effects on visual acuity. The import of the apparently greater progression of retinopathy in the intensively treated groups in relation to the longer-term prognosis for the eyes is uncertain, and it remains possible that the differences represent chance fluctuations in the progression of retinopathy. However, these controlled studies confirm the clinical experience that the degree of metabolic control attainable with CSII is not associated with arrest or retarded progression of established background retinopathy in IDDM within one year of such treatment, and even that relative worsening may occur in the intensively treated group. These results cannot be taken to exclude possible longer-term beneficial effects of intensive treatment on the progression of retinopathy. Without speculation regarding the possible mechanisms, it is clear that there may be a momentum in established background retinopathy, so that progression might continue for an undetermined period of time, irrespective of possible subsequent effects of improvement in glycemic control. These findings have to be reconciled with long-term prospective studies suggesting that relatively poor control of glycemia is associated with earlier development and more rapid progression of diabetic retinopathy (53). In this context it is of interest to note that analysis of the results of the Steno Group's Study in terms of the relation-

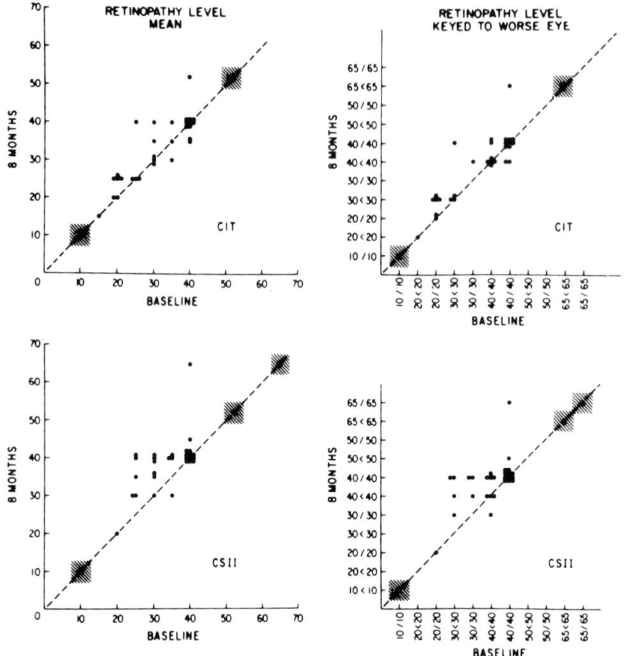

FIG. 4. *Retinopathy levels at base line and at 8 months in subjects undergoing conventional therapy (CIT) and CSII in the KROC Study Group Trial. Values falling on the broken identity line indicate no change, those falling to the left of the line indicate deterioration, and those falling to the right indicate improvement. Values obtained by both methods used to assess the retinopathy level (mean level and the system keyed to the worse eye) are shown for comparison. Note that units of severity are arbitrary and that intervals with the same numerical value may represent different degrees of clinical change. Retinopathy levels in patients initially selected for the trial but not meeting the eligibility criteria with respect to retinopathy are denoted by the shaded areas. Reproduced from KROC Study Group (6), by courtesy of the Editors of the New England Journal of Medicine.*

ship of glycemic control to progression of retinopathy irrespective of the mode of therapy showed a correlation between superior control of metabolism and relative worsening of retinopathy. This apparent difference between the relationship of glycemic control and retinopathy in long-term diabetes, and in studies of short-term improvement of glycemic control, supports speculation that this feature of the response to initiation of CSII may constitute a transient effect.

These results of the Steno and KROC Groups' studies are also apparently at variance with those earlier reported from France, based on observations of the effects of improved metabolic control achieved by means of multiple injection regimens in a comparison of such treatment with continued conventional treatment in IDDM (54). These studies suggested that intensified conventional treatment with multiple injection therapy (MIT) results in a reduced rate of development of microaneurysms. However, the study with MIT in France and the studies with CSII of the Steno Hospital and KROC Collaborative Groups are not comparable, since the demonstrated difference in glycemic control between the conventionally treated groups and the intensified forms of therapy in the two more recent studies was substantially greater than that achieved in the French study, and because the techniques of assessment of retinopathy were quite different in the French study and in the studies with CSII. The significance of the assessment of retinopathy in terms of microaneurysm counts with respect to progression towards functional impairment of vision remains uncertain. The same is also true of the assessments employed in the Steno and KROC studies. These problems, and the fact that to date no objective methods for assessment of the results of fluorescence angiography or vitreous fluorophotometry have been agreed, limit the present usefulness of the fluorescence dye techniques. However, since these methods provide permanent records which can be related to visual acuity, it is suggested that such studies can be conducted concurrently with development of methods for improving their interpretation and relating the results to clinical retinopathy.

Controlled studies of effects of CSII on diabetic nephropathy

In the KROC Collaborative Study the degree of proteinuria permissible in subjects entering the program was somewhat lower than that in the Steno Study. The progression of nephropathy in the KROC Collaborative Study was assessed in terms of albumin excretion rates (AER). Comparable numbers of subjects in the two treatment groups exhibited pathologic degrees of AER, and it was found that the subjects with pathologic elevation of AER in the CSII-treated group showed significant reduction of the AER, whereas this did not occur in the conventionally treated group of subjects (Fig. 5). Those subjects in both groups with normal AER at entry showed no significant deterioration through the period of study. These findings encourage the belief that intensified insulin therapy with the attainable improvement in glycemic control can lead to longer-term improvement on albuminuria, as suggested by the effects of short-term CSII (55).

Other evidence of effects of open-loop insulin therapy on complications of IDDM

The effects of the improvement of glycemic control attainable with CSII on functional derangements of the eyes and nerves, as well as of the kidneys as described, have been examined. These have included studies with electroretinography, nyctometry, and posterior vitreous fluorophotometry,

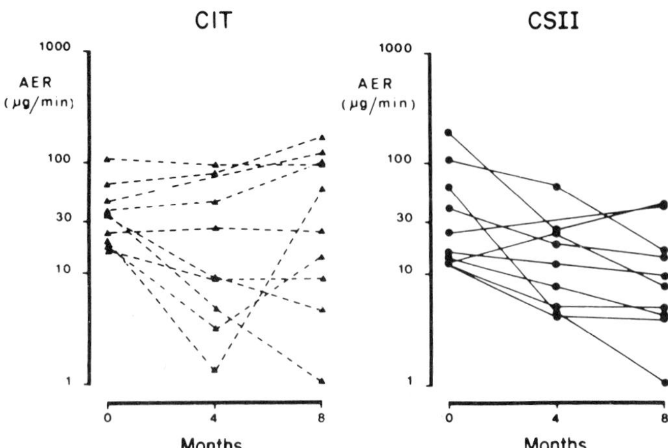

FIG. 5. *Changes in albumin excretion rates in subjects with supranormal baseline values (12 μg/min) receiving conventional insulin therapy (CIT) or CSII for eight months during the KROC Study Group Trial (n = 10 in each group). AER = albumin excretion rate; CIT = conventional injection treatment; CSII = continuous subcutaneous insulin infusion. Reproduced from KROC Study Group (6), by courtesy of the New England Journal of Medicine.*

while studies of nerve conduction, and assessments of proteinuria, during CSII have been reported (5, 6, 56). The implications of these findings for progression of clinical retinopathy, nephropathy and neuropathy, remain uncertain but the responses can clearly be interpreted as beneficial. In terms of biochemical risk factors for the complications of diabetes, in addition to the potential for correction of hyperlipidemia described above, it has been shown that abnormalities characteristic of platelet function in IDDM are not reproducible during long-term CSII (57). In terms of histopathological findings associated with long-term diabetes mellitus, studies of capillary basement membrane thickness have suggested that the increases documented in long-term diabetes under conventional therapy are reduced in the course of treatment by CSII (58). While these several indices of adverse effects of diabetes in different organ systems encourage the expectation of benefit from improvement in control of metabolism, their relationship to the clinical expression of the long-term complications of the disease remains uncertain.

The apparent failure of counter-regulatory responses to hypoglycemia in long-term IDDM must be regarded as a complication of the disease. In the case of the demonstrable disorder of glucagon secretion the possible relationships to insulin deficiency or neuropathy are obscure. The possible prevention or amelioration of this defect by means of long-term open-loop insulin infusion therapy has yet to be excluded (59).

CONCLUSIONS

The results of short-term controlled studies show that open-loop CSII is capable of superior metabolic control by comparison with once- or twice-daily injection therapy as employed under conventional conditions. These trials have also demonstrated that established diabetic retinopathy progresses through periods of treatment up to two years in duration with CSII. While this preliminary evidence also indicates a trend towards relative worsening of retinopathy through the course of 8–12 months of CSII, by comparison with conventional therapy, consideration of the available evidence suggests that this trend may represent a transient difference of response. At the same time the improvement of results of functional tests applied to the eyes and kidneys supports the notion that longer-term benefits through amelioration of the clinical expression of the complications of the disease may accrue. The metabolic effects observed with alternative routes of open-loop delivery of insulin, particularly the intravenous route and the intraperitoneal route, appear to be comparable with those attainable with CSII. It may be concluded that open-loop CSII represents a therapeutic option capable of improving control of metabolism in IDDM, by comparison with conventional depot injection therapy. It is not inconsistent to argue also that it is more than ever important to undertake controlled studies of the effects of available intensive insulin replacement treatment on the complications of diabetes. It now appears that such studies are feasible, that the comparative treatment regimens are acceptable under clinical conditions, and that the available techniques for assessment of retinopathy, nephropathy and neuropathy, while needing further development and refinement, are capable of application to these problems.

References

1. Pickup JC, Keen H, Parsons JA, Alberti KGMM (1978): Continuous subcutaneous insulin infusion: an approach to achieving normoglycemia. *Br. Med. J.*, *1*, 204.
2. Tamborlane WV, Sherwin RS, Genel M, Felig P. (1979): Administration of insulin to juvenile diabetics via portable pump. *N. Engl. J. Med.*, *300*, 573.
3. Champion MC, Shepherd GAA, Rodger NW, Dupré J (1980): Continuous subcutaneous infusion of insulin in the management of diabetes mellitus. *Diabetes*, *29*, 212.
4. Mecklenberg R, Benson J, Becker N, Brazel P, Fredlund P, Metz R, Nielsen R, Sannar C, Steenrod W (1982): Clinical use of the insulin infusion pump in 100 patients with Type I diabetes. *N. Engl. J. Med.,*, *307*, 513.
5. Lauritzen T, Larsen HW, Frost-Larsen K, Deckert T and The Steno Study Group (1983): Effect of 1 year of near-normal blood glucose levels on retinopathy in insulin-dependent diabetics. *Lancet*, *1*, 200.

6. The KROC Study Group (1984): Blood Glucose Control and the Evolution of Diabetic Retinopathy and Albuminuria. *N. Engl. J. Med.*, *311*, 365.
7. Dupré J, Champion M, Rodger NW (1983): Continuous infusion of insulin in diabetes mellitus: metabolic aims and effects in long-term studies of intensive insulin regimens. In: *Diabetes 1982*, pp 303–314. Editor: E.N. Mngola. Excerpta Medica, Amsterdam.
8. Dupré J, Champion MC, Rodger NW (1982): Replacement treatment with insulin in diabetes mellitus: problems and promise. *Clin. Invest. Med.*, *5*, 109.
9. Clarke W, Haymond M, Santiago J (1980): Overnight basal insulin requirements in fasting insulin-dependent diabetics. *Diabetes*, *29*, 78.
10. Service F, Rozza R, Westland R, Hall L, Nelson R, Haymond M, Clemens A, Gerich J (1980): Considerations for the programming of an open-loop insulin infusion device from the Biostator glucose controller. *Diabetes Care*, *3*, 278.
11. Skor DA, White NH, Thomas L, Shaw SD, Cryer PE, Santiago JV (1983): Examination of the role of the pituitary-adrenocortical axis, counterregulatory hormones, and insulin clearance in variable nocturnal insulin requirements in insulin-dependent diabetics. *Diabetes*, *32*, 403.
12. Skor DA, White NH, Thomas L, Santiago JV (1984): Relative roles of insulin clearance and insulin sensitivity in the prebreakfast increase in insulin requirements in insulin-dependent diabetic patients. *Diabetes*, *33*, 60.
13. Kerner W, Navascues I, Torres AA, Pfeiffer EF (1984): Studies on the pathogenesis of the dawn phenomenon in insulin-dependent diabetic patients. *Metabolism*, *33*, 458.
14. Duncan JA, Malone JI (1984): Continuous basal insulin infusion: an effective means to achieve good glycemic control without premeal boluses. *Diabetes Care*, *7*, 114.
15. Levy-Marchal C, Albisser AM, Zinman B (1983): Overnight metabolic control with pulsed intermittent versus continuous subcutaneous insulin infusion. *Diabetes Care*, *6*, 356.
16. Murray FT, Zinman B, McClean PA, Denoga A, Albisser AM, Leibel BS, Nakhooda AF, Stokes EF, Marliss EB (1977): The metabolic response to moderate exercise in diabetic man receiving intravenous and subcutaneous insulin. *J. Clin. Endocrinol. Metab.*, *44*, 708.
17. Dupré J, Radziuk JM, Rodger NW, Champion M (1981): Glucose turnover in insulin-dependent diabetes mellitus (IDDM) treated by continuous subcutaneous infusion of insulin (CSII): effect of exercise or interruption of treatment. *Diabetes*, *30*, 15A.
18. Zinman B, Marliss EB, Hanna AK, Minuk HL, Vranic M (1982): Exercise in diabetic man: glucose turnover and free insulin responses after glycemic normalization with intravenous insulin. *Can. J. Physiol. Pharmacol.*, *60*, 1236.
19. Koivisto VA, Tronier B (1983): Postprandial blood glucose response to exercise in Type 1 diabetes: comparison between pump and injection therapy. *Diabetes Care*, *6*, 436.
20. Nelson JD, Poussier P, Marliss EB, Albisser AM, Zinman B (1982): Metabolic response of normal man and insulin-infused diabetics to postprandial exercise. *Am. J. Physiol.*, *5*, E309.

21. Poussier P, Zinman B, Marliss EB, Albisser AM, Perlman K, Caron D (1983): Open-loop intravenous insulin waveforms for postprandial exercise in Type I diabetes. *Diabetes Care*, *6*, 129.
22. Lauritzen T, Frost-Larsen K, Larsen H-W et al (1983): Continuous subcutaneous insulin. *Lancet*, *1*, 1445.
23. Pickup JC, Keen H, Parsons JA, Alberti KGMM, Rowe AS (1979): Continuous subcutaneous insulin infusion: improved blood-glucose and intermediary-metabolite control in diabetics. *Lancet*, *1*, 1255.
24. Tamborlane WV, Sherwin RS, Genel M, Felig P (1979): Restoration of normal lipid and aminoacid metabolism in diabetic patients treated with a portable insulin-infusion pump. *Lancet*, *1*, 1258.
25. Pietri AO, Dunn FL, Grundy SM, Raskin P (1983): The effect of continuous subcutaneous insulin infusion on very-low-density lipoprotein triglyceride metabolism in Type I diabetes mellitus. *Diabetes*, *32*, 75.
26. Champion M, Shepherd G, Rodger NW, Dupré J (1980): The management of NIDDM by continuous subcutaneous insulin infusion. *Diabetes*, *29*, 29.
27. Rodger NW, Dupré J (1983): Comparison of metabolic effects of continuous subcutaneous insulin infusion (CSII) and itensified conventional insulin therapy (ICIT) in diabetes mellitus (DM): a crossover study. *Clin. Res.*, *32*, 407A.
28. Reeves ML, Seigler DE, Ryan EA, Skyler JS (1982): Glycemic control in insulin-dependent diabetes mellitus. *Amer. J. Med.*, *72*, 673.
29. Schiffrin AD, Desrosiers M, Aleyassine H, Belmonte MM (1984): Intensified insulin therapy in the Type I diabetic adolescent: a controlled trial. *Diabetes Care*, *7*, 107.
30. Irsigler K, Kritz H (1979): Long-term continuous intravenous insulin therapy with a portable insulin dosage-regulating apparatus. *Diabetes*, *28*, 196.
31. Irsigler K, Kritz H, Hagmuller G, Franetzki M, Prestele K, Thurow H, Geisen K (1981): Long-term continuous intraperitoneal insulin infusion with an implanted remote-controlled insulin infusion device. *Diabetes*, *30*, 1072.
32. Schade D, Eaton R, Spencer W, Goldman R, Corbett W (1979): The peritoneal absorption of insulin in diabetic man: A potential site for a mechanical insulin delivery system. *Clin. Exp. Metab.*, *28*, 195.
33. Walter H, Bachmann W, Mehnert H (1984): Continuous intraperitoneal (ip) insulin infusion (CIPII) in Type I diabetics: kinetics of insulin and comparison with intravenous (iv) infusion. *Diabetes*, *33*, 22A.
34. Pickup JC, Home PD, Bilous RW, Alberti KGMM, Keen H (1981): Management of severely brittle diabete by continuous subcutaneous and intramuscular insulin infusion: evidence for a defect in subcutaneous insulin absorption. *Br. Med. J.*, *282*, 347.
35. Home PD, Massi-Benedetti M, Gill GV, Capaldo B, Shepherd GAA, Alberti KGMM (1982): Impaired subcutaneous absorption of insulin in 'brittle' diabetics. *Acta Endocrinol. (Copenhagen)*, *101*, 414.
36. Buysschaert M, Marchand E, Ketelslegers JM, Lambert AE (1983): Comparison of plasma glucose and plasma free insulin during CSII and intensified conventional insulin therapy. *Diabetes Care*, *6*, 1.
37. Horwitz D, Zeidler A, Gonen B, Jaspan J (1980): Hyperinsulinism complicating control of diabetes mellitus by an artificial beta-cell. *Diabetes Care*, *3*, 274.

38. Behme MT, Dupré J (1984): Insulin-binding to erythrocytes in Type I diabetes mellitus: effects of continuous subcutaneous infusion of insulin. *Clin. Invest. Med.*, *7*, 109.
39. Pickup JC, Viberti GC, Bilous RW, Keen H, Alberti KGMM, Home PD, Binder C (1982): Safety of continuous subcutaneous insulin infusion: metabolic deterioration and glycaemic autoregulation after deliberate cessation of infusion. *Diabetologia*, *22*, 175.
40. Scheen AJ, Krzentowski G, Castillo M, Lefebvre PJ, Luyckx AS (1983): 1. A 6-hour nocturnal interruption of a continuous subcutaneous insulin infusion: 2. Marked attenuation of the metabolic deterioration by somatostatin. *Diabetologia*, *24*, 319.
41. Peden NR, Braaten JT, McKendry JBR (1984): Diabetic ketoacidosis during long-term treatment with continuous subcutaneous insulin infusion. *Diabetes Care*, *7*, 1.
42. Raskin P, Pietri AO, Unger R, Shannon WA (1983): The effect of diabetic control on the width of skeletal-muscle capillary basement membrane in patients with Type I diabetes mellitus. *N. Engl. J. Med.*, *309*, 1546.
43. Lougheed WD, Woulfe-Flanagan H, Clement JR, Albisser AM (1980): Insulin aggregation in artificial delivery systems. *Diabetologia*, *19*, 1.
44. Freeman DJ, Wolfe BM, Mascarenhas M (1983): Ketoacidosis resulting from precipitation of insulin in syringe used to delivery of constant subcutaneous insulin infusion. *Lancet*, *1*, 828.
45. Albisser AM, McAdam KPWJ, Perlman K, Carson S, Bahoric A, Wlliamson JR (1983): Unanticipated amyloidosis in dogs infused with insulin. *Diabetes*, *32*, 1092.
46. Brownlee M, Cerami A, Li JJ, Vlassara H, Martin TR, McAdam KPWJ (1984): Association of insulin pump therapy with raised serum amyloid A in Type 1 diabetes mellitus. *Lancet*, *1*, 411.
47. Koivisto VA, Teppo A-M, Maury CPJ, Taskinen M-R (1983): No evidence of amyloidoses in Type I diabetics treated with continuous subcutaneous insulin infusion. *Diabetes*, *32*, 88.
48. Teutsch SM, Herman WH, Dwyer DM, Lane JM (1984): Mortality among diabetic patients using continuous subcutaneous insulin-infusion pumps. *N. Engl. J. Med.*, *310*, 361.
49. Puklin JE, Tamborlane WV, Felig P, Genel M, Sherwin RS (1982): Influence of long-term insulin infusion pump treatment of Type I diabetes on diabetic retinopathy. *Ophthalmology*, *89*, 735.
50. Lawson PM, Champion MC, Canny C, Kingsley R, White MC, Dupré J, Kohner EM (1982): Continuous subcutaneous insulin infusion (CSII) does not prevent progression of proliferative and preproliferative retinopathy. *Br. J. Ophthalmol.*, *66*, 762.
51. Public Health Service (1980): *Early Treatment Diabetic Retinopathy Study: Manual of Operations*. Public Health Service, Bethesda, MD.
52. Klein BEK, Davis MD, Segal P, Long J, Harris A, Haug H, Magli Y, Syrjala S (1984): Diabetic retinopathy: assessment of severity and progression. *Ophthalmology*, *91*, 10.
53. Pirart J (1978): Diabetes mellitus and its degenerative complications: a prospective study of 4,400 patients observed between 1947 and 1973. *Diabetes Care*, *1*, 168.

54. Tchobroutsky G (1978): Relation of diabetic control to development of microvascular complications. *Diabetologia*, *15*, 143.
55. Viberti GC, Pickup JC, Jarrett RJ, Keen H (1979): Effect of control of blood glucose on urinary excretion of albumin and β:microglobulin in insulin-dependent diabetes. *N. Engl. J. Med.*, *300*, 638.
56. Boulton AJM, Drury J, Clarke B, Ward J (1982): Continuous subcutaneous insulin infusion in the management of painful diabetic neuropathy. *Diabetes Care*, *5*, 386.
57. McDonald JWD, Dupré J, Rodger NW, Champion MC, Webb CD, Ali M (1982): Comparison of platelet thromboxane synthesis in diabetic patients on conventional insulin therapy and continuous insulin infusions. *Thromb. Res.*, *28*, 705.
58. Raskin P, Pietri AO, Unger R, Shannon WA Jr (1983): The effect of diabetic control on the width of skeletal-muscle capillary basement membrane in patients with Type I diabetes mellitus. *N. Engl. J. Med.*, *309*, 1546.
59. Bolli G, De Feo P, De Cosmo S, Perriello G, Angeletti G, Ventura MR, Santeusanio F, Brunetti P, Gerich JE (1984): Effects of long-term optimization and short-term deterioration of glycemic control on glucose counterregulation in Type I diabetes mellitus. *Diabetes*, *33*, 394.

The Diabetes Annual/1
K.G.M.M. Alberti and L.P. Krall, editors

ISBN 0444 90 343 7
$0.85 per article per page (transactional system)
$0.20 per article per page (licensing system)

9 Implanted devices and the artificial pancreas

DAVID S. SCHADE AND R. PHILIP EATON

The development of artificial organs has been made possible by major advances in electronic technology and biocompatible materials during the last two decades. Although the external artificial kidney (hemodialysis) has received the most attention in prolonging the lives of patients with chronic renal disease, a multitude of prosthetic devices are now available for implantation. These devices range from the sophisticated electronic circuitry of pacemakers with defibrillation capability to the non-electrical prosthetic heart valves and artificial joints. Thus, it is inevitable that researchers in the area of diabetes have been examining the feasibility of an artificial pancreas (or more accurately, an artificial pancreatic islet B-cell). A functional definition of an artificial pancreas is an implanted device which releases insulin in response to an elevation in blood glucose concentration. It should be emphasized that this is a simplistic approach, since the normal pancreas (or more specifically, the B-cells of the islets of Langerhans) responds by altering the secretion of insulin after exposure to many stimuli, including amino acids, fatty acids and ketone bodies, and other hormones such as glucagon, somatostatin, and even insulin itself. However, because of the complexity of the B-cell and the rudimentary state of the development of an artificial pancreas, to date glucose has been chosen by all investigators to be the determinant of insulin release. The reason fot this choice is threefold. First, much evidence in animals and man implicates glucose as a causative factor for diabetic microangiopathy; second, glucose, in most physiological situations, is the major stimulus for endogenous insulin secretion; and third, the extremes of glucose concentration (hyperglycemia and hypoglycemia) can have rapid adverse effects in man and must be avoided.

This review will focus on implantation devices (or potentially implantable devices) which release insulin in response to a rise in blood glucose concentration. For the devices with mechanical pumping action, feedback as to the concurrent blood glucose level must be provided by the patient, utilizing home blood glucose monitoring described elsewhere in this volume (Chap-

This investigation was supported by NIH Grant No. 1 RO1 AM31973, The Clinical Research Center Program Grant No. RR-99, The Biomedical Research Support Grant No. 2 SO7 RR05583, and The Shiley Corporation.

ter 10). In contrast, other devices which release insulin non-mechanically may be designed to respond to endogenous glucose levels without the need for external control.

Non-electrical implanted pumps

The first category of artificial pancreata is the liquid-to-gas-driven non-electrical implantable pump manufactured by the Infusaid Corporation, Norwood, Mass. (Fig. 1) which has been implanted by several investigators

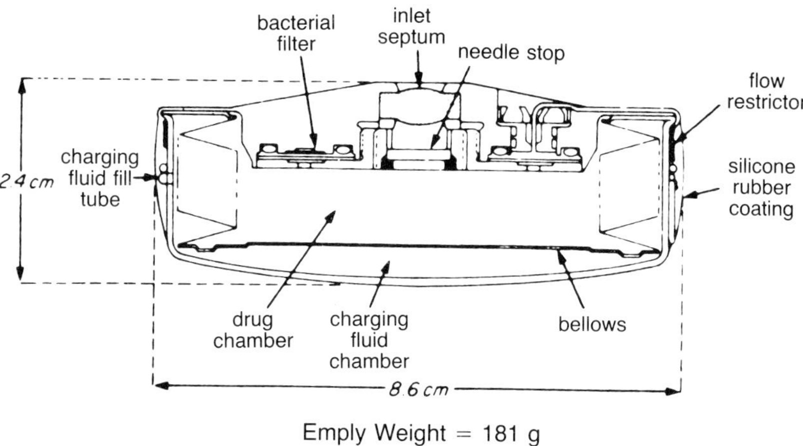

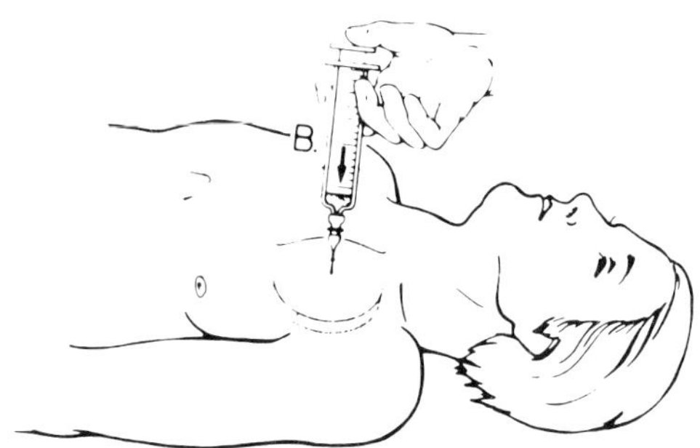

FIG. 1. *The components of the Infusaid pump. Implanted subcutaneously in the chest, the pump is 'charged' by fluid pressure from the refill syringe into the drug chamber. Its construction does not permit a change in basal rate or meal dose once the insulin concentration has been chosen. Reproduced from Schade et al. (5), by courtesy of the publisher.*

(1–3). This ingenious device utilizes the pressure necessary to refill the insulin pump's internal reservoir to subsequently pump the insulin into the patient. The major advantage of this approach is that no batteries (or non-renewable power source) are required, and thus a long pump lifespan is anticipated. The first Infusaid pump was implanted in September, 1980 by Buchwald and colleagues (1), with many thereafter. This pump has advantages and disadvantages, and its ultimate place in the therapy of diabetic patients has not yet been defined. The major advantages include a relatively low cost (comparable to some of the new external insulin pumps) and a potentially long lifespan. Major drawbacks include the difficulty of refilling the device (it cannot be done easily by the patient, unlike the implantable electromechanical pumps), the positive pressure in the reservoir which, in case of a mechanical rupture of the reservoir, could release large amounts of insulin into the patient, and the difficulty of changing the amount of insulin delivered to the patient (usually done by changing the concentration of insulin in the reservoir). Minor problems include changes in the flow rate of insulin when the patient's body temperature increases, as with a febrile episode, and during changes in altitude, as might be experienced during air travel.

Long-term clinical experience (mean of 7.0 months) with this pump was first reported in five Type 2 (NIDDM) diabetic patients (3). Although this report was encouraging in that glucose control improved in all patients, it must be emphasized that there was no randomized control group, nor were other modalities of treatment utilized as comparisons, such as oral hypoglycemic agents or optimized insulin therapy. Thus, as the authors point out, this report should be considered a feasibility study in which the implantation and delivery of insulin from the implanted pump was shown not only to be possible, but to result in good glucose control. However, conclusions should not be made relative to the usefulness of this approach compared with other, less expensive and less invasive, treatments for Type 2 diabetes, such as oral antidiabetic agents or optimized insulin therapy. More recently, this pump has been implanted into Type 1 (insulin-dependent) diabetic patients (4). Since this pump cannot currently be used to deliver a meal bolus of insulin, although a mechanical–magnetic switch which will allow this option is under development, Type 1 diabetic patients must still take injections of regular insulin before meals (usually before breakfast and supper). In this report, 4 Type 1 diabetic patients and 1 pancreatectomized patient were studied over a cumulative time period of 530 patient days. All patients had been trained with external pumps to simulate insulin delivery rates of the implanted pump. The data from this study would suggest that all modes of pump therapy (external or internal) were superior to two daily doses of mixed short and long-acting insulin, but the number of patients (five) is too small to conclude that the implanted pump with external injections of regular insulin is superior to an external pump alone. It should be emphasized that other investigators have not observed the superiority of an insulin pump to multiple daily injections of insulin when comparable insulin delivery algorithms are utilized and when home blood glucose monitoring is done four times per day (5). Enthusiasm for this approach has been stated, but again appropriate control groups are not available to assess its benefits versus risks in the care of Type 1 diabetic patients. Since these pumps cannot be 'turned off' by the patient, the danger of continuous insulin delivery during hypoglycemia is real, although not yet reported. Since the basal rate of insulin needed to control glycemia changes throughout the day and night (6), the single continuous basal rate delivered by the Infusaid pump cannot make fine adjustments in glucose control. The importance of these adjustments is not yet resolved in attaining improved glucose control in Type 1 diabetic patients.

Programmable electro-mechanical pump

The second category of devices developed to serve as an artificial pancreas are the remotely programmable electro-mechanical pumps. A component diagnostic prototype of this device, which has been implanted intro three insulin-dependent diabetic patients, is shown in Fig. 2 (7–9). At least three other prototypes are also being developed, including a device manufactured by the Siemens Company in Europe (10), Medtronics, Inc. (11), and Johns Hopkins University Applied Physics Laboratory (APL) in the United States (12). Of these latter devices, only the Siemens pump has been implanted into human diabetics to pump insulin, whereas the Medtronics pump has been utilized to deliver morphine for chronic pain. The APL device has not been tested in man but has been implanted into diabetic animals. Although each of these devices has several unique characteristics, they all consist of four basic parts: (1) an external remote programmer to control the implanted pumping unit; (2) a pump to regulate the flow of insulin from an internal reservoir into the patient; (3) batteries and electronics to control the pump and interact with the remote programmer; and (4) an internal reservoir to store the insulin prior to delivering it to the patient. Details of the individual characteristics of these pumps are given in the cited references.

The first implantation of a remotely programmable insulin pump took place in January, 1981, with additional implantations by other investigators soon after (8, 13–15). Although these initial reports were enthusiastic, it should be stressed that they all consisted of patient case reports without paired patient control groups (the patient usually served as his own control), and that they all covered only limited periods of time (months). Electromechanical problems were experienced by all investigators in that the pumps frequently required re-implantation of the insulin delivery catheter or reservoir revision (13, 14). The longest experience has been reported in a patient who received insulin for 12 months continuously (16). In this study, glucose control was similar to that achieved with an external pumping device, but the lifestyle of the patient, including lack of hypoglycemia, was improved. Much additional experience will be required before the benefits and risks of these devices are known with any degree of certainty.

Miniaturized glucose sensor

The availability of a miniaturized glucose sensor would be a great asset to the electromechanical implanted pumps. Many investigative groups are developing such a sensor, the most popular approach being immobilized glu-

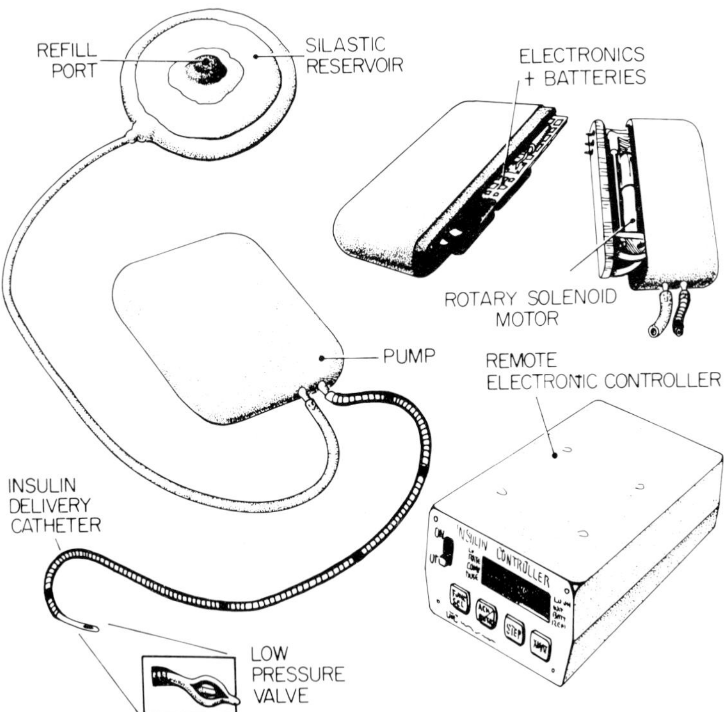

FIG. 2. Component parts of an implantable, remotely programmable insulin delivery system. The key features are a stepping motor that provides safety from pump runaway and extensive programming capability with multiple safety features. The entire unit is remotely controlled by an external portable controller that interacts with the implanted pump. The insulin is delivered from a refillable reservoir, through an insulin delivery catheter, into either the intraperitoneal space or the central venous circulation (7). Reproduced from Schade et al. (7), by courtesy of the American Diabetes Association, Inc.

cose oxidase on an implantable platinum electrode (17–19). Shichiri and co-workers have demonstrated the feasibility of this approach by attaching an external miniaturized electromechanical pump to an implanted electrode glucose sensor in dogs (20, 21). This technical advance is encouraging, but the major problem of enzyme stability and tissue isolation remains unresolved. Thus, after 4 days, not only does the glucose sensor become unstable, but it may become isolated from the surrounding blood or tissue by platelets or fibroblasts, respectively. This isolation is a major problem in the development of all insulin delivery devices and glucose sensors, and has required frequent replacement of the glucose sensor. Hopefully, more biocompatible materials will become available in the future to negate the isolation of the glucose sensor. Until this problem is resolved, patients will have to perform home blood glucose monitoring to regulate insulin delivery by their implantable pump.

Carrier-bound insulin

The third category of implantable artificial pancreata utilize insulin bound to a 'carrier' which slowly releases the insulin into the patient. One approach is the implantation of *insulin bound to albumin*, which slowly releases the hormone (22). This approach could be potentially effective in the Type 2 diabetic patient who has some endogenous insulin. The albumin–insulin bound complex is biodegradable, and has been implanted into diabetic rats. These complexes worked well for one week, with some animals remaining aglycosuric for up to one month. Since the albumin–insulin complex does not 'respond' to changes in blood glucose by releasing more insulin, the future usefulness of this approach in Type 1 diabetic patients remains in doubt. An additional problem is that the release of insulin was not constant, tending to peak at 10 days post-implantation, which has the potential for producing severe hypoglycemia at this time.

A different approach utilizing a reversible insulin binding complex is the use of *concanavalin A* (Fig. 3). These studies, which are still limited to in-vitro experiments, describe a potentially useful approach to an artificial pancreas with no need for a glucose sensor (23). Insulin is first attached chemically to an oligosaccharide, resulting in a glycosylated insulin molecule. In spite of the glycosylation, the insulin still retains full biological potency. The oligosaccharide–insulin complex is then reversibly bound to the glucose-binding lectin concanavalin A, which then serves as an insulin reservoir. Glucose added to the medium displaces the oligosaccharide from the concanavalin A, thereby liberating insulin to act at its target tissue. Although several problems still exist, such as formation of high molecular weight insulin complexes at 37 °C with loss of biological potency, these problems will probably be overcome with changes in the insulin molecule

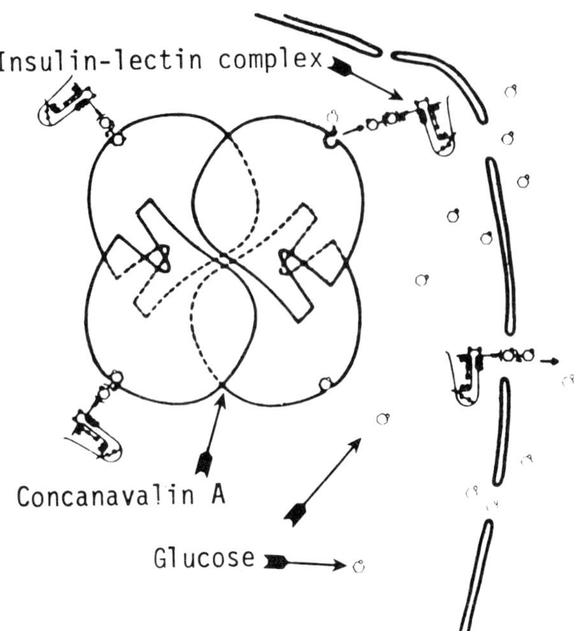

FIG. 3. *Schematic representation of glycosylated insulin bound to concanavalin A. Binding site on lower right subunit of the lectin is shown occupied by a glucose molecule. At the upper right binding site, a glucose molecule is shown displacing a glycosylated insulin molecule. Pores in the membrane of the container would permit bidirectional passage of glucose molecules and displaced oligosaccharide-insulin molecules (modified from Brownlee and Cerami (23)).*

(e.g. sulfation). The major problem will be the same which now faces the development of a glucose sensor – i.e. the implantation of the concanavalin A complex in vivo and preventing isolation by the body of the container holding the concanavalin A, thereby preventing insulin diffusion.

Other devices

A third approach to a non-electrical or non-mechanical artificial pancreas is the use of *osmotic insulin pumps* to deliver insulin (24). However, these pumps do not respond to glucose and they would only provide a 'basal' rate of insulin delivery. They have been implanted into diabetic rats with only short-term success (one week) in maintaining plasma glucose concentration. Although Lopaschuk et al. (24) were not enthusiastic about this approach compared to subcutaneous injection of insulin, theoretically a large osmotic pump might be suitable in specialized short-term applications of insulin delivery.

A fourth approach to a non-mechanical artificial pancreas is the use of *porcine islets of Langerhans held in artificial capillaries*. This device could be anastomosed between an arterio-venous shunt in the arm, thereby providing continuous plasma flow to support the islets and receive the secreted insulin. Although conceptually attractive, this device faces major biocompatibility problems which have not yet been resolved (25).

Conclusions

Three general approaches have been utilized in the development of an artificial pancreas. The first approach employs a fixed infusion of insulin from an implantable pump to supplement the Type 2 diabetic patient's own endogenous insulin or, in the case of Type 1 diabetic patients, to provide a background dose of insulin which is supplemented by external injections of short-acting insulin. The second approach utilizes a remotely controlled implantable insulin pump which is activated by the patient to deliver additional insulin at appropriate times, such as meals or illness. Both of these approaches require the patient to monitor his own blood glucose concentration, since an implantable glucose sensor is still in the developmental stages. A third approach to an artificial pancreas is the development of insulin complexed to a foreign substance which is either degraded *in situ* or which releases insulin in response to elevated glucose concentrations. This latter approach is still in the animal testing stage, whereas the first two approaches have been utilized on an experimental basis in diabetic man.

If one considers the major obstacles that confront the investigators, rapid progress has been made in the development of an artificial pancreas. It is still too early to tell what approach will ultimately succeed or be applicable to the majority of diabetic patients. Most probably, there will be a choice of devices from which the patient can choose one that fits his lifestyle and resources. As present problems are solved, new ones will become apparent. However, it is likely that an artificial pancreas which includes a glucose sensor will become a reality within the next decade.

References

1. Buchwald H, Varco R, Rupp WM, Goldberg FJ, Barbosa J, Rohde TD, Schwartz RA, Rublein T, Blackshear PJ (1981): Treatment of a Type 2 diabetic by a totally implantable insulin device. *Lancet*, *1*, 1233.
2. Kritz H, Hagmuller G, Buchwald H, Denck H, Najemnik C, Irsigler K (1983): Constant basal rate infusion of insulin with an implanted drug infusion device in insulin-dependent maturity-onset diabetics. In: *International Symposium on Artificial Systems for Insulin Delivery*. Editor: P. Brunetti. Raven Press, New York.

3. Rupp WM, Barbosa JJ, Blackshear PJ, McCarthy HB, Rohde TD, Goldenberg FJ, Rublein TG, Dorman FD, Buchwald H (1982): The use of an implantable insulin pump in the treatment of Type II diabetes. *N. Engl. J. Med.*, *307*, 265.
4. Kritz H, Hagmuller G, Lovett R, Irsigler K (1983): Implanted constant basal rate insulin infusion devices for Type I (insulin-dependent) diabetic patients. *Diabetologia*, *25*, 78.
5. Schade DS, Santiago JV, Skyler JS, Rizza RA (1983): In: *Intensive Insulin Therapy*, p 129. Excerpta Medica, New York.
6. Skor DA, White NH, Thomas L, Santiago JV (1984): Relative roles of insulin clearance and insulin sensitivity in the prebreakfast increase in insulin requirements in insulin-dependent diabetic patients. *Diabetes*, *33*, 60.
7. Schade DS, Eaton RP, Carlson GA, Bair RE, Gaona JI Jr, Love JT, Urenda RS, Spencer WJ (1981): Future therapy of the insulin-dependent diabetic patient – the implantable insulin delivery system. *Diabetes Care*, *4*, 319.
8. Schade DS, Eaton RP, Edwards WS, Doberneck RC, Spencer WJ, Carlson GA, Bair RE, Love JT, Urenda RS, Gaona JI Jr (1982): A remotely programmable insulin delivery system. Successful short-term implantation in man. *J. Am. Med. Assoc.*, *247*, 1848.
9. Schade DS, Eaton RP, Spencer W (1981): Implantation of an artificial pancreas. Current perspectives. *J. Am. Med. Assoc.*, *245*, 709.
10. Prestele K, Funke H, Moschl R (1983): Development of remotely controlled implantable devices for programmed insulin infusion. *Life Support Syst.*, *1*, 23.
11. Personal communication, Dr. Kent Van Kampen, Medtronics, Inc., Minneapolis, Minnesota, USA.
12. Fischell RE, Radford WE, Saudek CD (1983): Programmable implantable medication system: application to diabetes. *Med. Electron.*, *Dec.*, 114.
13. Irsigler K, Kritz H (1979): Long-term continuous intravenous insulin therapy with a portable insulin dosage-regulating apparatus. *Diabetes*, *28*, 196.
14. Selam JL, Slingeneyer A, Chaptal PA, Franetzki M, Prestele K, Mirouze J (1982): Total implantation of a remotely controlled insulin minipump in a human insulin-dependent diabetic. *Artif. Organs*, *6*, 315.
15. Walter H, Kemmler W, Kronski D (1982): Treatment of a Type I diabetic patient with an implanted program-controlled insulin infusion device. *Akt. Endokrinol. Stoffw.*, *3*, 48.
16. Schade DS, Eaton RP (1984): Remotely controlled, implantable versus manually controlled, external insulin pump. *West. J. Med.*, *140*, 948–951.
17. Christenssen SE, Schmitz O, Hansen AP, Orskov H (1983): The glucose sensor. Some results and applications. *Acta Med. Scand.*, *213*, *Suppl. 671*, 121.
18. Updike SJ, Shults M, Ekman B (1982): Implanting the glucose enzyme electrode: problems, progress, and alternative solutions. *Diabetes Care*, *5*, 207.
19. Wingard LB Jr (1983): Immobilized enzyme electrodes for glucose determination for the artificial pancreas. *Fed. Proc.*, *42*, 288.
20. Shichiri M, Kawamori R, Goriya Y, Yamasaki Y, Nomura M, Hakui N, Abe H (1983): Glycaemic control in pancreatectomized dogs with a wearable artificial endocrine pancreas. *Diabetologia*, *24*, 179.

21. Shichiri M, Yamasaki Y, Abe H, Kawamori R, Hakui N (1982): Wearable artificial endocrine pancreas with needle-type glucose sensor. *Lancet*, *2*, 1129.
22. Goosen MFA, Leung YF, O'Shea GM, Chou S, Sun AM (1983): Long-acting insulin. Slow release of insulin from a biodegradable matrix implanted in diabetic rats. *Diabetes*, *32*, 478.
23. Brownlee M, Cerami A (1983): Glycosylated insulin complexed to concanavalin A. Biochemical basis for a closed-loop insulin delivery system. *Diabetes*, *32*, 494.
24. Lopaschuk GD, Tahiliani AG, McNeill JH (1983): Continuous long-term insulin delivery in diabetic rats utilizing implanted osmotic minipumps. *J. Pharmacol. Meth.*, *9*, 71.
25. Buchs JB, Von Segesser L (1983): Biotechnical aspects of a new hybrid artificial endocrine pancreas. *Life Support Syst.*, *1*, 189.

The Diabetes Annual/1
K.G.M.M. Alberti and L.P. Krall, editors

ISBN 0444 90 343 7
$0.85 per article per page (transactional system)
$0.20 per article per page (licensing system)

10 Self-monitoring of blood glucose – 1978–1984

R.B. TATTERSALL

Insulin-dependent diabetes (IDDM) is a dynamic disease in which patients have always been given much responsibility for their own treatment and are expected to carry out tasks such as injections and urine testing which traditionally have been the preserve of professionals. Management has changed during the past five years with an increasing emphasis on normoglycemia with new forms of insulin delivery capable of achieving this goal. Many groups using closed- and open-loop infusion devices or multiple subcutaneous injections have reported improved diabetic control. Home blood glucose monitoring (HBGM) has become a *sine qua non* of all these strategies because it is the only way of documenting blood glucose concentrations in the physiological range and also of giving warning of abnormally low levels.

That diabetic patients might be capable of taking a blood sample from themselves several times daily first appeared to be realistic as long ago as 1962 (1) but the additional step of getting them to measure blood glucose as well had to await the development of glucose oxidase based strips and reflectance meters. It was not until 1978 that four groups (2–5) more or less simultaneously reported their experience in teaching insulin-treated diabetics to measure their own blood glucose concentrations with a reflectance meter. The general conclusions of the four studies were that: (1) patients had little difficulty obtaining the blood sample by pricking their fingers; (2) their results were sufficiently accurate for ordinary clinical practice; and (3) self-monitoring of blood glucose levels led to increased motivation and better control in most patients.

Since 1978 there has been an explosion in the use of HBGM, the development of hardware for it and, inevitably, of publications on its use. Several reviews have been published to which the reader is referred for an overview of the subject (6–10).

Does HBGM work?

Many articles on HBGM start with a statement that 'HBGM has made a major contribution to the improved management of the patient with

IDDM' (11) or 'HBGM has been shown to improve blood glucose control in many diabetic subjects which may result in reducing complications of the disease' (12). While it is true that HBGM has improved the quality of life of many patients with insulin-dependent diabetes, it is by no means self-evident that HBGM per se will lead to better blood glucose control although several early studies seemed to support this conclusion. For example, Peterson et al. (13) reported that ten patients had been able to reduce their hemoglobin A1c concentration from a mean of 10.4% to a mean of 5.7% (within the normal range) over five months and had then maintained this level for another four months. All these patients measured blood glucose concentrations six times a day and additionally were switched to four daily insulin injections, given intensive dietary advice and also exposed to unusual enthusiasm and feedback from their doctors. In an uncontrolled trial of this sort, it is impossible to say which factor was the major contributor to improved diabetic control. Surprisingly, only one study, that of Worth et al. (14) has considered the role of HBGM as an independent variable. In their study 46 patients on twice daily mixtures of regular and intermediate acting insulins were enrolled in an experiment which began with a six-month 'optimization period' during which they tested their urine four times daily before meals and were seen every two weeks by one of only two physicians. During this long 'run-in' period control improved from a mean hemoglobin A_1 (HbA_1) level of 11.4% at the beginning to 10.4% after 18 weeks but worsened again to 11% after 24 weeks. HBGM produced no further improvement and another dispiriting observation was that after 18 months the patients on average had reverted to their pre-study mean level of control. An initial improvement followed by reversion to the mean has been a common observation in most long-term (1 or 2 years) studies to evaluate almost any new aspect of the management of insulin-dependent diabetes. This probably demonstrates that most patients could achieve normoglycemia given sufficient motivation and hard work (15). Any new device tends to refocus the patient's attention on management of their diabetes. However, when the interest of the technical novelty wears off with time, control deteriorates unless other measures are taken to bolster motivation. The results of the Worth study (14) have been challenged on a number of grounds:

1. It has been suggested that since the patients were already 'moderately well controlled' any major change was unlikely whatever innovation was tried. In an uncontrolled study, Harrad et al. (16) showed that HBGM 2 to 4 times daily for 18 months together with regular meetings with a diabetes research nurse led to a fall of HbA_1 from 13% to a mean of 9% after 9 months and 8.2% after 18 months. In the first 12 months of this study only 5 of the 28 patients had never achieved a glycosylated hemoglobin of 8.5% or less on at least one occasion. Another possible explanation for the difference between the two studies lies in patient selec-

tion. The 46 patients of Worth et al. were unselected volunteers from a total of 154 aged 16 to 60 on the diabetic clinic register whereas Harrad et al. studied only 28 patients with no indication of how they were selected.

2. In the study of Harrad et al. (16) there did not appear to be a tendency to revert back to the previous poor level of control even after 18 months. One possible explanation is that the diabetes research nurse was able to maintain better rapport and motivation in the patients than were the two physicians in the study of Worth et al. That this might be the case is supported by the fact that in the former study, patients were frequently contacted by telephone whereas in the latter they hardly ever telephoned or asked questions between routine visits. In a New Zealand study (17) 39 patients with IDDM were supplied with HBGM equipment but remained under the care of their general practitioner without any advice from medical or nursing diabetes specialists. There was little improvement in control and it was noteworthy that patients saw their doctors only once every 92 days. The importance of patient selection was shown in Holland (18) where in a randomized trial of 87 patients who had failed to respond satisfactorily to a single daily insulin injection, the only ones who benefited from self-monitoring in terms of improved control were cooperative patients prepared, if necessary, to switch to a combination of short- and medium-acting insulins twice daily. The conclusion must be that HBGM is ineffective in improving control unless backed up with education and continuing advice.

3. Patients in the Worth study tested blood glucose only 4 times daily pre-prandially on 2 days each week with a seven-point profile, including one hour post-prandial values, once every 2 weeks. There is evidence that HBGM only leads to improved control when done intensively at least 5 times a day, every day. Schiffrin and Belmonte (19) achieved near-normoglycemia for 6 months in 16 patients with no endogenous insulin secretion. Their patients measured blood glucose 7 times every day but when blood sampling was reduced to twice daily there was a deterioration in control which was rectified when more frequent sampling was resumed. It might be argued that this is an unrealistic frequency of blood sampling for the average patient and that the 16 patients of Schiffrin and Belmonte were probably carefully selected for their enthusiasm and compliance.

One can conclude that HBGM does not necessarily lead to improved diabetic control. However, in almost every study so far reported, even in those in which it did not improve control, most (usually over 80%) of the patients chose blood in preference to urine testing. It may be that urine testing is seen as messy, unhygienic and old-fashioned but furthermore HBGM seems to have considerable advantages in improving the quality of life of the patient with IDDM. Its advantages can be summarized as follows:

a) It is the only logical method of monitoring if the target is to keep blood glucose within the normoglycemic range where, by definition, all values will be below the renal threshold.

b) HBGM is the only method of self-monitoring which can be used to confirm hypoglycemia. In this context one should note that its use before going to bed 'to ensure that blood sugar levels are high enough to make it safe to sleep' is illogical although widely practised as was the habit of having something extra to eat if a pre-bed urine test was sugar-free.

c) Patients who use HBGM often understand diabetes better and are able to take more responsibility for their own management. This educational value is not confined to patients since HBGM has furthered the education of many diabetologists by showing them what actually happens to blood glucose concentrations in their patients' real life. It has led, for example, to the realization that twice daily regimens of Actrapid and Semitard insulin produce undesirable blood glucose fluctuations in most patients. There is a strong impression that most patients who use HBGM end by reducing the proportion of fast acting insulin in their regimen.

d) HBGM has a valuable role in problem solving and it seems likely, (although not proven) that it has greatly reduced the number of hospital days for 'stabilisation'. In one Australian study (20) it was claimed that before the introduction of HBGM, 181 hospital admissions were recorded for 28 patients (2.1 admissions/person/year) for problems related to diabetic control but that with the introduction of HBGM this was reduced to 0.1 admissions/person/year.

Complications of HBGM: potential and actual

Inaccuracy

Many studies have shown that paramedical personnel and patients can measure blood glucose accurately under test conditions with either visually read strips or a meter. However, there is a nagging suspicion in many quarters that 'free range' patients obtain less accurate results or, if the results are accurate, that they are not used appropriately. Published results differ widely.

Schiffrin et al. (21) used Sarstedt tubes to check the result obtained at home by 16 adolescents using either visually read strips (BM 20-800) or a meter (Glucometer). With both methods there was an excellent correlation ($r = 0.96$) with laboratory measurements. The patients' accuracy was as good after 8 months as it had been after 2 months. However, the authors stress that to guarantee good performance the patient must be taught the technique correctly from the outset which in their experience requires several days of individual instruction with frequent follow-ups during the first weeks. Others have found less reassuring results. Fairclough et al. (22) evaluated the performance of 50 insulin-dependent patients using BM 20-800 sticks, Dextrostix-Dextrometer, and Reflotest-Reflomat. With all systems they found patient performance sub-optimal when compared with that of paramedical personnel. With the exception of the Reflomat, a third of determinations differed from the laboratory value by more than 20%. Only 75% of patients could perform accurately with any system and the factors which correlated with inaccuracy were youth, lack of higher education and low socio-economic class. In a New Zealand study (23) 43% of insulin-dependent patients used their meters in an unsatisfactory manner and 15% never wrote down the results. Patients who had used the meters for longest showed a significant trend to more inefficient use of the devices. Nearly half the patients still relied on their doctor for treatment changes, although most attended as infrequently as once every 3 months. The depressing conclusions from this study were that (1) many patients do not use home glucose monitoring devices in a manner likely to allow rational modification of therapy; (2) neither patients nor family physicians react appropriately to high blood glucose values; and (3) chronic use of home monitoring has not resulted in good glycemic control in many patients. In a multi-center study in Germany, Schöffling et al. (24) found an acceptable degree of accuracy in over 1500 samples from 105 patients who estimated their own blood sugar with BM 20-800 sticks and at the same time took a sample for analysis in a clinical laboratory. Below 11 mmol/l the mean difference of the two corresponding values was ± 1 mmol/l while above 11 mmol/l the difference rose to 2.5 mmol/l. Levels obtained by patients were correct in 69% of samples.

Many other conflicting studies could be cited showing that patients either do or do not measure their blood glucose concentrations accurately and do or do not use the results appropriately. There seems no need for further publications of this sort. It has been established beyond peradventure that within certain limits all home blood glucose monitoring systems available on the market are accurate if used properly. Conversely, they can all be inaccurate if used improperly. It is up to each clinic to do an audit of its own patients to make sure that this expensive equipment is being used appropriately and, if it is not, steps should be taken to improve training or ensure that HBGM is only given to appropriate patients. A single training session is likely to be inadequate. Most patients will need their technique checking two or three times at clinic visits. Perhaps patients and staff should be formally evaluated and not allowed to practice 'instant' blood glucose measurement without a certificate of competence?

Meters and sticks are now standard equipment on many hospital wards, both medical and surgical. Our experience suggests that nurses' technique and accuracy are rarely tested and at least one study (25) confirms this. Potential sources of error by nurses or patients are legion and range from contamination of the fingertips by glucose (26) to the more common failures to get a large enough drop of blood, or time accurately. One might think that defective color vision would be a bar to the use of visually read strips but the one study which has investigated this (27) did not find it so. However, there was an association between increasing age and poorer performance with visually read blood glucose strips.

Infection

Apart from some coarsening and loss of sensitivity of the skin of the fingertips, which might matter to a violinist, pricking of the fingertips for HBGM has been remarkably free of complications. However, Ryan et al. (28) have reported severe infection, osteomyelitis and ulceration in the fingers of two patients with renal failure, calcified vessels and hemodialysis shunts.

Psychological complications

It has been suggested that the frequent blood glucose determinations and multiple injections of insulin required to attain near-physiological control would be incompatible with a normal life style and might have adverse psychological effects (29). Patients might become so preoccupied with controlling diabetes that the rest of their life suffered. So far the few relatively short-term studies which have been done do not support this. Dupuis et al. (30) measured depression with the Hamilton rating scale and found a substantial and significant improvement after eight months in ten patients. They suggested that, as they learn to control their illness, patients develop feelings of competence, self-confidence and dependability which overcome the previous persistent sadness and despair. Similar conclusions were reached in two other studies (31, 32).

Special groups, childhood and pregnancy

HBGM in children

When HBGM was first introduced, there was concern among pediatricians that diabetic children would find the problems of finger pricking an additional and unwelcome assault. This apprehension appears to be groundless. When HBGM is presented to children (even those under 10 years old) as 'a new and better way of checking your diabetes', more than two-thirds prefer it to urine testing in the short-term (33–35). It has been reported (35) that, at first, children and adolescents are prepared to test 6 or more times daily although it would be unreasonable to expect such an intense long-term commitment from patients of this age and the chances are that, as with urine testing, compliance will drop with time. What one might expect is shown by a preliminary report from Spencer (36) who taught 10 adolescents to measure blood glucose at home with a meter 5 times a day.

They were encouraged to make changes in their regimen and over 6 months were able to reduce mean HbA_1 from 14.7 to 10.4%. However, during follow-up every 3 months by the same health care team, the frequency of testing was greatly reduced and HbA_1 levels reverted to a mean of 14.8%, the same as at the start of the study. This again emphasises that HBGM is only effective in improving control in the context of a high level of attention and feedback from the health care team.

Nevertheless, HBGM does have distinct advantages over urine testing in the management of childhood diabetes (37, 38):

1. Parents of very young children prefer it to the alternative of wringing out wet diapers to obtain a urine sample. Even if the child is older and toilet trained, it may still be hard to produce a urine specimen on request so that HBGM may be the only way of checking control at strategic times.
2. Up to half of apparent hypoglycemic reactions in children may be faked to obtain sugar, food or attention. Furthermore, it may be impossible to tell whether a child who is screaming and being naughty before lunch is hypoglycemic or just having a temper tantrum. In these situations HBGM is essential for a correct diagnosis.
3. Children may run extremely low blood sugar levels without being symptomatic (39) and these can only be detected by HBGM.
4. Parents of diabetic children are often encouraged to telephone the diabetic team with their problems. These may be impossible to interpret over the phone if only urine testing data are available whereas, if parents have a record of blood sugars, the call may be more constructive. Caution is necessary when advising over the telephone on the management of intercurrent illness using only HBGM since it is possible to be both ketoacidotic and have a relatively normal blood sugar level. Hence, it is probably wise to test the urine for ketones during an intercurrent illness.
5. HBGM gives children and their parents a sense of being in control, which is important in learning to live with a chronic illness (37).

Whatever means of monitoring a child is asked to use, it must be appropriate to its age and level of maturity (40), if it is not then non-compliance is almost inevitable.

Pregnancy

Most units now use only HBGM for monitoring their pregnant patients although its superiority over urine tests has been questioned (41). In a prospective study in which women were randomly allocated, Varner (42) found equally good glycemic control in women who monitored themselves at home with HBGM as in those who came to hospital each week for a profile to be done by the phlebotomist. Where HBGM scores in diabetic pregnancy is in its ability to document control without admitting or bringing patients up to hospital frequently for blood glucose profiles. This has considerable economic benefits. In Varner's study (42) the mean hospital stay for patients practising HBGM averaged only 28 days as compared to 42 days in the conventionally treated group which, after taking into account the capital expense of HBGM, resulted in an average saving of over 5000 dollars per pregnancy. Similar savings have been reported from New Zealand (43) and California (44).

Equipment for HBGM (see also Table 1)

Development in this field is explosive and any review is bound to be out of date before publication. When HBGM was first introduced in 1978, there were two types of glucose oxidase strip both designed to be read with a meter – Dextrostix (Ames) and Reflotest (Boehringer Mannheim). Many comparative studies have been done on these two products. A useful selection of papers was published as a symposium in the May-June 1981 issue of *Diabetes Care*. The main conclusions can be summarized as follows:

1. When used in accordance with the manufacturers' instructions both Dextrostix/Eyetone and Reflotest/Reflomat are sufficiently accurate for ordinary clinical purposes (45–48). Correlations between instant blood glucose measurements with a meter and values obtained with a laboratory blood glucose analyser are excellent and almost always exceed 0.90. Accuracy is best in the 'physiological' range of plasma glucose with greater percentage and absolute deviation when blood glucose exceeds 14 mmol/l (250 mg/dl). This inaccuracy in the high range is of interest to clinical chemists but of no great moment for patients or clinicians.

2. In general, Reflotest is more accurate and precise than Dextrostix because it is read close to 'endpoint' on the color development curve (48). As a result, timing inaccuracies produce a smaller error with Reflotest than Dextrostix. Furthermore, the color developed with Reflotest is more stable and the sticks can still be read accurately after several days if stored in their dry lightproof container (49). This is a cheaper method of checking a patient's accuracy and technique 'in the field' than for example using Sarstedt tubes (50). The developed color of Dextrostix stored at room temperature in desiccated bottles is unstable and fades rapidly in a non-uniform fashion. One rather impractical way of preserving the color of a Dextrostix for up to a week is to store it in a deep freeze (51).

The fact that Dextrostix is not read at endpoint can, in theory, be used to extend its useful range (52). If the blood glucose level is high, a more accurate measurement can be obtained by incubating for only 30 seconds and then multiplying the value by 2. Conversely, low blood glucose concentrations can apparently also be measured accurately by extending the incubation time to 120 or 180 seconds and dividing the result by 2 or 3. Glucose concentrations in the hypoglycemic range can also be measured

TABLE 1. *Reflectance meters*

UK name	US name	Manufacturer/distributor	Dimensions (mm)	Weight (g)	Power source	Strips	Blood glucose range (mmol/l)	Approx. price (UK £)	
Diagem	Diagem	Clinitron	125 × 110 × 40	380	Mains or rechargeable batteries	Dextrostix BM test BG BM test BG 20–800 Diagem BG Glucoscan			
GMI	GMI	Graseby Medical					1–20	80	
Not available	Dextrometer	Ames/Miles	160 × 100 × 44	300	Mains or rechargeable batteries				No longer manufactured
Hypocount II	Hypocount II	Hypoguard Ltd.	170 × 100 × 30	280	Rechargeable batteries	BM test BG Dextrostix	0–22	80	Audio version available for visually handicapped
Glucochek II	Glucochek II	Medistron (Larken Industries in USA)	162 × 70 × 23		Rechargeable batteries	BM test BG Dextrostix	0.5–22		
Not available	Glucoscan II		127 × 76 × 13	135		Glucoscan II	2–33		
Glucometer		Miles/Ames	170 × 85 × 38	270	4 AA alkaline batteries	Dextrostix	0–22	80	
Glucometer II		Miles/Ames	128 × 65 × 24	189	Battery (sufficient for 1000 tests)	Blot off strip			Also available is memory glucometer which can be linked to either a programmable calculator or microcomputer
Reflochek			160 × 110 × 53	360	9 V DC battery or mains adapter	Reflocheck® Glucose	1.1–25		
Reflolux	Accu-chek ™bG		180 × 98 × 35	270	6 V DC 4 × 1.5 V batteries	Haemoglukotest® 20–800	2.2–22	104	

with Reflotest-Hypoglycaemie – a stick with a range from 0.5 to 8 mmol/l which is very suitable for monitoring blood glucose during an insulin tolerance test, labor, or in patients on a pump. My own prejudice is that, while it may be appropriate to monitor very high or very low blood glucose concentrations with an 'instant' method, *diagnosis* (possible hypo- or hyperglycemic coma) ought to be undertaken with standard laboratory equipment.

3. Blood is removed from Reflotest by blotting and from Dextrostix with a wash bottle. The former is generally regarded as more convenient as is the smaller test area on Reflotest which requires less blood. Against this Dextrostix are quicker (one minute as against two for Reflotest).

Visually read sticks

The cost of a meter is a bar to HBGM for many patients. Both Dextrostix and Reflotest can be read by eye but visual inspection of Dextrostix is too limited in range and too inaccurate to be of real practical value (45). Hence, the development of the double-pad visually read test strip (Chemstrip BG or BM Test Glycaemie 20-800, Boehringer Mannheim) was an important advance in that it provided a reliable and convenient means of HBGM which could be used without a meter. The ability of patients, nurses and doctors to measure blood glucose with the BM 20-800 strips has been extensively evaluated and shown to be as good as or slightly inferior to the accuracy obtained with a meter (45–48, 53–55). Because of the discontinuous scale and the difficulty many patients have in interpolation, there is a tendency for clustering of blood glucose values which leads to a certain degree of imprecision. Most studies have suggested that patients who use BM 20-800 strips tend to underestimate their blood glucose perhaps because of a natural tendency, when the value is intermediate between two color blocks, to subconsciously choose the lower. Meters are inherently less prone to this type of 'cheating' since altering a number on a digital readout requires a more conscious and deliberate action than 'misjudging' a color. The main advantage of visually read strips is that they are cheaper and more portable than sticks which need a meter. Nevertheless, the cost is still much higher than urine testing and it is standard practise in many units to attempt to reduce this by asking patients to cut the strips lengthwise into either halves or thirds (56).

The first competitor to BM 20-800 in the field of visually read strips was Visidex I (Ames Division, Miles Laboratories, Elkhart, Indiana) which in most published reports before mid-1984 is merely called Visidex. It differed (past tense is used because it has now been withdrawn) from BM 20-800 in a number of ways; it had more reference pads (9 versus 8), and separate pads for low (20–180 mg/dl) and high (200–800 mg/dl) glucose levels rather than two pads throughout the entire range as with BM 20-800. Blood was removed from the Visidex strip by washing as with Dextrostix. Visidex was read at 60 seconds compared to 120 for the BM 20-800 (57). The correlation with the reference method of blood glucose concentration measured with Visidex was reasonably good with correlation coefficients varying from 0.81 to 0.97 over a full range of blood glucose values (11, 12, 58–60). However, Visidex appeared, in most instances, to be slightly but significantly less accurate than BM 20-800 (11, 59, 60). In most studies Visidex over-estimated the actual blood glucose concentration, particularly in the hypoglycemic range. On one study (11) 53% of values in the 'hypoglycemic' range would have been read as 'euglycemic' by the Visidex strip compared to only 16.7% with BM 20-800. The general conclusion (57) was that BM 20-800 scored over Visidex in being more accurate, having a more stable color, being more tolerant to minor technical errors and not needing a wash set. The manufacturers obviously agreed with these conclusions since Visidex has now been discontinued worldwide and replaced with Visidex II, a strip in which blood is blotted rather than washed off and in which color development is said to be more stable. At the time of writing (June 1984) Visidex II is already being marketed in the United Kingdom but no evaluation has been published in a refereed journal. When these evaluations do appear, it is likely that they will show Visidex II to be as accurate as BM 20-800 in which case the choice between the two sticks will probably be dictated solely by cost. A caveat on the use of visually read strips is in order; Rizza (57) appropriately states that blood glucose measurements with both Visidex and BM 20-800 serve as 'indicators' rather than as actual measurements of the prevailing blood glucose concentration since an individual blood glucose of 150 mg/dl may range from 100 to 200 mg/dl using a visually read strip. These results are the range to be expected from trained professionals under 'optimal' conditions rather than by patients in their less controlled environment.

Meters

In the early days of HBGM the only two meters available were Eyetone and Reflomat, both expensive, bulky mains-operated instruments designed basically for use in a lab or ward side-room. The second generation of meters (see Table 1) has been purpose-designed for use by patients and are, as one would expect, smaller and cheaper. Most are battery-operated, self-calibrating and have built-in timers and digital displays. All (except Diagem and Glucoscan II) have been compared and assessed in published trials and found to be adequate for the purpose for which they were designed. A gap in the literature is the sort of long-term surveys of reliability such as consumers associations carry out on cars and washing machines. It is my impression that, in practice, none are as reliable as comparable mass-produced electronic equipment such as pocket calculators. At the time of writing, it seems probable that a third generation of meters will be launched which will be smaller, more power-efficient and will include such features as a memory and the ability to be interfaced with a home computer.

Miscellaneous aspects of HBGM

Capillary blood can be obtained either from the fingers, ear lobes or – in infants – the side of the heel. Nerve endings in the fingers are concentrated in the pad over the distal phalanx and it is less painful to prick the side of the fingers although they bleed less efficiently. There are now at least five spring-loaded lancets on the market which make the finger prick virtually painless. Cleaning of the skin with an antiseptic wipe is not generally recommended and, if the alcohol from the wipe is not allowed to dry, it may react with reagents in the pad and lead to an artificially low reading.

Conclusions

With conventional insulin treatment, where blood glucose concentrations change rapidly, HBGM is superior to urine testing as a means of monitoring short- or long-term control and is the method preferred by most patients. However, control will only be improved if blood glucose is measured sufficiently often and if patients take action either on their own initiative or in consultation with the health care team. For patients treated with pumps, HBGM is the only method of monitoring which can measure, as opposed to infer, low blood glucose concentrations and is the only satisfactory method of monitoring for these and other patients whose blood glucose is always within the normal range. The use of HBGM in non-insulin-dependent diabetes has been relatively little explored. It has been suggested (61) that it is indicated for overweight patients, for checking suspected hypoglycemia and in patients with an altered renal threshold. The use of an 'instant' method of blood sugar measurement in conjunction with regular weighing seems to be a logical, cheap and effective way for the General, or Family Practitioner to monitor his patients with non-insulin-dependent diabetes (62).

Major problems in the use of HBGM remain its expense and the fact that its use on a regular long-term basis is monotonous and unlikely to be followed diligently unless motivation is constantly reinforced. Future advances are likely to include the development of personal blood glucose measuring machines with an inbuilt memory or machines which can be interfaced with a personal microcomputer (63). However, the ultimate goal must remain an implantable continuous glucose sensor (64).

References

1. Keen H, Knight RK, (1962): Self sampling for blood sugar. *Lancet*, *1*, 1037.
2. Sonksen PH, Judd SL, Lowy C (1978): Home monitoring of blood glucose. *Lancet*, *1*, 729.
3. Walford S, Gale EAM, Allison SP, Tattersall RB (1978): Self monitoring of blood glucose. *Lancet*, *1*, 732.
4. Danowski TS, Sunder JH (1978): Jet injection of insulin during self monitoring of blood glucose. *Diabetes Care*, *1*, 27.
5. Peterson CM, Jones RL, Dupuis A, Bernstein R, O'Shea M (1978): Feasibility of tight control of juvenile diabetes through patient monitored glucose determinations. *Diabetes*, *27*, 437.
6. Editorial (1980): Home blood glucose monitoring: revolution, revelation or rip off? *Lancet*, *2*, 187.
7. Skyler JS (1982): Self monitoring of blood glucose. *Med. Clin. N. Am.*, *66*, 1227.
8. Peacock I, Tattersall RB (1982): Methods of self-monitoring of diabetic control. *Clinics Endocrinol. Metab.*, *11*, 485.
9. Jovanovic L, Peterson CM (1982): Home blood glucose monitoring. *Compr. Ther.*, *8*, 10.
10. Bell PM, Walshe K (1983): Benefits of self-monitoring of blood glucose. *Br. Med. J.*, *286*, 1230.
11. Clarke AJL, Cudd RD, Newey C, Brooke D, Newall RG, Keen H (1983): Assessment of a new visual blood glucose strip. *Diabetes Care*, *6*, 540.
12. Frindik JP, Kassner DA, Pirkle DA, Kemp SF, Hoff C (1983): Comparison of visidex and chemstrip BG with Beckman Glucose Analyser determination of blood glucose. *Diabetes Care*, *6*, 536.
13. Peterson CM, Jones RL, Dupuis A, Levine BS, Bernstein R, O'Shea M (1979): Feasibility of improved blood glucose control in patients with insulin-dependent diabetes mellitus. *Diabetes Care*, *2*, 329.
14. Worth R, Home PD, Johnston DG, Anderson J, Ashworth L, Burrin JM, Appleton D, Binder C, Alberti KGMM (1982): Intensive attention improves glycaemic control in insulin-dependent diabetics without further advantage from home blood glucose monitoring: a controlled trial. *Br. Med. J.*, *285*, 1233.
15. Tattersall RB (1983): Diabetes, the young person, their family and the doctor. *Int. Diabetes Fed. Bull.*, *27*, 1.
16. Harrad RH, Plumb AP, Prickett S, Alford FP, Sonksen PH (1983): Intensive attention improves glycaemic control in insulin dependent diabetes without further advantage from home blood glucose monitoring. *Lancet*, *1*, 59.
17. Cox R, Beaven DW, Helm AM (1980): Home monitoring of blood glucose: a retrospective assessment in 38 insulin requiring diabetics. *N.Z. Med. J.*, *92*, 193.
18. Van Ballegooie E, Reitsma WD, Simter WJ, Doorenbos H (1983): Improvement of diabetes mellitus in patients practicing self-monitoring and self-management under out-patient supervision. *Ned. Tijdschr. Geneeskd.*, *127*, 44.
19. Schiffrin A, Belmonte M (1982): Multiple daily self-glucose monitoring: its

essential role in long-term glucose control in insulin-dependent diabetic patients treated with pump and multiple subcutaneous injections. *Diabetes Care*, *5*, 479.
20. Cohen M, Zimmet P (1980): Home blood glucose monitoring. *Med. J.Aust.*, *2*, 713.
21. Schiffrin A, Desrosiers M, Belmonte M (1983): Evaluation of two methods of self-blood glucose monitoring by trained insulin-dependent diabetic adolescents outside the hospital. *Diabetes Care*, *6*, 166.
22. Fairclough PK, Clements RS, Filer DV, Bell DSH (1983): An evaluation of patient performance of and their satisfaction with various rapid blood glucose measurement systems. *Diabetes Care*, *6*, 45.
23. Mountier VM, Scott RS, Beaven DW (1982): Use and abuse of glucose reflectance meters. *Diabetes Care*, *5*, 542.
24. Schöffling K, Bachmann W, Drost H et al (1982): How reliable are ambulatory patient-monitored blood sugar measurements: a multicentre trial. *Deutsch. Med. Woch.*, *107*, 605.
25. Hilton BA (1982): Nurse's performance and interpretation of urine testing and capillary blood glucose monitoring measures. *J. Adv. Nursing*, *7*, 509.
26. Kinmonth AL (1981): Home blood glucose monitoring: a sticky artefact. *Br. Med. J.*, *282*, 272.
27. Graham K, Kesson CM, Kennedy HB, Ireland JT (1980): Relevance of colour vision and diabetic retinopathy to self-monitoring of blood glucose. *Br. Med. J.*, *281*, 971.
28. Ryan EA, Miller J, Skyler JS (1983): Finger sepsis: possible complication of self-monitoring of blood glucose concentrations. *Br. Med. J.*, *286*, 1614.
29. Bradley C (1982): Psychophysiological aspects of the management of diabetes mellitus. *Int. J. Ment. Health*, *11*, 117.
30. Dupuis A, Jones RL, Peterson CM (1980): Psychological effects of blood glucose self-monitoring in diabetic patients. *Psychosomatics*, *21*, 581.
31. Rudolph MC, Ahern JA, Genel M, Bates S, Harding P, Hochsta DTJ, Quinlan D, Tamborlane W (1982): Optimal insulin delivery in adolescents with diabetes: impact of intensive treatment on psychosocial adjustment. *Diabetes Care*, *5*, *Suppl 1*, 53.
32. Tajima N, Ide Y, Minami N et al (1982): Psychological status and diabetic control in home blood glucose monitoring patients. *J. Jpn. Diabet. Soc.*, *25*, 1191.
33. Baumer JH, Edelsten AD, Howlett BC et al (1982): Impact of home blood glucose monitoring on childhood diabetes. *Arch. Dis. Child.*, *57*, 195.
34. Burghen GA (1983): Therapy in childhood diabetes. *J. Am. Med. Assoc.*, *249*, 2938.
35. Geffner ME, Kaplan SA, Lippe BM, Scott ML (1983): Self-monitoring of blood glucose levels and intensified insulin therapy. Acceptability and efficacy in childhood diabetes. *J. Am. Med. Assoc.*, *249*, 2913.
36. Spencer ML (1981): Home blood glucose monitoring six months later. *Diabetes*, *30*, *Suppl. 1*, 68A. 269.
37. MacDonald MJ (1983): Personal blood glucose testing in children. *Primary Care*, *10*, 565.
38. Miller PFW, Stratton C, Tripp JH (1983): Blood testing compared with urine

testing in the long-term control of diabetes. *Arch. Dis. Child.*, *58*, 294.
39. Darlow BA, Abbott GD, Beaven DW (1980): Assessment of an insulin regime and monitoring techniques in juvenile diabetes. *Aust. Pediat. J.*, *16*, 109.
40. Kohler E, Hurwitz LS, Milan D (1982): A developmentally staged curriculum for teaching self-care to the child with insulin-dependent diabetes mellitus. *Diabetes Care*, *5*, 300.
41. Stubbs SM, Brudenell JM, Pyke DA, Watkins PJ, Stubbs WA, Alberti KGMM (1980): Management of the pregnant diabetic: home or hospital, with or without glucose meters? *Lancet*, *1*, 1122.
42. Varner MW (1983): Efficacy of home glucose monitoring in diabetic pregnancy. *Am. J. Med.*, *75*, 592.
43. Cox R, Scott RS, MacLean AB, Beaven DW (1981): Home monitoring of blood glucose in diabetic pregnancy. *N.Z. Med. J.*, *94*, 371.
44. Goldstein A, Elliott J, Lederman S, Worcester B, Russell P, Linzey EM (1983): Economic effects of self-monitoring of blood glucose concentrations by women with insulin-dependent diabetes during pregnancy. *J. Reprod. Med.*, *21*, 449.
45. Clements RS, Keane NA, Kirk KA, Boshell BR (1981): Comparison of various methods for rapid glucose estimation. *Diabetes Care*, *4*, 392.
46. Shapiro B, Savage PJ, Lomatch D, Gniadek T, Forbes R, Mitchell R, Hein K, Starr R, Nutter M, Scherdt B (1981): A comparison of accuracy and estimated cost of methods for home blood glucose monitoring. *Diabetes Care*, *4*, 396.
47. Reeves ML, Forhan SE, Skyler JS and Peterson CM (1981): Comparison of methods for blood glucose monitoring. *Diabetes Care*, *4*, 404.
48. Worth RC, Harrison K, Anderson J, Johnston DG, Alberti KGMM (1981): A comparative study of blood glucose test strips. *Diabetes Care*, *4*, 407.
49. Howe-Davis S, Holman RR, Phillips M, Turner RC (1978): Home blood glucose sampling for plasma glucose assay in control of diabetes. *Br. Med. J.*, *2*, 596.
50. Clark AJL, Bilous RW, Keen WL, Keen H (1982): Capillary tubes for blood glucose sampling. *Diabetologia*, *23*, 539.
51. Dean BR, North SE, Harrison LC, Martin FIR (1982): Properties of Dextrostix. *Diabetes Care*, *5*, 554.
52. Scobie IN, Son HY, Tey BH, Sonksen PH (1983): Extending the range of blood glucose measurements with Dextrostix and a meter. *Diabetologia*, *25*, 123.
53. Birch K, Hildebrandt P, Marshall MO, Sestoft L (1981): Self monitoring of blood glucose without a meter. *Diabetes Care*, *4*, 414.
54. Ferguson SD, Prosser R (1980): Are reflectance meters necessary for home blood glucose monitoring? *Br. Med. J.*, *281*, 912.
55. Walford S, Clarke P, Paisey R, Hartog M, Allison SP (1980): Home blood glucose measurements without a reflectance meter. *Lancet*, *1*, 653.
56. Fahlen M, Lapidus L, Stromblad G, Stuart-Beck R (1983): Home monitoring of blood glucose and insulin therapy without a photometer. *Acta Med. Scand.*, *213*, *Suppl. 671*, 37.
57. Rizza RA (1983): Editorial: Use of Visidex for self-blood glucose monitoring. *Diabetes Care*, *6*, 614.

58. Aziz S, Hsiang Y (1983): Comparative study of home blood glucose monitoring devices: Visidex, chemstrip BG, glucometer and accu-chek BG. *Diabetes Care*, *6*, 529.
59. Silverstein JH, Rosenbloom AL, Clarke DW, Spillar R, Pendergast JF (1983): Accuracy of two systems for blood glucose monitoring without a meter (chemstrip/visidex). *Diabetes Care*, *6*, 533.
60. Marshall SM, Alberti KGMM (1983): Assessment of new visual test strip for blood glucose monitoring. *Diabetes Care*, *6*, 543.
61. Cohen M, Zimmet P (1983): Self-monitoring of blood glucose levels in non-insulin dependent diabetes mellitus. *Med. J. Aust.*, *8*, 377.
62. Howe-Davies S, Simpson RW, Turner RC (1980): Control of maturity-onset diabetes by monitoring fasting blood glucose and body weight. *Diabetes Care*, *3*, 607.
63. Wilson DE, Clarke DH (1983): Profiling self-monitored blood glucose results with the personal micro-computer. *Diabetes Care*, *6*, 604.
64. Shichiri M, Kawamori R, Yumasaki Y, Hakui N, Abe H (1982): Wearable artificial endocrine pancreas with needle-type glucose sensor. *Lancet*, *2*, 1129.

The Diabetes Annual/1
K.G.M.M. Alberti and L.P. Krall, editors

ISBN 0444 90 343 7
$0.85 per article per page (transactional system)
$0.20 per article per page (licensing system)

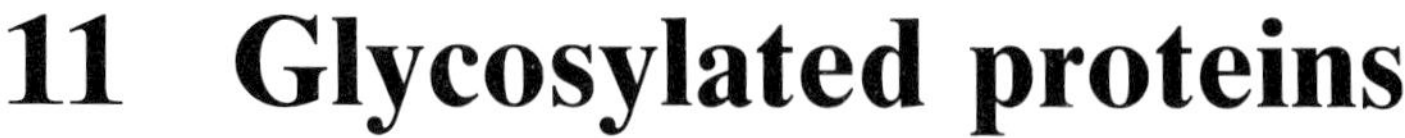

11 Glycosylated proteins

CHARLES M. PETERSON AND BENT FORMBY

In the past two years there have been over 500 publications related to the topic under review. Among these are a number of excellent reviews or symposia (1–7). As originally hypothesized (8), the measurement of glycosylated proteins has been increasingly defined as a clinical tool and the role of these types of reactions in the protean sequelae of diabetes is under intense study. One of the major developments during the past year has been the convening of an 'Expert Committee' under the auspices of the National Diabetes Data Group of the National Institutes of Health of the United States, whose charge is to standardize nomenclature and investigate the possibility of references and standards for glycosylated protein measurement. The recommended nomenclature is summarized in Table 1. The clinical utility of glycosylated hemoglobin or serum protein measurement will not achieve its full potential until appropriate references, standards, and degrees of accuracy and precision of these measurements are agreed upon. Considerable progress has been made in methods development. The potential for automated systems of measurement with acceptable precision and accuracy appears clear. The increased interest in glycosylation reactions on the part of biochemists has led to insight into the potential import of post-translational modification of proteins in the pathophysiology of diabetes mellitus. While the functional changes which occurred concomitant with glucosylation were appreciated relatively early as perhaps being important in the initiation or propagation of the manifestations of hyperglycemia, more recent work has focused on the influence of these reactions on the rate of catabolism of various structural or functional proteins.

Studies of the biochemistry of glucosylation

Adducts of hemoglobin A (HbA) are formed spontaneously with reducing sugars and measurement of the resulting minor hemoglobins $HbA_{1a\text{-}c}$ has been used increasingly in monitoring hyperglycemia in diabetes mellitus. The glucosylation of HbA is a non-enzymatic reaction between the aldehyde group of glucose and the N-terminal valine as well as intra-chain lysine residues of the β-chains of HbA with initial formation of a Schiff-base adduct which is stabilized by a subsequent Amadori rearrangement from

TABLE 1. *Glossary of terms*

Hemoglobin A (HbA): The major adult form of hemoglobin. A tetramer consisting of two α- and two β-chains (α_2, β_2)

Hemoglobin A_0 (HbA_0): The major component of hemoglobin A identified by its chromatographic and electrophoretic properties. Post-translation modifications including glycosylation do exist, but do not significantly affect the charge properties of the protein.

Hemoglobin A_1 (HbA_1): Post-translationally modified, more negatively charged forms of hemoglobin A_0 (primarily glucosylation at the β-chain terminal valine residue). Separable from HbA_0 by chromatographic and electrophoretic methods.

Hemoglobin A_{1a}, HbA_{1a2}, HbA_{1b}, HbA_{1c}: Chromatographically distinct stable components of HbA_1.

'Fast' hemoglobin: The total of HbA_1 fractions (HbA_{1a}, HbA_{1a2}, HbA_{1b}, HbA_{1c}) which, because of more negative charge, migrates toward the anode on electrophoresis and elutes earlier on cation exchange chromatography than HbA_0.

Glucosylated hemoglobin: Hemoglobin modified by glucose at β-chain valine residues and ε amino groups of lysine residues.

Glycosylated hemoglobin (glyco-hemoglobin): A generic term for hemoglobin containing glucose and/or other carbohydrate at either valine or lysine residues thus the sum of glycosyl adducts.

Hemoglobin A_{1a}, HbA_{1a2}, HbA_{1b}: 'Fastest' most anionic forms of hemoglobin consisting primarily of adducts of phosphorylated glycolytic intermediates with HbA_0.

Hemoglobin A_{1c}: Component of HbA_1 which consists of 50 to 90% hemoglobin (depending on the quality of resolution of the chromatographic system) glucosylated by a ketoamine linkage at the β-chain terminal valine residue.

Pre-hemoglobin A_{1c}: A labile form of glucosylated Hb containing glucose bound in aldimine linkage to the β-chain terminal valine residue.

the aldimine to a ketoamine. Since the initial step involves the condensation of an amine moiety with the aldehyde form of a particular sugar, it is important to note that only a very small fraction of the most common sugars is present in the aldehyde form in solution. Thus, for glucose 62% will be in the β-pyranose form, 38% in the α-pyranose form and only 0.001% in the aldehyde form. The relative reactivity for the most common sugars with a simple amine nucleophile such as hydroxylamine is ribose >

arabinose > mannose > galactose > glucose (9). Although HbA is exposed to glucose during the lifespan of the erythrocyte (120 days), how can the low expected percentage of solubilized glucose in the aldehyde form produce measurable concentrations of glucosylated HbA?

Mortensen et al. (10) studied the stability of HbA_{1c} using an isoelectric focusing method. They found that prolonged saline incubation of purified HbA_{1c} followed by renewed isoelectric focusing gave rise to an increase in the HbA concentrations and concluded that the non-enzymatic glucosylation of HbA to HbA_{1c} is a reversible process with an equilibrium constant K of 8.4 M^{-1}. Using this information and assuming a monomer hemoglobin concentration in the erythrocyte of about 20 mM and a concentration of glucose in the aldehydic form of 5.10^{-5} mM, then the calculated concentration of formed ketoamine adduct i.e. HbA_{1c} would be less than 0.02% of the total hemoglobin concentration. Since in non-diabetics 3–6% of hemoglobin is glucosylated, it seems unlikely that adduct formation in vivo only involves glucose in the aldehydic form. This has been confirmed experimentally by Stevens et al. (11), who could not demonstrate a reaction between glucose and hemoglobin in vitro. How does one explain the in-vivo formation of hemoglobin adducts? Non-enzymatic glucosylation of hemoglobin in vitro has been demonstrated with phosphorylated carbohydrates containing a free carbonyl-group and resulting in HbA_{1b}-like molecules. Thus, 72-hour incubation of hemoglobin A (Table 2) with phosphorylated hexoses and trioses resulted in 7–12% modification of the hemoglobin. By

TABLE 2. *Percentage of HbA adduct formed after 72 hours*

Intermediate	HbA adduct (72 hrs) (%)
Glucose-6-P	7.12
Fructose-6-P	4.21
Fructose-1-P	9.75
Fructose-1,6-P_2	8.86
Glyceraldehyde-3-P	11.22
Dihydroxyacetone-P	8.36
Glucose	<0.05
Fructose	<0.05
Glucose-1-P	<0.05
Glucose-1,6-P_2	<0.05
UDP-glucose	<0.05

Reprinted from Stevens et al. (11), by courtesy of the Editors of the *Journal of Biological Chemistry*.

ion exchange chromatography and isoelectric focusing all of the HbA adducts were indistinguishable from HbA_{1b} (11). Since 2,3-DPG inhibits the adduct formation it appears that the phosphate group of the phosphorylated carbohydrates is mandatory to orient the carbonyl-group in the 2,3-DPG pocket of the hemoglobin molecule to allow the adduct formation (11–14). It might be expected that HbA_{1b} in vivo is dephosphorylated to form HbA_{1c}. Significantly elevated values of glycosylated intermediates are found in the erythrocytes of diabetics (Table 3), which presumably explains the increased values of HbA_{1b} in diabetics as compared with normal controls (11, 14). However, no phosphatases have been implicated in such a reaction and a satisfactory quantitative theory of hemoglobin A_{1c} formation has yet to be advanced.

1-(N^5-lysino)-1-deoxy-D-fructose (fructose lysine) arises from the reaction between glucose and lysine ε-NH_2 groups in the vicinity of carboxyl groups on a protein surface. Since no direct correspondence between the pKa of the amino groups and its extent of glucosylation exists, the kinetics of the Amadori rearrangement rather than the pKa of the amino group may be the crucial factor in determining sites of glucosylation in proteins. Non-enzymatic glucosylation occurs primarily at intra-chain lysine residues. Non-enzymatic glucosylation in vitro of the most abundant serum protein, albumin, has been reported (15–17), but interestingly Eble et al. (18) and others (15, 19) were unable to detect any effects on the biological properties of glucosylated albumin, including its circulating half-life or

TABLE 3. *Glycolytic intermediates in erythrocytes*

Intermediate	Diabetics (n = 14)		Controls (n = 4)	
	$\bar{x}$	± S.E.	$\bar{x}$	± S.E.
	μM		μM	
Glucose-6-P	42.82	2.22	28.94	4.05
Fructose-6-P	17.59	1.09	12.50	0.40
Fructose-1,6-P_2	8.21	0.64	2.59	0.76
Glyceraldehyde-3-P	4.21	0.46	1.62	0.86
DHAP*	20.94	2.51	7.18	1.07

Hemoglobin A_{1c} concentrations, which provide a measure of blood control, ranged from 4.8 to 7.3% in the diabetics and 3.5 to 4.1% in the controls at the time blood samples were taken.

* DHAP = dihydroxyacetone phosphate.

Reprinted from Stevens et al. (11), by courtesy of the Editors of the *Journal of Biological Chemistry*.

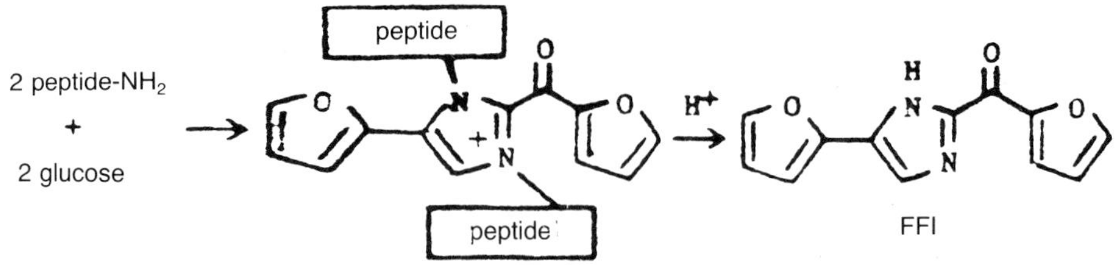

FIG. 1. *Structure of 2-furoyl-4(5)-(2-furanyl)-1H-imidazole. Reproduced from Ulrich et al. (21), by courtesy of the Editors of Federation Proceedings.*

ligand binding capacity. However, it is recognized that non-enzymatic glucosylation of proteins is only the late step in a complex series of so-called Maillard or browning reactions (20) where the products are denatured cross-linked protein polymers and protein-bound fluorescent pigments, which may contribute to the development of the pathophysiology of diabetes through effects on the structure function and metabolism of protein.

To learn more about the mechanisms of cross-linking reactions, Eble et al. (18) studied the kinetics and products of non-enzymatic glucosylation of RNase A. The role of glucosylation under physiological in-vitro conditions was first order with glucose and accompanied by a comparable decrease in primary amino-groups in the protein and lysine recoverable by amino acid analysis. Of interest was the observation that when glucosylated protein was separated from glucose, the protein continued to polymerize even in the absence of glucose, suggesting that the primary mechanism of cross-linking involves the reaction between a glucosylated amino acid i.e. lysine on one protein and an unmodified amino acid on the same or another protein.

Using long-term exposure of proteins to glucose, Ulrich et al. (21) observed the formation of brown fluorescent pigments or advanced glucosylation end-products (AGE). Chemical analysis of acid hydrolysates of AGE-poly-L-lysine or AGE-albumin (21) showed the formation of the novel structure 2-furoyl-4(5)-(2-furanyl)-1H-imidazole (FFI) (Fig. 1).

Incorporation of two peptidic amine nitrogens and two glucose residues in FFI could account for cross-linking of proteins observed in vivo and thereby provide an important key to the understanding of glucose mediated protein modifications such as occur in collagens and lens crystallins (22–26) in diabetes and aging.

Studies on methods of measurement

Table 4 summarizes the clinically used measurements of glucosylation and their relative advantages and disadvantages. The major problem with all

TABLE 4. *Clinical methods employed for measurement of glycosylation*

A. Physical methods based on changes in pI

1. Cation exchange chromatography
   PRO: Inexpensive and rapid
   CON: Sensitive to small changes in resin packing, ionic strength, pH, temperature, column loading, and affected by the labile fraction

2. High-performance liquid chromatography (HPLC)
   PRO: Dedicated instruments avoid many problems in 1
   CON: Relatively expensive and still affected by the labile fraction

3. Agarose gel electrophoresis
   PRO: Inexpensive, low technician time, standardized plates and conditions in kits, less sensitive to pH, triglyceride concentrations, and temperature
   CON: Precision problems induced by scanner and loading variation; sensitive to labile fraction

4. Isoelectric focusing
   PRO: Separates most minor hemoglobin variants
   CON: Precision over time dependent on use of same batch of ampholines on standardized plates; scanning effects precision

B. Methods based on chemical principles

1. Thiobarbituric acid/colorimetric assay
   PRO: Minimally effected by storage condition, fructose or 5-hydroxy-methyl furfural standards may be incorporated
   CON: Difficult to establish, large amount of technical time required, and affected by labile fraction

2. Affinity chromatography with immobilized m-phenyl-boronate
   PRO: Rapid, inexpensive, minimally effected by chromatographic conditions, eliminates labile adduct
   CON: Resins vary within and between manufacturers

3. Fructosamine determination by nitroblue tetrazolium reduction
   PRO: Inexpensive, standards incorporated, may be automated, not effected by labile adduct
   CON: Only for serum, lipids may interfere, reducing substances (e.g. ascorbate) may interfere

C. Radioimmunoassay

PRO: Inexpensive, rapid, sensitive, specific, not effected by labile adduct
CON: Antibodies difficult to raise and not commercially available

methods is that as yet there are no agreed upon references and standards. The recently constituted committee of the National Diabetes Data Group may be able in part to speak to this need. The other major problem in terms of the clinical utility of these measurements lies in the problem of accuracy (difficult to approach without standards) and precision. Acceptable precision for assays of glycosylated proteins should be preferably less than 2%. The necessity of such precision for intra- and inter-assay measurements becomes clear when one considers that for hemoglobin A_{1c} measurements, a change of 1% represents a mean blood glucose change of approximately 30–35 mg/dl or 2 mM. Methods which achieve these levels of precision generally have relatively narrow ranges for 'normal' populations. This observation was recently confirmed by Blouquit et al. (27) using high-performance liquid chromatography (HPLC) methodologies and Bio-rex-70 columns. The normal level was 5.4 $\pm$ 0.04%. Four new potentially useful methods of quantitating glucosylated proteins have been described: (1) affinity chromatography; (2) fructosamine quantification; (3) monoclonal antibodies specific for glucosylated ε amino groups of lysine; and (4) spectrophotometric assay dependent on the change in absorbance when phytic acid binds to HbA (28–40). All these methods are now in the process of being tested in clinical situations.

Affinity chromatography has received the most attention. The resins bind cis-diols and therefore bind glucosylated amino acids, peptides, and proteins (41–43). Therefore, both serum protein and hemoglobin glucosylation can be measured by this method in human as well as animal specimens. Hemoglobinopathies do not affect the measurement unless accompanied by a shortened erythrocyte survival (28, 33). The measurement is minimally affected by the labile fraction of hemoglobin (30, 36). Samples may be stored for as long as 21 days at room temperature without affecting the value (32) although storage properties may change if the cells are washed and the hemoglobin refrigerated or frozen (44). The precision of these methods in general appears good, although it may vary greatly depending on the source of the resin or prepacked columns (32, 35, 44).

The other three methods have been less well evaluated. Murine monoclonal antibodies have been raised (37) with the dominant epitope recognized being glucitol-lysine, the reduced hexose alcohol form of glucose conjugated to the ε amino group of lysine. The antibody recognized glucitol lysine epitopes in reduced high-density lipoprotein, albumin, hemoglobin, transferrin, and plasma proteins. Whether this method will have the desired precision for clinical use remains to be determined. Furthermore, reducing agents may be selective in their relative reactivity with various glucosylated ε amino groups of lysine (34). Previous attempts at raising polyclonal antibodies have only rarely been successful (35).

The use of phytic acid to bind to HbA and produce a change in absorbance which does not occur when hemoglobin is glucosylated appears attractive since it could be automated if problems with standards and calibration are solved (40). Even more appealing is the estimation of serum fructosamine utilizing the principle that the Amadori rearrangement product formed by the condensation of glucose and proteins acts as a reducing agent in alkaline solution (46). An assay has been described which uses nitroblue tetrazolium and 1-deoxy,1-morpholinofructose standards (38). As described, the method is rapid, relatively inexpensive, amenable to automation and appears useful as a screening test for diabetes with 88% sensitivity and 9% false positives (39). The assay can only be used on sera. Reducing substances such as ascorbate or glutathione may interfere.

A number of investigators have now evaluated measurement of serum glucosylated proteins as a means of monitoring hyperglycemia (38, 39, 47–54). The measurements should have the same constraints in terms of accuracy and precision as for quantitation of glucosylated hemoglobins to be clinically useful. Most authors agree that serum or plasma protein glucosylation measurement provides an 'intermediate' index of hyperglycemia, whereas normalization of blood glucose is followed by normalization of HbA_{1c} in approximately 8 weeks (55), glucosylated serum protein values reach a stable plateau in 3–5 weeks (39, 51, 53).

A number of studies have been performed comparing one method with another (27, 30, 32, 33, 35, 38, 40, 44, 53, 54, 56–61). Almost all methods perform with the appropriate precision if conditions and handling are optimized. Storage conditions markedly affect the values obtained especially in methods which rely on physical property changes induced by glucosylation (44, 62, 63). Proper handling of specimens with appropriate controls is therefore mandatory. Without references or standards, accuracy cannot be evaluated. Nevertheless, each method correlated well with others and therefore can be used clinically. An automated method with references and standards preferably expressed as moles of glucose bound per mole hemoglobin or protein is sorely needed.

A number of investigations have been performed regarding the significance and elimination of the labile fraction (64–69). The labile fraction affects the results in methods which separate hemoglobin by charge except for isoelectric focusing (69) where the labile glucopyranose ring is more anodal than HbA_{1c}. Dialysis for 4 hours at 37 °C, 18 hours at 4 °C, lysis at pH 5 with or without semicarbazide and aniline all appear to be successful means of eliminating the labile adduct. Dialysis at 22 °C for 18 hours was also recommended (67) but found to lead to small differences and therefore was not felt to be worth the effort in clinical situations. However, under these latter conditions artefactual increases in HbA_{1a+b} will occur compensating for the decrease in HbA_{1c} (44) and therefore measurements of HbA_1 will not change as dramatically as anticipated. Elimination of the labile fraction becomes most important where the values are elevated since the amount of labile fraction is proportional to the total fast fraction and the mean amplitude of glycemic excursion (70–72). This has led some authors to recommend elimination of the labile adduct only if values are above 12% (72) or not at all (67, 68, 71). Since the labile adduct provides information which is different from the stable fraction and failure to eliminate the adduct provides a 'yea or nea' test of glucose 'control', the clinical situation will determine the best way of handling this adduct. Certainly for studies which are using the measurement of glucosylated hemoglobin to document long-term glycemia the elimination of the labile adduct would appear wise.

Studies on the role of glycosylation in the secondary sequelae of diabetes mellitus

A number of studies have shown that glucosylation of various proteins or tissues occurs in vitro. The documentation that these reactions occur concomitant with or are causative of pathological consequences has been more difficult.

Since the observation that serum triglyceride and cholesterol levels correlate with HbA_{1c} levels and decrease with improved glucose control in Types 1 and 2 diabetes mellitus (73), these observations have been confirmed and extended by a number of investigators (74–81) such that it has become clear that with improved glucose levels, LDL levels decrease and HDL levels increase. In addition, a correctable defect in lipoprotein lipase occurs which may contribute to the elevation in plasma triglyceride concentration by limiting triglyceride removal from plasma (81). However, experiments with continuous subcutaneous insulin infusion (CSII) giving rise to peripheral hyperinsulinemia, showed no change in the mean fractional clearance rate and suggested that the decrease may be due to suppression of hepatic VLDL-TG synthesis (82).

More provocative are the demonstrations that in vitro non-enzymatic glucosylation stabilized by reduction with sodium borohydride of LDL, HDL, and albumin alters the catabolism of these molecules in animal systems (83–86). The importance of these findings remains to be determined since reduction with sodium borohydride may alter protein structure and it is not surprising that the altered molecules are treated as 'foreign'. Thus, studies of fibroblast binding of LDL particles obtained from normals and Type 2 diabetic subjects were found to be similar and there was no difference in their degradation by mouse peritoneal macrophages (87). Another problem lies in the fact that the sodium borohydride reduced adduct of glucose plus a protein (glucitollysine) is not the chemical species found in vivo. Steinbrecher and Witzum (88) attempted to examine this problem by studying reduced and non-reduced glucose reacted LDL molecules and found that receptor mediated catabolism was still impaired with only 5% of lysine residues being modified.

Improved diabetic control as documented by glucosylated protein levels continues to be associated with an improvement in abnormalities associated with diabetes mellitus. Thus, Holman and colleagues (89) showed that improved insulin treatment in patients with Type 1 diabetes resulted in better preservation of sensory-nerve function, lower LDL-cholesterol levels, and lower whole blood low-shear viscosity.

The role of glucosylation in the etiology of renal disease in diabetes remains controversial. The previous report that glucosylated albumin injected into rats (90) led to diabetic renal disease has not been confirmed (91). Hypertension even in the presence of improved glucose levels exerts an independent and deleterious effect on the development of renal disease since hypertensive patients were noted to have progressive proteinuria despite improved glucose levels achieved with CSII whereas normotensive patients showed a reduction in proteinuria (92). The levels of urinary β-hexosaminidase have been documented to be a sensitive indicator of early renal damage and to be elevated in the plasma and urine of patients with Type 1 diabetes (93). Whether elevated levels of this enzyme reflect compensatory responses to increased levels of glucosylated proteins remains to be established.

A number of studies have documented changes in the erythrocyte coincident with glucosylation of hemoglobin. The hypothesis that glucosylation of hemoglobin might contribute to pathology through an effect on oxygen affinity (94) does not appear to be applicable since the whole blood oxygen affinity in persons with diabetes was not increased when compared with normals (95). A number of studies have confirmed glucosylation of erythrocyte membrane proteins (96, 97) and altered physical properties of the erythrocyte and blood viscosity in diabetes (96-100). Whether these phenomena are related remains conjectural since insulin infusion seems to improve erythrocyte deformability within hours (100).

Glucosylation reactions may play a role in the hyperaggregation of platelets seen in diabetes. Erythrocytes from diabetic individuals led to increased aggregation of platelets from controls (100) and in rat studies, platelets stimulated with glucosylated collagen showed hyperaggregation when compared with controls (101).

The role of glucosylation reactions in ocular pathology is under intense study. Muntoni et al. (102) found a direct correlation between glucosylated hemoglobin levels and a dyschromatopsia in the yellow–blue axis which improved with improvement in glycemia. The ocular lens is vulnerable to glucosylation which occurs concomitant with high molecular weight aggregate formation of crystallins and opacification (22). The observations that aspirin dosing by patients with rheumatoid arthritis or in animal systems may retard cataract formation either by inhibiting aldose reductase or lens protein glucosylation are extremely provocative (103, 104).

Collagen has been found to undergo increased non-enzymatic glucosylation in patients with diabetes and to have changed physical properties such as decreased flexibility and solubility (24–26). The thermal stability of collagen is also altered concomitant with non-enzymatic glucosylation (25). Whether these observations can be related to the limited joint mobility which correlated with growth retardation and elevated hemoglobin A_{1c} levels seen in diabetic children (105) remains to be determined.

Scleroderma-like changes in the skin of children with Type 1 diabetes has been correlated with non-enzymatic glucosylations of skin collagen (106). There was increased accumulation of collagen in the lower dermis in the skin biopsies of children with scleroderma-like changes and the authors hypothesize that non-enzymatic glucosylation alters the turnover of collagen, thus contributing to the scleroderma-like syndrome of skin, joints and lungs seen in Type 1 diabetes mellitus. Placental collagen has also been found in humans to have increased glucosylation when obtained following gestation characterized by hyperglycemia. Glucosylated human placental collagen showed increased platelet aggregating potency (107). Glycosylation of glomerular basement membrane appears to be increased in diabetic children (108) and Vogt et al. observed increased ε amino lysine bound glucose in tendon, aorta, coronary artery, femoral nerve, glomerular basement membrane and lung parenchyma in autopsy tissue obtained from diabetic subjects when compared with controls (109). The role of glucosylation of nervous tissue may play a role in the physiological abnormalities seen in nerve conduction in persons with diabetes which correlate with glucose levels as quantitated by glucosylated hemoglobin (110–112).

Studies of the clinical utility of glucosylated protein measurements

Clinical studies in general agree that glucosylated serum or hemoglobin measurements correlate with hyperglycemia over time as noted above. Confounding clinical conditions may arise in the form of (1) compounds such as aspirin, cyanate (uremia), acetaldehyde (alcoholism), or galactose which modify the chromatographic properties of hemoglobin, (2) lactescent plasma in hypertriglyceridemia which alters spectrophotometric readings, (3) hemoglobinopathies which alter the chromatographic properties of hemoglobin (S, C, F, Wayne, or Hijiyama), or (4) conditions which alter erythrocyte survival such as iron deficiency, chronic disease, or uremia (113–124). Nevertheless, although disputed (123), most authors find that measurements of glucosylated hemoglobin are moderately useful in discriminating a diabetic from a non-diabetic group and therefore of perhaps use in the diagnosis of diabetes (126, 127), even post-mortem (128). In addition, the test is useful in distinguishing ‘stress hyperglycemia’ from diabetes in the presence of acute myocardial infarction (129). Hyperglycemia commonly precedes stroke and may be a risk factor and/or predictor of the extent of stroke even in the 'non-diabetic' population (130).

Some clinicians have begun to use glucosylated protein measurements as a predictor of outcome. Thus, Brunner et al. found that in patients with retinopathy, those who maintained a HbA_1 level of less than 8% remained stable, those with levels of 8–10% showed moderate progression of retinopathy which could be stabilized by laser treatment, and those with levels higher than 10% showed a marked progression (131). The greatest correlation with outcome appears to be in pregnancy where an elevated blood glucose during pregnancy tends to be predictive of higher risk in terms of malformation, fetal wastage (132), macrosomia (133), and pre-eclampsia (134). Roberts et al. suggest that fructosamine determination may be a useful diagnostic test for gestational diabetes as well (135).

References

1. Mayer TK, Freedman ZR (1983): Protein glycosylation in diabetes mellitus: a review of laboratory measurements and of their clinical utility. *Clin. Chim. Acta*, *127*, 147.
2. Nathan DM (1983): Glycosylated hemoglobin: What it is and how to use it. *Clin. Diabetes*, *1*, 2.
3. Peterson CM (Ed) (1982): Proceedings of a conference on nonenzymatic glycosylation and browning reactions: their relevance to diabetes mellitus. *Diabetes*, *31*, *Suppl. 3*, 1.
4. Wieland OH (1983): Late diabetic damage and non-enzymatic glucosylation of proteins (in German). *Med. Klin.*, *78*, 107.
5. Gabbay KH (1982): Glycosylated hemoglobin and diabetes mellitus. *Med. Clin. N. Am.*, *66*, 1309.
6. Monnier VM, Cerami A (1982): Non-enzymatic glycosylation and browning of proteins in diabetes. *Clin. Endocrinol. Metab.*, *11*, 431.
7. Kennedy L, Baynes JW (1984): Non-enzymatic glycosylation and the chronic complications of diabetes: an overview. *Diabetologia*, *26*, 93.
8. Peterson CM, Jones RL (1977): Minor hemoglobins, diabetic 'control' and diseases of postsynthetic protein modification. *Ann. Intern. Med.*, *87*, 489.
9. Capon B (1969): Mechanism of carbohydrate chemistry. *Chem. Rev.*, *69*, 407.
10. Mortensen HB, Christophensen C (1983): Glycosylation of human hemoglobin A in red blood cells studied in vitro. Kinetics of the formation and dissociation of hemoglobin A_{1c}. *Clin. Chim. Acta*, *134*, 317.
11. Stevens VD, Vlassara H, Abati A, Cerami A (1977): Nonenzymatic glycosylation of hemoglobin. *J. Biol. Chem.*, *252*, 2998.
12. McDonald MT, Bleichman M, Bunn HF, Noble H (1979): Functional properties of the glycosylated minor components of human adult hemoglobin. *J. Biol. Chem.*, *254*, 702.
13. Snider RJ, Koenig RJ, Binnertz A (1982): Regulation of hemoglobin A_{1c}

formation in human erythrocytes in vitro. Effects of physiologic factors other than glucose. *J. Clin. Invest.*, *69*, 1164.
14. Abraham EC, Stallings CR, Abraham A (1983): Demonstration of a minor hemoglobin with modified alpha chains and additional modified hemoglobins in normal and diabetic adults. *Biochim. Biophys. Acta*, *744*, 335.
15. Day JF, Thornburg RW, Thorpe SR, Baynes JW (1979): Nonenzymatic glycosylation of rat albumin. *J. Biol. Chem.*, *254*, 9394.
16. Day JF, Thorpe SR, Baynes JW (1979): Nonenzymatically glycosylated albumin. *J. Biol. Chem.*, *254*, 595.
17. Doelhoefer R, Wieland OH (1979): Glycosylation of serum albumin: elevated glycosyl-albumin in diabetic patients. *Fed. Eur. Biol. Soc. Lett.*, *103*, 282.
18. Eble AS, Thorpe SR, Baynes JW (1983): Nonenzymatic glycosylation and glucose dependent cross linking of protein. *J. Biol. Chem.*, *258*, 9406.
19. Poffenbarger PL, Megna AT (1979): In: *Red Blood Cell and Lens Metabolism*, p. 485. Editor: S.U. Strivastava. Elsevier/North-Holland, New York.
20. Friedman M (1982): Chemically reactive and unreactive lysine as an index of browning. *Diabetes*, *31*, *Suppl. 3*, 5.
21. Ulrich P, Ponger S, Benesader A, Cerami A (1984): Aging of proteins, the Furoyl imidazole crosslink as a key advanced glycosylation event (Abstract). *Fed. Proc.*, *43*, 1487.
22. Monnier VM, Cerami A (1982): Nonenzymatic glycosylation and browning in diabetes and aging: studies on lens proteins. *Diabetes*, *31*, *Suppl. 3*, 57.
23. Dasai K, Nakamura T, Kase N et al (1983): Increased glycosylation of proteins from cataractous lenses in diabetes. *Diabetologia*, *25*, 36.
24. Kohn RR, Schnider SL (1982): Glucosylation of human collagen. *Diabetes*, *31*, *Suppl. 3*, 47.
25. Yue DK, McLennan S, Delbridge L et al (1983): The thermal stability of collagen in diabetic rats: Correlation with severity of diabetes and non-enzymatic glycosylation. *Diabetologia*, *24*, 282.
26. Kohn RR, Cerami A, Monnier VM (1984): Collagen aging in vitro by nonenzymatic glycosylation and browning. *Diabetes*, *33*, 57.
27. Blouquet Y, Senan C, Rosa J (1983): An automatic method for determination of glycosylated hemoglobins using low-pressure liquid chromatography. *J. Chromatogr. Biomed. Appl.*, *275*, 41.
28. Yue DK, McLennan S, Church DB, Turtle JR (1982): The measurement of glycosylated hemoglobin in man and animals by aminophenylboronic acid affinity chromatography. *Diabetes*, *31*, 701.
29. Gould BJ, Hall PM, Cook JGH (1982): Measurement of glycosylated haemoglobins using an affinity chromatography method. *Clin. Chim. Acta*, *125*, 41.
30. Klenk DC, Hermanson GT, Krohn RI et al (1982): Determination of glycosylated hemoglobin by affinity chromatography: Comparison with colorimetric and ion-exchange methods, and effects of common interferences. *Clin. Chem.*, *28*, 2088.
31. Vlassara H, Brownlee M, Cerami A (1982): Assessment of diabetic control by measurement of urinary glycopeptides. *Diabetologia*, *23*, 252.

32. Little RR, England JD, Wiedmeyer HM, Goldstein DE (1983): Glycosylated hemoglobin measured by affinity chromatography: Microsample collection and room-temperature storage. *Clin. Chem.*, *29*, 1080.
33. Abraham EC, Perry RE, Stallings M (1983): Application of affinity chromatography for separation and quantitation of glycosylated hemoglobins. *J. Lab. Clin. Med.*, *102*, 187.
34. Garlick RL, Mazer JS, Higgins PJ, Bunn HF (1983): Characterization of glycosylated hemoglobins. Relevance to monitoring of diabetic control and analysis of other proteins. *J. Clin. Invest.*, *71*, 1062.
35. Herold DA, Boyd JC, Bruns DE et al (1983): Measurement of glycosylated hemoglobins using boronate affinity chromatography. *Ann. Clin. Lab. Sci.*, *13*, 482.
36. Middle FA, Bannister A, Bellingham AJ, Dean PDG (1983): Separation of glycosylated haemoglobins using immobilized phenylboronic acid. Effect of ligand concentration, column operating conditions, and comparison with ion-exchange and isoelectric focusing. *Biochem. J.*, *209*, 771.
37. Curtiss LK, Witztum JL (1983): A novel method for generating region-specific monoclonal antibodies to modified proteins. Application to the identification of human glucosylated low density lipoproteins. *J. Clin. Invest.*, *72*, 1427.
38. Johnson RN, Metcalf PA, Baker JR (1982): Fructosamine: a new approach to the estimation of serum glycosylprotein. An index of diabetic control. *Clin. Chim. Acta*, *127*, 87.
39. Baker JR, O'Connor JP, Metcalf PA, Lawson MR, Johnson RN (1983): Clinical usefulness of estimation of serum fructosamine concentration as a screening test for diabetes mellitus. *Br. Med. J.*, *287*, 863.
40. Walinder O, Ronquist G, Fager PJ (1982): New spectrophotometric method for the determination of hemoglobin A_1 compared with a microcolumn technique. *Clin. Chem.*, *28*, 96.
41. Duncan RW, Gilham PT (1975): Isolation of transfer RNA iso-acceptors by chromatography on dihydroxy-boryl-substituted cellulose, polyacrylamide, and glass. *Anal. Biochem.*, *66*, 532.
42. Weith HL, Wiebers JL, Gilham PT (1980): Synthesis of cellulose derivatives containing the dihydroxyboryl group and a study of their capacity to form specific complexes with sugars and nucleic acid components. *Biochemistry*, *9*, 4396.
43. Malia AK, Hermanson GT, Krohn RI et al (1981): Preparation and use of a boronic acid affinity support for separation and quantitation of glycosylated hemoglobins. *Anal. Lett.*, *14*, 649.
44. Peterson CM, Jovanovic L, Raskin P, Goldstein DE (1984): A comparative evaluation of glycosylated hemoglobin assays: Feasibility of references and standards. *Diabetologia*, *26*, 214.
45. Javid J, Pettis, PK, Koenig RJ, Cerami A (1978): Immunological characterization and quantification of HbA_{1c}. *Br. J. Haematol.*, *38*, 329.
46. Hodge JE (1955): The Amadori rearrangement. *Adv. Carbohydr. Chem.*, *10*, 169.
47. Kennedy L, Mehl TD, Elder E et al (1982): Nonenzymatic glycosylation of serum and plasma proteins. *Diabetes*, *31*, *Suppl. 3*, 52.

48. Nakayama H, Manda N, Komori K et al (1982): Studies on the determination of glucosylated albumin using affinity chromatography. *J. Jpn. Diabetes Soc.*, *25*, 963.
49. Nakayama H, Manda N, Komori K et al (1982): Measurement of glucosylated serum proteins using affinity chromatography. *J. Jpn. Diabetes Soc.*, *25*, 1011.
50. Gragnoli G, Tanganelli I, Signorini AM et al (1982) Non-enzymatic glycosylation of serum proteins as an indicator of diabetic control. *Acta Diabetol. Lat.*, *19*, 161.
51. Manda N, Nakayama H, Aoki S et al (1982): Determination of glucosylated albumin and its clinical significance in diabetes mellitus. *J. Jpn. Diabetes Soc.*, *25*, 691.
52. Murtiashaw MH, Young JE, Strickland AL et al (1983): Measurement of nonenzymatically glucosylated serum protein by an improved thiobarbituric acid assay. *Clin. Chim. Acta*, *130*, 177.
53. Mehl TD, Wenzel SE, Russell B et al (1983): Comparison of two indices of glycemic control in diabetic subjects: Glycosylated serum protein and hemoglobin. *Diabetes Care*, *6*, 34.
54. Jones IR, Owens DR, Williams S et al (1983): Glycosylated serum albumin: An intermediate index of diabetic control. *Diabetes Care*, *6*, 501.
55. Jovanovic L, Peterson CM, Saxena BB et al (1980): Feasibility of maintaining normal glucose profiles in insulin-dependent pregnant diabetic women. *Am. J. Med.*, *68*, 105.
56. Yatscoff RW, Braidwood JL (1982): Comparison of column chromatographic, colorimetric and electrophoretic methods for determination of glycosylated hemoglobin (HbA). *Clin. Biochem.*, *15*, 302.
57. Lee LPK, Arnott B, Feng M, Hynie I (1982): Comparison of four commercial methods for the determination of fast hemoglobins. *Clin. Biochem.*, *15*, 230.
58. Dahl-Jorgensen K, Larsen AE (1982): HbA1 determination by agar gel electrophoresis after elimination of labile HbA1: A comparison with ion-exchange chromatography. *Scand. J. Clin. Lab. Invest.*, *42*, 27.
59. Hammons GT, Junger K, McDonald JM, Ladenson JH (1982): Evaluation of three minicolumn procedures for measuring hemoglobin A1. *Clin. Chem.*, *28*, 1775.
60. Castagnola M, Caradonna P, Salvi ML et al (1983): The chromatographic separation of glycosylated haemoglobins: A comparison between macro- and micromethods. *J. Clin. Chem. Clin. Biochem.*, *21*, 233.
61. Mortensen HB, Nielsen L, Soegaard U et al (1983): Comparison of six assays for glycosylated haemoglobin determination. *Scand. J. Clin. Lab. Invest.*, *43*, 357.
62. Cachon AM, Ghaddab M, Ketzis A et al (1982): Fast fluctuations of glycosylated hemoglobins. I. Implications for the preparation and storage of samples for hemoglobin A1c determinations. *Clin. Chim. Acta*, *121*, 125.
63. Little RR, England JD, Wiedmeyer HM, Goldstein DE (1983): Effects of whole blood storage on results for glycosylated hemoglobin as measured by ion-exchange chromatography, affinity chromatography, and colorimetry. *Clin. Chem.*, *29*, 1113.
64. Nathan DM, Avezzano E, Palmer JL (1982): Rapid method for eliminating

labile glycosylated hemoglobin from the assay for hemoglobin A1. *Clin. Chem.*, *28*, 512.

65. Bisse E, Berger W, Fluckiger R (1982): Quantitation of glycosylated hemoglobin. Elimination of labile glycohemoglobin during sample hemolysis at pH 5. *Diabetes*, *31*, 630.
66. Maquart FX, Poynard JP, Leutenegger M, Borel JP (1982): On the importance of a prolonged dialysis for haemoglobin A1c determination. *Clin. Chim. Acta, 121*, 393.
67. Shenouda FS, Cockram CS, Baron MD (1982): Importance of short-term changes in glycosylated haemoglobin. *Br. Med. J., 284*, 1084.
68. Jury DR, Baker JR, Bunn PJ (1983): Clinical importance of the reversible fraction of haemoglobin A1c in type 2 (non-insulin-dependent) diabetes. *Diabetologia*, *25*, 313.
69. Mortensen HB, Marshall MO (1983): Effect of saline incubation on red cell content of glucosylated haemoglobins studied by iso-electric focusing. *Clin. Chim. Acta, 132*, 213.
70. Daneman D, Luley N, Becker DJ (1982): Diurnal glucose-dependent fluctuations in glycosylated hemoglobin levels in insulin-dependent diabetes. *Metab. Clin. Exp.*, *31*, 989.
71. Tibi L, Young RJ, Smith AF (1982): Clinical implications of labile HbA1 as assayed by the electrophoretic method. *Clin. Chim. Acta*, *126*, 257.
72. Ukena T, Merrill E, Morgan C (1982): An analysis of the importance of the 'labile' fraction of glycosylated hemoglobin as determined by a minicolumn method. *Am. J. Clin. Pathol.*, *78*, 724.
73. Peterson CM, Koenig RJ, Jones RL et al (1977): Correlation of serum triglyceride levels and hemoglobin A_{1c} concentrations in diabetes mellitus. *Diabetes*, *26*, 507.
74. Schmitt JK, Poole JR, Lewis SB et al (1982): Hemoglobin A_1 correlates with the ratio of low- to high-density-lipoprotein cholesterol in normal weight type II diabetics. *Metab. Clin. Exp.*, *31*, 1084.
75. Richard L, Delaunay J, Dorleac E, Gillet P (1983): Apolipoproteïnes et hémoglobine glycosylée chez le jeune diabètique insulino-dépendant. *Arch. Fr. Pédiatr.*, *40*, 11.
76. Jialal I, Joubert SM, Asmal AC (1982): Cholesterol, triglyceride and high-density lipoprotein cholesterol levels in non-insulin-dependent diabetes in the young. *S. Afr. Med. J.*, *61*, 393.
77. Bachem MB, Paschen K, Strobel B et al (1982): Correlations between lipoproteins and glycosylated hemoglobins in juvenile diabetes mellitus. *Klin. Wochenschr.*, *60*, 497.
78. Agardh CD, Nilsson-Ehle P, Schersten B (1982): Improvement of the plasma lipoprotein pattern after institution of insulin treatment in diabetes mellitus. *Diabetes Care*, *5*, 322.
79. Currington PN (1982): Serum high density lipoprotein cholesterol subfractions in type I (insulin-dependent) diabetes mellitus. *Clin. Chim. Acta*, *120*, 21.
80. Sosenko JM, Breslow J, Miettinin OS, Gabbay KH (1982): Hyperglycemia and plasma lipid levels: Covariations in insulin-dependent diabetes. *Diabetes Care*, *5*, 40.

81. Pfeifer MA, Brunzell JD, Best JD et al (1983): The response of plasma triglyceride, cholesterol, and lipoprotein lipase to treatment in non-insulin-dependent diabetic subjects without familial hypertriglyceridemia. *Diabetes*, *32*, 525.
82. Pietri AO, Dunn FL, Grundy SM, Raskin P (1983): The effect of continuous subcutaneous insulin infusion on very-low-density lipoprotein triglyceride metabolism in type I diabetes mellitus. *Diabetes*, *32*, 75.
83. Kim HJ, Kurup IV (1982): Nonenzymatic glycosylation of human plasma low density lipoprotein. Evidence for in vitro and in vivo glucosylation. *Metab. Clin. Exp.*, *31*, 348.
84. Witzum JL, Mahoney EM, Branks MJ et al (1982): Nonenzymatic glucosylation of low-density lipoprotein alters its biologic activity. *Diabetes*, *31*, 283.
85. Witzum JL, Steinbrecher UP, Fisher M, Kesaniemi A (1983): Nonenzymatic glucosylation of homologous low density lipoprotein and albumin renders them immunogenic in the guinea pig. *Proc. Natl Acad. Sci. USA*, *80*, 2757.
86. Witzum JL, Fisher M, Pietro T et al (1982): Nonenzymatic glucosylation of high-density lipoprotein accelerates its catabolism in guinea pigs. *Diabetes*, *31*, 1029.
87. Kraemer FB, Chen YDI, Cheung RMC, Reaven GM (1982): Are the binding and degradation of low density lipoprotein altered in Type 2 (non-insulin-dependent) diabetes mellitus? *Diabetologia*, *23*, 28.
88. Steinbrecher UP, Witzum JL (1984): Glucosylation of low density lipoproteins to an extent comparable to that seen in diabetes slows their catabolism. *Diabetes*, *33*, 130.
89. Holman RR, Dornan TL, Mayon-White V et al (1983): Prevention of deterioration of renal and sensory-nerve function by more intensive management of insulin-dependent diabetic patients. A two-year randomised prospective study. *Lancet*, *1*, 204.
90. McVerry BA, Fisher C, Hopp A, Huehns ER (1980): Production of pseudodiabetic renal glomerular changes in mice after repeated injections of glucosylated proteins. *Lancet*, *1*, 738.
91. Jeraj KP, Michael A, Mauer SM, Brown DM (1983): Glucosylated and normal human or rat albumin do not bind to renal basement membranes of diabetic and control rats. *Diabetes*, *32*, 380.
92. Cataland S, O'Dorisio TM (1983): Diabetic nephropathy. Clinical course in patients treated with the subcutaneous insulin pump. *J. Am. Med. Assoc.*, *249*, 2059.
93. Hanseus K, Hultberg B, Isaksson A, Sjoblad S (1983): Plasma and urinary beta-hexosaminidase in juvenile diabetes mellitus. *Acta Paediatr. Scand.*, *72*, 77.
94. Ditzel J (1976): Oxygen transport impairment in diabetes. *Diabetes*, *25*, *Suppl. 2*, 832.
95. Samaja M, Melotti D, Carenini A, Pozza G (1982): Glycosylated haemoglobins and the oxygen affinity of whole blood. *Diabetologia*, *23*, 399.
96. McMillan DE, Brooks SM (1982): Erythrocyte spectrin glucosylation in diabetes. *Diabetes 31*, *Suppl. 3*, 64.
97. Compagnucci P, Crechini MG, Bolli G et al (1983): Hyperglycemia alters the

physico-chemical properties of proteins in erythrocyte membranes of diabetic patients. *Horm. Metab. Res.*, *15*, 263.

98. Kanada T, Otsuji S (1983): Lower levels of erythrocyte membrane fluidity in diabetic patients. A spin label study. *Diabetes*, *37*, 585.
99. Poon PYW, Dornan TL, Orde-Peckar C et al (1982): Blood viscosity, glycaemic control and retinopathy in insulin-dependent diabetes. *Clin. Sci.*, *63*, 211.
100. Juhan-Vagua I, Vague P (1982): Properties of eyrthrocytes and platelets and the degree of diabetic control. *Nouv. Rev. Fr. Hématol.*, *24*, 191.
101. Le-Pape A, Guitton JD, Gutman N et al (1983): Nonenzymatic glycosylation of collagen in diabetes: Incidence of increased normal platelet aggregation. *Haemostasis, 13*, 36.
102. Muntoni S, Serra A, Mascia C, Songini M (1982): Dyschromatopsia in diabetes mellitus and its relation to metabolic control. *Diabetes Care*, *5*, 375.
103. Cotlier E, Sharma YR, Niven T, Brescia M (1983): Distribution of salicylate in lens and intraocular fluids and its effect on cataract formation. *Am. J. Med.*, *74*, 83.
104. Cotlier E, Fagadau W, Cicchetti DV (1983): Methods for evaluation of medical therapy of senile and diabetic cataracts. *Trans. Ophthalmol. Soc. UK*, *102*, 416.
105. Rosenbloom AL, Silverstein JH, Lexotte DC et al (1982): Limited joint mobility in diabetes mellitus of childhood. Natural history and relationship to growth impairment. *J. Pediatr.*, *101*, 874.
106. Buckingham BA, Uitto J, Sandorg C et al (1984): Scleroderma-like changes in insulin dependent diabetes mellitus: clinical and biochemical studies. *Diabetes Care*, *7*, 63.
107. Le-Pape A, Gutman N, Guitton JD et al (1983): Non enzymatic glycosylation increases platelet aggregating potency of collagen from placenta of diabetic human beings. *Biochem. Biophys. Res. Commun.*, *111*, 602.
108. Schober E, Pollak A, Coradello H, Bubec G (1982): Glycosylation of glomerular basement membrane in type 1 (insulin-dependent) diabetic children. *Diabetologia*, *23*, 485.
109. Vogt BW, Schleicher ED, Wieland OH (1982): Epsilon-amino-lysine-bound glucose in human tissucs obtained at autopsy. Increase in diabetes mellitus. *Diabetes*, *31*, 1123.
110. Peterson CM, Jones RL, Dupuis A et al (1979): Feasibility of improved blood glucose control in patients with insulin dependent diabetes mellitus. *Diabetes Care*, *2*, 239.
111. Young RJ, Ewing DJ, Clarke BF (1983): Nerve function and metabolic control in teenage diabetics. *Diabetes*, *32*, 142.
112. Mabin D, Darragon T, Menez JF et al (1982): Influence of glycemic control on peripheral nerve conduction in insulin-dependent diabetic subjects. *Rev. EEG Neurol. Physiol. Clin.*, *12*, 72.
113. Nathan DM, Francis TB, Palmer JL (1983): Effect of aspirin on determinations of glycosylated hemoglobin. *Clin. Chim. Acta*, *29*, 466.
114. Falko JM, Dorisio TM, Cataland S (1982): Spurious elevations in glycosylated hemoglobin (HbA*1*) secondary to hypertriglyceridemia. *Arch. Intern. Med.*, *142*, 1370.

115. Lederman MM, Rodman HM, McLaren GD (1983): Measurement of glycosylated hemoglobins in black diabetic patients: A note of caution. *J. Natl Med. Assoc.*, *75*, 353.
116. Paukka R, Hekali R, Akerblom HK et al (1982): Haemoglobin Hijiyama: A haemoglobin variant found in connection with glycosylated haemoglobin estimation in a Finnish diabetic boy. *Clin. Chim. Acta*, *121*, 51.
117. Krause JR, Stolc V, Campbell E (1982): The effect of hemoglobin F upon glycosylated hemoglobin determinations. *Am. J. Clin. Pathol.*, *78*, 767.
118. Bernstein RM, Freedman DB, Liyanage SP, Dandona P (1982): Glycosylated haemoglobin in rheumatoid arthritis. *Ann. Rheum. Dis.*, *41*, 604.
119. Jialal I, Joubert SM, Kendall D (1982): Fasting plasma glucose and glycosylated haemoglobin levels in the assessment of diabetic control in non-insulin-dependent diabetes in the young. *S. Afr. Med. J.*, *62*, 889.
120. Davis RE, McCann VJ, Nicol DJ (1983): Influence of iron-deficiency anaemia on the glycosylated haemoglobin level in a patient with diabetes mellitus. *Med. J. Austr.*, *1*, 40.
121. Eschwege E, Saddi R, Wacjman H et al (1982): Haemoglobin A1c in patients on venesection therapy for haemochromatosis. *Diabète Métabol.*, *8*, 137.
122. Panzer S, Kronik G, Lechner K et al (1982): Glycosylated hemoglobins (GHb): An index of red cell survival. *Blood*, *59*, 1348.
123. Peer G, Graff E, Amir C, Aviram A (1982): Rapid changes in glycosylated hemoglobin induced by hemodialysis. *Isr. J. Med. Sci.*, *18*, 960.
124. Panzetta G, Bassetto MA, Feller P (1983): Micro-chromatographic measurement of hemoglobin A_1 in uremia. *Clin. Nephrol.*, *20*, 259.
125. Orchard TJ, Daneman D, Becker DJ et al (1982): Glycosylated hemoglobin: A screening test for diabetes mellitus? *Previews in Med.*, *11*, 595.
126. Verillo A, De-Teresa A, Golia R, Nunziata V (1983): The relationship between glycosylated haemoglobin levels and various degrees of glucose intolerance. *Diabetologia*, *24*, 391.
127. Kesson CM, Young RE, Talwar D et al (1982): Glycosylated hemoglobin in the diagnosis of non-insulin dependent diabetes mellitus. *Diabetes Care*, *5*, 395.
128. Chen C, Glagov S, Mako M et al (1983): Post-mortem glycosylated hemoglobin (HbA_{1c}): Evidence for a history of diabetes mellitus. *Ann. Clin. Lab. Sci.*, *13*, 407.
129. Husband DJ, Alberti KGMM, Julian DG (1983): 'Stress' hyperglycaemia during acute myocardial infarction: An indicator of pre-existing diabetes. *Lancet*, *2*, 179.
130. Riddle MC, Hart J (1982): Hyperglycemia, recognized and unrecognized, as a risk factor for stroke and transient ischemic attacks. *Stroke*, *13*, 356.
131. Brunner H, Schmut O, Gaschinger C (1982): HbA_1 as a parameter of progression of diabetic retinopathy. *Klin. Monatsbl. Augenheilkd.*, *181*, 326.
132. Wright AD, Nicholson HD, Pollock A et al (1983): Spontaneous abortion and diabetes mellitus. *Postgrad. Med. J.*, *59*, 295.
133. Sosenko JM, Kitzmiller JL, Fluckiger R et al. (1982) Umbilical cord glycosylated hemoglobin in infants of diabetic mothers: relationship to neonatal hypoglycemia, macrosomia, and cord serum c-peptide. *Diabetes Care*, *5*, 566.

134. Cardonna P, Piccaro M, Castagnola M, Moneta E (1982): Glycosylated hemoglobin in preeclampsia. *G. Ital. Diabetol. 2*, 117.
135. Roberts AB, Baker JR, Court DJ et al (1983): Fructosamine in diabetic pregnancy. *Lancet*, *2*, 998.

The Diabetes Annual/1
K.G.M.M. Alberti and L.P. Krall, editors

ISBN 0444 90 343 7
$0.85 per article per page (transactional system)
$0.20 per article per page (licensing system)

12 Pancreas transplantation in man

DAVID E.R. SUTHERLAND, DAVID KENDALL, FREDERICK C. GOETZ AND JOHN S. NAJARIAN

The application of pancreas transplantation for the treatment of diabetes mellitus has increased dramatically in recent years (1). More pancreas transplants were performed in the 2-year period from January 1, 1982 to December 31, 1983 than in the preceding 16 years since the first transplant performed by Kelly and Lillehei and associates in 1966 (2).

There is convincing evidence that the complications of diabetes are secondary to disordered metabolism (3), and many diabetologists are now making intense efforts to maintain euglycemia in diabetic patients (4). New methods of exogenous insulin delivery are currently being employed in attempts to maintain nearly constant euglycemia. However, these techniques have risks, specifically hypoglycemia (5). Pancreas transplantation is the most physiological approach to the treatment of diabetes and maintenance of euglycemia. Clinical transplantation has had limited application because of technical and immunological problems, but these problems are gradually being overcome, and the number of successful transplants has increased in recent years.

The American College of Surgeons/National Institutes of Health (ACS/NIH) Organ Transplant Registry received information on 57 pancreas transplants in 55 diabetic patients from December 17, 1966 to June 30, 1977 when the Registry closed (6). Three additional pancreas transplants (one primary, two secondary) performed in 1976 were not reported to the ACS/NIH Registry, but to the new International Human Pancreas Transplant Registry (7). The new Registry has also compiled data on all known cases of pancreas transplantation since July 1, 1977 (1) (Table 1). The information on vascularized pancreas transplant cases reported to the Registry from December 17, 1966 through December 31, 1983 is summarized in the following section. The experience at the University of Minnesota, where more than 25% of the transplants have been performed (8), is described in a subsequent section.

TABLE 1. *Pancreas transplant experience of individual institutions reporting ⩾ 10 cases between July 1, 1977 and December 31, 1983*

Institution	No. of transpl. performed (pts)	Reported to be functioning[a]	
		No. pts	No. of months (technique[b])
Minnesota	86 (75)	23	54, 59, 70 (open peritoneal); 8, 12, 18, 20, 28, 41 (duct-inj.); 5, 5, 9, 10, 10, 10, 13, 13, 15, 19, 22, 29, 31, 33 (enteric)
Lyon	43 (41)	12	2, 4, 5, 6, 9, 10, 10, 10, 15, 23, 27, 35 (duct-inj.)
Stockholm	23 (22)	3	13, 26, 30 (enteric)
Munich	22 (21)	11	3, 5, 7, 7, 7, 9, 12, 13, 13, 23, 33 (duct-inj.)
Cambridge	17 (16)	3	7, 16 (enteric); 55 (duct-inj.)
Detroit	17	4	5 (ligation; 5, 6, 14 (duct-inj.)
Zurich	15	4	4, 5, 35, 44 (duct-inj.)
Cincinnati	12 (10)	3	3, 19 (urinary); 27 (duct-inj.)
Birmingham	12	3	26, 32, 36 (duct-inj.)
Wisconsin	10	3	3, 10, 13 (urinary)
⩽ 8 cases	81 (78)	16	5, 5, 7, 7, 12, 13, 13, 14, 18 (enteric); 12 (urinary); 5, 6, 8, 10, 15, 41 (duct-inj.)
Total	338 (317)	85	2–71 months

[a] Recipients insulin-independent, assuming continuous function, of cases reported to be functioning between March 1984 and May 1984.
[b] For drainage or occlusion of exocrine secretion.

Pancreas transplant registry

Number of transplants and overall results

From December 17, 1966 to December 31, 1983, 398 pancreas transplants were performed in 373 diabetic patients at 48 institutions (Fig. 1). Of these, 361 transplants were from cadaver (336 primary, 23 secondary and 2 tertiary grafts) and 37 were from living related donors (all primary grafts). The 338 transplants performed since July 1, 1977 were placed in 317 patients (Table 1). One patient each from Stockholm and Lyon had had previous transplants recorded by the ACS/NIH Registry.

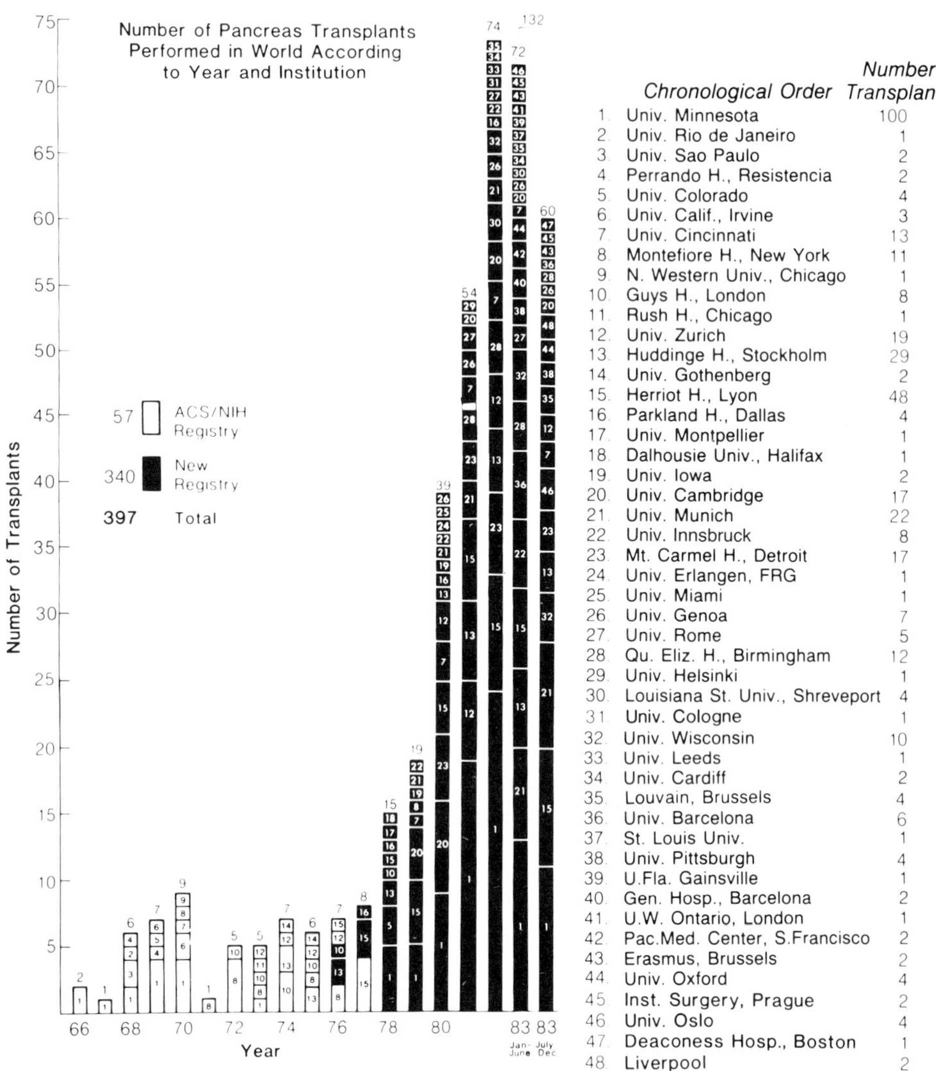

FIG. 1. *Number of pancreas transplants by year and institution reported to the Registries between December 17, 1966 and December 31, 1983. Each institution is assigned a number according to the chronological order by which they did their first transplant. One transplant performed at institution No. 37 in the last half of 1983 is not included in this figure.*

The institutions with the largest and most recent experiences, Minnesota (9, 10), Lyon (11), Stockholm (12), Munich (13), Cambridge (14), Detroit (15), Zurich (16), Cincinnati (17), Birmingham (18), and Wisconsin (19), have published the details on all except their latest cases of pancreas transplantation. Published reports on pancreas transplants at most other institutions are referenced in an earlier comprehensive review article (20).

Eighty-five patients are currently (May, 1984) listed in the Registry as having functioning grafts. Of these, at least 46 have been insulin-independent for more than one year. Twelve other grafts have functioned for more than one year, and then either failed and the patients resumed exogenous insulin, or the recipients died with functioning grafts. The other 295 grafts ceased to function at less than one year because of either technical complications, rejection or death of the recipients. All the grafts that are currently functioning were transplanted since 1978.

The actuarial patient and graft survival rate curves for all pancreas transplant cases performed between 1966–1983 are shown in Figure 2A. Overall,

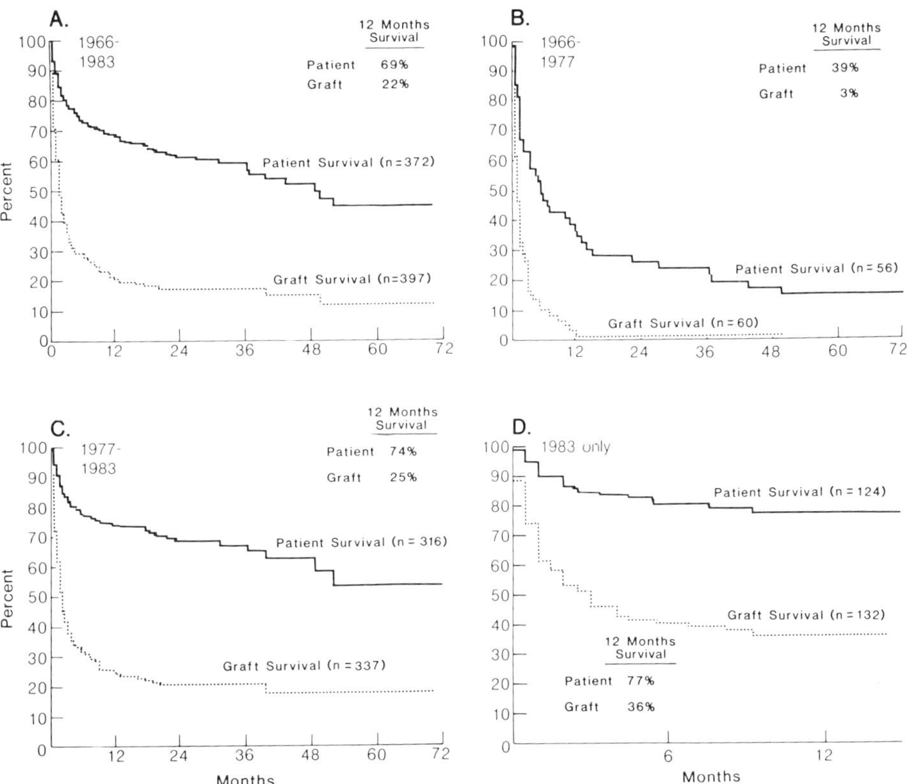

FIG. 2. *Patient and graft functional survival rates for Pancreas Transplant Registry cases according to era. (A) 1966–83; (B) 1966–77; (C) 1977–83; and (D) 1983 only.*

69% of the recipients were alive and 22% were insulin-independent at 1 year post-transplant. The results have improved in recent years, and transplantation has definitely become safer. Of 60 grafts placed in 56 patients before July 1, 1977, the one year actuarial patient survival rate was 39% and the graft survival rate was only 3% (Fig. 2B). In contrast, of the 317 patients who received transplants from July 1, 1977 to December 31, 1983, 226 are currently said to be alive, and the 1-year patient survival rate was 74%; the 1-year graft survival rate during this period was 25% (Fig. 2C). For 1983 only (133 transplants in 125 recipients), the 1-year patient survival rate was 77% and the graft survival rate was 36% (Fig. 2D).

Most recipients of successful pancreas transplants are euglycemic. The metabolic test results can, however, be quite variable (21–23). Examples of the types of test results in individual pancreas transplant recipients are given with the University of Minnesota experience in a following section.

Pancreas transplant results according to association with kidney grafts

The majority of pancreas transplant recipients have had diabetic nephropathy and/or other far advanced complications of diabetes. Kidney transplants were performed in 248 of the 317 recipients (78%) of 338 pancreas grafts transplanted since July 1, 1977.

The pancreas transplant success rates have been approximately the same in non-uremic, non-kidney-transplant recipients and in kidney transplant recipients (Fig. 3). There also were no differences in the functional survival rates of pancreas grafts transplanted simultaneously with or after a kidney transplant. One-year actuarial graft survival rates were 27% in recipients

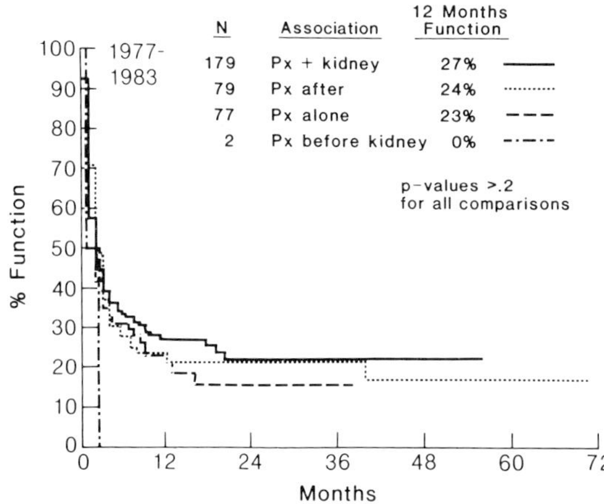

FIG. 3. *Registry data on functional graft survival rates for 337 pancreas transplants performed between July 1, 1977 and December 31, 1983 according to association with kidney transplants.*

of simultaneous kidney transplants, 24% in recipients of previous kidney transplants, and 23% for non-uremic, non-kidney-transplant patients (P > 0.2). Both recipients of kidney grafts after a pancreas transplant lost pancreas graft function before the kidney transplant.

There is no evidence that pancreas transplants have improved the outcome of kidney transplants in uremic diabetic patients. In fact, the patient and kidney graft survival rates in pancreas transplant recipients with end-stage diabetic nephropathy (24) are less than those reported for diabetic uremic recipients of kidney transplants alone (25, 26). Thus, correction of uremia by kidney transplantation is more beneficial and more important than total endocrine replacement therapy in diabetic patients with renal failure.

Pancreas transplant results according to technique

Twenty-nine of the transplants performed in the world between July 1, 1977 and December 31, 1983 were whole pancreas grafts (5 with and 24 without the duodenum). The other 309 were segmental (hemi-pancreas) grafts (Fig. 4). The provisions made for the management of the exocrine secretions form the most important issue in pancreas transplantation. Several methods for duct management have been used. Suppression of exocrine function and obstruction of residual excretions by polymer injection of the duct (27) has been the most widely used technique; 198 of 337 grafts transplanted since July 1, 1977 were duct-injected (59%). The complication rate for polymer injection remains relatively low, but fibrosis, induced by the injected agent, can involve the islets and might lead to graft failure (28). Duct ligation was used in the first pancreas transplant case (2) and has been used sporadically since July 1, 1977 (11 cases). The pancreatic duct has also been left open to drain freely into the peritoneum (29), and the secretions are absorbed if the pancreatic enzymes are not activated (16 cases since July 1, 1977). Currently, pancreatico-enterostomy (12, 30, 31) or urinary drainage (19) are gaining in popularity (82 and 25 cases, respectively, since July 1, 1977). Except for duct ligation, all techniques have been associated with long term graft function (Fig. 5). The 1-year actuarial functional survival rates of pancreas grafts transplanted since July 1, 1977 were 28% with enteric drainage, 25% with duct injection, 21% for urinary drainage (12 bladder, 13 ureter) and 16% for open duct, but the differences are not statistically significant (P > 0.1).

Pancreas transplant results according to immunosuppression

Before June 30, 1977 all pancreas transplant recipients were treated with azathioprine. Since July 1, 1977, cyclosporin has been the principal immunosuppressant in 156 recipients of pancreas allografts, and 49 currently

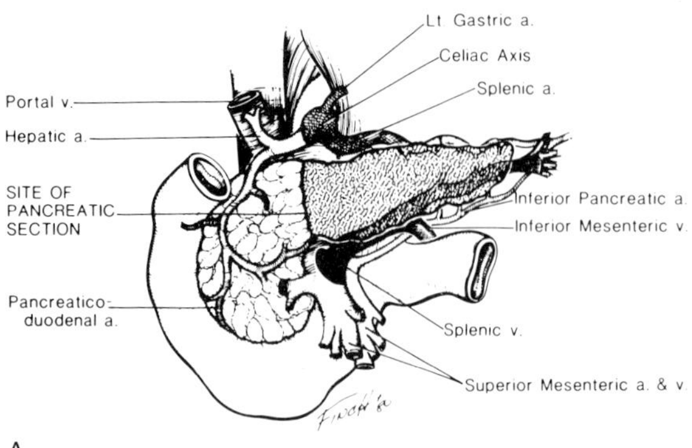

A

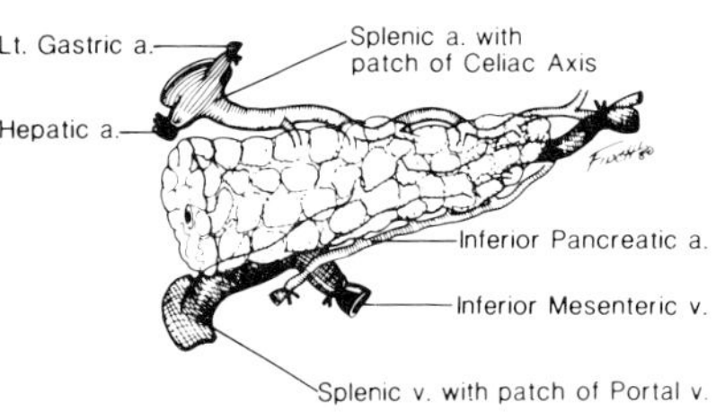

B

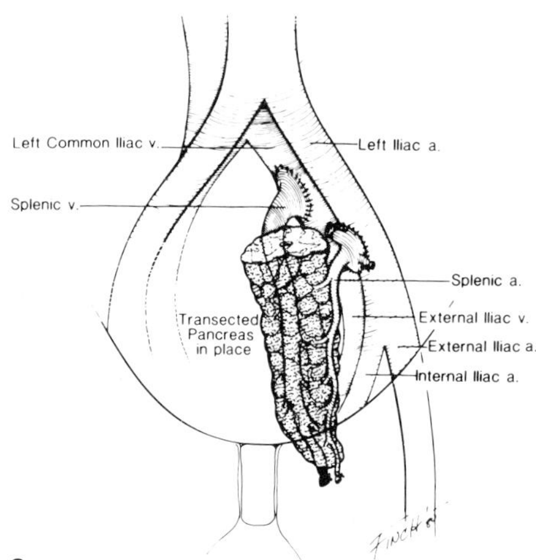

C

FIG. 4. *Basic technique of segmental pancreas transplantation: (A) Donor anatomy. (B) Graft after excision from cadaver donor. (C) Graft after implantation in recipient. See text and Table 2 for methods to handle exocrine secretions. Reproduced from Sutherland (Diabetologia, 20, 435, 1981) by courtesy of the Editors.*

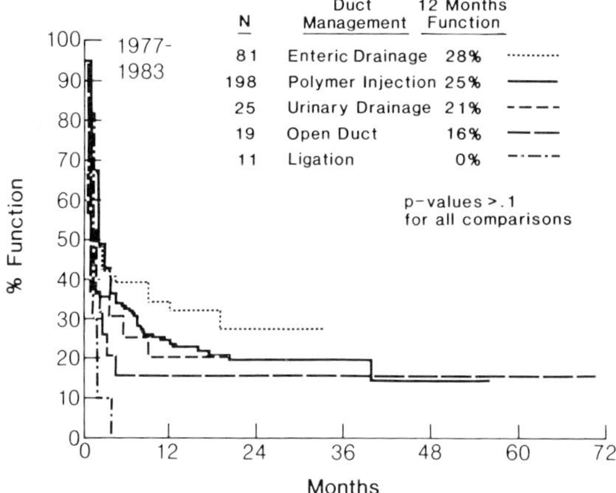

FIG. 5. *Registry data on pancreas graft functional survival rates according to technique of duct management in 337 transplants performed between July 1, 1977 and December 31, 1983.*

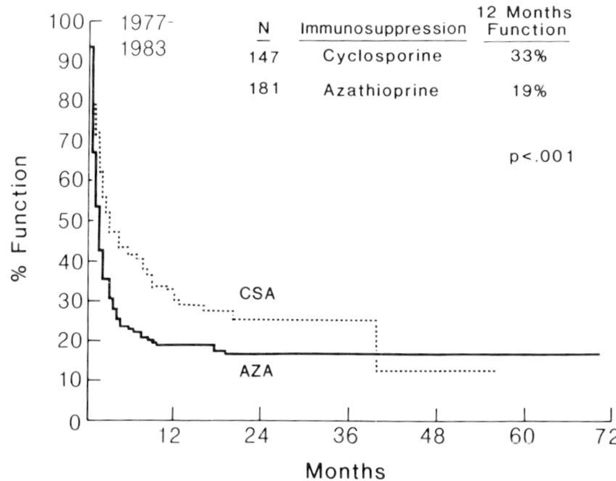

FIG. 6. *Functional graft survival rates for pancreas transplants according to recipient immunosuppression (cyclosporin vs. azathioprine) for cases reported to the Registry between July 1, 1977 and December 31, 1983.*

have functioning grafts. Azathioprine has been the basic immunosuppressant in 182 patients transplanted since July 1, 1977, and 36 currently have functioning grafts. An actuarial analysis according to immunosuppression (Fig. 6) showed that 1-year pancreas allograft functional survival rates were significantly higher ($P < 0.001$) in all patients treated with cyclosporin (33%) than with azathioprine (19%). When technically successful transplants only were considered, the 1-year allograft function rates in cyclosporin (n = 143) and azathioprine (n = 151) treated recipients were 37% and 23% respectively ($P < 0.001$).

Pancreas transplant results according to graft preservation

Many of the pancreas grafts have been transplanted immediately following removal from the donor. However, the interval between removal from the donor and transplantation to the recipient was reported on 224 grafts preserved by hypothermic storage in electrolyte solutions. An actuarial analysis showed a statistically higher functional survival rate (P = 0.021) for grafts preserved less than 6 hours than for those stored more than 6 hours (Fig. 7). The longer storage times were associated with a higher percentage of early (less than 7 days) graft failures, but late losses were nearly equivalent. Thus, at one year the differences in graft survival rates were insignificant, 19% for the <6 hour and 20% for the >6 hour preservation groups. Indeed an earlier analysis showed that the immediate function rates were similar for all storage times up to 24 hours (32). The capacity to preserve pancreas grafts has greatly facilitated the logistical aspects of pancreas transplantation (33).

Pancreas transplant experience at the University of Minnesota

Transplants of immediately vascularized pancreas grafts or of free grafts of islet tissue have been made almost continuously at the University of Minnesota since 1966 (34, 35). There have been two series of pancreas transplants and two series of islet transplants. In both islet transplant series (10 cases each) no recipients became insulin-independent (36, 37).

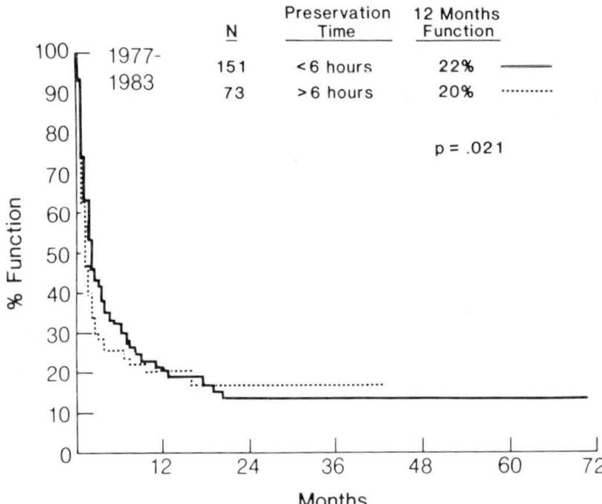

FIG. 7. *Registry data on pancreas graft functional survival rates according to duration of preservation time for transplants performed between July 1, 1977 to December 31, 1983.*

The first series of pancreas transplants was between 1966 and 1983 (9). Only one recipient survived for more than one year with a functioning pancreas graft (38). The most recent series began in July 25, 1978 (29), and through December 31, 1983, included 86 pancreas transplants performed in 75 diabetic patients. The results in this series have been periodically reported (8, 10, 30, 39, 40).

Patient population, transplant technique and immunosuppression

Of the 75 patients undergoing pancreas transplantation in the most recent University of Minnesota series, 41 had functioning renal grafts (40 allografts, 1 isograft) placed 6 months to 9 years previously for treatment of end-stage diabetic nephropathy. Thirty-four patients were non-uremic and had not received kidney grafts at the time of the pancreas transplant. Fifty-one of the 86 pancreas grafts (59%) came from cadaver donors and 35 came from living related donors. Sixty-seven grafts were segmental (all the living-related and 32 cadaveric), while 19 were cadaveric grafts of the whole pancreas as previously described (41).

All of the transplanted pancreas grafts were placed intraperitoneally. Four different techniques were used for management of exocrine secretions (Table 2). Enteric drainage into a Roux-en-Y limb of recipient jejunum is now preferred.

The immunosuppressive protocols used in our patients have been previously described (8, 42, 43). Twenty-three recipients of pancreas allografts were treated with azathioprine (AZA), prednisone and antilymphocyte globulin (ALG); 7 were treated with AZA and prednisone only; 9 were treated with cyclosporin (CSA) (and usually prednisone) after an initial course of conventional (AZA, prednisone, ALG) immunosuppression; 36 were treated with CSA and prednisone beginning immediately after transplantation, and five patients received a combination of CSA, AZA and prednisone (triple therapy) (see Table 2). Four patients, treated initially with CSA were switched to AZA between 3 and 6 months post-transplant. One of these patients had no change in graft function and is currently insulin-independent with a functioning graft longer than 2 years after transplantation. The other three had decline of graft function and resumed exogenous insulin 2 to 6 months after conversion. Fifteen grafts in the conventionally immunosuppressed patients failed for technical reasons, while 5 grafts in the CSA group were lost to technical failure.

Current status of pancreas transplant recipients at the University of Minnesota

As of May, 1984, 61 of 75 patients were alive (81%) and 23 had full (20 cases, receive no exogenous insulin) or partial (3 cases, have C-peptide

TABLE 2. *Outcome after pancreas transplantation in recent Minnesota cases according to technique, donor source and immunosuppression*

Technique	No. of transpl. (r/c)	Immuno-suppr.[a] C/A/T	Technical failures	Late loss[b] of function	Currently functioning*	
					No. of grafts	Duration in months
Duct ligation	3 (0/3)	0/3/0	3 (100%)	0 (0%)	0 (0%)	–
Open peritoneal	15 (5/10)	1/14/0	8 (53%)	4 (27%)	3 (20%)	55 (A)[c], 60 (A)[r], 71 (A)[c]
Enteric	29 (25/4)	15/8/4	8 (28%)	5 (17%)	14 (48%)	5 (T)[c], 5(T)[r], 9 (T)[c], 10 (T)[c], 10 (A)[r], 10 (C)[r], 13 (C)[r], 13 (A)[r], 15 (A)[r], 19 (C)[r], 22 (C)[r], 29 (C)[r], 31 (A)[r], 33 (C)[r]
Duct injection	39 (5/34)	29/8/1	3 (8%)	28 (72%)	6 (15%)	8 (C)[r], 12 (T)[c], 18 (A)[r], 20 (C)[c], 28 (C)[c], 42 (A)[r]
Total	86 (35/51)	43/29	22 (26%)	34 (42%)	23 (27%)	5–71

[a] All patients received prednisone in addition to either cyclosporin (C), azathioprine (A) or triple therapy (T = combination of cyclosporin and azathioprine).

[b] Does not include 4 patients with technically successful transplants (2 duct-inj., 2 enterically drained) who died with functioning grafts. As of May, 1983, 15/35 (43%) related and 8/51 (16%) cadaver grafts were functioning. Of technically successful allografts, 8/16 (50%) treated with azathioprine, 8/39 (21%) with cyclosporin, and 5/5 (100%) with triple therapy are functioning.

* Immunosuppression in parenthesis (C, A or T), and donor source: cadaver (c) or related (r), as superscripts.

levels along baseline and are no longer ketosis-prone, but require supplemental insulin to maintain normoglycemia) function of their pancreas grafts (31%). Seventeen grafts have functioned for longer than 1 year, of which 15 are still functioning, the longest for 5.9 years. Sixteen of the 23 currently functioning grafts are from living related donors (40). In 35 instances the pancreas grafts functioned for 1 to 12 months before hyperglycemia recurred and the recipients had to resume exogenous insulin. Graft biopsies performed in 16 cases at the time of or a few months after loss of function showed rejection in 13 instances (44). In 3 instances (including 2 isografts with insulitis) it appeared that diabetes and β-cell destruction had recurred independent of rejection (30, 45, 46), most likely because of an autoimmune insulitis (45, 46).

Hyperglycemia that occurred weeks or months after transplantation was presumptively diagnosed as rejection in 22 graft recipients (8 from related, 14 from cadaver donors). Rejection was treated with either an increase in prednisone dose or with administration of antilymphocyte globulin (8, 62). Three recipients of related and three recipients of cadaver grafts reverted to euglycemia after anti-rejection treatment and are currently insulin-independent.

Most of the insulin-independent patients with functioning grafts have normal or nearly normal glucose tolerance test results (8, 21, 40). However, there is great variability in the response of individual patients (Fig. 8). The patient whose graft has functioned the longest (now 71 months post-transplant) had normal glucose tolerance test results at 2, 3, and 4 years, while the results were abnormal at 1 and 5 years (Fig. 8C).

The 35 related donors of segmental pancreas grafts are currently alive. Two donors (6%) required reoperation, one for a splenectomy and one to ligate the pancreatic duct at the line of transection. Changes in glucose tolerance occurred in some donors postoperatively, but were physiologically significant only in one obese donor (47).

Comments

The current protocol for pancreas transplantation at the University of Minnesota has been derived from lessons learned during 120 attempts at endocrine replacement therapy in 102 patients since 1966. The experience includes 12 pancreaticoduodenal, 20 islet, 20 whole and 68 segmental pancreas transplants. We now offer pancreas transplantation to patients whose diabetic complications are, or potentially will be, more serious than the possible side effects of chronic immunosuppression. Thirty-four of the 75 patients transplanted since 1978 were non-uremic (45%), including 16 of 22 in 1983 (73%). Early nephropathy, or progressive retinopathy or neuropathy, were indications for pancreas transplantation in these patients. Thirteen of the 23 patients whose grafts are currently functioning (57%) had not received previous kidney grafts.

Most of our efforts have been focused on simply achieving an acceptable pancreas graft functional survival rate with a low morbidity and mortality rate. Our preference at this time is to drain exocrine pancreas secretions into a hollow viscus, and enteric drainage is the most physiologic method.

Diagnosis of rejection is particularly difficult, as noted by other groups (48). Close monitoring of plasma glucose levels and early use of a graft biopsy have been the most useful indicators of rejection in our series (8, 44).

It is important to follow recipients closely for the effect of the procedure on secondary complications. Unpublished observations on kidney biopsies in two patients followed for over 4 years following successful pancreas transplantation, suggest that progression of renal lesions can be prevented

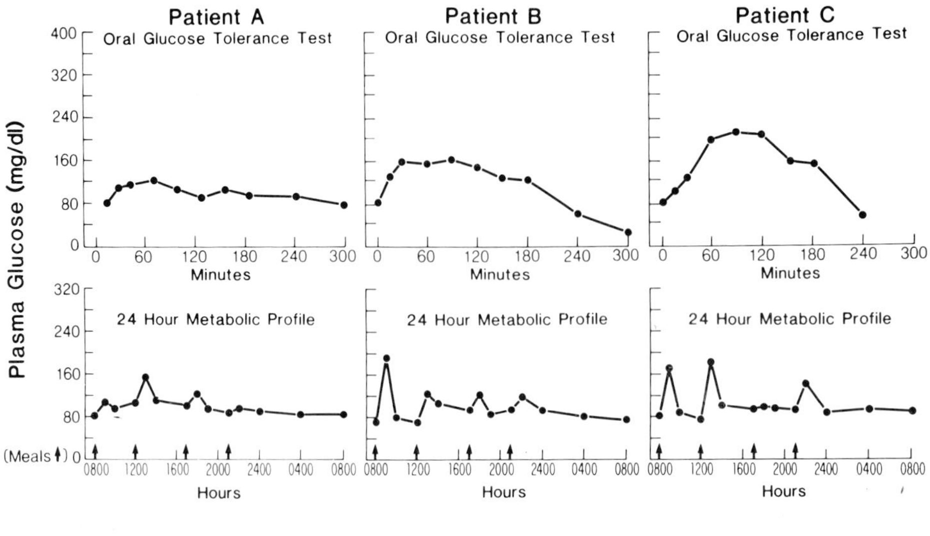

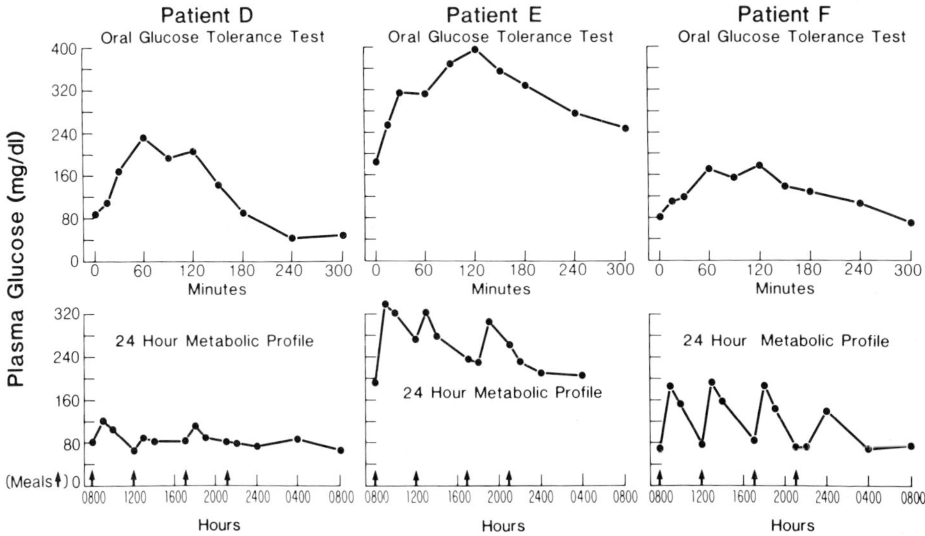

FIG. 8. *Results of metabolic studies (glucose tolerance tests and 24 hour profiles) in the absence of exogenous insulin in six recipients of segmental pancreas transplants functioning at > 12 months, illustrating the variability in response of individual patients.*

Patient A, 12 months post-transplant, has both a normal glucose tolerance test (GTT) results and a normal metabolic profile during a day of normal meals and activity. Patient B, 36 months post-transplant, is normal except for a slight hypoglycemic trend at 4–5 hours during the GTT. Patient C, at 60 months post-transplant, has an abnormal GTT with elevated 2 hour glucose value, but is *euglycemic through a day of standard meals and activity. Patient D, 24 months post-transplant, has abnormal GTT (with both hyperglycemia and hypoglycemia), but displays a normal 24 hour glucose profile. Patient E, 36 months post-transplant, has highly abnormal GTT as well as fasting and postprandial hyperglycemia during a day of normal meals and activity. Patient F, 12 months post-transplant, has a normal GTT, but an abnormal profile with elevated postprandial glucose during 24-hour profile.*

and early lesions may actually regress. Certain aspects of our program, including the use of cyclosporin for recipient immunosuppression (43) and either polymer injection (39) or pancreatico-enterostomy (30) for management of exocrine function are similar to those of other groups (12, 14, 27) applying pancreas transplantation to the treatment of diabetes. However, treatment of uremic diabetic patients at Minnesota differs from most groups performing pancreas transplantation. Kidney and pancreas grafts are not placed simultaneously. Kidney transplantation alone rehabilitates most uremic diabetics (26), and simultaneous pancreas and kidney grafting does not improve renal graft survival rates (24). Thus we delay pancreas transplantation until the renal graft is well established.

Pancreas transplantation should, if possible, be accomplished earlier in the course of the disease. However, since generalized immunosuppression is required to prevent rejection, this approach can not be taken unless the patients clearly have, or are developing, serious secondary complications.

In summary, of 86 pancreas transplants performed in 75 diabetic patients at the University of Minnesota since 1978, 23 patients currently (May 1984) have functioning pancreas grafts. Fifteen patients have functioning grafts at longer than 1 year post-transplant. Advances in immunosuppressive therapy, in surgical technique and in patient selection criteria, have been associated with a progressive increase in the success rate of pancreas transplantation at our institution (11 of 24 grafts placed in 1983 are currently functioning).

Conclusions

Nearly one-third of the pancreas transplants performed since 1966 were done in 1983, emphasizing the fact that there has been a renewed interest in pancreas transplantation in recent years. The success rate is steadily improving and long-term graft function with normal or near-normal glucose tolerance has been sustained in several patients. Eventually, pancreas transplantation could have the same impact on the treatment of diabetes as kidney transplantation has had on the treatment of end-stage renal disease. Also pancreas transplants should allow many fundamental questions related to diabetes to be answered (49).

Most pancreas transplant recipients have far advanced secondary complications. Ideally, pancreas grafting could be performed early in the stages of the disease. There is some tendency in this direction, particularly in the most recent Minnesota series.

Immunologic factors have been the greatest hindrance to successful pancreas transplantation. The use of cyclosporin has been associated with an improvement in the results of pancreas transplantation (see Fig. 6). The success rate is still much less than that reported for kidney transplantation

(14). CSA is also a generalized immunosuppressive agent with potentially adverse side effects. Nevertheless, the patient population that can be considered for pancreas transplantation has been expanded by the use of cyclosporin.

Clinical attempts at islet allotransplantation have not been successful (1). The manipulations that lead to a relatively high success rate in experimental animal models (50) have not been applied in the clinical situation. Islet transplantation is not simpler for the transplant team; it is difficult to procure a sufficient quantity of viable islet tissue from a single donor pancreas, and techniques to alter graft immunogenicity need to be made practical. If the methods currently being used in animals are effective for isolation and reduction of immunogenicity of human islets (51), a rational basis for attempts at clinical islet transplantation will be established, but it is unlikely that clinical islet transplantation will be successful in the immediate future.

Pancreas transplantations are being performed in selected diabetic patients at this time. Because generalized immunosuppression is needed to prevent rejection, pancreas transplantation is currently restricted to patients whose secondary complications of diabetes are, or predictably will be, more serious than the potential side effects of anti-rejection therapy. Patients who have had, or who require a kidney transplant, and in whom immunosuppressive therapy is obligatory meet this criterion. However, some non-uremic, non-kidney-transplant patients are also in this category, such as those with pre-proliferative retinopathy and who are thus at great risk of loss of vision.

When abrogation of a specific immune response in humans is possible, and the risks of transplantation are minimal, the limiting factor will be the availability of donor pancreases. This problem can be solved. In the United States approximately 5000 kidney transplants are done each year (52). The incidence of new cases of Type 1 diabetes is approximately 10,000 per year in the United States, and less than half of the patients with the disease develop serious complications (53).

Thus, the current kidney transplant rate is similar to the yearly incidence of complications for Type 1 diabetes. Only a small proportion of potential donors are currently used as a source of organs (54), but there is no inherent reason why donor procurement should be any more difficult for pancreas transplantation than for kidney transplantation. Measurement of joint stiffness (55) or of insulin-like growth factors (56) may identify diabetic patients who are at high risk to develop secondary complications. It could also be possible to identify diabetics who are at high risk for hypoglycemic reactions while on insulin pump or other intensified insulin therapy regimens (5). Patients with these characteristics (5, 54, 55) are the ones who are most likely to benefit from a pancreas transplant, and a sufficient number of pancreases from cadaver and related donors should be available for this select group.

In conclusion, pancreas transplantation is being applied with increasing effectiveness for the treatment of human diabetes. Islet transplantation is still only successful in the laboratory. Until islet yield can be improved and methods to reduce immunogenicity can be made practical, pancreas transplantation is the only method of total endocrine replacement therapy in diabetes that can succeed. Pancreas transplantation potentially could be applied on as large a scale as renal transplantation. Ultimately pancreas transplantation could be performed at a stage sufficiently early to prevent the development of diabetic nephropathy, and supercede kidney transplantation in the management of complication-prone diabetic patients.

Note added in proof

One transplant performed at institution No.37 (seeFig. 1), on enteric-drained graft in a recipient of a previous kidney graft, was not included in the data for Figures 1–7. It failed for technical reasons; its exclusion does not alter the results reported.

References

1. Sutherland DER (1984): Pancreas and islet transplantation registry data. *World J. Surg.*, *8*, 270.
2. Kelly WD, Lillehei RC, Merkel FK, Idezuki Y, Goetz FC (1967): Allotransplantation of the pancreas and duodenum along with the kidney in diabetic nephropathy. *Surgery*, *61*, 827.
3. Brownlee MC, Cahill GF (1979): Diabetic control and vascular complications. In: *Atherosclerotic Reviews*, *Vol. 4*, p. 29. Editors: R. Paoletti and A.M. Gatto. Raven Press, New York.
4. Ungar RH (1982): Meticulous control of diabetes: Benefits, risks and precautions. *Diabetes*, *31*, 479.
5. White N, Skor DA, Cryer PE, Levandoski PA, Bier DM, Santiago JV (1983): Identification or Type I diabetic patients at increased risk for hypoglycemia during intensive therapy. *N. Engl. J. Med.*, *308*, 485.
6. Gerrish EW (1977): *Final Newsletter, American College of Surgeons/National Institutes of Health Organ Transplant Registry*, June 30, 1977.
7. Sutherland DER (1980): International human pancreas and islet transplant registry. *Transpl. Proc.*, *12/4*, *Suppl. 2*, 229.
8. Sutherland DER, Goetz FC, Najarian JS (1984): 100 pancreas transplants at a single institution. *Ann. Surg.*, *200*, 414.
9. Lillehei RC, Ruiz JO, Acquino C, Goetz FC (1976): Transplantation of the pancreas. *Acta Endocrinol.*, *83*, *Suppl. 205*, 303.
10. Sutherland DER, Chinn PL, Goetz FC et al (1984): Minnesota experience with 85 pancreas transplants between 1978 and 1983. *World J. Surg.*, *8*, 244.
11. Dubernard JM, Traeger J, Bodi E et al (1984): Transplantation for the treat-

ment of insulin-dependent diabetes: Clinical experience with polymer-obstructed pancreatic grafts using Neoprene. *World J. Surg.*, *8*, 262.

12. Groth CG, Tyden G, Lundgren G et al (1984): Segmental pancreas transplantation with enteric exocrine diversion. *World J. Surg.*, *8*, 257.
13. Landgraf R, Abendroth D, Land W (1983): Mechanical and hormonal blockade of the pancreatic transplant function in man. *Horm. Metab. Res., Suppl.*, *13*, 57.
14. Calne RY, White DJG (1982): The use of cyclosporine in clinical organ grafting. *Ann. Surg.*, *196*, 330.
15. Toledo-Pereyra LH (1983): Pancreas transplantation. *Surg. Gynecol. Obstet.*, *157*, 49.
16. Baumgartner D, Largiader F (1984): Simultaneous renal and intraperitoneal segmental pancreatic transplantation. *World J. Surg.*, *8*, 267.
17. McMaster P, Michael J, Adu D et al (1984): Experience in human segmental pancreas transplantation. *World J. Surg.*, *8*, 253.
18. Munda R, First MR, Webb CB, Alexander JW (1984): Clinical experience with segmental pancreatic allografts. *Transpl. Proc.*, *16*, 692.
19. Cook K, Sollinger HW, Warner J et al (1983): Pancreaticocystostomy: an alternative method for exocrine drainage of segmental pancreatic allografts. *Transplantation*, *35*, 634.
20. Sutherland DER, Goetz FC, Najarian JS (1982): Pancreas organ transplantation. *Clin. Endocrinol. Metab.*, *11*, 549.
21. Sutherland DER, Najarian JS, Greenberg BZ, Senske BJ, Anderson GE, Francis RS, Goetz FC (1981): Hormonal and metabolic effects of an endocrine graft: Vascularized segmental transplantation on the pancreas in insulin-dependent patients. *Ann. Intern. Med.*, *95*, 537.
22. Chinn PL, Sutherland DER, Goetz FC, Elick BA, Najarian JS (1983): Metabolic studies in patients with long-term functioning pancreas grafts. *Diabetes*, *32*, *Suppl. 1*, 37A.
23. Pozza G, Traeger J, Dubernard JM, Serdri A, Pontiroli AE, Boss E, Malik MC, Ruitton A, Blanc N (1983): Endocrine responses of Type I (insulin-dependent) diabetic patients following successful pancreas transplantation. *Diabetologia*, *24*, 244.
24. Sutherland DER, Kendall D (1984): Clinical pancreas and islet transplant registry report. *Transpl. Proc.*, *17*, in press.
25. Standards Committee of the American Society of Transplant Surgeons (1981): Current results and expectations of renal transplantation. *J. Am. Med. Assoc.*, *246*, 133.
26. Sutherland DER, Morrow CE, Fryd DS, Ferguson RM, Simmons RL, Najarian JS (1982): Improved patient and primary renal allograft survival in uremic diabetic recipients. *Transplantation*, *34*, 319.
27. Dubernard JM, Traeger J, Neyra P, Touraine JL, Traudiant D, Blanc-Brunat N (1978): A new method of preparation of segmental pancreatic grafts for transplantation: Trials in dogs and in man. *Surgery*, *84*, 633.
28. Blanc-Brunat N, Dubernard JM, Touraine JL et al (1983): Pathology of the pancreas after intraductal neoprene injection in dogs and diabetic patients treated by pancreatic transplantation. *Diabetologia*, *25*, 97.

29. Sutherland DER, Goetz FC, Najarian JS (1979): Intraperitoneal transplantation of immediately vascularized segmental pancreatic grafts without duct ligation: A clinical trial. *Transplantation*, *28*, 485.
30. Sutherland DER, Goetz FC, Elick BA, Najarian JS (1982): Experience with 49 segmental pancreas transplants in 45 diabetic patients. *Transplantation*, *34*, 330.
31. Calne RY, White DJG, Rolles K et al (1982): Renal and segmental pancreatic grafting with drainage of exocrine secretions and initial continuous intravenous cyclosporin A in patients with insulin-dependent diabetes and renal failure. *Br. Med. J.*, *285*, 677.
32. Sutherland DER (1983): Current status of clinical pancreas and islet transplantation with comments on need for and complications of cryogenic and other preservation techniques. *Cryobiology*, *20*, 245.
33. Florack G, Sutherland DER, Chinn PL et al (1984): Clinical experience with transplantation of hypothermically preserved pancreas grafts. *Transplant. Proc.*, *16*, 153.
34. Lillehei RC, Ruiz JO, Acquino C, Goetz FC (1976): Transplantation of the pancreas. *Acta Endocrinol.*, *83*, *Suppl. 205*, 303.
35. Najarian JS, Sutherland DER, Matas AJ, Steffes MW, Goetz FC (1977): Human islet transplantation: A preliminary experience. *Transpl. Proc.*, *9*, 233.
36. Sutherland DER, Matas AJ, Najarian JS (1978): Pancreatic islet cell transplantation. *Surg. Clin. North Am.*, *58*, 365.
37. Sutherland DER, Matas AJ, Goetz FC, Najarian JS (1980): Transplantation of dispersed pancreatic islet tissue in humans: Autografts and allografts. *Diabetes*, *29*, *Suppl. 1*, 34.
38. Sutherland DER, Goetz FC, Carpenter AM et al (1979): Pancreaticoduodenal grafts: Clinical and pathological observations in uremic versus nonuremic recipients. In: *Transplantation and Clinical Immunology*, *Vol. 10*, pp. 90–195. Editors: J.L. Touraine et al. Excerpta Medica, Amsterdam.
39. Sutherland DER, Goetz FC, Rynasiewicz JJ, Baumgartner D, White DC, Elick BA, Najarian JS (1981): Segmental pancreas transplantation from living related and cadaver donors: A clinical experience. *Surgery*, *90*, 159.
40. Sutherland DER, Goetz FC, Najarian JS (1984): Pancreas transplants from related donors. *Transplantation*, in press.
41. Sutherland DER, Chinn PL, Elick BA et al (1984): Maximization of islet mass in pancreas grafts by near total or total whole organ excision without duodenum from cadaver donors. *Transplant. Proc.*, *16*, 115.
42. Sutherland DER, Chinn PL, Goetz FC et al (1983): Experience with cyclosporine vs. Azathioprine for pancreas transplantation. *Transplant. Proc.*, *15*, 2606.
43. Rynasiewicz JJ, Sutherland DER, Ferguson RM et al (1982): Cyclosporin A for immunosuppression: Observations in rat heart, pancreas and islet allograft models and in human renal and pancreas transplantation. *Diabetes*, *31*, *Suppl. 4*, 92.
44. Sibley RK, Mukai K (1983): Pathological features in 29 segmental pancreas transplants in 27 diabetic patients. *Lab. Invest.*, *48*, 78A.

45. Sutherland DER, Sibley RK, Chinn PL et al (1984): Identical twin pancreas transplants: Reversal and recurrence of pathogenesis in Type I diabetes. *Clin. Res., 32/2*, 561A.
46. Sibley RK, Sutherland DER, Goetz FC (1984): Recurrence of Type I diabetes mellitus in pancreatic allografts and isografts. *Lab. Invest., 50*, 54A.
47. Chinn P, Sutherland DER, Goetz FC, Elick BA, Najarian JS (1984): Metabolic effects of hemipancreatectomy in living related graft donors. *Transplant. Proc., 16*, 11.
48. Secchi A, Pontiroli AE, Traeger J et al (1983): A method of detection of graft failure in pancreas transplantation. *Transplantation, 35*, 344.
49. Barker CF, Naji A, Perloff LJ, Dafoe DC, Bartlett S (1982): Invited commentary: An overview of pancreas transplantation – biologic aspects. *Surgery, 92*, 113.
50. Faustman D, Hauptfeld V, Lacy P, Davie J (1981): Prolongation of murine islet allograft survival by pretreatment of islets with antibody directed to Ia determinants. *Proc. Natl Acad. Sci. USA 78, 8*, 5156.
51. Clark WH (Ed) (1982): Proceedings of a workshop on Preventing Rejection of Transplanted Pancreas or Islets. *Diabetes, 31, Suppl. 4*, 1.
52. Health Care Financing Administration (HCFA) Office of Special Programs (1981): *End-Stage Renal Disease Program Medical Information System, Facility Survey Tables. January 1–December 31*, 1981. Department of Health and Human Services, USA, HCFA.
53. West KM (1978): *Epidemiology of Diabetes and its Vascular Lesions.* Elsevier, New York.
54. Bart KJ, Macon EJ, Whittier FC, Baldwin PJ, Blaunt JH (1981): Cadaveric kidneys for transplantation. A paradox of shortage in the face of plenty. *Transplantation, 31*, 374.
55. Rosenbloom AL, Silverstein JH, Lezotte DC, Richardson K, McCallum RN (1981): Limited joint mobility in childhood diabetes mellitus indicates increased risk for microvascular disease. *N. Engl. J. Med., 305*, 191.
56. Merimee TJ, Zapf J, Froesch ER (1983): Insulin-like growth factors. Studies in diabetes with and without retinopathy. *N. Engl. J. Med., 309*, 527.

The Diabetes Annual/1
K.G.M.M. Alberti and L.P. Krall, editors

ISBN 0444 90 343 7
$0.85 per article per page (transactional system)
$0.20 per article per page (licensing system)

13 Diabetes in the young

DONNELL D. ETZWILER

Diabetes mellitus in the young continues to be a puzzling complex of diseases whose causes, treatments, and outcomes are poorly understood. In developing nations this is frequently described as a non-insulin-dependent illness whose incidence, prevalence and etiology are ill-defined. In developed nations it is regarded as the most severe form of diabetes and is associated with insulin dependence and ketoacidosis.

Increasing evidence is accumulating which demonstrates an association between the HLA histocompatibility complexes and environmental factors as a possible cause of this disease. Major efforts are now being made to identify individuals who are (1) 'at risk' so that preventative measures can be initiated, (2) in the prodromal stage so that therapeutic interventions can reverse the process, and (3) diagnosed as having the disease in an attempt to attain euglycemia or ultimately provide a cure. The past decade has been particularly stimulating as increased interest and funds are being directed towards diabetes in youth. The future of this disease appears both exciting and promising.

Etiology

Undoubtedly, hereditary factors play an important role in the etiology of insulin-dependent diabetes mellitus (IDDM). Identical twin studies among individuals with Type 1 and Type 2 diabetes show that the genetic factors are of much lesser importance in Type 1 disease than previously thought and that there may be a variety of environmental factors which contribute to disease onset.

The recent discovery and ability to identify the HLA histocompatibility complex has stimulated increased interest in the genetic/immunologic/environmental question. The identity of 'at risk' patients may increase our ability to intervene before the onset of the disease and thus enhance our preventative capability.

Specific HLA types may relate to individual susceptibility to B-cell damage by viruses or other environmental toxins or to an immunologic response to such factors. The detection of insulitis or islet cell antibodies (ICA) may permit intervention with immunotherapy and reversal of this process (1).

The HLA complexes have been found to vary among the differing diabetic population groupings around the world. Initially these studies concerned the detection of A, B and C loci. More recently the evidence has favored the presence of two separate susceptibility chains in strong linkage disequilibrium with HLA-DR3 and HLA-DR4. It is thought by some that the mode of action of these particular chains is in response to environmental factors capable of initiating damage to the pancreatic islet B-cell membrane. It is suggested that this may be a relatively slow immune-mediated destruction of B-cells involving both humeral and cell-mediated immunological processes. Using monoclonal antibodies and human pancreatic islet cell tissue knowledge of these mechanisms is developing rapidly and focusing on lymphocyte subtypes with cytotoxic activity. Recent studies have even suggested that there may be an even more generalized autoimmune endocrine disturbance in the early pathogenesis of Type 1 diabetes. The high frequency of antibodies reacting with different cells in anterior pituitary have been found in subjects who are genetically at risk and have complement fixing ICA. It could possibly be interpreted that certain viruses may be capable of initiating damage to more than one endocrine organ at a time (2).

Among the Chinese, HLA-Bw22, B17, and Aw33 have been found to be increased in the diabetic population in contrast to some of the HLA-B8, B15 and B18 found in Caucasian groupings (3). In this study the DR3 and DR4 antigens were not addressed. Among the Japanese there has been an increased focus on the HLA-DR antigens and a significant increase in the frequency of HLA-DR4 was found in patients. This was 56.3% of the patients versus 32.6% of the unaffected persons (4). There has been some interest concerning whether DR2 might be a protective antigen among the Japanese population. However, the negative correlation between DR2 and the patients was not statistically significant. Goldman (5), however, states that HLA-DR2 carriers appear to be resistant to the disease and that the HLA-DR3-associated disease probably arises from an autoimmune process and that HLA-DR4 is possibly a form of human intolerance to certain viruses.

Evidence continues to accumulate, which emphasizes the importance of the DR3 and DR4 loci and their subgroupings.

The importance of these HLA-immune complexes is suggested by Cudworth and Wolfe (2), who state the risk of developing the disease is approximately 90 times increased in HLA-identical siblings of Type 1 diabetics.

Gorsuch et al. (6) reported that HLA-identical siblings (both haplotypes in common) have an approximately 100 times greater risk of developing the disease than the general population. They suggest these findings may carry implications for genetic counseling and research.

The role viruses play in initiating the onset of diabetes in school-aged children is suggested in many studies which demonstrate peak incidences of the disease occurring during certain seasons of the year when schools are in session. This is in contrast to the lack of peaks among the 0–5-year-old preschoolers. Several viruses, e.g. mumps, rubella, coxsackie, have been implicated and the general feeling is that there is probably a group of viruses which may be contributors. The hope is that if these agents could be identified, an appropriate vaccine might be developed and administered to the 'at risk' population.

Mertens et al. (7), in a search for Coxsackie B virus-induced insulin-dependent diabetes among 166 patients, reported all had a history of recent infectious illnesses. 80% of the patients had antibodies against at least 1 Coxsackie B virus type. Among the children studied with antibody titers higher than 256, in only 44% could a recent Coxsackie B virus infection be demonstrated serologically by determining specific neutral antibodies. The result again strengthened the notion that IDDM includes several different etiologic groups among which some are possibly induced by Coxsackie B viruses.

One consideration at present is that the viral particles themselves may initiate the disease by directly attacking the islet cells in an unimpeded manner. Among those patients who are HLA-DR3, it seems likely that minor damage to the islets may initiate an autoimmune-like response which in turn may destroy the B-cells. The presence of ICA in the serum of those with diabetes and their family members has been of increasing interest.

Salardi et al. (8) reported that in 101 children from 18 months to 15 years of age, ICA were positive in 92.3% of the cases at the time of onset, falling to 60% between the 2nd and 6th month of the disease. The presence of ICA showed no relationship with anti-Coxsackie antibodies. Mustonen et al. (9) reported in a study of 184 children that 53% were positive with respect to the ICA.

Borsey and co-workers (10) demonstrated that among 153 insulin-dependent diabetics studied at diagnosis and, subsequently, in 88 of these patients for intervals up to 3 years the presence of ICA positively declined from 50% at the time of diagnosis to 45, 38, 36, 31, 26, 19 and 17% at 1, 3, 6, 9, 12, 24, and 36 months after diagnosis, respectively. Circulating immune complexes seem to parallel that of ICA in the early stage of diabetes and both phenomena may be primarily or secondarily involved in the development of the disease.

A study was conducted among 22 insulin-dependent diabetes patients to investigate the possibility of an additional target of autoimmunity (11). The sera were examined for antibodies to insulin receptors. The sera obtained before treatment with exogenous insulins of 10 of the patients demonstrated the occurrence of anti-insulin receptor antibodies of the IgM class. These findings suggest that autoimmunity to insulin receptors may possibly contribute to the pathophysiology of diabetes.

Serrano-Rios et al. (12) in 1983 reported the case of a 16-year-old boy with persistent hyperglycemia and acanthosis nigricans with insulin resistance up to 2800 units of short-acting insulin per day. The number and affinity of insulin receptors in this patient were markedly decreased and no significant insulin binding to IgG could be detected. It was felt that the severe insulin resistance in this patient was probably caused by a receptor defect associated with marked increase of B-cell function.

Another possible etiology of diabetes occurring in children is steroid diabetes, reported by Perlman and Ehrlich (13). Among the 17 patients studied, insulin therapy was necessary in 15 episodes in 11 patients. Permanent insulin dependence developed immediately in 1 patient and eventually in 3 other patients. The steroid-precipitated diabetes must be anticipated and they felt it should not interfere with the treatment of the primary disease.

Incidence and prevalence

A prospective study by Dahlquist et al. (14) reported all newly diagnosed cases from all over Sweden among children 0–14 years of age. The yearly incidence was found to be a little over 22 per 100 000 children. The mean prevalence of diabetes in 1980 was 1.48 per 1000 children. Peak incidence was at 11 years of age among girls, and at 4 and 13 years of age among boys. Peak incidences of new cases occurred in January, March, and July–October for older age groupings. There appeared to be no seasonal variation among children 0–4 years of age.

In another study from Sweden (15) the incidence of diabetes was reported to be 14.2 cases per 100,000 between the years 1938 to 1942. The lowest incidence (10.2 per 100,000) was reported during the war years and rose to 37.9 per 100,000 between 1973 and 1977. The increasing incidence in the past decade was particularly notable among children under 5 years of age. The peak incidence of new cases were seen during the winter and summertime and varied with geographic distribution. In Vasterbotten the prevalence among 0–14-year-old children was 3 per 1000.

A Scottish study (16) showed the annual incidence of the disease in the period 1968–1976 to be about 13.8 per 100,000 children under 19 years of age with the highest incidence of 20 per 100,000 among the 0–14 age grouping. The first admission rates showed seasonal variation for those of 5 years and older, with a peak in October–November and January–February. It was felt that these observations were compatible with the disease having a viral etiology. It was estimated that during this study period there was an 80% increase in the annual incidence of diabetes mellitus from about 10 per 100,000 in 1968 to about 18 per 100,000 in 1976.

Reunanen et al. (17) reported the incidence of IDDM in children and adolescents in Finland, using a national register of drug-treated diabetics and hospital records. At the end of 1979, the prevalence of diabetes in children 0–14 years of age was 1.91 per 1000 and among those aged 0–19 the prevalence was 2.62 per 1000. The annual incidence of diabetes was 27.3 per 100,000 in the 0–19 age group and 28.6 per 100,000 in those 0–14 years of age. The peak incidence of diabetes in girls was at 12 years of age and at 14 in boys. There was seasonal variation with peaks in April and September. The prevalence of diabetes mellitus increased clearly during the observation period and the incidence has tended to increase especially during the past few years. Both the prevalence and incidence rates of diabetes mellitus in Finnish children are high by international standards and it is felt that they could possibly be the highest in the world.

In Italy, Salardi et al. (8) reported a peak incidence of diabetes in the 2nd and 11th year, with a significant prevalence in males between 0–2 years. February was found to be the month of maximum incidence, with high peaks also found in November and December in school-aged children, but not in the preschoolers.

Data from the recently established registry for IDDM in Rhode Island (18) showed that young adults aged 20–29 had the onset of diabetes as frequently as adolescents and teenagers aged 10–19. The overall incidence in persons less than 30 years of age was 14 per 100,000 with the peak incidence occurring at 10–14 years with 19 per 100,000 population.

The prevalence of diabetes mellitus among cohorted children in the Child Health and Education Study in England at age 10, was 1.3 per 1000 (19). Compared with two previous cohort studies this suggested that the prevalence of diabetes is doubling roughly every decade.

Flood et al. (20) demonstrated an increase of incidence in children born to older mothers. Diabetes was also much more frequent in the late birth order siblings, which appeared to be an alternative expression of advanced maternal age. Their observations suggest that the development of Type 1 diabetes by some children may be at increased risk by virtue of being born to older mothers. Wagener et al. (21) reported there was no increased risk to siblings of diabetics who had had an early age of onset of diabetes. There was increased risk to siblings of diabetes (10.5%) in families where at least one parent had IDDM and also an increased risk to siblings of diabetics (8.8%) when at least one parent had non-insulin-dependent diabetes (NIDDM). Average age of onset of the second case in the family is significantly older than the age of onset in single families.

Wagener and co-workers (22) also reported on the series of juvenile diabetes having the onset of their diabetes before age 17. The prevalence of the disease differed by birth order with, unexpectedly, the greater number among the first born. There was also increased prevalence among children born to mothers older than 35 as well as increased prevalence among children of very young mothers.

Management

At the present time insulin-dependent diabetes in youth cannot be cured. It can, however, be controlled. The goal of therapy is the restoration of euglycemia at all times. It is assumed that if the body's ability to properly use carbohydrate is restored, normal metabolism of fat and protein follows. The importance of control versus the psychosocial repercussions among the children has been debated for decades. In 1976 the American Diabetes Association issued a policy statement saying: 'The goals of appropriate therapy should thus include a serious effort to achieve levels of blood glucose as close to those in the non-diabetic as feasible ... This concept is particularly applicable to the diabetics at greatest risk of developing the microvascular complications – the young and middle-aged' (23). Although this has been disputed by some, the definitive study, the Diabetes Control and Complications Trial, now being conducted by the National Institutes of Health, may resolve this discussion.

Control still depends on balance of insulin, food, and activities. The importance of diet continues to be not only the quantity of food eaten but also the quality and timing of its ingestion. Frequent review and updating of the diet of children is encouraged. Their rapid growth and development makes this imperative. All too frequently children may be given an appropriate dietary prescription at the onset of their disease which is rarely updated despite their increasing height, weight and development. Most diabetologists feel that dietary reassessment should be made at intervals of at least 6 months. Diets must be compatible with and acceptable to patients for which they are prescribed, and the range of 45–60% carbohydrate appears to be appropriate. The percentage of carbohydrate has gradually been increasing in most developed nations in the past few years. According to Hadden (24), improvement of blood glucose control due to fiber supplements appears marginal in children and the side effects of excess fiber are unacceptable.

Baumer and co-workers (25) demonstrated in a group of 21 children that a low fiber diet resulted in the highest blood glucose concentration after breakfast. A medium and a high fiber diet, which were as popular as the low fiber diet, showed lower blood glucose levels. Their conclusion was that the more acceptable cereal fibers produced a smaller but important benefit on morning hyperglycemia after breakfast.

Kinmonth et al. (26) felt that glycemic control was significantly better on an unrefined diet. Six months after the study, the children were eating appreciably more dietary fiber than before. It was felt that attention to the food type and structure can improve blood glucose control in diabetic children and should provide an acceptable, more rational basis for dietary prescription than one based on carbohydrate quantity alone.

Insulin remains a mainstay for the treatment of these diabetics and in the past few years there has been marked improvement in insulin purity, which has drastically reduced the occurrence of hypertrophy and atrophy at injection sites. The use of these more purified preparations is vigorously encouraged.

Concern for the availability of insulin in the world of increasing diabetes has stimulated the development of new methods of producing the hormone. Human-like insulin is now derived from recombinant DNA techniques by Lilly. Human-like insulin has also been produced by Novo by a transpeptidation process using purified porcine insulin. This process removes the terminal amino acid (alanine) on the β-chain, replacing it with threonine. The insulin obtained from these two techniques appear to be chemically identical with that of insulin obtained from the human pancreas. The time of onset of regular human insulin appears to be slightly more rapid than their counterparts derived from porcine and mixed bovine insulin. Duration of action of human-like NPH insulin has been reported to be slightly shortened. In general, these preparations can be substituted for the traditional insulins on a unit to unit basis. Insulin antibodies have been shown to be drastically reduced when patients previously on mixed bovine/porcine insulin were switched to the human insulin. There has been little change in insulin antibody levels among patients who had been on highly purified porcine products and then switched to human insulin. Human-like insulin appears to be the insulin of the future and assurance of sufficient quantity in years to come is encouraging. Reports about these insulins have been numerous (27–33). The use of human compared with porcine insulin in the treatment of diabetic ketoacidosis and severe non-ketotic hyperglycemia showed that they were equally effective (34). DeLeeuw et al. (35) reported successful use of human insulin in two insulin-dependent patients whose treatment with bovine and porcine insulins has been discontinued because of severe insulin allergic reactions.

Dimitriadis and Gerich (36) reported on the appropriate timing for preprandial insulin injections. The comparison of administering subcutaneous insulin *immediately*, *30* and *60* minutes before meals demonstrated that the 60-minute-before-the-meal injection provided plasma glucose and insulin profiles closest to normal and permitted less insulin to be used. This suggests that the timing as well as the amount of insulin used may be important in attaining good control.

Schneider (37) reported on efforts to start juvenile diabetics on insulin using an ambulatory program, thus eliminating 'unnecessary hospitalization' for 52 children, 11 months to 16 years of age. Forty-four were sent home 1–4 hours after instruction. This approach was apparently well received by the patients, parents and referring physicians, and may be the technique of the future in view of increased concern for cost containment.

The manner in which insulin is delivered has also changed drastically within the past decade. In the past, a single injection of intermediate insulin

seemed to suffice for reasonable diabetes care but with better means of monitoring blood glucose levels and estimating the degree of control, such as self blood glucose monitoring and hemoglobin A_{1C} determinations, increasing interest and concern for the timing and frequency of insulin administration has resulted. Consequently, most patients treated in diabetes centers are given mixed doses of regular and intermediate insulins on a twice-a-day basis, usually before breakfast and before dinnertime.

Introduction of the insulin pump represents an attempt to deliver insulin in a more physiological manner. These efforts began in the 1970s and a great deal of literature has been published on this. The enthusiasm for using pumps has diminished somewhat since it has been demonstrated by crossover studies that comparable control of glucose levels can be obtained by multiple-dose therapy.

Continuous subcutaneous insulin infusion (CSII) therapy consists of a basal infusion of Regular (soluble) insulin and 3–4 boluses of Regular usually 30 to 60 minutes before each main meal and the evening snack. Pump technology is advancing rapidly and although the size of the instruments is diminishing, the capabilities are increasing. Their cost remains a significant factor in their use and they require frequent blood glucose monitoring. Efforts are being made to perfect implantable instruments which would eliminate their visibility and decrease the risk of infection. The elusive 'implantable glucose sensor', when developed, would permit a major advance in the field.

Most pump studies have been carried out among adults. Skyler et al. (38) have reported a study in which 10 ambulatory patients were compared on three intensive treatment regimens: (1) twice daily Regular and Lente, (2) multiple preprandial injections of Regular insulin accompanied by Ultralente insulin, and (3) CSII with a portable insulin pump. All groups improved and no differences were noted among the groups. Skyler et al. (39) also described the importance of education, cooperation and negotiation necessary to achieve control with infusion devices along with the algorithms for subcutaneous injection. Schiffrin (40) also reported that a regimen of multiple subcutaneous insulin (MSI) injections can provide comparable glycemic control to that achieved with more expensive and sophisticated methods of administration such as open-loop and closed-loop systems.

Schiffrin and Belmonte (41) carried out a similar study among 20 insulin-dependent diabetics participating in a 1-year protective randomized crossover study comparing MSI and CSI devices. No significant difference in degree of metabolic control was achieved as measured by mean fasting blood sugar, preprandial, postprandial capillary blood glucose levels and glycosylated hemoglobin, cholesterol and triglycerides were seen between the 16 patients who completed the study. After completion of the study 2 patients went back to conventional therapy, 7 remained on the pump and

7 choose to stay on MSI. It was concluded that on a long-term basis the two methods can produce comparable levels of blood glucose glycosylated hemoglobins. Calabrese et al. (42) demonstrated similar effects.

Dahlquist et al. (43) demonstrated that in juvenile-onset diabetics endogenous insulin secretion, as reflected by immunoreactive C-peptide levels, is the best factor to correlate with low levels of hemoglobin A_{1C}. After cessation of endogenous insulin secretion there was a progressive deterioration of metabolic control. Multiple injections of insulin rather than one or two per day may be necessary to reach optimal control in these patients.

White et al. (44) demonstrated that certain Type 1 diabetic patients were particularly at risk for hypoglycemia during intensive therapy. Nine of 22 patients with insulin-requiring diabetes had neurological signs and symptoms of hypoglycemia with plasma glucose concentrations that were below 35 mg/ml and continued to decline. The inadequate glucose counterregulation resulted from a combined effect of deficient glucagon and epinephrine response. In 8 of the 9 patients with inadequate counterregulation severe hypoglycemia developed during subsequent intensive therapy, whereas only 1 of 13 patients with adequate counterregulatory mechanisms experienced this. Thus, an intravenous insulin infusion test can prospectively identify a patient who might be at increased risk. This test is not conducted as a routine procedure when trying an intensive control program.

The development of a practical means of frequent self blood glucose monitoring by the patient has made possible all of the recent intensified efforts to attain control of diabetes. The discrepancy between urinary glucose and blood glucose monitoring at times are immense. Schiffrin and Belmonte (45) reported that diabetes control was significantly better during periods of frequent self blood glucose monitoring. They concluded that in compliant, motivated young adults with insulin-dependent diabetes, frequent self blood glucose monitoring is critical for long-term maintenance of glycemic control.

Carney et al. (46) also demonstrated the effect of blood glucose testing versus urine testing on metabolic control in insulin-dependent diabetes in children. When the explanation for the improved hemoglobin A_{1C} was noted, 81% of the trained children accepted and continued to use the blood glucose monitoring for at least 9 months after training.

Schiffrin et al. (47) also studied the accuracy of Chemstrip bG and Glucometer measuring systems in self blood glucose monitoring in trained adolescents. Simultaneous collection of whole blood in capillary tubes was obtained and later analyzed. In both cases there was excellent correlation between both methods and the determinations. There was a tendency toward greater deviation with higher plasma glucose values. Well-trained patients can achieve sufficient accuracy to permit the use of either of these methods as tests with similar results.

Fahlen et al. (48) reported the use of self glucose monitoring among a population of diabetic patients, and a questionnaire showed 25 of the 29 preferred blood glucose monitoring. This seems a highly acceptable task in patient groups. Skyler (49) also reports that self blood glucose monitoring is now an integral component of treatment rather than an end point in assessing outcome. The attainment of excellent glycemic control facilitated by this technique has initiated a new era in diabetes management with potential promises of lessening the frequency and severity of chronic complications of the disease.

The frequent determinations of blood glucose have become burdensome to patients and health professionals alike. Wilson and Clarke (50) have pointed out that personal microcomputers are becoming readily available and have great potential for the identification of long-term trends in blood glucose regulation (see also Chapter 9).

The recent use of glycosylated hemoglobin levels as an index of long-term blood glucose levels also represents a significant tool in research and improved therapeutic attainment. Gabbay (51) has written extensively about this and the importance of proper collection and processing methods. It is advisable that the specimen be washed prior to a determination being made. This removes a labile glucose fraction which does not reflect the longer control period. The glycosylated hemoglobin provides a good indication of the mean blood glucose levels over the previous 4–6-week period and should be part of the control program when quality and reliable determinations are available (see also Chapter 10).

In studies published by Tamborlane et al. (52), the restoration of near normal blood glucose in insulin pump therapy without retinopathy at the start of the study remained without retinopathy after 15–23 months of therapy. One of the 11 eyes with background retinopathy developed proliferative disease and in 3 of 13 eyes proliferative retinopathy progressed during pump therapy. Reports over longer periods of time suggest that the changes noted in early reports are not necessarily sustained over a prolonged period of time.

Major intervention therapy includes pancreatic transplantation, plasmapheresis and the use of immunosuppressive agents. Sutherland et al. (53) have been major contributors in the field of pancreatic transplantation. The need for antirejection therapy is still a major cause of graft failure. In a certain number of patients, a pancreas transplant has been successful for a period, thus eliminating the need for exogenous insulin (see also Chapter 11).

The possibility of immune mechanisms being associated with the etiology of insulin-dependent diabetes in youth suggests the possible use of plasmapheresis in the early treatment of the disease. This was performed 4 times over 1–2 weeks in 17 age-matched children (54). The C-peptide concentrations at the onset were the same in the two groups but after 1 month the children treated with plasmapheresis had significant higher values. This difference became more pronounced after 3, 6 and 18 months. The same group also had a significantly more stable metabolism, and longer partial remissions. Insulin requirements in the groups were approximately the same. In the 10 treated children islet cell plasmic antibodies were present in 7 before plasmapheresis and in 9 during treatment. The antibodies remained detectable in 6 out of the 9 patients at 6 months after plasmapheresis. Although mechanisms were obscure, plasmapheresis was performed at the onset of diabetes in an attempt to preserve B-cell function.

The possible use of cyclosporin has been reported by Stiller et al. (55). Of 30 patients treated with cyclosporin for 2–12 months (starting within 6 weeks of diagnosis), 16 became insulin-independent during this period (see also Chapter 4).

Acute, intermediate and long-term complications

Despite low mortality rates in children experiencing diabetic ketoacidosis it remains a potentially fatal condition. In the young individuals rapid decrease in serum potassium, cerebral edema and severe hypoglycemia are the most frequent complications to be avoided. Burger and Weber (56) recommend that the intravenous insulin be administered in a continuous infusion at a rate of 0.1 unit/kilogram body weight per hour following initial bolus injection of 0.1 unit. As blood glucose decreases to 250 mg/dl or below, the infusion rate can be reduced. Intravenous saline solution is initiated and bicarbonate was shown to be hardly ever necessary in their study. Potassium replacement begins after assurance that urinary flow is going well, and must be closely monitored. At our clinic bicarbonate is used whenever the serum pH is 7.0 or lower.

The comparison of the treatment of diabetic acidosis using subcutaneous and intravenous therapy continues. Results indicate that perhaps strict monitoring of patients is more important than the specific route of insulin administration.

In children with diabetes under the age of 10, diabetic ketoacidosis accounts for 70% of the diabetes-related deaths (57) although this varies greatly in different parts of the world. Those caring for these children must have a good understanding of the condition and its treatment. One complication of therapy is the possible occurrence of cerebral edema which may be fatal. Franklin et al. (58) reported that the edema may be reversed by the administration of mannitol. The patient had experienced ophthalmoplegia but improved immediately after treatment, and the problems completely resolved within 2 weeks. It was concluded that mannitol is beneficial if instituted promptly.

Of considerable interest in the literature have been the numerous reports of limited joint mobility in the hands of Type 1 diabetics. Starkman and Brink (59) reported this phenomenon in 32 of 100 subjects 3–22 years of age. It appeared to be independent of age but to increase with duration of diabetes, with the peak occurrence in individuals who had diabetes for more than 5 years. There was no correlation of limited joint mobility with insulin type, allergy, family history of arthritis or growth retardation, nor with control parameters including the number of hypoglycemic and ketoacidosis episodes, hemoglobin A_{1C}, fasting triglycerides or cholesterol values.

Rosenbloom et al. (60), in a follow-up study over 7 years, reported that 30% of 309 patients with juvenile diabetes experienced limited joint mobility. They felt its appearance was influenced more by age than duration of diabetes. Of 142 patients with onset before puberty and of longer than 3 years duration, 74 had limited joint mobility. They described a disproportionate distribution of height percentiles for age characterizing this entire group. Those with limited joint mobility had 4 times the skewing of those without these signs (74% vs. 37% were below the 25th percentile). The presence or absence of thyroid microsome antibodies or ICA did not relate significantly to the limited joint mobility. Subjective diabetes control by clinical estimation and by hemoglobin A_{1C} levels was generally unrelated to joint findings.

Brice et al. (61) described that 42% of diabetic children had limited joint mobility with 14% of them having a more severe form. He correlated the findings with increasing age, early presentation and long duration of diabetes. The first-degree relatives of affected diabetic children had a higher incidence (35%) with limited joint mobility compared with relatives of non-affected diabetic children (13%). Other articles have described various aspects of this question (62–66). An attempt was made by Chapple et al. (66) to correlate it with early signs of retinopathy; however, it was concluded that joint contractures (cheirarthropathy) are not a predictor of early retinopathy.

Although the acute and intermediate problems associated with diabetes are significant, it is the dread of long-term complications which most concern patients, their families and health professionals. Neuropathy, micro- and macroangiopathy spell out an ominous future for these children. The Report of the National Commission (67) pointed out that renal failure would be the cause of death in over 50% of the young insulin-dependent diabetics.

A long-term study (68) from the Steno Memorial Hospital in Denmark indicated that 41% of the 1303 patients evaluated developed nephropathy. Two incidence peaks of proteinuria were noted, one after 10 years and one after 32 years, and a male predominance was noted. An association between daily insulin requirement and nephropathy incidence was found.

The worsening of some long-term complications of diabetes with the attainment of good control has been reported. Ellis et al. (69) reported 2 patients with diabetes of 7 and 9 years duration who exhibited overt and persistent proteinuria after improved glycemic control. One patient also experienced a deterioration of non-proliferative retinopathy after 6 weeks of strict control.

Frank et al. (70) studied retinopathy in 173 children with IDDM and determined the prevalence increased with the duration of diabetes. The overall prevalence of retinopathy was 18% with 1% from 0–4 years after diagnosis, 25% from 5–9 years, and 67% from 10–16 years after the onset of the disease. Little retinopathy was seen before the age of 15 and a 48% prevalence was found in older persons. Retinopathy appeared to be independently associated with diabetes control, lens opacities and frequency of daily insulin injections. They stated that the study supported the hypothesis that long-term hyperglycemia as well as changes (possibly hormonal) in nature associated with puberty are causally related to diabetes retinopathy.

Retinal studies reported by Jackson et al. (71) were carried out among 181 post-pubescent insulin-dependent diabetics who developed their diabetes before the age of 20. Retinal studies included serial and direct ophthalmoscopic examinations, stereoscopic fundus photography, and fluorescein angiopathy. Muscle biopsies were also done to obtain capillary membrane thickness as an index of early microvascular changes in skeletal muscles. No retinopathy was detected in patients who were known to have been continuously in excellent metabolic control. Twenty-five of the patients with worse control for extended periods had retinopathy. The capillary basement membrane thickening was found to be variable and to progress or regress within a year depending upon the degree of control. The study was felt to demonstrate that very good metabolic control delays and may prevent microvascular changes.

In a study by Bodansky et al. (72) among 133 subjects with Type 1 diabetes and severe microvascular disease, it was concluded that HLA genetic factors, insulin-binding capacity, and autoimmunity were unrelated to the pathogenesis of microvascular disease. However, raised levels of circulating immune complexes may be associated with proliferative retinopathy.

Capillary basement membrane width (CBMW) studies conducted among monozygotic twins by Ganda et al. (73) demonstrated that the CBMW of IDDM twins is frequently but not invariably thicker than that of their non-diabetic twin. No mention or validation of the degree of disease control was included. Among 8 pairs of identical twins discordant for IDDM for 11–29 years, reported by Barnett et al. (74), the absence of CBMW in all of the non-diabetic twins and in 4 of the IDDM twins argues against the existence of hereditary determinants of diabetic vascular disease being linked to those governing susceptibility to diabetes, and indicates diabetic microangiopathy is not an inevitable consequence of the disease.

Kaar et al. (75) reported on a study among 161 children with diabetes that the greatest impairment of nerve conduction was found in the peroneal motor conduction velocity and was present in 30% of the patients. There was a correlation between the control of diabetes based on hemoglobin A_{1C} and glucosuria and median and peroneal motor conduction velocities.

In a study (76) of 19 IDDM patients 7–25 years of age compared with 15 normal controls, diabetic autonomic dysfunction seemed to be rare, and the authors felt routine testing for this sequela would not be justified.

Studies to detect early cardiomyopathy have included a study (77) of 10 young IDDM patients by M-mode echocardiography. The findings did not correlate with either duration of disease or glucose control as assessed by hemoglobin A_{1C} and plasma glucose concentrations at the time of the study. The results did show a high prevalence of abnormalities in young diabetics which may represent preclinical cardiomyopathy.

Education

Patient education is now considered to be an integral part of quality health care. Quality care for chronic illness such as diabetes cannot be provided without informed patients cooperating with concerned and knowledgeable health professionals in planned systems of health care. The National Diabetes Advisory Board established a steering committee on patient education and in November 1983 the Standards for Patient Education were published (78). The importance of education and its cost savings in diabetes have been validated not only in studies in the 1970s but more recently in Kentucky and Maine, where third-party payment is now attainable for that service.

A recent study (79) reported a model for autonomous decision-making and deliberate action in diabetes self-management. A conceptual model that has stressed health/wellness, underlining deliberate action as a function of development capabilities of individual choice, is presented in the frame of personal values and social norms. It is felt that the application of knowledge, decision-making and taking deliberate action can be more effectively taught in diabetic patients by encouraging deliberate action based on informed decisions and reinforced through appropriate feedback mechanisms. The view of health in terms of individual surveillance and autonomy is supported. The challenge presented to diabetes educators is to facilitate in their patients' competent and autonomous behavior powered by purpose and commitment.

Increasing numbers of people are recognizing that the transference of knowledge alone does not necessarily improve patient performance and disease management (80).

Warren-Boulton et al. (81) have described the Washington University Diabetes Research Training Program where health professionals participate in a 4-day simulation exercise and are required to adhere to a diabetes regimen. The mean scores for adherence over the 4-day period for each component of the regimen were injections 82%, diet 67%, urine testing 58% and record recording results 56%. Of the total number of adherence problems encountered by the participants, 52% were diet-related, 17% involved urine testing, 17% involved constraints and 10% loss of spontaneity, and 4% injection. Analysis of the impact of the experience has indicated an improved participant sensitivity and has provided an increased ability to effectively counsel patients and family members.

Psychosocial concerns

The diagnosis and management of a chronic illness in a child provokes numerous concerns and psychosocial difficulties within each family. Rodin (82) demonstrated that lower self-esteem and feelings of depression are common among diabetics and particularly among those with poor control of their illness. Poor control in children appears to be associated with pathological interactions in the families. Hamburg and Inoff (83) studied 211 IDDM children 5–19 years of age at a camp. The poorer the control, the higher the degree of knowledge was found to be, and acquisition of a high level of knowledge was viewed as a coping effort in response to the stress of poor control.

The importance of early use of a special crisis intervention program offered to every family of a newly diagnosed patient was demonstrated in a comparative study by Galatzer et al. (84). Three times the amount of time and effort in counseling and psychotherapeutic measures was necessary to achieve comparable levels of adjustment. The importance of psychosocial problems in these children must be recognized and appropriate services made available.

Conclusions

Diabetes mellitus is a serious chronic disease which is affecting an increasing number of children each year. The genetic/environmental causes of the disease are not clearly defined but early identification of individuals at risk or those in the presymptomatic phases may soon be possible. The attainment of continuous euglycemia is rarely possible at the present time but newer insulins, means of insulin delivery and glucose monitoring have made major impacts on control within the past 5 years. The value of optimal control upon the acute and intermediate complications of the disease is agreed upon. Its influence upon the chronic complications appears favorable and the current Diabetes Control and Complications Trial by the National Institutes of Health hopes to finally resolve the question.

Increasing recognition of the spectrum of care required by these patients and their families transcends the medical field and includes education, communications, support, reward, family and community involvement. The need for comprehensive care of those children challenges us all.

References

1. Albin J, Rifkin H (1981): Etiologies of diabetes mellitus. *Med. Clin. North Am.*, *23*, 1209.
2. Cudworth AG, Wolfe E (1982): The genetic susceptibility of Type I (insulin dependent) diabetes mellitus. *Clin. Endocrinol. Metab.*, *11*, 389.
3. Lee BW, Chan SH, Tan SH, Wong HB, Tan CL (1983): HLA system in Chinese children with insulin-dependent diabetes mellitus. *Aust. Pediatr. J.*, *19*, 34.
4. Sakurami T, Ueno Y, Nagaoka K, Iwaki Y, Park MS, Terasaki PI, Saji H (1982): HLA-DR specifications in Japanese with juvenile onset insulin-dependent diabetes mellitus. *Diabetes*, *31*, 105.
5. Goldmann SF (1982): The chief histocompatibility system, HLA, and the genetics of diabetes. *Dtsch. Ärztebl.*, *79*, 41.
6. Gorsuch AN, Spencer KM, Lister J, McNally JM, Dean BM, Bottazzo GF, Cudworth AG (1982): Can future type 1 diabetes be predicted? A study in families of affected children. *Diabetes*, *31*, 862.
7. Mertens T, Gruneklee D, Eggers HJ, Schurmann W, Kruppenbacher J, Rheingans K, Kellermann K, Maas G (1983): Neutralizing antibodies against Coxsackie B viruses in patients with recent onset of type 1 diabetes. *Eur. J. Pediatr.*, *140*, 293.
8. Salardi S, Villa MP, Frejavilla E (1982): Seasonal onset of insulin dependent diabetes in relation to sex, age, anti-coxsackie and islet cell antibodies titers, and HLA phenotype. *Riv. Ital. Pediatr.*, *8*, 175.
9. Mustonen A, Knip M, Akerblom HK (1983): An association between complement-fixing cytoplasmic islet cell antibodies and endogenous insulin secretion in children with insulin-dependent diabetes mellitus. *Diabetes*, *32*, 743.
10. Borsey DQ, DiMario U, Irvine WJ, Gray RS, Guy K, Weston J, Peutherer J, Duncan LJ (1983): Humoral immunity in type I diabetes mellitus: a prospective study. *J. Clin. Lab. Immunol.*, *11*, 9.
11. Maron R, Elias D, DeJongh BM (1983): Antibodies to the insulin receptor in juvenile onset insulin dependent diabetes. *Nature (London)*, *303*, 817.
12. Serrano-Rios M, Dela-Vina S, Carbo ME (1983): Pancreatic A and B cell hyperfunction in the Mendenhall syndrome. *Diabetologia*, *25*, 8.
13. Perlman K, Ehrlich RM (1982): Steroid diabetes in childhood. *Am. J. Dis. Child.*, *136*, 64.
14. Dahlquist G, Gustavsson KH, Holmgren G, Hagglof B, Larsson Y, Nilsson KO, Samuelsson G, Sterky G, Thalme B, Wall S (1982): The incidence of

diabetes mellitus in Swedish children 0–14 years of age. A prospective study 1977–1980. *Acta Paediatr. Scand.*, *71*, 7.
15. Hagglof B, Holmgren G, Wall S (1982): Incidence of insulin-dependent diabetes mellitus among children in a North-Swedish population 1938–1977. *Hum. Hered.*, *32*, 408.
16. Patterson CC, Thorogood M, Smith PG, Mann JI, Heasman MA, Clarke JA (1983): Epidemiology of type I (insulin dependent) diabetes in Scotland 1968–1976: evidence of an increasing incidence. *Diabetologia*, *24*, 238.
17. Reunanen A, Akerblom HK, Kaar ML, Takkunen H, Aromaa A (1982): Prevalence and ten-year (1970–1979) incidence of insulin-dependent diabetes mellitus in children and adolescents in Finland. *Acta Paediatr. Scand.*, *71*, 893.
18. Fishbein HA, Faich GA, Ellis SE (1982): Incidence and hospitalization patterns of insulin-dependent diabetes mellitus. *Diabetes Care*, *5*, 630.
19. Stewart-Brown S, Haslum M, Butler M (1983): Evidence for increasing prevalence of diabetes mellitus in childhood. *Br. Med. J.*, *286*, 1855.
20. Flood TM, Brink SJ, Gleason RE (1982): Increased incidence of type I diabetes in children of older mothers. *Diabetes Care*, *5*, 571.
21. Wagener DK, Sacks JM, LaPorte RE, MacGregor JM (1982): The Pittsburgh study of insulin-dependent diabetes mellitus. Risk for diabetes among relatives of IDDM. *Diabetes*, *31*, 136.
22. Wagener DK, LaPorte RE, Orchard TJ (1983): The Pittsburgh diabetes mellitus study. III. An increased prevalence with older maternal age. *Diabetologia*, *25*, 82.
23. American Diabetes Association (1976): *Policy Statement on Patient Education*. American Diabetes Association, New York.
24. Hadden DR (1982): Food and diabetes: the dietary treatment of insulin-dependent and non-insulin-dependent diabetes. *Clin. Endocrinol. Metab.*, *11*, 503.
25. Baumer JH, Drakeford JA, Wadsworth J, Savage DCL, Edelsten AD, Howlett BC, Owens C, Pennock CA (1982): Effects of dietary fibre and exercise on mid-morning diabetic control – a controlled trial. *Arch. Dis. Child.*, *57*, 905.
26. Kinmonth AL, Angus RM, Jenkins PA, Smith MA, Baum JD (1982): Whole foods and increased dietary fibre improve blood glucose control in diabetic children. *Arch. Dis. Child.*, *57*, 187.
27. Clark AJL, Adeniyi-Jones RO, Knight G, Leiper JM, Wiles PG, Jones RH, Keen H, MacCuish AC, Ward JD, Watkins PJ, Cauldwell JM (1982): Biosynthetic human insulin in the treatment of diabetes. A double-blind crossover trial in established diabetic patients. *Lancet*, *2*, 354.
28. Weinges K, Ehrhardt M, Nell G, Enzmann F (1982): Pharmacodynamics of human insulin (recombinant DNA) – regular, NPH, and mixtures – obtained by the Gerritzen method in healthy volunteers. *Diabetes Care*, *5*, *Suppl. 2*, 67.
29. Greene SA, Smith MA, Cartwright B, Baum JD (1983): Comparison of human versus porcine insulin in treatment of diabetes in children. *Br. Med. J.*, *287*, 1578.
30. Howey DC, Fineberg SE, Nolen PA (1982): The therapeutic efficacy of

human insulin (recombinant DNA) in patients with insulin-dependent diabetes mellitus: a comparative study with purified porcine insulin. *Diabetes Care*, *5*, *Suppl. 2*, 71.
31. Lotz N, Bachmann W, Mehnert H, Walter H (1982): Human insulin (recombinant DNA) in the treatment of patients with newly diagnosed insulin dependent diabetes mellitus (IDDM). *Diabetes Care*, *5*, *Suppl. 2*, 149.
32. Beyer J, Benzmann F, Lauerbach M (1982): Treatment with human insulin (recombinant DNA) in diabetic subjects pretreated with pork or beef insulin: first results of a multicenter study. *Diabetes Care*, *5*, *Suppl. 2*, 140.
33. Lyngsoe, J, Vestermark S (1983): The efficacy and safety of human insulin (Novo) in insulin-dependent diabetic patients. *Diabetes Care*, *6*, *Suppl. 1*, 53.
34. Bachmann W, Walter H, Lotz N, Mehnert H (1982): Efficiency of human insulin (recombinant DNA) in the treatment of diabetic ketoacidosis and severe nonketoacidotic hyperglycemia. *Diabetes Care*, *5*, *Suppl. 2*, 161.
35. DeLeeuw I, Delvigne C, Bekaert J, Vanderwoude M, Van Elst F (1982): Insulin allergy treated with human insulin (recombinant DNA). *Diabetes Care*, *5*, *Suppl. 2*, 168.
36. Dimitriadis SD, Gerich JE (1983): Importance of timing of preprandial subcutaneous insulin administration in the management of diabetes mellitus. *Diabetes Care*, *6*, 374.
37. Schneider AJ (1983): Starting insulin therapy in children with newly diagnosed diabetes. An outpatient approach. *Am. J. Dis. Child.*, *137*, 782.
38. Skyler JS, Seigler DE, Reeves ML, Forhan SE, Peterson CM (1982): A comparison of insulin regimens in insulin-dependent diabetes mellitus. *Diabetes Care*, *5*, *Suppl. 2*, 11.
39. Skyler JS, Seigler DE, Reeves ML (1982): Optimizing pumped insulin delivery. *Diabetes Care*, *5*, 135.
40. Schiffrin A (1982): Treatment of insulin dependent diabetes with multiple subcutaneous insulin injections. *Med. Clin. North Am.*, *66*, 1251.
41. Schiffrin A, Belmonte MM (1982): Comparison between continuous subcutaneous insulin infusion and multiple injection of insulin. A one year prospective study. *Diabetes*, *31*, 255.
42. Calabrese G, Bueti A, Santeusanio F (1982): Continuous subcutaneous insulin infusion treatment in insulin-dependent diabetic patients: a comparison with conventional optimized treatment in a long term study. *Diabetes Care*, *5*, 457.
43. Dahlquist G, Blom L, Bolme P, Hagenfeldt L, Lindgren F, Persson B, Thalme B, Theorell M, Westin S (1982): Metabolic control in 131 juvenile-onset diabetic patients as measured by HbA_1C: relation to age, duration, C-peptide, insulin dose, and one or two insulin injections. *Diabetes Care*, *5*, 399.
44. White NH, Skor DA, Cryer PE, Levandoski LA, Bier DM, Santiago JV (1983): Identification of Type I diabetic patients at increased risk for hypoglycemia during intensive therapy. *N. Engl. J. Med.*, *308*, 485.
45. Schiffrin A, Belmonte M (1982): Multiple daily self-glucose monitoring: its essential role in long term glucose control in insulin-dependent diabetic patients treated with pump and multiple subcutaneous injections. *Diabetes Care*, *5*, 479.

46. Carney RM, Schechter K, Homa M (1983): The effects of blood glucose testing versus urine sugar testing on the metabolic control of insulin-dependent diabetic children. *Diabetes Care*, *6*, 378.
47. Schiffrin A, Desrosiers M, Belmonte M (1983): Evaluation of two methods of self blood glucose monitoring by trained insulin-dependent diabetic adolescents outside the hospital. *Diabetes Care*, *6*, 196.
48. Fahlen M, Lapidus L, Stromblad G, Stuart-Beck R (1983): Home monitoring of blood glucose and insulin therapy without a photometer. *Acta Med. Scand.*, *213*, S37.
49. Skyler JS (1982): Self-monitoring of blood glucose. *Med. Clin. North Am.*, *66*, 1227.
50. Wilson DE, Clarke DH (1983): Profiling self-monitored blood glucose results with the personal microcomputer. *Diabetes Care*, *6*, 604.
51. Gabbay KH (1982): Glycosylated hemoglobin and diabetes mellitus. *Med. Clin. North Am.*, *66*, 1309.
52. Tamborlane WV, Puklin JE, Bergman M, Hintz RL, Horst RL (1982): Long-term improvement of metabolic control with the insulin pump does not reverse diabetic microangiopathy. *Diabetes Care*, *5*, *Suppl. 2*, 58.
53. Sutherland DER, Goetz FC, Najarian JS (1982): Pancreas transplantation. *Clin. Endocrinol. Metab.*, *11*, 549.
54. Ludvigsson J, Heding L, Lieden G (1983): Plasmapheresis in the initial treatment of insulin-dependent diabetes mellitus in children. *Br. Med. J.*, *286*, 176.
55. Stiller CR, Dupré J, Gent M, Jenner MR, Keown PS, Laupacis A, Martell R, Rodger NW, Graffenried BV, Wolfe BMJ (1984): Effects of Cyclosporin immunosuppression in insulin-dependent diabetes mellitus of recent onset. *Science*, *223*, 1362.
56. Burger W, Weber B (1983): Treatment of diabetic ketoacidosis in children and adolescents. *Monatsschr. Kinderheilk.*, *131*, 694.
57. Foster DW, McGarry JD (1983): The metabolic derangements and treatment of diabetic ketoaçidosis. *N. Engl. J. Med.*, *309*, 159.
58. Franklin B, Liu J, Ginsberg-Fellner F (1982): Cerebral edema and ophthalmoplegia reversed by mannitol in a new case of insulin-dependent diabetes mellitus. *Pediatrics*, *69*, 87.
59. Starkman H, Brink S (1982): Limited joint mobility of the hand in type I diabetes mellitus. *Diabetes Care*, *5*, 534.
60. Rosenbloom AL, Silverstein JH, Lezotte DC (1982): Limited joint mobility in diabetes mellitus of childhood. Natural history and relationship to growth impairment. *J. Pediatr.*, *101*, 874.
61. Brice JEH, Johnston DI, Noronha JL (1982): Limited finger joint mobility in diabetes. *Arch. Dis. Child.*, *57*, 879.
62. Scott DL, Melamere JP, Mackintosh LP, Jobson S (1982): Familial cheiroarthropathy without juvenile onset diabetes mellitus. *Rheumatol. Int.*, *2*, 141.
63. Zick R, Hurter P, Berger M, Lange P, Mitzkat HJ (1983): Diabetes specific hand alterations in diabetes mellitus type I. *Dtsch. Med. Wochenschr.*, *108*, 1178.
64. Hurter P, Berger M, Kubel R, Stolzenback K, Von Schutz W, Zick R (1983):

Diabetes mellitus specific hand changes (cheiropathy) in children and adolescents with insulin dependent diabetes (type I). *Monatsschr. Kinderheilk.*, *131*, 582.
65. Rosenbloom AL, Silverstein JH, Riley WJ, Lezotte DC, MacLaren NK (1983): Limited joint mobility in childhood diabetes: family studies. *Diabetes Care*, *6*, 370.
66. Chapple M, Jung RT, Francis J, Webster J, Kohner EM, Bloom SR (1983): Joint contractures and diabetic retinopathy. *Postgrad. Med. J.*, *59*, 291.
67. National Commission on Diabetes (1975): *Vol. I: The Long-Range Plan to Combat Diabetes*. U.S. Department of Health, Education and Welfare, National Institutes of Health, Bethesda, MD.
68. Andersen AR, Sandahl-Christiansen J, Andersen JK (1983): Diabetic nephropathy in type I (insulin-dependent) diabetes: an epidemiological study. *Diabetologia*, *25*, 496.
69. Ellis D, Avner ED, Transue D, Jaffe R (1983): Diabetic nephropathy in adolescence: appearance during improved glycemic control. *Pediatrics*, *71*, 824.
70. Frank RN, Hoffman WH, Podgor MJ (1982): Retinopathy in juvenile onset type I diabetes of short duration. *Diabetes*, *31*, 874.
71. Jackson RL, Ide CH, Guthrie RA, James RD (1982): Retinopathy in adolescents and young adults with onset of insulin-dependent diabetes in childhood. *Ophthalmology*, *89*, 7.
72. Bodansky HJ, Wolf E, Cudworth AG, Medback S, Drury PL (1982): Genetic and immunologic factors in macrovascular disease in Type I insulin-dependent diabetes. *Diabetes*, *31*, 70.
73. Ganda OP, Williamson JR, Soeldner JS (1983): Muscle capillary basement membrane width and its relationship to diabetes mellitus in monozygotic twins. *Diabetes*, *32*, 659.
74. Barnett AH, Spillopoulos AJ, Pyke DA, Stubbs WA, Burrin J, Alberti KG (1983): Muscle capillary basement in identical twins discordant for insulin dependent diabetes. *Diabetes*, *32*, 857.
75. Kaar ML, Saukkonen AL, Pitkanen M, Akerblom HK (1983): Peripheral neuropathy in diabetic children and adolescents. A cross-sectional study. *Acta Paediatr. Scand.*, *72*, 373.
76. Koepp P, Hamm H (1983): Testing for autonomous nervous function in children and adolescents with insulin dependent diabetes mellitus. *Monatsschr. Kinderheilk.*, *131*, 273.
77. Lababidi ZA, Goldstein DE (1983): High prevalence of echocardiographic abnormalities in diabetic youths. *Diabetes Care*, *6*, 18.
78. National Diabetes Advisory Board (1983): *National Standards for Diabetes Patient Education Programs*. National Diabetes Advisory Board, Bethesda, MD.
79. Strowig S (1982): Patient education: a model for autonomous decision-making and deliberate action in diabetes self-management. *Med. Clin. North Am.*, *66*, 1293.
80. Korhonen T, Huttunen JK, Aro A, Hentinen M, Ihalainen O, Majander H, Siitonen O, Uustupa M, Pyorald K (1983): A controlled trial on the effects

of patient education in the treatment of insulin-dependent diabetes. *Diabetes Care*, *6*, 256.
81. Warren-Boulton E, Auslander WF, Gettinger JM (1982): Understanding diabetes routines: a professional training exercise. *Diabetes Care*, *5*, 537.
82. Rodin GM (1983): Psychosocial aspects of diabetes mellitus. *Can. J. Psychiatry*, *28*, 219.
83. Hamburg BA, Inoff GE (1983): Relationships between behavioral factors and diabetic control in children and adolescents: a camp study. *Psychosom. Med.*, *44*, 321.
84. Galatzer A, Amir S, Gil R, Nofar E, Beit-Halachmi N, Aran O, Shalit M, Roitman A, Laron Z (1982): Crisis intervention program in newly diagnosed diabetic children. *Diabetes Care*, *5*, 414.

The Diabetes Annual/1
K.G.M.M. Alberti and L.P. Krall, editors

ISBN 0444 90 343 7
$0.85 per article per page (transactional system)
$0.20 per article per page (licensing system)

14 Pregnancy and diabetes

LARS MØLSTED-PEDERSEN

In some respects the results of pregnancy in women with diabetes mellitus have improved greatly during the last two decades. Meticulous control of diabetes in the mother, careful monitoring of the fetus and fetal-placental unit and advances in perinatal nursing care have led to a highly significant reduction in the perinatal mortality and morbidity rate. Despite this improvement the incidence of congenital malformations has not decreased over the past five decades (1) (Table 1).

Congenital malformations

Several animal studies have been performed in recent years defining the relationship between diabetes and fetal malformation. Two excellent papers were published from Uppsala, Sweden, dealing with congenital malformation in the diabetic rat (2, 3). Female virgin rats made diabetic with a single injection of streptozotocin were mated about two weeks later. About 20% of 135 viable fetuses in a non-insulin-treated group showed skeletal malformations comprising either micrognathia or caudal dysgenesis compared to only two cases of caudal dysgenesis and no micrognathia among 233 offspring in an insulin-treated group. These defects were not found in 314 offspring of control rats (2).

In the second study (3) streptozotocin-diabetic rats (MDI) were randomly divided into groups, each of which was left without insulin treatment during

TABLE 1. *Congenital malformations (CM) during 4 periods in relation to White's classification: Copenhagen series*

Period	No. of infants	Infants with CM (%) according to White's classification		
		A	B + C	D + F
1926–56	489	3.9	4.2	9.7
1957–65	514	7.3	5.2	12.9
1966–72	484	3.6	7.9	13.3
1973–78	553	3.6	5.7	13.2

gestational days 2–3, 4–5, 6–7, 8–9 and 10–11 respectively. Skeletal malformations occurred in 2 of 52 viable fetuses (3.8%) with interruption of maternal insulin treatment on gestational days 2–3, in 7 of 118 fetuses (5.9%) with interruption of insulin on Days 4–5, and in 4 of 77 fetuses (5.2%) with interruption on Days 6–7. No skeletal malformations were seen in a total of 75 MDI fetuses after interruption of insulin treatment on either Days 8–9 or 10–11.

Both studies showed that untreated manifest diabetes mellitus in the pregnant rat induced a decrease in fetal weight and viability, a high rate of fetal resorption as well as retardation of skeletal development. Furthermore a significant increase in skeletal malformations comprising either micrognathia or caudal dysgenesis was found. These congenital malformations could be prevented by maternal insulin treatment and the second study strongly suggested that in rats, the teratogenic impact of maternal diabetes on embryonic skeletal development manifests itself at an unexpectedly early embryonic age.

The recent results of Sadler and Horton (4) corroborates this. They used the whole embryo culture system and in that way investigated the effects of insulin on early mouse embryogenesis. The results demonstrated that serum from diabetic rats receiving insulin therapy was effective in reduction of malformations and growth retardation produced by serum from diabetic rats receiving no hormone supplement. However, addition of insulin directly to serum from diabetic rats was not effective in reducing the rate of abnormalities produced by this method. In the same study (4) it was shown that addition of insulin at extremely high concentrations produced no abnormal embryos.

In summary, the results of these three studies support the impression that careful insulin therapy with strict control of the diabetic state reduces the risk of occurrence of congenital anomalies in the offspring of diabetic rats, and furthermore that early periods of gestation are particularly sensitive.

The excellent paper by Norbert Freinkel and co-workers with the colorful title 'Honeybee syndrome' (5) gives a broader view of teratogenesis. Through their interest in diabetes in pregnancy and especially the heightened incidence of congenital lesions in the offspring of diabetic mothers, the authors tested the effects of high glucose concentrations on the rat embryo in culture. Mannose was one of five hexoses chosen as controls. It proved to be a more potent teratogen at 1.5 mg/ml than glucose at 12 mg/ml in the culture medium; mannose at this concentration caused growth retardation and faulty neural-tube closure in approximately two-thirds of the embryos. Further experiment indicated that mannose depressed glycolysis, and that high glucose concentrations restored glycolysis to normal and prevented the teratogenic effects. It seemed that mannose and glucose competed for entry to the glycolytic pathway, possibly at hexokinase (6). The fact that extra oxygen could have a similar effect suggested that the production of high-energy phosphate was a more critical factor than any other more direct effect of a glycolytic pathway intermediate (7). The finding further highlights the metabolic vulnerabilities that exist during early organogenesis and should focus the attention of teratologists upon the possibility that major congenital lesions may occur coincidently with relative minor disturbances in glycolyses before oxidative maturation in the embryo unit.

The morphogenetic events that occur in cultured embryos fortuitously correspond to those observed in human embryos during the 4th–6th weeks of gestation, i.e. the susceptible period of teratogenesis in diabetics (8). In this context the observation of an early fetal growth delay introduced in the earliest gestational weeks of human diabetic pregnancy (9) was notable. The same authors later showed that these delayed fetuses were at a higher risk of being malformed (10, 11), suggesting a common mechanism behind early growth delay and induction of abnormal embryogenesis and maybe even fetal death.

The cause of these high malformation rates among offspring of diabetics is unknown. During the latest years more attention has been directed towards 'the metabolic' hypothesis, i.e. that incomplete metabolic compensation at nidation and during the first trimester might be important (12).

This hypothesis has been substantially elucidated by the essential study from Karlsburg by Kurt Fuhrmann and coworkers (13) (Table 2). Intensive treatment was begun before conception in 128 diabetic women planning pregnancy and only one malformation was found in this group (0.8%). In contrast, the malformation rate was 7.5% in a group of insulin-dependent diabetic women in whom strict metabolic control was begun after 8 weeks gestation. These observations indicate that good metabolic control, started before conception and continued during the first weeks of pregnancy, can prevent malformations in infants of diabetic mothers.

TABLE 2. *Prevention of congenital malformation in infants of insulin-dependent diabetic mothers by strict metabolic control started before conception and continued during the first weeks of gestation: Karlsburg series*

Groups	No. of women	Infants with congenital malformation (%)
Non-diabetic women	420	1.4
Diabetic women with strict metabolic control *before* conception	128	0.8
Diabetic women with strict metabolic control *after* 8th week of gestation	292	7.5

Adapted from Fuhrmann et al. (13).

The question of how strict metabolic control should be in early pregnancy in order to prevent malformations in infants of diabetic mothers has not yet been answered. However, from July 1981 to July 1984, 125 infants of insulin-dependent diabetic mothers (birthweight ⩾ 1000 g) were born in our department in Copenhagen with only one of these (0.8%) having congenital malformations. The frequency of planned pregnancies was 72% in this period but intensive treatment before conception was begun in only 10% of the diabetic women. In this unselected group of insulin-dependent pregnant women the average glucose profile in the first trimester was above 8 mmol/l in around 60% of the pregnancies (14).

During our prospective study of congenital malformations in infants of diabetic mothers in Rigshospitalet, Copenhagen, the decrease in number of malformations has now achieved statistical significance. The figure from the latest 5 year-period was 2.8% (Table 3), a figure not different from that in the non-diabetic population (15). Also the severity of congenital malformations (CM) has changed remarkably during the latest period, indicating that the frequency of lethal and multiple CM is similar to that in the control series (Table 4) (15).

Studies from other centers still give a high frequency of CM in diabetic pregnancies (16) and thus far no studies other than those from Copenhagen have reported significant decreases in the number of CM in infants of diabetic mothers from unselected groups. What is the explanation of these satisfactory data from the diabetic pregnancies in Copenhagen? No single answer is apparent and the cause may be non-specific but some points of possible relevance should be mentioned.

Firstly: as in other centers (17) an out-patient clinic for supervision of

TABLE 3. *Congenital malformations in infants of diabetic mothers during 2 periods: Copenhagen series*

Period	No. of infants	Infants with CM (%)
1926–78	2041	7.6
1979–83	547	2.8

TABLE 4. *Fatal and multiple malformations during 2 periods: Copenhagen series*

Period	No. of infants	Infants with CM (%) fatal	multiple
1926–78	2041	2.7	2.3
1979–83	547	0.4	0.4

contraception and planning for future pregnancies in diabetic women was organized in our hospital in 1976. The purpose of the clinic was to improve the contraceptive guidance for all diabetic women in the area and especially to give optimal post-partum contraceptive advice to all diabetics discharged from our obstetric department. A few years after the opening of this clinic a significant increase in the frequency of planned pregnancies was seen (18).

Secondly: as recently stated by Milunsky and co-workers (19), a tenfold increase of neural tube defects was observed in the offspring of diabetic patients. During the past six years serum alpha-fetoprotein determinations have been included in the standard care for diabetic pregnancies in Copenhagen and in some cases early amniocentesis has been performed. This regimen has led to second-trimester interruption of pregnancy in two cases with neural tube defects. Furthermore we have induced abortions in diabetic women from White's classes D and F who had unregulated diabetic metabolism during conception and the first gestational weeks and moreover had a significant ultrascan-verified growth delay during early pregnancy and thereby a risk of major CM of 27% (10). Finally it is a personal impression that during recent years improved treatment of young diabetics has taken place in our country. In conclusion, our advice for prevention of congenital malformations in infants of diabetic mothers is as follows:
(1) Planned pregnancy requires effective contraceptive advice. (2) Fully compensated diabetes metabolism is required at conception, nidation and throughout pregnancy. (3) Vascular complications in young diabetic females should be avoided. (4) Serum alpha-fetoprotein must be monitored in early pregnancy and, if necessary, early amniocentesis is indicated. (5) Ultrasonic scanning in early pregnancy is recommended.

Control of maternal blood glucose level

During the past decade, beginning with the paper of Karlsson and Kjellmer (20) followed by Roversi and co-workers in 1973 (21) many reports dealing with the management of pregnancy in the diabetic patient emphasized the importance of 'strict' control of the maternal blood glucose level, indicating that this significantly affects neonatal outcome (22, 23). However, 'strict' is a vague term, which varies with each author (24, 25, 26). As a result of this confusion, many investigators advocated that euglycemia during pregnancy was vital (27, 28). The most impressive results have been obtained by Lois Jovanovic and Charles Peterson of New York (28). They have developed successful programs that utilize home blood glucose monitoring, physiologic delivery of insulin, and quantitation of caloric intake carefully matched to insulin dosage. The pregnant diabetic patients in their study seemed to be highly motivated and well selected and exposed to extensive and time-consuming instruction and teaching during the first trimester of pregnancy. In a group of 53 insulin-dependent diabetic women in whom normoglycemia was established throughout gestation the rates for mortality and morbidity for both infant and mother approached normal (non-diabetic) rates (Table 5). There were no complications, as shown by the absence of pre-eclampsia.

This is in keeping with a recent study dealing with the hypothesis that pre-eclampsia in pregnant diabetics may be related to the adverse influence of relatively poor diabetic control on the pregnancy-induced changes in the spiral arteries (29). This hypothesis was examined by comparing mean blood glucose and glycosylated hemoglobin levels throughout the second and third trimesters of pregnancy in two relatively small groups of pregnant diabetics. One group was composed of patients who developed pre-eclampsia and the other of patients who did not. Differences showing poorer control between 11 and 14 weeks in the pre-eclamptic patients were found and this coincided with the time of endovascular trophoblastic invasion of the myometrial segments of these vessels.

In a paper from East Germany it was shown recently that maintenance of normal glycemic metabolism throughout pregnancy would have a favorable impact not only upon perinatal mortality and morbidity but it would also cause significant reduction of placental maturation disorders (30).

It seems obvious, especially from the New York results (28), that normalization of the maternal blood glucose level throughout pregnancy can avoid nearly all the fetal problems related to diabetes occurring in diabetic pregnancies. But most obstetric clinics have unselected patient groups and

TABLE 5. *Neonatal data from the offspring of euglycemic diabetic women*

White class.	No. of infants	Percentile body weight*	Gestational age (wk)	Congenital malformations		Apgar at 5 min
				Major	Minor	
B	12	60 ± 10.0	39.0	0	0	9.9
C	11	60 ± 7.0	39.5	0	0	10.0
D	8	54 ± 2.0	38.0	0	0	10.0
R	4	54 ± 4.0	37.5	0	0	10.0
F	1	51	37.0	0	0	10.0
G	17	60 ± 4.0	39.5	0	0	10.0
Mean		58.2 ± 5.5	39.0			
Non-diabetic comparison group						
Mean	53	61.8 ± 21.4	39.2 ± 1 (SD)	5	2	9.7

* Mean ± SD.
Adapted from Jovanovic and Peterson (28).

normalization of the maternal blood glucose level is difficult, if not impossible, with many diabetic pregnancies in these clinics.

However, in well-controlled diabetic pregnancies deliveries of macrosomic infants with the appearance typical of a baby born after a badly controlled diabetic pregnancy may still occur (31, 32). These remind one of 1971, when there was a discussion concerning the weight of the newborn baby in relationship to the hyperglycemia-hyperinsulinemia theory (33). Based on our observations of the disappearance rate of glucose (k-value) in newborn infants of both diabetic and non-diabetic mothers, we suggested that a growth impulse, common to all infants, operates through the glycemia-insulin system. In the normal fetus and newborn a close connection between growth and insulinism exists. In infants of diabetic women this glycemia-insulin factor is increased, but the correlation to growth and weight is weaker. Because of their hyperinsulinism these infants are larger than normal, in fact, the theory should account for excess weight – consisting mainly of fat – of about 500 g 3 weeks before term. Therefore, if it is possible to keep the blood glucose completely normal throughout pregnancy, it might be possible to reduce the birth weight from about 4800 to 4300, but not to 3500 g.

When the maternal blood glucose level is outside the normal boundaries the growth stimulus is weakened and paradoxically disturbed: In White classes A–F, the mean birth weight decreases and class F infants are underweight, while, most likely, the maternal pregnancy level of glucose increases throughout the White classes (34). Several factors may account for these observations. These include the placenta, its blood flow and membrane functions. Untill now, very few investigations on utero-placental blood flow in diabetic pregnancies have been performed and the results have been conflicting. The most convincing study on this topic comes from Sweden (35) where Nyland and co-workers with indium 113m and a computer-linked gamma-camera measured the utero-placental blood flow in 26 women with diabetes mellitus and in 41 healthy normal control subjects. In the last trimester the maternal-placental blood flow index was reduced 35% to 45% compared to that in healthy women. The blood flow index tended to be further impaired in those diabetic women who had higher blood glucose values.

A reduction of the intervillous space might affect the utero-placental blood flow and in fact recent histomorphometric studies of the placental villi showed that in diabetics only 25% of the villus surface is taken up by capillary surface as contrasted to about 50% in placentas from non-diabetics (36).

In order to achieve normalization of maternal blood glucose level in diabetic pregnancy insulin infusion pumps have been used in both in- and outpatient programs (37, 38). Thus far the number of pregnant diabetics on pump treatment is small and the experience therefore is limited. Our own knowledge of pump treatment of pregnant women with diabetes is also restricted (39) and agrees with recently published results from the Netherlands (32). In both studies near-normal blood glucose levels were achieved two months prior to conception and continued throughout the entire pregnancy. The preliminary results of these two studies are a bit disappointing in two respects: in Copenhagen the strict metabolic control at the time of conception and in early pregnancy did not normalize fetal growth in every case, as assessed by ultrasonic scanning in the 7th to 14th gestational week (11) and in the Netherlands the pump-treated patients had several obstetric complications including one 'unexplained' intrauterine death at the 37th week. Possibly the metabolic control might have been even more rigorous in these two studies.

Diabetic retinopathy in pregnancy

It is still not known whether pregnancy in women with insulin-dependent diabetes influences the spontaneous course of diabetic retinopathy. It is also uncertain as to what extent it is justified to treat retinopathy with photocoagulation during pregnancy or after delivery. Until recently the general impression was that worsening as well as amelioration could take place but most of the pregnant diabetics with retinopathy showed no changes during pregnancy (40).

Recently four papers dealing with prospective studies of diabetic retinopathy during pregnancy have been published (41–44). The conclusion of these four papers could be summarized as follows: the spontaneous course of retinopathy is influenced by pregnancy. Deterioration is observed in about 20% of women with background retinopathy, however, regression is common at delivery. Also some patients with proliferative changes deteriorate during pregnancy with some regression after delivery. Treatment with photocoagulation is most effective when applied *before* pregnancy, and there is no significant evidence that it may be particularly so during pregnancy. Proliferative eye changes are associated with increased obstetrical complications and poorer fetal outcome. However, proliferative retinopathy is not considered an absolute indication for termination of pregnancy.

In a retrospective investigation (45) Carstensen et al. studied 22 pairs (44 patients) of female insulin-dependent diabetics in order to evaluate the effect of one or two pregnancies on the prevalence and severity of late diabetic complications. Each pair consisted of one patient who had completed one or two pregnancies and one who had not. No difference in prevalence or severity of retinopathy was found.

Since 1979 a prospective study on eye changes during pregnancy in women with insulin-dependent diabetes has been conducted at Rigshospitalet, Copenhagen. A total of 145 women are participating in the study. Forty women have been followed until one year and 73 until two months after delivery (46). Our preliminary conclusions of the study are as follows: women with no retinopathy at the onset of pregnancy do not develop persistant retinopathy. About 50% of diabetic women with background retinopathy deteriorate during pregnancy, but they all regress to some extent after delivery. A few women with background retinopathy at the beginning of pregnancy develop proliferative retinopathy, which commonly disappears during the first month after delivery. No severe changes with respect to vitreous hemorrhages or severe proliferative changes have been observed and in only one case photocoagulation 8 months after delivery was necessary to arrest retinal proliferative changes at the optic disc. As a consequence of these conclusions, treatment with photocoagulation during pregnancy or the first month after delivery needs to be used only exceptionally since spontaneous regression is to be expected. It is thus justified to postpone photocoagulation therapy with close ophthalmological control until 8–12 months after delivery.

Ante-partum fetal surveillance

Assessment of fetal wellbeing in diabetic pregnancies includes antepartum non-stress fetal heart rate (FHR) recording, maternal monitoring of fetal movement (FM) backed up by a fetal biophysical profile (47, 48). No specific patterns of FHR in diabetic pregnancies have until now been demonstrated but a suspicious or pathological FHR recording was significantly more frequent in women with poor metabolic control of their diabetes than in pregnant diabetics with good metabolic control (49). The major benefit of the antepartum fetal surveillance techniques in diabetic pregnancies seems to be in determining when not to intervene, thus allowing safe prolongation of pregnancy (50).

Whether fetal activity in diabetic pregnancies differs from non-diabetic pregnancies is not yet settled (51). An important observation made by Sadovsky et al. (52) suggested that in diabetic pregnancies severe fetal distress should be suspected following 6 to 8 hours of fetal movement cessation and not after 12 hours, as previously described for other high-risk conditions.

During the last decade many obstetric centers around the world have investigated the value of registering the intrauterine fetal respiratory movements. The most common way to measure fetal respiration is by the fetal breathing index, which is the time during which the fetus is breathing, expressed in percentage of the observation period. Fetal breathing immediately following lunch and dinner showed significantly lower indices in diabetics than in normals (53). However, the variation in the fetal breathing index is substantial and for this reason a method has been worked out in our department by which it is made possible to measure qualitatively the amplitude of the fetal thoracal and abdominal wall (54). The respiratory amplitude was found to be significantly correlated with gestational age, but unrelated to weight (54). In diabetic pregnancies as a group, the respiratory amplitude increased earlier in gestation (Fig. 1) and was also significantly correlated to gestational age (47).

For more than four decades elective termination of diabetic pregnancies between 34 and 37 weeks gestation has been performed in most obstetrical departments in order to avoid sudden and often unexplained intrauterine

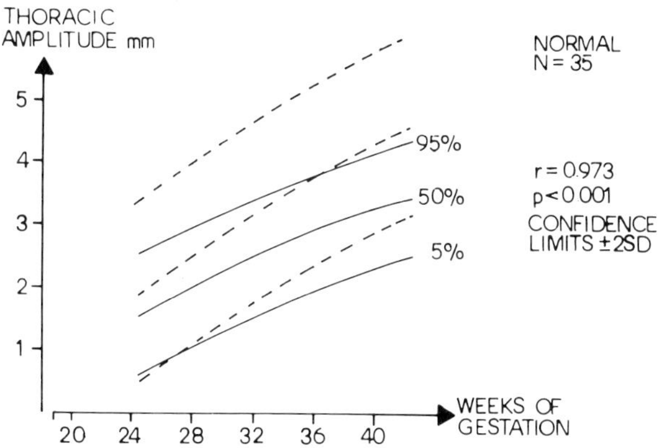

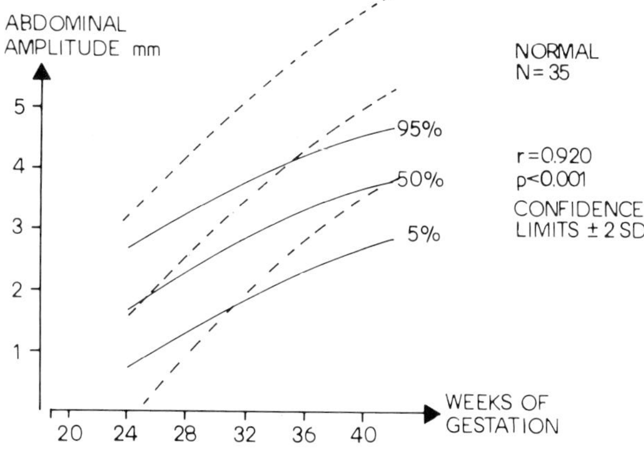

FIG. 1. *Correlation between fetal thoracic and abdominal respiratory amplitude and gestational age (—— = normal pregnancies; --------- = insulin-dependent diabetic pregnancies).*

death (40). This policy has gradually changed over recent years whereby in uncomplicated diabetic pregnancies it is not uncommon to await spontaneous delivery or postpone induction of labour until term.

Obstetric complications occur, however, more often in diabetic than in non-diabetic pregnancies and prediction of fetal lung maturation by amniocentesis in order to avoid respiratory distress syndrome (RDS) therefore should still be useful. In this respect the value of amniotic fluid lecithin/sphingomyelin (L/S) ratio in diabetic pregnancies is controversial (55). In a recent paper James and co-workers have described the levels of phosphatidyl choline (PC), phosphatidyl inositol (PI) and phosphatidyl glycerol (PG) in amniotic fluid from diabetic and normal pregnancies and, compared to determination of L/S ratio, the prediction of fetal lung maturity was improved dramatically by measuring these three phospholipid concentrations. Surprisingly no evidence of delayed appearance of fetal surfactant phospholipids in either well- or poorly controlled diabetic pregnancies was found (56). Measurement of PC levels alone was the most accurate method of predicting RDS (55).

Contraception in diabetics

As previously pointed out, a diabetic woman should become pregnant only by plan and therefore requires specific advice concerning contraceptive agents that are not only reliable, but acceptable to her. The intrauterine contraceptive devices (IUCDs) have traditionally been considered preferable to oral contraception because they do not influence carbohydrate tolerance. However, the efficacy of the IUCDs in women with diabetes has been disputed (57). A surprisingly high pregnancy rate of 37% within the first year was found in this retrospective study of copper as well as plastic IUCD insertion in 30 insulin-dependent diabetic women.

We have, however, recently investigated the clinical performance of a T Cu-200 model in 105 insulin-dependent diabetic women and in 119 non-diabetic controls. The events and overall efficacy rates were compared by life table analysis and the main results are presented in Table 6. No difference in accidental pregnancy rate, removal rate or total continuation rate could be demonstrated (58). In the Diabetes Center in Copenhagen the IUCD method is therefore still considered a reliable and acceptable contraceptive practice in diabetic women.

The influence of oral contraceptives on carbohydrate metabolism has been thoroughly investigated during the last fifteen years and some of these data have recently been reviewed by Spellacy (59). In users of the combination oral contraceptives containing 50 μg of estrogen, most of the carbohydrate studies performed have demonstrated elevations of blood glucose and similarly plasma-insulin levels were elevated in oral glucose tolerance

TABLE 6. *Net cumulative rates per 100 women for different events in diabetics fitted with copper T 200 devices*

	Insulin-dependent diabetes		Controls	
	3 mths	12 mths	3 mths	12 mths
Rates				
Accidental pregnancy	0.0	1.0	0.0	0.8
Expulsion	2.9	3.9	0.0	0.8
Removals				
Bleeding/pain	1.0	3.9	3.4	7.6
Infection	1.0	1.0	1.7	1.7
Other medical indication	1.0	1.0	0.0	0.0
Planned pregnancy	0.0	1.9	0.0	0.8
Continuation rate	94.1	87.3	94.9	88.3
No. of first insertions		105		119

tests (OGTT). Investigations of progestogen preparations have disclosed that the influence of the combined compounds with 50 μg estrogen can be reproduced with 19-nortestosterone derivatives. The synthetic estrogen compounds (ethinyl estradiol, mestranol) alone have no influence on glucose metabolism, but they act in a synergistic way with progestogens. Whether or not oral contraceptives of the combined low-dosage type can be administered to women with previous abnormal glucose tolerance, without increasing the risk of developing overt diabetes, is still subject to discussion.

We have studied the effect of 30 μg ethinyl estradiol (EE) and 150 μg levonorgestrel (LNg) in women with a previous gestational diabetes (60). After a 6-month treatment period the plasma insulin levels were significantly elevated during an OGTT, but the glucose tolerance remained unchanged. The effect of a triphasic compound containing low doses of EE and LNg has also been examined and the effect on glucose tolerance was very much like the effect of the monophasic EE plus LN_g compound (61). During intake of the triphasic compound plasma lipoprotein levels have also been measured. The HDL-cholesterol/total cholesterol ratio for the previous gestational diabetic women and for a control group was determined, and no changes were seen in either group, nor was any difference observed between the groups (61).

In insulin-dependent diabetic women there are reports of difficulties with diabetes control and increased insulin requirements during intake of compounds containing 50 μg estrogen (62). There are as yet no data concerning the influence of low-dose compounds on diabetic control. Progestogens of the 19-norethisterone type may in low dosage be administered to diabetic women without inducing changes in insulin requirements (63). Quite recently we have examined the effects of a contraceptive compound containing 4 mg estradiol plus 2 mg estriol in a monophasic combination with 3 mg norethisterone on diabetes control and lipid metabolism. The results showed no difference in insulin requirement, 24-hour urinary glucose excretion or body weight during treatment, and the HDL-cholesterol/total cholesterol ratio remained constant (61).

In conclusion, we consider the IUCD method safe and effective in diabetic women. Oral contraceptives of the low-dose type apply well to non-insulin-dependent diabetic women and in insulin-dependent diabetic women only the low-dosage progestogen pill or a combined compound containing natural estrogen may be administered.

Gestational diabetes

In normal pregnant women several physiological changes take place, the sum of which tends to reset the homeostasis of carbohydrate metabolism in the direction of diabetes; in this sense pregnancy may be called 'diabetogenic'. In about 1% of all pregnancies an abnormal OGTT develops, but still there is no general agreement concerning the screening procedure to be used, the choice of glucose tolerance test, and the diagnostic criteria of a diabetic curve (64). In our center in Copenhagen we find it worthwhile to try to detect the 1% with, most often, very mild diabetes. The screening procedure used in Copenhagen has been previously described (40) and the aim of this screening is: (1) to diagnose diabetes in pregnancy with reference to treatment and thereby reduce the perinatal mortality and morbidity, and (2) to screen for future diabetes. Ten per cent of the women with diabetes diagnosed during pregnancy had to be treated with insulin and in a recent follow-up study from Copenhagen including the period from 1966 to 1980, 65 women belonged to this category (65). Among these women 4 intrauterine deaths occurred during Weeks 32 to 36 of gestation and these could probably have been avoided if screening for diabetes had been performed earlier in pregnancy, since all four women were potential diabetics.

As a possible new screening test for gestational diabetes glycohemoglobin (HbA_{1C}) has been investigated and HbA_{1C} does not appear to be a sensitive enough screening tool for the detection of gestational diabetes mellitus (66, 67). Also fructosamine as an indicator of glycosylated serum protein has been proposed as a possible screening tool for gestational diabetes (68); however, there are objections to this method as a screening test for diabetes in pregnancy (69).

The diabetogenicity of pregnancy which has been studied for some years in the Copenhagen Center cannot be ascribed to diabetes-like changes in the secretory function of the endocrine pancreas, hypersecretion of the biologically almost inactive proinsulin, or enhanced insulin degradation. The insulin secretory reserve of gestational diabetics seems, however, to be considerably less than that of healthy pregnant women. The reason for the diabetogenicity of pregnancy must be sought outside the endocrine pancreas, and it is probably primarily due to a diminished tissue sensitivity to the biological action of insulin (70). An impaired gastrointestinal stimulation of insulin secretion might play a minor contributory role (71) and the elevation of cortisol levels in pregnancy might possibly also be associated with the diabetogenicity of pregnancy (72).

In normal non-diabetic pregnancy a significant decrease in HbA_{1C} concentration takes place during the 20th week of gestation (28) or even earlier (73) while also a biphasic pattern has been described (74). In diabetic pregnancies HbA_{1C} also decreases during gestation, but HbA_{1C} was found to be a poor predictor of the average blood glucose concentration in the individual patient (75).

In two recent studies glycosylated hemoglobin levels were determined in maternal and cord blood at delivery in normal and diabetic pregnancies. Total glycosylated hemoglobin was lower in cord than in maternal blood but higher following diabetic pregnancies both in cord and maternal samples (76). In the other study, HbA_{1C} was measured in diabetic and non-diabetic pregnant women at delivery and hemoglobin F adducts in paired cord blood of their infants. The conclusion was that diabetes in pregnancy probably increases both hemoglobin F adduct formation in the fetus and the birthweight ratio, but control during pregnancy efficiently keeps the increase at low or statistically non-significant levels (77).

Conclusions

The incidence of congenital malformations in newborn infants of diabetic mothers is still high. However, it is now evident that congenital malformations can be decreased by insulin therapy in animal models and in humans by planning of pregnancy, including careful preconceptional diabetes control continued during pregnancy.

Besides a lower rate of congenital malformations, better metabolic control will decrease neonatal morbidity, reduce obstetric complications, including pre-eclampsia and placental maturation disorders. Also the risk of decreased placental blood flow and of a pathological fetal heart rate pattern will be diminished.

Treatment of diabetic proliferative retinopathy with photocoagulation during pregnancy or the first month after delivery should only be used exceptionally since spontaneous regression is to be expected.

Measurement of phosphatidyl choline in amniotic fluid was the most accurate method of predicting respiratory distress syndrome.

The IUCD method is safe and effective in diabetic women; oral contraceptives of the low-dose type apply well to non-insulin-dependent diabetic women and in insulin-dependent diabetics low-dose progesteron or a combined compound containing natural estrogen may be administered.

References

1. Mølsted-Pedersen L (1980): Congenital malformations in the offspring of diabetic women. In: *Diabetes 1979: Proceedings, 10th Congress of IDF, Vienna, Austria, September 1979*. Editor: W.K. Waldhäusl. Excerpta Medica, Amsterdam.
2. Eriksson UJ, Dahlström E, Larsson KS, Hellerstrøm C (1982): Increased incidence of congenital malformations in the offspring of diabetic rats and their prevention by maternal insulin therapy. *Diabetes*, *31*, 1.
3. Eriksson UJ, Dahlström E, Hellerstrøm C (1983): Diabetes in pregnancy. Skeletal malformations in the offspring of diabetic rats after intermittent withdrawal of insulin in early gestation. *Diabetes*, *32*, 1141.
4. Sadler TW, Horton Jr WE (1983): Effect of maternal diabetes on early embryogenesis. The role of insulin and insulin therapy. *Diabetes*, *32*, 1070.
5. Freinkel N, Lewis NJ, Akazawa S, Roth SI, Gorman L (1984): The honeybee syndrome – implications of the teratogenicity of mannose in rat-embryo culture. *N. Engl. J. Med.*, *310*, 223.
6. Villee CA (1984): Birth defects and glycolysis. *N. Engl. J. Med.*, *310*, 254.
7. Editorial (1984): Honeybees: energy supply and birth defects. *Lancet*, *1*, 886.
8. Mills JL, Baker L, Goldman AA (1979): Malformations in infants of diabetic mothers occur before the seventh gestational week. Implications for treatment. *Diabetes*, *28*, 292.
9. Pedersen JF, Mølsted-Pedersen L (1979): Early growth retardation in diabetic pregnancy. *Br. Med. J.*, *1*, 18.
10. Pedersen JF, Mølsted-Pedersen L (1981): Early fetal growth delay detected by ultrasound marks increased risk of congenital malformation in diabetic pregnancy. *Br. Med. J.*, *283*, 269.
11. Pedersen JF, Mølsted-Pedersen L (1982): Early growth delay predisposes the fetus in diabetic pregnancy to congenital malformation. *Lancet*, *1*, 737.
12. Pedersen J, Mølsted-Pedersen L (1979): Congenital malformations: the possible role of diabetes care outside pregnancy. In: *Pregnancy Metabolism, Diabetes and the Fetus*. Ciba Foundation Series 63 (new series), p 265. Excerpta Medica, Amsterdam.
13. Fuhrmann K, Reiher H, Semmler K, Fisher F, Fisher M, Glöckner E (1983): Prevention of congenital malformations in infants of insulin-dependent diabetic mothers. *Diabetes Care*, *6*, 219.

14. Mølsted-Pedersen L, Hansen PK, Hansen T (1982): Maternal blood-glucose profile and neonatal mortality. Paper presented at: XIII Annual Meeting, Diabetic Pregnancy Study Group, September 1982, Villars, Switzerland.
15. Mølsted-Pedersen L (1983): Congenital malformations and growth delay in diabetic pregnancies. *State of the Art Lecture, 19th Annual Meeting, European Association for the Study of Diabetes, September 14, 1983, Oslo, Norway.*
16. Simpson JL, Sherman E, Martin AO, Palmer MS, Ogata EA, Radvany RA (1983): Diabetes pregnancy. Northwestern University series (1977–81). I. Prospective study of anomalies in offspring of mothers with diabetes mellitus. *Am. J. Obstet. Gynecol.*, *146*, 263.
17. Steel JM, Johnstone FD, Smith AF, Duncan LJP (1982): Five years experience of a 'prepregnancy' clinic for insulin-dependent diabetics. *Br. Med. J.*, *285*, 353.
18. Mølsted-Pedersen L, Skouby SO (1984): Contraception in Diabetics. In: *Carbohydrate Metabolism in Pregnancy and the Newborn, Vol. 3.* Editors: H.W. Sutherland and J.M. Stowers. Churchill/Livingstone, Edinburgh.
19. Milunsky A, Alpert E, Kitzmiller JL, Yonger MD, Raymond KN (1982): Prenatal diagnosis of neural defects. VIII. The importance of serum alphafetoprotein screening in diabetic pregnant women. *Am. J. Obstet. Gynecol.*, *142*, 1030.
20. Karlsson K, Kjellmer I (1972): The outcome of diabetic pregnancies in relation to the mothers blood sugar level. *Am. J. Obstet. Gynecol.*, *112*, 213.
21. Roversi GD, Cammisio V, Gargiulo M, Candiani GB (1973): The intensive care of perinatal risk in pregnant diabetics (136 cases): A new therapeutic scheme for the best control of maternal disease. *J. Perinatal Med.*, *1*, 114.
22. Wright AD, Nicholson HO, Taylor KG, Insley J, Evans SE (1982): Maternal blood glucose control and outcome of diabetic pregnancy. *Postgrad. Med. J.*, *58*, 411.
23. Artal R, Golde SH, Dorey F, McClellan SN, Gratacos J, Lirette RNT, Montoro M, Wu PYK, Anderson B, Mestman J (1983): The effect of plasma glucose variability on neonatal outcome in the pregnant diabetic patient. *Am. J. Obstet. Gynecol.*, *147*, 537.
24. Adashi EY, Pinto H, Tyson JE (1979): Impact of maternal euglycemia on fetal outcome in diabetic pregnancy. *Am. J. Obstet. Gynecol.*, *133*, 268.
25. Leveno KS, Hauth JC, Gilstarp LC, Whalley PJ (1979): Appraisal of 'rigid' blood glucose control during pregnancy in the overthy diabetic women. *Am. J. Obstet. Gynecol.*, *135*, 853.
26. Constan DR, Berkowitz RL, Hobbins JC (1980): Tight metabolic control of overt diabetes in pregnancy. *Am. J. Med.*, *68*, 845.
27. Roversi GD, Garginto M, Nicolini U, Ferrazzi E, Pedretti E, Gruft L, Tronconi G (1980): Maximal tolerated insulin therapy in gestational diabetes. *Diabetes Care*, *3*, 489.
28. Jovanovic L, Peterson CM (1982): Optimal insulin delivery for pregnant diabetic patient. *Diabetes Care*, *5 Suppl. 1*, 24.
29. Bromham DR (1983): The increased risk of pre-eclampsia in pregnant diabetics. *J. Obstet. Gynaecol.*, *3*, 212.
30. Semmler K, Emmrich P, Fuhrmann K, Godel E (1982): Relationship between placental maturation disorders and standards of metabolic monitoring

of pregnant patients with insulin-dependent and gestational diabetes. *Zbl. Gynäkol.*, *104*, 1494.

31. Knight G, Worth RC, Ward JD (1983): Macrosomy despite a well-controlled diabetic pregnancy. *Lancet*, *2*, 1431.
32. Visser GHA, Van Ballegooie E, Sluiter WJ (1984): Macrosomy despite well-controlled diabetic pregnancy. *Lancet*, *1*, 284.
33. Pedersen J, Mølsted-Pedersen L (1971): Diabetes mellitus and pregnancy. The hyperglycaemia-hyperinsulin theory and the weight of the newborn baby. In: *Diabetes: Proceedings, VII Congress of the International Diabetes Federation*, p 678. Editors: R.R. Rodriques and J. Vallance-Owen. Excerpta Medica, Amsterdam.
34. Pedersen J (1977): Birth weight of newborn infants of diabetic women. In: *Diabetes: Proceedings, IX Congress of the International Diabetes Federation*, p 353. Editor: J.S. Bajaj. Excerpta Medica, Amsterdam.
35. Nylund L, Lunell N-O, Lewander R, Persson B, Sarby B, Thornstrøm S (1982): Uteroplacental blood flow in diabetic pregnancy: Measurements with indium 113m and a computer-linked gamma camera. *Am. J. Obstet. Gynecol.*, *144*, 298.
36. Geppert M, Peters FD, Geppert J (1982): Histomorphometry of the vascularization of the placental villi in diabetic pregnant women. *Geburtsh. Frauenheilk.*, *42*, 628.
37. Potter JM, Reckless JPD, Cullen DR (1980): Subcutaneous continuous insulin infusion and control of blood glucose concentration in diabetics in third trimester of pregnancy. *Br. Med. J.*, *1*, 1099.
38. Rudolf MCJ, Coustan DR, Sherwin RS, Bates SE, Felig P, Genel M, Tamborlane WV (1981): Efficacy of the insulin pump in the home treatment of pregnant diabetics. *Diabetes*, *30*, 891.
39. Kühl C, Jensen BM, Pedersen JF, Mølsted-Pedersen L (1983): Influence of intensified pre- and postconceptional metabolic control on early fetal growth in diabetic pregnancy. *Diabetologia*, *25*, 173.
40. Pedersen J (1977): *The Pregnant Diabetic and Her Newborn, 2nd ed*, Chapter VII, p 96. Munksgaard, Copenhagen.
41. Moloney JBM, Drury MI (1982): The effect of pregnancy on the natural course of diabetic retinopathy. *Am. J. Ophthalmol.*, *93,* 745.
42. Dibble CM, Kochenour NK, Worley RJ, Tyler FH, Swart M (1982): Effect of pregnancy on diabetic retinopathy. *Obstet. Gynecol.*, *59*, 699.
43. Gerke E, Meyer-Schwikerath G (1982): Proliferative diabetic retinopathy and pregnancy. *Klin. Monatsbl. Augenheilk.*, *181*, 170.
44. Prica JH, Hadden DR, Archer DB, Harley JMG (1984): Diabetic retinopathy in pregnancy. *Br. J. Obstet. Gynaecol.*, *91*, 11.
45. Carstensen LL, Frost-Larsen K, Fuglebjerg S, Nerup J (1982): Does pregnancy influence the proposes of uncomplicated insulin-dependent diabetes mellitus? *Diabetes Care*, *5*, 1.
46. Serup L (1984): Influence of pregnancy on diabetic retinopathy. *Acta Endocrinol. (Copenh.)*, *Suppl.* (in press).
47. Mølsted-Pedersen L (1982): Control fetal en la diabetes. In: *Perinatologia clinica 5, Diabetes y Embarazo*. Chapter 5, p 43. Editors: J. Esteban-Altirriba and L. Cabero Roura. Salvat Editors, Barcelona-Madrid.

48. Golde SH, Good-Anderson B, Broussard P, Jacobs N, Loesser C, Trujillo M, Walla C, Phelan J, Platt LD (1984): The role of nonstress test, fetal biophysical profile and contraction stress test in the out-patient management of insulin-requiring diabetic pregnancies. *Am. J. Obstet. Gynecol.*, *148*, 269.
49. Teramo K, Ammala P, Ylinen K, Raivio KO (1983): Pathologic fetal heart rate associated with poor metabolic control in diabetic pregnancies. *Obstet. Gynecol.*, *61*, 559.
50. Jorge CS, Artal R, Paul RH, Goebelsmann U, Gratacos J, Yeh S, Golde SH, Mestermann JH (1981): Antepartum fetal surveillance in diabetic pregnant patients. *Am. J. Obstet. Gynecol.*, *141*, 641.
51. Dierker Jr LJ, Pillay S, Sorokin Y, Rosen MG (1982): The change in fetal activity periods in diabetic and non-diabetic pregnancies. *Am. J. Obstet. Gynecol.*, *143*, 181.
52. Sadovsky E, Brzezinski A, Mor-Yosef S (1983): Fetal activity in diabetic pregnancy. *J. Foetal Med.*, *3*, 1.
53. Wladimiroff JW, Roodenburg PS (1982): Human fetal breathing and gross body activity relative to maternal meals during insulin-dependent pregnancy. *Acta Obstet. Gynaecol. Scand.*, *61*, 65.
54. Neldam S (1980): Fetal body and respiratory movements. In: *Current Status of EPH Gestosis*. Editors: A. Kurjak, E.T. Rippmann, V. Sulovic. Excerpta Medica, Amsterdam.
55. James DK, Chiswick ML, Harkes A, Williams M, Tindale VR (1984): Maternal diabetes and neonatal respiratory distress. II. Prediction of fetal lung maturity. *Br. J. Obstet. Gynaecol.*, *91*, 325.
56. James DK, Chiswick ML, Harkes A, Williams M, Tindal VR (1984): Maternal diabetes and neonatal respiratory distress. I. Maturation of fetal surfactant. *Br. J. Obstet. Gynaecol.*, *91*, 316.
57. Gosden C, Steel J, Ross A, Springbelt A (1982): Intrauterine contraceptive devices in diabetic women. *Lancet*, *1*, 530.
58. Skouby SO, Mølsted-Pedersen L (1982): Intrauterine contraceptive devices for diabetics. *Lancet*, *1*, 968.
59. Spellacy WN (1982): Carbohydrate metabolism during treatment with estrogen, progestogen, and low-dose oral contraceptives. *Am. J. Obstet. Gynecol.*, *142*, 732.
60. Skouby SO, Mølsted-Pedersen L, Kühl C (1982): Low dosage oral contraception in women with previous gestational diabetes. *Obstet. Gynecol.*, *59*, 325.
61. Skouby SO, Mølsted-Pedersen L, Kühl C (1984): Contraception in diabetic women. *Acta Endocrinol.* (*Copenh.*), *Suppl.* (in press).
62. Steel JM, Duncan LJP (1978): The effect of oral contraceptives on insulin requirements in diabetics. *Br. J. Fam. Plann.*, *3*, 77.
63. Rådberg T, Gustafson A, Skryten A, Karlsson K (1982): Metabolic studies in women with previous gestational diabetes during contraceptive treatment: effects on serum lipids and high density lipoproteins. *Acta Endocrinol.* (*Copenh.*), *101*, 134.
64. Jarret RJ (1981): Reflections on gestational diabetes mellitus. *Lancet*, *2*, 1220.
65. Kühl C, Buschard K, Mølsted-Pedersen L (1983): Study of newly developed insulin-dependent diabetes mellitus in pregnancy. *Diabetes*, *32*, *Suppl. 1*, 109A.

66. Shah BD, Cohen AW, May C, Gabbe SG (1982): Comparison of glycohemoglobin determination and the one-hour oral glucose screen in the identification of gestational diabetes. *Am. J. Obstet. Gynecol.*, *144*, 774.
67. Artal R, Mosley GM, Dorey FJ (1984): Glycohemoglobin as a screening test for gestational diabetes. *Am. J. Obstet. Gynecol.*, *148*, 412.
68. Roberts AB, Court DJ, Henley P, Baker JR, James AG, Ronayne ID (1983): Fructosamine in diabetic pregnancy. *Lancet*, *2*, 998.
69. Kennedy L, Hadden DR (1983): Fructosamine in diabetic pregnancy. *Lancet*, *2*, 1193.
70. Kühl C, Hornnes PJ (1984): Plasma insulin, proinsulin and pancreatic glucagon in gestational diabetes. In: *Recent Advances in Obesity and Diabetes Research*, p 129. Editor: N. Melchionda. Raven Press, New York.
71. Hornnes PJ, Kühl C, Lauritsen KB (1982): Gastro-enteropancreatic hormones in gestational diabetes: Response to a protein rich meal. *Horm. Metabol. Res.*, *14*, 335.
72. Hornnes PJ, Kühl C (1984): Cortisol and glucosetolerance in normal pregnancy. *Diabète Métab.*, *10*, 1.
73. Hanson U, Hagenfeldt L, Hagenfeldt K (1983): Glycosylated hemoglobins in normal pregnancy: Sequential changes and relation to birth weight. *Obstet. Gynecol.*, *62*, 741.
74. Phelps RL, Honig GR, Green D, Metzger BE, Frederiksen MC, Freinkel N (1983): Biphasic changes in hemoglobin A_1C concentrations during normal human pregnancy. *Am. J. Obstet. Gynecol.*, *147*, 651.
75. Madsen H, Ditzel J, Hansen P, Hahnemann N, Andersen OP, Kjaegaard JJ (1981): Hemoglobin A_1C determinations in diabetic pregnancy. *Diabetes Care*, *4*, 54.
76. Worth R, Ashworth L, Home PD, Gerrard J, Lind T, Anderson J, Alberti KGMM (1983): Glycosylated haemoglobin in cord blood following normal and diabetic pregnancies. *Diabetologia*, *25*, 482.
77. Olesen HA, Sørensen S, Hansen PK, Mølsted-Pedersen L (1984): Haemoglobin A_1C in pregnant diabetic patients at delivery and haemoglobin F_1 in cord blood from their newborns. *Scand. J. Clin. Lab. Invest.*, *44*, 329.

The Diabetes Annual/1
K.G.M.M. Alberti and L.P. Krall, editors

ISBN 0444 90 343 7
$0.85 per article per page (transactional system)
$0.20 per article per page (licensing system)

15 Recent advances in diabetic retinopathy

EVA M. KOHNER

In the 1970s for the first time an effective treatment for diabetic retinopathy became available. This treatment, photocoagulation, could be applied to a large number of patients and as a local treatment did not depend on the patient's age and general health, as did the only previous effective treatment, pituitary ablation. Photocoagulation has been found effective in preserving vision in some 70% of patients with proliferative retinopathy who otherwise would have lost vision (1–4). It has also been found to be effective in non-proliferative diabetic retinopathy with macular edema, diabetic maculopathy (5–7). Recent advances in technology also allow for saving of eyes which have become blind already from complications of proliferative retinopathy such as vitreous hemorrhage and retinal detachment. Vitrectomies now save or restore sight in patients who had no hope before (8, 9).

Improvements in our understanding of normal insulin production in non-diabetics, and the introduction of continuous infusion of insulin together with valid assessments of short- and long-term diabetic control now enable us to evaluate the role of 'good' diabetic control in the evolution of diabetic retinopathy. Great advances have been made in this field. The effectiveness of a new treatment has to be established by valid methods of assessment of retinopathy. New treatments resulted in the increased interest in diabetic retinopathy, epidemiological studies increased as did studies on risk factors for diabetic retinopathy.

Finally ophthalmologists have become interested in the pathogenic mechanisms in diabetic retinopathy. Together with basic scientists the mechanisms leading to diabetic retinopathy have been attacked seriously.

For this summary of recent advances, over 500 articles have been reviewed. Not all will be quoted, but it is hoped that the present state of the knowledge about diabetic retinopathy is adequately and critically presented.

Assessment of diabetic retinopathy

For the study of the natural history of diabetic retinopathy as well as for evaluation of treatment effects, valid methods of assessment are required.

These include assessment of the anatomical lesions and their severity and, more recently, functional changes which may predict development or change in severity of retinopathy.

Quantitative assessment

Retinopathy can be quantitated from color photographs and fluorescein angiograms. Many grading systems have been developed in the past relating mainly to specific treatment trials, such as pituitary ablation (10) or photocoagulation (11) or, more recently, to the study of early treatment of diabetic retinopathy (ETDRS) (12). A new system has been added to these recently (13). It is based on the retinopathy features of 191 patients studied in 1970–71 and again 2 and 6 years later. The assessment uses stereo color photographs of 7 standard retinal fields and attempts to group retinopathy features into prognostically significant categories, covering the range of severity, from no retinopathy to proliferative lesions in 6 separate levels. Some of these levels are defined by description alone, while in others some lesions are described while others are graded by comparison with standard photographs. The system has many advantages. These include the possibility of assessing the two eyes separately, e.g. by 'worse' eye, or of studying the two eyes together. It is sufficiently sensitive to allow for study in changes as seen in early diabetic retinopathy – at present probably the most interesting and most studied form of diabetic retinopathy – and it is also reproducible. Out of 382 eyes graded by 4 different observers, 339 were graded identically. Like all work coming from Madison, it is carefully thought out and reliable, though not entirely without its difficulty; indeed the grades have already been increased to 8 (14).

Fluorescein angiograms of good quality may visualize lesions not discerned on color photographs or by ophthalmoscopy (15). Quantitation of fluorescein angiograms may be a more valid test of changes in really early diabetic retinopathy. However, quantitation is difficult and attempts at evaluation of the Diabetic Retinopathy Study Group's fluorescein angiograms quantitatively did not seem possible. The reason for the difficulty lies in the necessity to obtain high-quality fluorescein angiograms of the same field repeatedly. This is only possible if the patient is cooperative, the media clear, the circulation adequate and the photographer well-trained. A method for counting microaneurysms in the central 20° field focused on the macula has been developed (16). The method subdivides microaneurysms by size into definite and possible ones. The definite ones are over 25 μm in diameter, the possible ones smaller, between about 20 and 25 μm. Very good correlation between two separate readings was observed by individual observers (0.987–0.99) for definite aneurysms. The identity of location including all aneurysms was, however, on average only 70% reproducible, though the percentage was again much higher for the definite ones. The method at present is entirely by hand and therefore very time-consuming. It is quite sensitive and it was found to differentiate between patients on conventional treatment and those treated by continuous subcutaneous insulin infusion (17). At present, methods are being developed which allow computer-assisted analysis (18) or complete computerization (19). Lesions other than microaneurysms, such as non-perfused areas, can also be quantitated (18). The importance of detailed studies of this sort, even in research, is argued, especially as it has not been clearly established what the role of change in microaneurysm numbers in the evolution of retinopathy is. However, it can be stated that in early retinopathy an increase in microaneurysms indicates deterioration while a decrease may also either indicate deterioration (enlarged non-perfused areas) or improvement, when capillaries get remodelled and the capillary bed becomes normal.

Functional assessment

Functional changes in the retinal circulation and in the visual function accompany and even precede anatomical changes. Thus Riva and associates, using blue light entoptoscopy (20), showed reduced autoregulation to raised intraocular pressure. Measuring blood flow by laser Doppler velocimetry, they showed in diabetics reduced response to increased oxygen in the inspired air, as compared with normals (21). They also showed that panretinal photocoagulation improves markedly the reduced response to oxygen, suggesting that the altered autoregulation in diabetes may be at least in part reversible. These results need further investigations and validation. At present there is no study available which correlates the perifoveal capillary circulation as obtained by blue light entoptoscopy with laser Doppler velocimetry. These tests which measure retinal blood flow and its adaptation, are of utmost importance in understanding the underlying mechanisms in the development of diabetic retinopathy.

Vitreous fluorophotometry is a measure of the blood retinal barrier function and has been in use since 1975 (22). This technique offered the possibility of detecting functional abnormalities manifest by leakage of fluorescein from the retinal vessels into the vitreous, before the development of diabetic retinopathy. However, there were some misgivings about the technique from the beginning and contradictory results were obtained by different observers, the major differences and their causes being reviewed by Kohner and Alderson (23). The major problem was the wide variety of sensitivity of equipment used and the different techniques employed. These prevented valid comparison between centers, though carefully performed studies could give scientifically valid results (24).

In 1982, new commercially available, simple-to-use equipment became available, and this allows for valid, repeatable measurements (25–27).

Studies using eyes of rats which have only 2 mm vitreous (28) and other studies using the old equipment (29–31) can no longer be regarded as valid. The lack of meaningful correlation with retinopathy has been amply proven in the Steno study (31) of continuous subcutaneous insulin infusion, where functional improvements, i.e. reduced leakage was observed in eyes which anatomically became worse (32). Use of the new equipment produced unexpected results. No difference in permeability between normals and diabetics without or with early retinopathy was found by Chahal et al (33). Kritz and Irsigler (34) also found no difference between diabetics without retinopathy and normal subjects. Their patients with mild background retinopathy could be subdivided into those who show little or no leakage into the posterior vitreous (Group A) and those who show extensive leakage (Group B). These authors state that the anatomical features of retinopathy as seen on the color photos in the two groups was similar, though the method of examination is not detailed. If confirmed it could indicate patients who have more rapidly advancing retinopathy. At present it appears that vitreous fluorophotometry does not predict the development of retinopathy, but when retinopathy is present it quantitates leakage and therefore gives a measure of change in the retinopathy.

Of other functional tests, many have been reported to be of importance in predicting deterioration or no retinopathy or mild background retinopathy to proliferative retinopathy. Nyctometry, a test used to evaluate adaptation of visual acuity to glare, is one of these. Frost-Larsen et al. (35) and Kritz and Irsigler (34) consider it a useful test. The former report on 6 out of 16 patients with reduced nyctometry who developed proliferative retinopathy within 3 years while no patient with a normal test developed such lesions. However, the finding of improved nyctometry with deteriorating lesions (31, 32) somewhat negates the validity of the results.

Frost-Larsen also found reduction in the oscillatory potential of the electro-retinogram to predict proliferative retinopathy (36). The study was confirmed recently by Bresnick (37), who found that when correcting for duration of diabetes, reduced oscillatory potentials did correlate with development of proliferative lesions. Brunette and Lafand (38) found oscillatory potential useful in differentiating stages of retinopathy. This expensive, time-consuming technique unfortunately does not reduce the importance of adequate retinal examination, and normal oscillatory potentials do not exclude the presence of proliferative lesions. Other functional tests, such as flicker tests (34), evoked potentials (39), Arden Grid readings and color discriminatory function (40) are often abnormal in diabetes. Their importance has not been established and a clear relationship to retinopathy has not been shown (41, 42).

Epidemiological studies

Epidemiological studies on diabetic retinopathy fall into two groups: those looking at prevalence of retinopathy, and those looking at visual impairment presumably due to diabetic retinopathy.

Prevalence of diabetic retinopathy

Diabetic retinopathy has been shown to occur in all forms of diabetes in all populations. Thus, Zimmet and co-workers (43) were able to show that in the Micronesian population of Nauru, where non-insulin-dependent diabetes (NIDD) is present in 24% of the population and 80% of those over 55 years have impaired glucose tolerance – retinopathy occurs in 24.2% of all diabetic subjects. Even in those with impaired glucose tolerance it was as high as 2.5%, and in newly diagnosed diabetics 5.9%. The majority of patients had background retinopathy of varying severity, only 1.2% of males and 2% of females having proliferative lesions.

In underdeveloped countries insulin dependent diabetics (IDD) rarely survive 15 years. If they do, they are liable to microvascular complications. In 84 patients who had diabetes for over 15 years in Ethiopia, Lester (44) found retinopathy in 38% of the patients. In 35% of patients fundus examination was not possible. Cataract was a more common cause of visual loss, even in young diabetics, than retinopathy.

Jialal et al. (45) reported on 85 NIDD young diabetics of Indian origin in South Africa and found 17% with retinopathy, but only one patient had proliferative lesions and the duration of diabetes on the whole was short.

Looking at Caucasian populations, Danielsen (46) reported on insulin-treated patients of Iceland. Of the total of 266 eligible patients, 212 were seen. Retinopathy was present in 27.4% with 6.1% having proliferative retinopathy. Retinopathy was less frequent in the first 20 years of diabetes in those who were diagnosed between 0–19 years, than in those whose diabetes was diagnosed later in life.

The best of many prevalence studies comes from Wisconsin where R. Klein and associates performed a large epidemiological study in 11 counties of South Wisconsin. They reported separately on those diagnosed under 30 years (14) and those diagnosed when 30 years or older (47). Of the 9283 evaluable patients, 1210 had diabetes diagnosed under the age of 30 and were on insulin. Investigations included some general information and eye examination was detailed, including corrected visual acuity, slit-lamp biomicroscopy and both direct and indirect ophthalmoscopy. Stereo fundus photographs of 7 standard fields were taken. Details are available on 996 of the patients. Duration of diabetes was the most important determinant of retinopathy prevalence. This rose steeply from 2% after 2 years' diabetes duration to a staggering 97.5% in those with diabetes over 15 years. Proliferative retinopathy increased from 4% after 5 years to 25% after 15 years and 67% after 35 years. While retinopathy occurred with equal frequency in both sexes, proliferative lesions were more common in males ($P < 0.05$) in accordance with previous observations (48).

Of the 7887 diabetic patients diagnosed after the age of 30 years, 1370 were selected randomly after stratification by duration and treatment. Insulin takers had 30% prevalence of retinopathy after 2 years and 84.5% after 15 years. In non-insulin-takers, prevalence was lower, 23 and 57.5%, respectively. Proliferative retinopathy was also more common in insulin takers reaching 20% after 15 or more years diabetes duration. It never exceeded 4.5% in those not on insulin.

Only 2 studies of incidence are reported in the literature on Type 1 and Type 2 diabetics from the small island of Falster in Denmark (49, 50). The cohorts were small and only 1-year follow up was available. During this time the prevalence of background and proliferative retinopathy changed non-significantly (50 to 51.6% and 16.3 to 18.6%). In Type 1 diabetics the incidence of newly developed retinopathy was 5.7% and proliferative retinopathy 2.5%. In the non-insulin-treated patients the incidence for background retinopathy was the same but only 1.1% developed proliferative lesions.

Visual disability

Visual disability in most studies is from blind or partially sighted people's registration forms. Foulds (51), looking at blind registrations in the West of Scotland, found that 10% of all blindness was due to retinopathy and in the age group 45–64 years, diabetes was the commonest cause of blindness. In the UK Cullinan (52) estimated visual loss due to diabetic retinopathy to be 30/100,000 of the population. Two new blind patients are added each year for every 100,000 of the population. These figures are similar to the incidence of 2.2% of partial sightedness and 10% of blindness in the diabetic population of Falster (53). Nielson found legal blindness in 6.2% of diabetics and 9.9% were partially sighted when insulin-treated, but 10.5% when non-insulin-requiring. While diabetic maculopathy was the commonest cause in non-insulin-treated patients, non-diabetic macular disease was also common.

Checking blind certificates in the county of Tolna in Hungary, among 550 blind patients, diabetic retinopathy was the cause of visual loss in 8.6% (54). Again the best study is by Klein et al. (55). In the Wisconsin study 1.4% of insulin-treated diabetics diagnosed before the age of 30 had moderate visual impairment and 3.6% were blind. In the older age group the figures were higher. However, while diabetic retinopathy alone was the cause of visual loss in 86% of earlier-onset patients, this was so only in 33% of those diagnosed after 30 years.

These studies indicate that diabetic retinopathy is common in all populations and its prevalence, especially in Caucasians, is higher than was previously thought. In developed countries at least, blind certification should decrease, now that photocoagulation is available, and the lower figure of Klein et al. (55) may be due to this.

Risk factors for diabetic retinopathy

In order to prevent the development of diabetic retinopathy and to identify those at risk, large numbers of cross-sectional studies have been performed looking at correlates of diabetic retinopathy. Most of these studies are on small numbers of highly selected patients and only few on populations. Even looking at similar parameters different groups used different tests. The results obtained are profuse, sometimes confusing and only rarely helpful.

Genetic factors and retinopathy

Since genetic factors are important in the development of diabetes, such factors have also been sought to explain complications. Studying HLA-A and B series, neither Johnston et al. (56) nor Gray et al. (57), found significant differences between those with and those without retinopathy, though in the latter study HLA-B7 showed a reduced prevalence in those with retinopathy. Cudworth's group (58) also looked at HLA-DR antigens in over 130 patients with proliferative retinopathy and compared these with 50 patients without retinopathy after similar diabetes duration. Neither in their own group nor in reviewing the world literature (59) did they find a significant relationship between HLA and retinopathy. The only group which found a relationship with HLA-DR3 and DR4 was the Oxford group (60). However, their patients were highly selected (those without retinopathy had had diabetes for over 30 years, during which period a large proportion of the retinopaths would have died) and their numbers were small.

Nevertheless genetic factors may be important at least in NIDD, in whom Leslie and Pyke (61) showed that among 37 pairs of diabetic twins concordant for diabetes, 35 were in the same retinal category. In insulin-dependent twin pairs there was often a striking difference in retinopathy status.

Immunological factors

An immune basis for diabetic retinopathy has been proposed on the basis of experimental work in monkeys (62), but has never been substantiated in patients. Increased immune complexes in patients with proliferative retinopathy found by Cudworth's group (48, 58) could be related to coexistent renal involvement and did not correlate with insulin antibodies. Increased acute phase reactants in Dornan's (63) patients was not related to either retinopathy or to nephropathy. Van Oost and co-workers (64) also found this abnormality but more so in those with proliferative lesions.

Duration of diabetes, age and sex

There is little doubt that duration of diabetes is the most important risk factor in diabetic retinopathy. All the epidemiological studies support this view. It has also been found by Dornan et al. (60) and Gray et al. (57). In the epidemiological studies, proliferative retinopathy was even more strongly related to diabetes duration than background retinopathy (14, 47, 64). Frank et al. (65) found both duration and age to be important in the development of retinopathy in 173 juvenile onset young diabetics.

Actual age and age of onset of diabetes are less important, but severe retinopathy is rarely seen before the age of 18. In the large referral clinic at Hammersmith Hospital only 9 adolescents with severe proliferative retinopathy were seen in over 10 years (66). Klein found an association between retinopathy and younger age of onset only when the diabetes duration was longer than 5 years (47), while Barnett et al. (67) found no relation at all, although non-retinopaths had longer duration of diabetes.

While retinopathy of 'any type' occurs with equal frequency in both sexes and may even be more frequent in women, proliferative retinopathy is more common in males when the diabetes onset is before the age of 30 (14, 48, 64).

Diabetic control

The strongest correlation in almost all studies of risk factors is with diabetic control. Better control seems to protect patients from retinopathy even after 30 years diabetes duration (68). It must however be remembered that in the study showing this, patients' blood glucose levels were taken after lunch and it was the blood glucose which was different between retinopaths and non-retinopaths. The difference of HbA_1 levels was not significant. Dornan (68) thinks this is due to improved control after finding retinopathy. But since the clinics were after lunch it may indicate different eating habits, and distribution of meals, although with overall similar control. Control was found to be related to retinopathy by Klein et al. (17, 47), Dornan et al. (60), Gray et al. (57) and Rand et al. (69). Jackson et al. (70) found retinopathy among adolescents and young adults only in those who were poorly controlled. Retinopathy advance and change in basement membrane thickness was also associated with poorer control over a short period of time. In Japanese patients Nakayoshi et al. (71) found HbA_1 and fasting blood glucose levels to correlate with severity and progression of retinopathy. Looking at the level of control in young patients, Dorchy et al. (72) found no correlation between retinopathy and HbA_1 levels over a one-year follow-up; HbA_1 was related to the duration of diabetes. It is tempting to incriminate absent or reduced C-peptide levels early in the disease for worse control and hence for the development of retinopathy. However, Zick et al. (73) found no correlation between C-peptide levels and retinopathy in 70 children.

Worse control could also be the result of increased insulin resistance. Using the glucose clamp technique Vitelli et al. (74) found increased resistance to insulin in IDDs with retinopathy when the plasma glucose was 12 mmol, though only at 100 mU/ml of insulin, suggesting a receptor defect. In NIDD the same group (75) found insulin resistance in retinopaths compared with non-retinopaths, even at normal plasma glucose, and both at 100 and 1000 mU/ml of insulin.

It is probably acceptable, on reading the work of the last two years (and also many papers written in the previous 40 years), that diabetic control and retinopathy are related. However, the nature of the relationship has not yet been established.

Blood flow and coagulation

In the 1970s a number of communications suggested that abnormal viscosity resulted in reduced flow and increased coagulation in diabetes. This work is reviewed by one of its foremost exponents, H.L. Little (76). Increased viscosity has been reported by Torpe et al. (77) in those with proliferative retinopathy and large areas of non-perfusion, compared with those without these lesions. The increased viscosity was associated with increased fibrinogen levels. The higher hematocrit did not seem to be significant.

Importantly, no abnormalities of the red cell mechanical properties have been demonstrated by Sewchand and co-workers (78), supporting that red cell clumping and lack of deformity – if this occurs at all – is due to plasma rather than red cell factors.

Abnormalities of platelets and coagulation are common in diabetes (79). The question is what the abnormalities are and whether they are of pathogenic importance or whether they represent a reaction to endothelial cell damage. The findings are often contradictory. Plasma co-factor activity which correlates with platelet hyperaggregation was higher in adult diabetics than controls (80) and in diabetic children than controls, but did not correlate with retinopathy in the studies of Levin et al. (81). Factor VIII and all its components (pro-coagulant activities, ristocetin co-factor, and Factor VIII-related antigen) were all elevated in Dornan's studies (63) and the rise correlated with retinopathy severity. Similar findings were reported by Brooks et al. (82) in a small series of patients. Lamberton et al. (83) found both Factor VIII-related antigen and fibronectin elevated in patients with diabetes. There was, however, no correlation between Von Willebrand factor and retinopathy. These results are in agreement with the earlier reports of Porta et al. from the Hammersmith Hospital (84, 85), who also reported no relationship between ristocetin co-factor and severity of retinopathy, but an inverse correlation with platelet aggregation in insulin-dependent diabetes (86, 87). Increased platelet volume found by Cagliero et al. (88) would suggest increased platelet turnover. However, Porta et al. (86) found no real relationship between the different parameters of platelet function, platelet survival and diabetic retinopathy. Finally Lane et al. (89), using a very insensitive method, found increased levels of PGI_2 in patients with proliferative retinopathy. In view of these contradictory results, which nevertheless indicate that in-vitro platelet function is often abnormal in diabetes, it is probable that the endothelial cells are primarily affected in diabetes, and abnormalities of platelets and fibrinolysis (84) are secondary to this.

Other medical risk factors

Of other medical parameters measured, there are hardly any which have not been found to be abnormal by some investigators. Dornan et al. (90) found proliferative retinopathy associated with raised cholesterol, due almost entirely to raised LDL, while HDL was similar in those with and without retinopathy. Mohan et al. (91) whose Indian patients are NIDD also found raised cholesterol especially LDL in those with diabetic maculopathy. However, it has been known for over two decades that hard exudates are associated with raised levels of cholesterol (92).

Measurements of other factors all showed abnormalities. Thus, raised cortisol levels (93) and catecholamines (94) were reported with increasing severity of retinopathy. Plasma renin activity was increased in proliferative retinopathy (95) and did not correlate with blood pressure or diabetic control. Diabetics tend to have higher blood pressure (BP) than non-diabetics and this has been related to retinopathy. The findings are not really helpful. Drury (95) compared patients with proliferative retinopathy with others, without any microvascular complications and found BP to be higher in those with retinopathy. In a leading article Drury (96) found little support for a direct relationship. The answers will have to come from epidemiological studies. Klein et al. (14) found no relationship between systolic BP and 'any' retinopathy, but those with proliferative lesions had raised systolic and diastolic BP. In the older-onset group (47), these workers found a relationship between BP and retinopathy only in those whose diabetes was diagnosed 5–14 years previously.

Diabetic retinopathy is associated with other abnormalities. While neuropathy is common in those with retinopathy, the two conditions are not really related in severity and can occur independently (97). Coexisting abnormalities also include impaired joint mobility. Its prevalence depends on the method used to detect it and there is no agreement on its frequency and exact relationship to diabetic retinopathy (98–101). The highest correlation is that found by Rosenbloom (101) but in his young patients retinopathy was determined by fluorescein angiography by Malone, who seems to find more retinopathy than does any other group.

Pregnancy has an adverse effect on retinopathy (102–104), most patients showing deterioration even when control is good. The best of the studies comes from Dublin (104), which demonstrates the deterioration of retinopathy clearly and also the development of retinopathy during pregnancy, with some reversal after delivery. The authors also found increased infant morbidity in those with hemorrhages and proliferative lesions. Undoubtedly patients with proliferative retinopathy should be photocoagulated even during pregnancy.

Among the risk factors smoking looms large, but the evidence for the importance of smoking in the evolution of retinopathy was never strong. It is therefore important to note three large studies which deny any association between smoking and retinopathy (105–107). Again, the most important is from Wisconsin, where information is available on well over 2000 patients.

Ocular factors

It would be unexpected if local factors would not influence development of progression of retinopathy. Jalkh et al. (108) studied the vitreous to determine its effect on proliferative retinopathy. They found that vitreo-retinal traction was of major importance in the progression of proliferative retinopathy, even when photocoagulation was performed. These authors found that complete vitreous detachment was associated with less progression than partial detachment.

In maculopathy, as expected, interruption of over 50% of the perifoveal capillary arcade was associated with worse visual prognosis than when less of the capillary network was damaged (109).

A case control study from the Joslin Clinic confirmed the negative correlation between high myopia and proliferative retinopathy (110). Intraocular pressure was found to be similar in children without retinopathy and normals, while those with retinopathy had higher pressures (111). There was however, no relationship between the ocular hypertensive response to steroids and the development of severity of retinopathy (112).

Obviously, many factors interact in the development of diabetic retinopathy and in its proliferative complications. In spite of the many papers written, we still do not know which are the ones that really matter.

The treatment of diabetic retinopathy

The previous sections have shown that retinopathy is common: visual impairment, even complete loss, is frequent in the diabetic population. This section reviews evidence for successful treatment at all stages of retinopathy, whether directed at arrest, reversal or prevention and will also review the present studies of vitrectomy, which aims at restoring vision in those who had already lost it. Because of the large volume of literature on the subject the review will have to be very selective and reports of drug therapies in particular not based on randomized controlled clinical studies are omitted.

Insulin infusion – improved diabetic control

Continuous subcutaneous insulin infusion (CSII) has become available during the late 1970s and early 1980s. So, for the first time the role of good diabetic control can be evaluated more accurately. Reports of individual cases of retinopathy improving with continuous insulin infusion have been reported previously. Two large studies looked at a wide variety of patients. The Yale group studied patients with and without retinopathy (113, 114). No patient without retinopathy developed new lesions for the first time while on CSII, but those who already had retinopathy deteriorated or at best remained unchanged. Lawson et al. (115) studied a highly selected group in whom answer to the efficacy of CSII could be obtained quickly. These were 12 patients with preproliferative or early proliferative retinopathy with peripheral new vessels only, with only 'low risk' characteristics. A striking deterioration occurred in all patients over a relatively short period of time, some losing sight in spite of added photocoagulation. Improved control if anything caused a more rapid deterioration of the retinopathy. Other reports followed with variable results. In Waldhäusel's (116) series 2 patients without retinopathy developed lesions for the first time while on the pump, and one developed proliferative lesions progressing to blindness. Hooymas (117) noted deterioration in 11 out of 18 patients. Mirouze et al. (118), using intraperitoneal insulin, found 1 patient improving, 1 deteriorating and the other 5 remaining unchanged. In contrast, Segato et al. (119) found improvement in 5 patients with proliferative retinopathy. Looking at vitreous fluorophotometry only, White et al. (120) found reduced leakage in 8 pump-treated patients. However, they used the old equipment, the readings on which are suspect.

Lack of improvement in advanced retinopathy could have been due to the retinopathy being too advanced, the lesions being already irreversible. Therefore studies on early retinopathy were needed. The Steno Group reported a small randomized clinical trial on 30 patients, and found improvement in retinal function but deterioration in background retinopathy, both after 6 months and after 1 year (31, 32). The larger Kroc study (17, 121, 122) reporting on 68 patients, randomized in pairs to CSII and conventional treatment, obtained similar results, with more marked deterioration of retinopathy features especially cotton wool spots, hemorrhages and microaneurysms in the CSII group. The disappointing results have to be viewed in the light of long duration of diabetes with only short periods (8–12 months) of near normal blood glucose control. Indeed preliminary results after two years from the Steno Study Group showed that the deterioration had not continued: if anything, after 2 years the CSII patient's retinopathy improved in comparison with the original photographs. Conclusive answers for the role of CSII or rather really good diabetic control may eventually come from the American study now in progress.

Anti-platelet therapy

If increased aggregation of platelets is responsible for the development of retinopathy, reduction in the hyperaggregability may be of value. A most important step is improved diabetic control, since this may reduce β-thromboglobulin levels (123), thromboxane synthesis (123) and also reduce platelet aggregation (125). Even if the improved control works, lesions already developed and vessels already occluded would not be reversed, nor would active anti-platelet drugs do this. These drugs could, however, prevent occlusion of further capillaries. Acetylsalicylic acid has indeed been found to be effective in diabetic retinopathy in reducing collagen-induced hyperaggregation, though the tests did not return to normal after 2 days treatment with acetylsalicylic acid (126). Tindall et al. (127) studied patients with retinopathy for platelet survival after placebo treatment, treatment with high dose (1 g/day) acetylsalicylic acid and dipyridamole, or low dose acetylsalicylic acid and dipyridamole. They found that platelet survival increased significantly only with the high-dose acetylsalicylic acid, an important finding since most patients are now advised to have only very small doses of aspirin (50–75 mg/day). If the findings of this study are true, and abnormal platelet function contributes to the development of diabetic retinopathy, the INSERM and Boehringer supported DAMAD study (128, 129), which uses high-dose acetylsalicylic acid alone and in combination with dipyridamole, or placebo in early diabetic retinopathy, should be found to be effective. Results of this study should appear in the next year.

Several other drugs, gliclazide and calcium debosilate among them, have been reported to affect platelet aggregation and diabetic retinopathy favorably. These studies are largely uncontrolled, not masked, and the evaluation of the retinopathy is dubious. They do not deserve discussion in this section, since they have not really been shown to affect retinopathy.

Photocoagulation

Photocoagulation remains the main method of treatment in the sight-threatening forms of retinopathy. Its value has already been proven in previous years but in the last year the two final reports of the British Multicentre Study were published (130, 131).

Diabetic maculopathy, which affects mainly the middle aged and elderly Type 2 NIDD patients (130, 132), can be treated effectively by photocoagulation. In a randomized controlled clinical study, the British Group (130) demonstrated that treatment could maintain mean visual acuity while untreated eyes deteriorated significantly. Out of 99 untreated eyes, 39 were blind at the end of the study, only 19 treated eyes lost this degree of vision. Out of the 19 blind treated eyes, 7 had visual acuity of 6/36 or worse when first seen. The best results were obtained when the initial visual acuity was good, only 1 out of 20 such treated eyes became blind, while 10 out of 20 untreated ones did so, suggesting the need for early treatment. In an uncontrolled study Kelemen et al. (133) showed even better results, out of 136 treated eyes with diabetic maculopathy, 77% showed arrest of the retinopathy while 80% of 246 untreated eyes deteriorated. The British study used the xenon arc with all its disadvantages. The ETDRS (12) study now in progress in the US should show better results.

For proliferative retinopathy the British Multicentre Group (131) confirmed the findings of the American study reported in previous years (1, 4). It showed that especially for the 'high-risk' patients with new vessels on the disc, treatment was most effective. Three-and-a-half times as many untreated eyes became blind than treated ones. Photocoagulation caused regression of the new vessels and other retinal lesions, and prevented new vessel formation on the disc if there were only peripheral new vessels when first seen. Treatment was most effective when it was heavy, those with a large number of burns doing better than those with lighter treatment. This study too was using the xenon arc only. However, this is unlikely to alter the results since Plumb et al. (134) have shown that xenon arc and argon laser therapy is equally effective in causing disc vessel regression and maintenance of visual acuity. While some patients responded to peripheral treatment only, in many it was necessary to treat the mid-periphery as well. Indeed, today it is suggested that extensive treatment should be given approaching the disc, outside the temporal arcade (135). Inadequate treatment is one of the main causes of visual loss today in proliferative retinopathy. Photocoagulation can be given in single or in multiple sessions. Doft and Blankenship (136) found no significant difference in the two groups, though transient complications were more common in those who had all their treatment in one session. In the authors' experience, single sessions are sometimes successful in causing complete regression of retinopathy; in most patients several sessions are necessary. Several sessions should probably always be used when there is associated macular ischemia, as otherwise irreversible macular edema may negate the results of new vessel regression.

Photocoagulation is effective even if new vessels occur on the iris or in the angle, both being associated with profound retinal ischemia. In a well-conducted prospective controlled masked trial, Pavan et al. (137) demonstrated the efficacy of the treatment (which has been shown to be effective in iris rubeosis associated with central vein occlusion many years ago (139)).

In pregnant patients with proliferative retinopathy, photocoagulation is as effective as in non-pregnant patients, Gerke and Meyer-Schwickerath (139) felt that in some the retina was healthier than before pregnancy. Patients who had treatment before pregnancy fared best. Photocoagulation is a destructive form of treatment. Nevertheless, it is so effective in maintaining vision that at present and in the near future there is no other treatment for sight threatening forms of retinopathy that can take its place.

Vitrectomy

In spite of photocoagulation, many patients still lose vision from complications of proliferative diabetic retinopathy. The main cause is too little treatment, or delay in carrying out panretinal photocoagulation (140). Once the tractional complications, vitreous hemorrhage and traction retinal detachment have occurred, photocoagulation cannot restore vision, closed intraocular microsurgery, vitrectomy is often successful.

Vitrectomy for vitreous hemorrhage alone is most effective. Koerner (141) compared 110 untreated eyes with 80 which had vitrectomy. He found the operation to offer advantages over no treatment, but warned about severe complications which may cause complete loss of the eye (rare if vitreous hemorrhage alone is present). The best results come from centers which do large series. Michaels (142) obtained a good visual outcome (20/100 or better) in 115 out of 248 eyes. Traction retinal detachments are more difficult to treat and complications are more common. Rice et al. (143) obtained 6/60 or better vision in only 43 out of 168 eyes. The vitrectomies were done only for macular detachment when visual loss is catastrophic. In contrast Shea (144) performed the operation in patients with still good vision, when retinal detachment was absent or peripheral only, as a prophylactic measure. Nearly 10% of eyes with initially 20/40 or better vision lost vision to 20/200 and those with poorer preoperative vision faired worse. Because of complications which are common even in the best hands (145–147) prophylactic vitrectomy is probably not justified. In his review article on pars plana vitrectomy, the greatest expert, Steve Charles (9) clearly advises against operation until macular detachment occurs, not only because of the complications, but because of the slow extension of the detachment, less than 14% developing macular involvement each year. In order to improve results, Blankenship (148) tried to determine pre-operative prognostic factors. Although he did describe such factors, major operative complications still reduced the successful visual outcome from 53 to 22%. In the Moorfields Hospital series (149) 74% of eyes achieved surgical re-attachment of the macula, the extent of the pre-operative epiretinal membrane being the most important adverse risk factor. Another adverse factor is rubeosis iridis, but this may improve after successful reattachment of the macula (150). In macular detachment the duration of the detachment is also important. After a long period of detachment even if the surgical outcome is good, the functional result may be poor (9). Therefore, in contrast to simple vitreous hemorrhage, where optimal time for operation has not been determined in macular detachment, operation is always urgent.

Pathological mechanisms in the development of diabetic retinopathy and response to treatment

Among the many mechanisms which have been postulated to contribute to the development of retinopathy, most act locally. Of the many hormones found to be abnormal in diabetes, only growth hormone (GH) has been given a specific pathogenic role.

Growth hormone and diabetic retinopathy

That GH may be of importance in diabetic vascular disease stems from the work of Lundbaek and co-workers, summarized in a review article in 1978 (151). It has come to the fore again because of some recent studies which indicated abnormal response of GH in diabetics, especially those with retinopathy. Thus in the glucose clamp studies growth hormone levels increased when insulin was increased, in spite of steady glucose levels, most markedly in those with retinopathy (75, 152). Increase in GH levels following exercise was only seen in those with retinopathy (153). Recent work reported from the Hammersmith (154, 155) and from the Yale groups (156) showed that, while normal subjects suppress GH response to growth hormone releasing factor (GRF) in the presence of hyperglycemia, not all diabetics do so. It is tempting to speculate that breakdown of the blood–brain barrier allows access of glucose to hypothalamic centers and thus is responsible for abnormal GRF release. Preliminary studies do not support this hypothesis.

GH may exert its effects through insulin-like growth factors. Ashton et al. (157) found elevated somatomedin levels in patients with retinopathy using a bioassay. However, Lamberton et al. (83) could not differentiate between those with and those without retinopathy using an immunoassay.

The only group of retinopaths with elevated levels were those in whom the retinopathy was actively progressing (158). Tamborlane et al. (159) reported that with CSII and normalization of blood sugar, GH levels decreased in diabetic patients, but somatomedin levels rose, possibly accounting in part for the deterioration of the retinopathy. Certainly adequate insulinization seems to reduce GH levels (160, 161). The exact relationship between GH, insulin-like growth factors and retinopathy has not been established, but the field is new and fashionable and it is hoped that new information is going to be available soon.

Ischemia and hypoxemia

Ischemic retina is known to stimulate growth of new vessels even in the absence of diabetes. Ischemia and hypoxemia have been incriminated for many years. Why diabetic retina should be ischemic or hypoxemic prior to vascular occlusion is difficult to understand. Blair et al. (162), using mean transit time measurements, suggested increased blood flow with increasing retinopathy, but clearly they did not understand the importance of peripheral vascular occlusion which invalidates measurements in severe retinopathy. Oswald et al. (163) also using mean transit time measurement found both duration of diabetes and type of diabetes important. Increased flow was more marked in Type 1 diabetes and only with severe retinopathy and duration of 20 years or over did it reduce. How can increased flow be equated with hypoxemia and/or ischemia? In a series of articles, Wolbarsht and co-workers expand their views (164–166). They suggest that the vasodilation often seen in retinal vessels in diabetes is an autoregulatory adaptation to hypoxemia of the inner retina. This is due to the choroidal oxygen being taken up by the metabolically active photoreceptor cells, only little oxygen reaching the inner retina, which they measured in experimental animals by the use of oxygen electrodes. Following panretinal photocoagulation it is the outer retina which is damaged most severely, the inner retina often remaining intact. The authors found increased oxygen tension with their electrodes and state that this was due to the metabolically inactive fibrous tissue replacing photoreceptors, allowing adequate oxygenation of the inner retina. The retina, no longer very hypoxic will then stop releasing vasoproliferative factor, and new vessels regress. The narrowing of vessels seen after photocoagulation could be secondary to higher oxygen levels. This possibility of improved autoregulation after photocoagulation was also suggested by the laser Doppler velocimetry studies of Feke et al. (167). The original hypoxemia however, is still not fully explained. High blood glucose levels increase retinal and choroidal blood flow and impairs autoregulation (168, 169). This could be the first step in endothelial damage if it persists for long periods of time. High levels of HbA_1 reduce oxygen-releasing capacity, and this together with low 2,3-diphosphoglycerate (DPG) levels could shift the oxygen dissociation curve to the right. The finding by Ditzel (170) that etidronate disodium increases 2,3-DPG and stabilizes retinopathy possibly supports this. If the hypoxic theory is correct, a possible explanation for the deterioration of retinopathy with good control achieved by CSII can be explained. The blood flow hitherto increased is quickly normalized. The areas already damaged by narrowed or blocked capillaries become increasingly hypoxic, so much so that axoplasmic transport is interrupted, resulting in cotton wool spots, ischemic hemorrhages and increased number of microaneurysms. The diabetic retina already synthesizes less protein than the normal retina, at least in rabbits (171), so that axonal transport in ganglion cell axons is reduced. Only slight worsening in hypoxia is required to stop it completely.

The other, more widely accepted, theory is that the vascular occlusion results in ischemia, and ischemic retina produces an angiogenic factor which accumulates in the vitreous and is responsible for new vessel growth. Hill and co-workers (172) found only diabetic vitreous from patients with proliferative retinopathy stimulated angiogenesis in the chick chorioallantoic membrane, non-proliferative vitreous or normal vitreous failed to do so. Photocoagulation in this instance would then work by reducing the ischemic area. Unfortunately, the cause of the vaso-occlusion has still not been found.

Endothelial cells

Since it is the vessels which are abnormal in diabetes, it is likely that endothelial cells are the major cause of retinopathy, though the first cells to be damaged are the pericytes rather than the endothelial cells. In BB Wistar rats, which are spontaneously diabetic, Sima et al. (173) found pericyte loss and capillary occlusion by platelet thrombi and fibrin. The pericyte loss could be prevented in diabetic mice with islet cell transplants into the portal vein, provided it was done early after induction of diabetes. If the diabetes was present for over 4 months the pericyte loss could not be reversed (174). Endothelial cell damage in rats has been demonstrated by Ennis et al. (175), who measured glucose transport across the blood–retinal barrier. They showed at least two unidirectional glucose transport systems, unaffected by Na^+ or K^+ but influenced by Ca^{++}. The K_m for both systems was significantly increased in streptozotocin diabetes. Betz et al. (176) studied glucose transport across bovine retinal endothelial cells (REC) in tissue culture. They found facilitated uptake of 3-O-methyl-D-glucose, which was increased by preloading with glucose. Endothelial cells contained free sugar even when the glucose concentration in the medium was physiological. The authors felt that the free transport of sugar from blood to retina, though necessary in conditions of high glucose concentration – as seen in diabetes, could cause endothelial damage. That this may occur has been demonstrated by Tripathi and Tripathi (177), who were the first to culture cadaver

RECs. These cells grew normally under standard conditions, but when the glucose concentration in the culture medium was raised to 400 mg% the RECs got irreversibly damaged.

The endothelial cell changes in diabetes have been further investigated by Chronister's group (178) who found altered activation of adenylate cyclase to norepinephrine and dopamine in both retinal and cerebral microvessels which suggests altered response to a whole range of stimuli.

Paton et al. (179) used human umbilical vein endothelial cell culture. They observed that thrombin stimulated cells produced prostacyclin (PGI_1) and measured this by ADP-induced platelet aggregation and 6-keto-PGF_1 by immunoassay. Endothelial cells cultured in diabetic serum showed reduced PGI_2 and 6-keto-PGF_1 levels. The latter was also related to the HbA_1 level of the diabetics. Since RECs differ from all other capillaries in the body (with the exception of the brain), and both pericytes and RECs can be cultured (180) there is no longer a need for studying endothelial cells from other parts of the body to evaluate retinopathy.

Integrity of the blood-retinal barrier (BRB) is important for normal retinal function. It has been suggested that in early diabetes not only the inner BRB (capillary endothelium) is abnormal, but also the outer BRB, the pigment epithelium. This is based on animal work by Blair et al. (181), who showed increased permeability to horseradish peroxidase in diabetic rat pigment epithelium, which was associated with focal anatomical lesions. However, Tso (182), studying the pathology of macular edema, found no evidence for the involvement of the pigment epithelium in diabetic maculopathy. There may nevertheless be an important role played by the pigment epithelium. Marshall et al. (183) found that after photocoagulation in experimental animals there was no occlusion of retinal vessels, but pigment epithelial damage was consistently present. There was striking proliferation of the endothelial cells in the retinal capillaries and later the retinal veins as well (never in arteries). This endothelial cell proliferation occurred not only at the site of the burn, but also some distance away. It was accompanied by proliferation in the choriocapillaris and pigment epithelium. The full meaning of these findings is not yet clear, but it is possibly responsible for the response to photocoagulation at least in diabetic maculopathy. The reduction in antibody response to bovine retinal S antigen and rod outer segments some weeks after photocoagulation (184) could be the result of destruction of these cells, possibly already damaged, by treatment.

Finally, another possible cause of endothelial cell damage has been postulated, when Engerman and Kern (185) demonstrated that non-diabetic dogs fed on a high galactose diet developed a retinopathy indistinguishable from diabetic retinopathy. Galactose is metabolized to dolcitol in the tissues through the activity of aldose reductase, an enzyme which also converts glucose to sorbitol. These polyols are not readily metabolized nor do they penetrate cell membranes easily. They may therefore accumulate to high levels in cells, leading to hypertonicity and alteration of ion permeability, and eventually to cell damage and death. The problem is the presence of aldose reductase in endothelial cells. Kinoshita's group (186) could demonstrate dolcitol accumulation in endothelial cells cultured in galactose. They also showed that the aldose reductase inhibitor sorbinil prevented basement membrane thickening in galactose-fed rats (187). Kennedy et al. (188) were not convinced of sorbitol accumulation in endothelial cells, nor were they convinced that it was responsible for the development of retinopathy. Poulsom et al. (189–191) found sorbitol accumulation in the retina (and other tissues) of diabetic rats. Aldose reductase inhibitors reduced this accumulation and improved diabetic cataracts. These authors did not implicate any specific cell – they used whole retinas – but the accumulation of sorbitol in uncontrolled diabetes was confirmed.

It would be of interest if the studies starting in the US and UK on aldose reductase inhibitors would show a beneficial effect on diabetic retinopathy.

References

1. Diabetic Retinopathy Study Research Group (1976): Preliminary report on effects of photocoagulation therapy. *Am. J. Ophthalmol.*, *81*, 383.
2. British Multicentre Study Group (1977): Proliferative diabetic retinopathy treatment with xenon arc photocoagulation. *Br. Med. J.*, *1*, 739.
3. Diabetic Retinopathy Study Research Group (1979): Four risk factors for severe visual loss in diabetic retinopathy. *Arch. Ophthalmol.*, *97*, 654.
4. Diabetic Retinopathy Study Research Group (1981): Photocoagulation treatment of proliferative diabetic retinopathy. Diabetic Retinopathy Study Report No. 8. *Ophthalmology*, *88*, 583.
5. Patz A, Schatz H, Berkow JW, Gittelsohn AM, Ticho U (1977): Macular oedema, an overlooked complication of diabetic retinopathy. *Am. Acad. Ophthalmol. Otolaryngol.*, *77*, 34.
6. British Multicentre Study Group (1975): Photocoagulation in the treatment of diabetic maculopathy. *Lancet*, *2*, 110.
7. Whitelock RA, Kearns M, Blach RK, Hamilton AM (1979): The Diabetic Maculopathy's. *Trans. Ophthalmol. Soc. UK.*, *99*, 314.
8. Jack RL (1983): Vitreous surgery in diabetic retinopathy. In: *Diabetic Retinopathy*, Chapter 24, p. 299. Editors: H.L. Little, R.L. Jack, A. Patz and P.H. Forsham. Thieme-Stratton Inc., New York.
9. Charles S (1983): Pars plana vitrectomy for traction retinal detachment. In: *Diabetic Retinopathy*, Chapter 25, p. 305. Editors: H.L. Little, R.L. Jack, A. Patz and P.H. Forsham. Thieme-Stratton Inc., New York.
10. Oakley NW, Hill DW, Joplin GF, Kohner EM, Fraser TR (1967): Diabetic retinopathy: assessment of severity and progression with a set of standard photographs. *Diabetologia*, *3*, 402.
11. Diabetic Retinopathy Study Research Group (1981): Modification of the Airlie House classification of diabetic retinopathy. *Invest. Ophthalmol. Vis. Sci.*, *21*, 210.

12. Early Treatment of Diabetic Retinopathy Research Group (1980): *Manual of Operations*. Department of Health, Education and Welfare, Bethesda MD.
13. Klein BE, Davis MD, Segal P, Long JA, Harris WA, Haug GH, Magli YL (1984): Diabetic retinopathy. Assessment of severity and progression. *Ophthalmology*, *91*, 10.
14. Klein R, Klein BE, Moss SE, Davis MD, DeMets DL (1984): The Wisconsin epidemiologic study of diabetic retinopathy II, prevalence and risk of diabetic retinopathy when age and diagnosis is less than 30 years. *Arch. Ophthalmol.*, *102*, 520.
15. Yamana Y, Ohnishi Y, Taniguchi Y, Ikeda M (1983): Early signs of diabetic retinopathy by fluorescein angiography. *Jpn. J. Ophthalmol.*, *27*, 218.
16. Baudoin C, Maneschi F, Quentel G, Soubrane G, Hayes T, Jones G, Kohner EM (1983): Quantitative evaluation of fluorescein angiograms. *Diabetes*, *32*, *Suppl. 2*, 8.
17. Kohner EM, for the Kroc Study Group (1984): The effect of diabetic control on early diabetic retinopathy studied by fluorescein angiograms. *Invest. Ophthalmol. Vis. Sci.*, *25*, 128.
18. Sleightholm MA, Arnold J, Aldington SJ, Kohner EM (1984): Computer aided system for analysis of fundus photographs. *Diabetic Med.*, *1*, 157a.
19. Lay BJ, Baudoin CE, Klein JC (1984): Automatic detection of microaneurysms. In: *Applications of Digital Image Processing, VI, 432*, pp. 165-173. Editor: A.G. Tescher. Pub. SPIE, Washington, DC.
20. Sinclair SH, Grunwald JE, Riva CE, Braunstein SN, Nichols CW, Schwartz SS (1982): Retinal vascular autoregulation in diabetes mellitus. *Ophthalmology*, *89*, 748.
21. Riva CE, Grunwald JE, Sinclair SH (1983): Laser doppler velocimetry study of the effect of pure oxygen breathing on retinal blood flow. *Invest. Ophthalmol. Vis. Sci.*, *24*, 47.
22. Cunha-Vaz JG, De Abreau F, Campos AJ, Figo GM (1975): Early breakdown of the blood retinal barrier in diabetes. *Br. J. Ophthalmol.*, *59*, 649.
23. Kohner EM, Alderson AR (1981): Vitreous fluorophotometry. *Trans. Ophthalmol. Soc. UK*, *101*, 446.
24. Lund-Andersen H, Krogsaa B, Larsen J (1983): Computerised calculation of blood-retinal barrier permeability and vitreous body diffusion coefficient for fluorescein in man. In: *Acta, XXIV International Congress of Ophthalmology*, p. 458. Editor: P. Henkind. Lippincott and Co., Philadelphia.
25. Zeimer RC, Blair NP, Cunha-Vaz JG (1983): Vitreous fluorophotometry for clinical research. Description and evaluation of a new fluorophotometer. *Arch. Ophthalmol.*, *101*, 1753.
26. Zeimer RC, Blair NP, Cunha-Vaz JG (1983): Vitreous fluorophotometry for clinical research II. Methodology of data acquisition and processing. *Arch. Ophthalmol.*, *101*, 1757.
27. Zeimer RC, Blair NP, Cunha-Vaz JG (1983): Pharmacokinetic interpretation of vitreous fluorophotometry. *Invest. Ophthalmol. Vis. Sci.*, *24*, 1374.
28. Kernell A, Arnquist H (1983): Effect of insulin treatment on the blood retinal barrier in rats with streptozotocin induced diabetes. *Arch. Ophthalmol.*, *101*, 968.

29. Cunha-Vaz JG, Zeimer R, Wong WP, Kiani RZ (1982): Kinetic vitreous fluorophotometry in normals and non insulin dependent diabetics. *Ophthalmology*, *89*, 751.
30. Prager TC, Chu HH, Garcia CA, Anderson RE (1982): The influence of vitreous change on vitreous fluorophotometry. *Arch. Ophthalmol.*, *100*, 584.
31. The Steno Study Group (1982): Effect of 6 months of strict metabolic control on eye and kidney function in insulin dependent diabetics with background retinopathy. *Lancet*, *1*, 121.
32. Lauritzen T, Frost-Larsen K, Larsen HW, Deckert T (1983): Effect of one year normal blood glucose levels on retinopathy in insulin dependent diabetics. *Lancet*, *1*, 200.
33. Chahal P, Kohner EM (1984): Vitreous fluorophotometry in diabetes with and without retinopathy. Paper presented at: 2nd Vitreous Fluorophotometry Workshop, Sarasota. *Albrecht von Graefes Arch. Klin. Exp. Ophthalmol.* (in press).
34. Kritz H, Irsigler K (1983): Functional tests for diabetic retinopathy. In: *Diabetes Treatment with Implantable Insulin Infusion Systems*, Chapter 19, p. 160. Editors: K. Irsigler, H. Kritz and R. Lovett. Urban und Schwarzenberg, Munich-Berlin.
35. Frost-Larsen K, Larsen HW (1983): Nyctometry, a new screening method for selection of patients with simple diabetic retinopathy who are at risk of developing proliferative retinopathy. *Acta Ophthalmol.*, *61*, 353.
36. Frost-Larsen K, Larsen HW, Simonsen SE (1980): Oscillatory potential and nyctometry in insulin dependent diabetics. *Acta Ophthalmol.*, *58*, 879.
37. Bresnick GH, Korth K, Groo A, Palta M (1984): Electroretinographic oscillatory potentials predict progression of diabetic retinopathy. *Invest. Ophthalmol. Vis. Sci.*, *25*, 128.
38. Brunette JR, Lafond G (1983): Electroretinographic evaluation of diabetic retinopathy: sensitivity of amplitude and time response. *Can. J. Ophthalmol.*, *18*, 285.
39. Cirillo D, Gonfiantini E, De Grandis D, Borgiovanian L, Robert JJ, Pinelli L (1984): Visually evoked potentials in diabetic children and adolescents. *Diab. Care*, *7*, 269.
40. Levin RD, Kwaan H, Dobbie JG, Fetkanhour CL, Traisman HS, Kramer C (1982): Studies of retinopathy and plasma cofactor of platelet hyperaggregation in type 1 diabetic children. *Diabetologia*, *22*, 445.
41. Aspinall PH, Kinnear PR, Duncan LJP, Clarke BF (1983): Prediction of diabetic retinopathy from clinical variables and colour vision data. *Diab. Care*, *6*, 144.
42. Maloney J, Drury MI (1982): Retinopathy and retinal function in insulin dependent diabetes mellitus. *Br. J. Ophthalmol.*, *66*, 759.
43. Zimmet P, King H, Taylor R, Raper LR, Balkau B, Borger J, Heriot W, Thoma K (1984): The high prevalence of diabetes mellitus, impaired glucose tolerance and diabetic retinopathy in Nauru – the 1982 survey. *Diabetes Res.*, *1*, 13.
44. Lester FT (1983): Longstanding diabetes mellitus in Ethiopia: a survey of 105 patients. *Diabetologia*, *25*, 222.
45. Jialal J, Welsh NH, Joubert SM, Rajput MC (1982): Vascular complications

in non insulin dependent diabetes in the young. *S. Afr. Med. J.*, *62*, 155.
46. Danielsen R, Jonasson F, Helgason T (1982): Prevalence of retinopathy and proteinuria in type I diabetics in Iceland. *Acta Med. Scand.*, *212*, 527.
47. Klein R, Klein BE, Moss SE, Davis MD, Clemets DL (1981): The Wisconsin epidemiologic study of diabetic retinopathy III. Prevalence and risk of diabetic retinopathy when age at diagnosis is over 30 years. *Arch. Ophthalmol.*, *102*, 527.
48. Bodansky HJ, Drury PL, Cudworth AG, Kohner EM (1982): Risk factor associated with severe proliferative retinopathy in insulin dependent diabetes mellitus. *Diabetes Care*, *5*, 97.
49. Nielsen NV (1984): Diabetic retinopathy I. The course of retinopathy in insulin treated diabetics. *Acta Ophthalmol.*, *62*, 256.
50. Nielsen NV (1984): Diabetic retinopathy II. The course of retinopathy in diabetics treated with oral hypoglycaemic agents and diet regime alone. *Acta Ophthalmol.*, *62*, 266.
51. Foulds WS, McCuish A, Barrie T, Green F, Scobie IN, Ghafour IM, McCrure E, Barber JH (1983): Diabetic retinopathy in the west of Scotland, its detection and prevalence and the cost effectiveness of proposed screening programme. *Scott. Home Health Dept. Health Bull.*, *41*, 319.
52. Cullinan TR (1982): Diabetic retinopathy and visual disability. *Diabetologia*, *23*, 504.
53. Nielsen NV (1982): The prevalence and courses of impaired vision in diabetics. *Acta Ophthalmol.*, *60*, 677.
54. Vastag O, Sisak J (1983): Vaksagi statisztikak elemezese. *Szemeszet*, *120*, 57.
55. Klein R, Klein BE, Moss SE (1984): Visual impairment in diabetes. *Ophthalmology*, *91*, 1.
56. Johnston PB, Kidd M, Middleton D, Greenfield DH, Dicher DB, Maguire CJF, Kennedy L (1982): Analysis of HLA antigen association with proliferative diabetic retinopathy. *Br. J. Ophthalmol.*, *66*, 277.
57. Gray RS, Starkey IR, Rainbow S, Kurtz AB, Abdel-Khalik A, Urbaniak S, Elton RA, Duncan LJP, Clark BF (1982): HLA and other risk factors in the development of retinopathy in type I diabetes. *Br. J. Ophthalmol.*, *66*, 277.
58. Bodansky HJ, Wolf E, Cudworth AG, Dean BM, Nineham LJ, Botazzo GF, Matthews JP, Kurtz AB, Kohner EM (1982): Genetic and immunological factors in microvascular disease of type I insulin dependent diabetes. *Diabetes*, *31*, 70.
59. Cudworth AG, Bodansky HJ (1982): Genetic and immunological factors in diabetic complications. In: *Complications of Diabetics,* Ch. 1. Editors: H. Keen and J. Jarrett. Edward Arnold, London.
60. Dornan TL, Ting H, McPherson CK, Peckar CO, Mann JI, Turner RC, Morris PJ (1982): Genetic susceptibility to the development of retinopathy in insulin dependent diabetics. *Diabetes*, *31*, 226.
61. Leslie RDJ, Pyke DA (1982): Diabetic retinopathy in identical twins. *Diabetes*, *31*, 19.
62. Shabo A, Maxwell DS, Shintaku IP (1983): Immunogenic vasculitis and its role in diabetic ocular disease. In: *Diabetic Retinopathy*, Ch. 15. Editors: H.L. Little, R.L. Jack, H. Patz and P.H. Forsham. Thieme-Stratton Inc., New York.

63. Dornan TL, Rhymes IL, Cederholm-Williams A, Rizza CR, Pepys MB (1983): Plasma haemostatic factors and diabetic retinopathy. *Eur. J. Clin. Invest.*, *13*, 231.
64. Krolewski HS, Rand LI, Warram JH, Christlieb AR (1984): Development of proliferative retinopathy in juvenile onset IDDM (40 years follow up study). *Invest. Ophthalmol. Vis. Sci.*, *25*, 128.
65. Frank RN, Hoffman WH, Podgor MG (1982): Retinopathy in juvenile onset type 1 diabetes of short duration. *Diabetes*, *31*, 874.
66. Kingsley R, Gnosh GK, Lawson P, Kohner EM (1983): Severe diabetic retinopathy in adolescents. *Br. J. Ophthalmol.*, *67*, 73.
67. Barnett HH, Britton JR, Leatherdale BH (1983): Study of possible risk factors for severe retinopathy in non insulin dependent diabetes. *Br. Med. J.*, *287*, 529.
68. Dornan T, Mann JI, Turner R (1982): Factors protective against retinopathy in insulin dependent diabetics free of retinopathy for 30 years. *Br. Med. J.*, *285*, 1073.
69. Rand LI, Krolewski HS, Warram JH, Aiello LM (1984): Frequent hyperglycaemia is associated with proliferative diabetic retinopathy. *Invest. Ophthalmol. Vis. Sci.*, *25*, 128.
70. Jackson RL, Ide CH, Guthrie RH, James MD (1982): Retinopathy in adolescents and young adults with onset of insulin dependent diabetes in childhood. *Ophthalmology*, *89*, 7.
71. Nakayoshi N, Nuoni K, Ohnishi Y (1983): Diabetic retinopathy and haemoglobin A_1. *Jpn. J. Ophthalmol.*, *27*, 255.
72. Dorchy H, Despontin M, Haumont D, Poussant D, De Verdoc M, Loe LH (1982): Hémoglobine glycosylée et estimation clinique du degré du contrôle du diabète. *Ann. Paediatr. (Paris)*, *29*, 319.
73. Zick R, Lange P, Hoffman K, Hurter P, Mitzkat HJ (1983): Diabetische Retinopathie bei Kindern und Jugendlichen. Ihre Abhängigkeit von der Insulinrestsekretion. *Nat. Endokrinol. Stoffwechsel*, *4*, 132.
74. Vitelli F, Maneschi F, Foley K, Mashiter K, Kohner EM (1983): Insulin resistance in insulin dependent diabetes with and without retinopathy. *Clin. Sci.*, *64*, 2a.
75. Maneschi F, Mashiter K, Kohner EM (1983): Insulin resistance and insulin deficiency in diabetic retinopathy of non-insulin dependent diabetes. *Diabetes*, *32*, 82.
76. Little HL (1983): The role of blood elements in the pathogenesis of diabetic retinopathy. In: *Diabetic Retinopathy*, Ch. 13. Editors: H.L. Little, R.L. Jack, A. Patz and P.H. Forsham. Thieme-Stratton Inc., New York.
77. Torpe E, Lowe GDO, Ghafour IM, Foulds WS, Forbes CD (1983): Blood viscosity in proliferative diabetic retinopathy and complicated retinal vein thrombosis. *Trans. Ophthalmol. Soc. UK*, *103*, 108.
78. Sewchand LS, Hampel WL, Diddie KR, Meiselman HI (1982): Membrane mechanical properties of erythrocytes from patients with diabetic retinopathy. *Microcirculation*, *1*, 361.
79. Colwell JA (1983): Platelets and diabetic retinopathy. In: *Diabetic Retinopathy*, Ch. 10. Editors: H.L. Little, R.L. Jack, H. Patz and P.H. Forsham. Thieme-Stratton Inc., New York.

80. Koneti-Rao A, Goldberg RE, Walsh PN (1984): Platelet coagulant activities in diabetes mellitus. Evidence for platelet coagulant hyperactivity and platelet volume. *J. Lab. Clin. Med.*, *103*, 82.
81. Levin RD, Kwaan HC, Dobbie JG, Fetkenhour CL, Traisman HS, Kramer C (1982): Studies of retinopathy and plasma co-factor of platelet hyperaggregation in type I (Insulin dependent) diabetic children. *Diabetologia*, *22*, 445.
82. Brooks AMV, Hussein S, Chesterman CN, Martin JF, Alford FP, Penin DG (1983): Platelets coagulation and fibrinolysis in patients with diabetic retinopathy. *Thromb. Haemostasis*, *49*, 123.
83. Lamerton RP, Goodman AD, Kassoff A, Rubin CL, Treble DH, Siba TM, Merimee TJ, Dodds VJ (1984): Von Willebrand factor, fibronectin and insulin like growth factor I and II in diabetic retinopathy and nephropathy. *Diabetes*, *33*, 125.
84. Porta M, Townsend C, Clover G, Nanson M, Alderson AR, McCraw A, Kohner EM (1981): Evidence for functional endothelial cell damage in early diabetic retinopathy. *Diabetologia*, *20*, 597.
85. Porta M, Maneschi F, White MC, Kohner EM (1981): Twenty-four hour variations of Von Willebrand factor and factor VIII related antigen in diabetic retinopathy. *Metabolism*, *30*, 595.
86. Porta M, Peters AM, Cousins SH, Cagliero E, Fitzpatrick ML, Kohner EM (1983): A study of platelet relevant parameters in patients with diabetic microangiography. *Diabetologia*, *25*, 21.
87. Porta M, McCraw A, Kohner EM (1982): Inverse relationship between ristocetin co-factor levels and platelet aggregation in insulin dependent diabetes. *Thromb. Res.*, *25*, 507.
88. Cagliero E, Porta M, Cousins S, Kohner EM (1982): Increased platelet volume in diabetic retinopathy. *Homeostasis*, *12*, 293.
89. Lane LS, Jansen PD, Lahau M, Rudy CM (1982): Circulatory prostacycline and thromboxane levels in patients with diabetic retinopathy. *Ophthalmology*, *89*, 763.
90. Dornan TL, Carter RD, Bron HJ, Turner RC, Mann JI (1982): Low density lipoprotein, cholesterol and association with the severity of diabetic retinopathy. *Diabetologia*, *22*, 167.
91. Mohan R, Mohan V, Sushela L, Ramachandran A, Viswanathan M (1984): Increased LDL cholesterol in non-insulin dependent diabetics with maculopathy. *Acta Diabetol. Lat.*, *22*, 167.
92. Esman V, Lundback K, Madsen PH (1963): Exudates in diabetic retinopathy. *Acta Med. Scand.*, *174*, 375.
93. Bhatia RPS, Singh RH (1983): Cortisol in diabetic retinopathy. *Ann. Ophthalmol.*, *15*, 128.
94. Bhatia RPS, Singh RH (1983): Catecholamines in diabetic retinopathy. *Ann. Ophthalmol.*, *15*, 677.
95. Drury PL, Bodansky HJ, Oddie CJ, Cudworth AG, Edwards CR (1982): Increased plasma renin activity in type I diabetes with microvascular disease. *Clin. Endocrinol.*, *16*, 453.
96. Drury PL (1983): Diabetes and arterial hypertension. *Diabetologia*, *24*, 1.
97. Hoffman WH, Hart ZH, Frank RN (1983): Correlates of delayed motor

nerve conduction and retinopathy in juvenile onset diabetes mellitus. *J. Paediatr.*, *102*, 357.

98. Kennedy L, Archer DB, Campbell SL, Beacom R, Carson DJ, Johnston PB, Maguire CJ (1982): Limited joint mobility in type I diabetes mellitus. *Postgrad. Med. J.*, *58*, 481.
99. Chapple M, Jung RT, Francis J, Webster J, Kohner EM, Bloom SR (1983): Joint contractures and diabetic retinopathy. *Postgrad. Med. J.*, *59*, 291.
100. Lawson P, Maneschi F, Kohner EM (1983): The relationship of hand abnormalities to diabetes and diabetic retinopathy. *Diabetes Care*, *6*, 140.
101. Rosenbloom AL, Malone JI, Yucha J, van Cader TC (1984): Limited joint mobility and diabetic retinopathy demonstrated by fluorescein angiography. *Eur. J. Pediatr.*, *141*, 163.
102. Dibble M, Kochenour MK, Worley RJ, Taylor H, Swartz H (1982): Effect of pregnancy on diabetic retinopathy. *Obstet. Gynecol.*, *59*, 699.
103. Price JH, Hadden DR, Archer DB, Harley JMcDG (1984): Diabetic retinopathy in pregnancy. *Br. J. Ophthalmol. Gynecol.*, *91*, 11.
104. Maloney JBM, Drury MI (1982): The effect of pregnancy on the natural course of diabetic retinopathy. *Am. J. Ophthalmol.*, *93*, 745.
105. Lombartil P, Passa P, Thiboult N (1983): Prevalence of smokers among diabetics and influence of tobacco on diabetic retinopathy. *Presse Méd.*, *12*, 2677.
106. Telmer S, Christiansen JS, Anderson AR, Nerup J, Deckert T (1984): Smoking habits and prevalence of clinical diabetic microangiography in insulin dependent diabetics. *Acta Med. Scand.*, *215*, 63.
107. Klein R, Klein BE, Davis MD (1983): Is cigarette smoking associated with diabetic retinopathy? *Am. J. Epidemiol.*, *118*, 228.
108. Jalkh H, Takahashi M, Topilow HW, Trempe CL, McMeel W (1982): Prognostic value of vitreous findings in diabetic retinopathy. *Arch. Ophthalmol.*, *100*, 432.
109. Tamura T, Tamura M (1982): Perifoveal capillary network and visual prognosis in diabetic retinopathy. *Ophthalmologica*, *185*, 141.
110. Baker RR, Rand LI, Krolewski AS (1984): Myopia and proliferative retinopathy in insulin dependent diabetes. *Invest. Ophthalmol. Vis. Sci.*, *25*, 128.
111. Blanksma LJ, Rouwe C, Drayer NM (1983): Retinopathy and intraocular pressure in diabetic children. *Ophthalmologica*, *187*, 137.
112. Krupin T, Schock LH, Cooper D, Becker B (1983): Lack of correlation between ocular hypertensive response to topical steroids and progression of retinopathy in insulin dependent diabetes mellitus. *Am. J. Ophthalmol.*, *96*, 52.
113. Tamborlane WV, Puklin JE, Bergman M, Verdonk C, Rudolf MC, Felig P, Genel M, Sherwin R (1982): Long term improvement of metabolic control with the insulin pump does not reverse diabetic microangiopathy. *Diabetes Care*, *5*, *Suppl. 1*, 56.
114. Puklin JE, Tamborlane WV, Felig P, Genel M, Sherwin RS (1982): Influence of longterm insulin infusion pump treatment of type I diabetes with diabetic retinopathy. *Ophthalmology*, *89*, 735.

115. Lawson P, Champion M, Canny C, Kingsley R, White M, Dupré J, Kohner EM (1982): Continuous subcutaneous insulin infusion does not prevent progression of proliferative and preproliferative retinopathy. *Br. J. Ophthalmol.*, *96*, 762.
116. Waldhäusel W, Fryler H, Bratusch-Marrain P, Vierhapper H, Brunder H (1983): Kontinuierliche subkutane Insulin Infusion. *Dtsch. Med. Wochenschr.*, *108*, 570.
117. Hooymans JMN, Ballegoore EV, Schweitzer NMJ, Doorenbos H, Reitsman WD, Sluiter WJ (1982): Worsening of retinopathy with strict control of blood sugar. *Lancet*, *2*, 435.
118. Mirouze J, Selam JL, Millet P, Slingeneyer A, Mercadier B (1982): Diabetic retinopathy and prolonged strict metabolic control via insulin pump: variable effect with the degree of lesions. Presented at: Toronto International Workshop on Insulin and Portable Delivery Systems, June 9–11th 1982.
119. Segato T, Midena S, Piermarocchi G, Birani R, Mancinta R, Crepaldi C (1982): Evaluation of proliferative diabetic retinopathy in a group of 5 insulin dependent diabetics treated with continuous subcutaneous insulin infusion for one year. In: *Abstracts, 11th Congress of the International Diabetes Federation, November 10–17, 1982, Nairobi, Kenya*, p. 123. Editors: K.G.M.M. Alberti, T. Ogada, J.A. Aluoch and E.N. Mngola. Excerpta Medica, Amsterdam.
120. White MH, Waltman SR, Krupin T, Santiago J (1982): Reversal of abnormalities in ocular fluorophotometry in insulin dependent diabetics after 5 to 9 months of improved diabetic control. *Diabetes*, *31*, 80.
121. Kroc Collaborative Study Group (1983): Near normal glycaemic control does not slow progression of mild diabetic retinopathy. *Diabetes*, *32*, *Suppl. 1*, 10A.
122. The KROC Collaborative Study Group (1984): Blood glucose control and evaluation of diabetic retinopathy and albuminuria. A multicentre randomised feasibility trial. *N. Engl. J. Med.*, *311*, 365.
123. Voisin PJ, Rouselle D, Streiff F, Debry G, Stoltz JF, Drouin P (1983): Reduction of B thromboglobulin levels in diabetics controlled by artificial pancreas. *Metabolism*, *32*, 138.
124. McDonald JW, Dupré J, Rodger NW, Champion MC, Webb CD, Ali M (1982): Comparison of platelet thromboxane synthesis in diabetic patients on conventional insulin therapy and continuous insulin infusion. *Thromb. Res.*, *28*, 705.
125. Giugliamo D, Misso L, Tirelli A, Coppola L, Di Pinto P, Torella R (1982): Platelet aggregation after strict metabolic control using the artificial pancreas. *Diabetologia*, *23*, 104.
126. Khosla PK, Seth V, Tiwari HK, Saraya AK (1982): Effect of aspirin on platelet aggregation in diabetes mellitus. *Diabetologia*, *23*, 104.
127. Tindall H, Paton RC, McNicol GP (1982): Aspirin dipyridamol and platelet survival in patients with diabetes mellitus. *Clin. Sci.*, *63*, 205.
128. DAMAD Study Group (1982): Essai contrôle de l'aspirine et de l'association aspirine et dipyridamole sur l'évolution de la rétinopathie diabétique I. Protocol Générale. *Diabète Métab.*, *8*, 91.

129. DAMAD Study Group (1982): Essai Contrôle de l'aspirine et de l'association aspirine et dipyridamole sur l'évolution de la rétinopathie diabétique II. Protocol Ophthalmologique. *Diabète Métab.*, *8*, 307.
130. British Multicentre Study Group (1983): Photocoagulation for diabetic maculopathy. A randomised controlled clinical trial using the xenon arc. *Diabetes*, *32*, 1010.
131. British Multicentre Study Group (1984): Photocoagulation for proliferative diabetic retinopathy: a randomised controlled clinical trial using the xenon arc. *Diabetologia*, *26*, 109.
132. Bodansky HJ, Cudworth HG, Whitelock RAF, Dobrec JH (1982): Diabetic retinopathy and its relation to type of diabetes: review of a retinal clinical population. *Br. J. Ophthalmol.*, *66*, 496.
133. Kelemen UM, Fryler H, Ghad HD (1982): Photocoagulation in diabetic maculopathy. *Klin. Monatsbl. Augenheilkd.*, *181*, 329.
134. Plumb AP, Swan AV, Chignell AH, Shilling JS (1982): A comparative trial of xenon arc and argon laser photocoagulation in the treatment of proliferative diabetic retinopathy. *Br. J. Ophthalmol.*, *66*, 213.
135. Kohner EM, Barry PJ (1984): Prevention of blindness in diabetic retinopathy. *Diabetologia*, *26*, 173.
136. Doft BH, Blankenship GW (1982): Single versus multiple treatment sessions of argon laser panretinal photocoagulation for proliferative diabetic retinopathy. *Ophthalmology*, *89*, 772.
137. Pavan PR, Folk JC, Weingeirst TA, Hermsen VM, Watzke RC, Montague PR (1983): Diabetic rubeosis and panretinal photocoagulation in prospective controlled masked trial using iris fluorescein angiography. *Arch. Ophthalmol.*, *101*, 882.
138. Laatikainen L (1977): Preliminary report on the effect of retinal panphotocoagulation on rubeosis iridis and neovascular glaucoma. *Br. J. Ophthalmol.*, *61*, 278.
139. Gerke E, Meyer-Schwickerath G (1982): Proliferative diabetic retinopathy and pregnancy. *Klin. Monatsbl. Augenheilkd.*, *181*, 170.
140. Scheiber S, Bischoff P, Speiser P (1982): Progression of diabetic retinopathy despite panretinal photocoagulation. *Klin. Monatsbl. Augenheilkd.*, *180*, 391.
141. Koerner F (1982): Diabetic vitreous haemorrhage. Comparison of vitrectomy results and natural history. *Klin. Monatsbl. Augenheilkd.*, *180*, 394.
142. Michaels RG, Rice TA, Rice EF (1983): Vitrectomy for diabetic traction detachment involving the macula. *Am. J. Ophthalmol.*, *95*, 22.
143. Rice TA, Michaels RG, Rice EF (1983): Vitrectomy for diabetic traction detachment involving the macula. *Am. J. Ophthalmol.*, *95*, 22.
144. Shea M (1983): Early vitrectomy in proliferative diabetic retinopathy. *Arch. Ophthalmol.*, *101*, 1204.
145. Oyakawa RF, Schachat AP, Michaels RG, Rice T (1983): Complications of vitreous surgery for diabetic retinopathy I. Intraoperative complications. *Ophthalmology*, *90*, 517.
146. Schachat AP, Oyakawa RT, Michaels RG, Rice TA (1983): Complications of vitreous surgery for diabetic retinopathy II. Postoperative complications. *Ophthalmology*, *90*, 522.

147. Blankenship GW (1983): Posterior retinal holes secondary to diabetic retinopathy. *Arch. Ophthalmol.*, *101*, 885.
148. Blankenship GW (1982): Preoperative prognostic factors in diabetic pars plana vitrectomy. *Ophthalmology*, *89*, 1246.
149. Barrie T, Feretis E, Leaver PK, McLeod D (1982): Closed microsurgery for diabetic traction macular detachment. *Br. J. Ophthalmol.*, *66*, 754.
150. Scuderi JJ, Blumenkranz MG, Blankenship GW (1982): Regression of diabetic rubeosis iridis following successful surgical reattachment of the retina by vitrectomy. *Retina*, *2*, 193.
151. Christensen NJ, Hansen AP, Lundbaek K (1978): Metabolic and hormonal factors in diabetic retinopathy. In: *International Ophthalmology Clinics*, *18*, p. 55. Editor: E.M. Kohner. Little Brown and Co., Boston.
152. Sharp PS, Foley K, Vitelli F, Maneschi F, Kohner EM (1984): Growth hormone to hyperinsulinaemia in insulin dependent diabetics: comparison of patients with and without retinopathy. *Diabetic Med.*, *1*, 55.
153. Sundkuist G, Almer L, Lilja H, Pandolfi M (1984): Growth hormone and endothelial function during exercise in diabetes with and without retinopathy. *Acta Med. Scand.*, *215*, 55.
154. Sharp PS, Foley R, Chahal P, Kohner EM (1984): The effect of plasma glucose on the growth hormone response to human pancreatic growth hormone releasing factors in normal subjects. *Clin. Endocrinol.*, *20*, 497.
155. Sharp PS, Foley K, Kohner EM (1984): Evidence for abnormal central regulation of growth hormone secretion in insulin dependent diabetics. *Diabetic Med.*, *1*, 140a.
156. Press M, Tamborlane WV, Thorner MO, Vale W, Rivers J, Sherwin RS (1984): Growth hormone hypersecretion in diabetes: hypothalamic or pituitary? *Diabetic Med.*, *1*, 140a.
157. Ashton IK, Dornan TL, Pocock AE (1983): Plasma somatomedin activity and diabetic retinopathy. *Clin. Endocrinol.*, *19*, 105.
158. Merimee TJ, Zapf J, Froesch ER (1983): Insulin like growth factors: studies in diabetics with and without retinopath. *N. Engl. J. Med.*, *309*, 527.
159. Tamborlane WV, Hintz RL, Bagman M, Genel M, Felig P, Sherwin RS (1980): Insulin infusion pump treatment of diabetes: influence of improved metabolic control on plasma somatomedin levels. *N. Engl. J. Med.*, *305*, 303.
160. Mayfield RK, Sullivan FM, Colwell JH, Wohltman HJ (1983): Predicting insulin requirements for a portable insulin pump using the biostator. Evidence for reversible insulin resistance in poorly controlled type I diabetes. *Diabetes*, *32*, 908.
161. Sharp P, Vitell F, Foley K, Kohner EM (1984): Improvement in insulin resistance with long term insulin therapy is related to copeptide level. *Clin. Sci.*, *67*, 45p.
162. Yoshida A, Feke GT, Morales-Stopello J, Collas GD, Goger DG, McMeel W (1983): Retinal blood flow alterations during progression of diabetic retinopathy. *Arch. Ophthalmol.*, *101*, 225.
163. Oswald B, Vieser W, Oswald H, Jutte H, Konigsdorffer E, Schweitzer D (1983): Messung strömungsphysiologischer Grossen der Netzhautzirkulation bei Diabetikern Typ 1 und 2. *Albrecht von Graefes Arch. Klin. Exp. Ophthalmol.*, *220*, 42.

164. Landers MB, Stefansson E, Wolbarsht ML (1982): Panretinal photocoagulation and retinal oxygenation. *Retina*, *2*, 167.
165. Stefansson E, Landers MB, Wolbarsht ML (1982): Vitrectomy, lensectomy and ocular oxygenation. *Retina*, *2*, 159.
166. Stefansson E, Landers MB, Wolbarsht ML (1983): Oxygenation and vasodilation in relation to diabetic and other proliferative retinopathy. *Ophthalmic Surg.*, *14*, 209.
167. Feke GT, Green GJ, Goger DG, McMeel JW (1982): Laser-doppler measurements of the effect of panretinal photocoagulation on retinal blood flow. *Ophthalmology*, *89*, 757.
168. Ernest JT, Goldstick TK, Engerman RL (1983): Hyperglycaemia impairs retinal oxygen autoregulation in normal and diabetic dogs. *Invest. Ophthalmol. Vis. Sci.*, *24*, 985.
169. Ernest JT, Goldstick TK (1983): Response of choroidal vascular resistance to hyperglycaemia. *Int. Ophthalmol.*, *6*, 119.
170. Nielsen NV, Ditzel J, Jensen S, Kjaergaara JJ (1982): The effect of etidronate disodium (EHDP) on retinopathy in insulin dependent diabetic patients. *Albrecht von Graefes Arch. Klin. Exp. Ophthalmol.*, *219*, 60.
171. Chihara E, Sakugawa M, Entan S (1982): Reduced protein synthesis in diabetic retina and secondary reduction of slow axonal transport. *Brain Res.*, *250*, 363.
172. Hill CR, Kissun RD, Weiss JB, Garner A (1983): Angiogenic factor in vitreous from diabetic retinopathy. *Experientia*, *39*, 583.
173. Sima AAF, Garcia-Salinas R, Basu PK (1983): The BB Wistar rat: an experimental model for the study of diabetic retinopathy. *Metab. Clin. Exp.*, *32*, *Suppl.*, 136.
174. Naeser P, Andersson A (1983): Effect of pancreatic islet transplantation on the morphology of retinal capillaries in alloxan diabetic mice. *Acta Ophthalmol.*, *61*, 30.
175. Ennis SR, Johnson JE, Pautler EL (1982): In situ kinetics of glucose transport across the blood retinal barrier in normal rats and rats with streptozotocin induced diabetes. *Invest. Ophthalmol. Vis. Sci.*, *23*, 447.
176. Betz AL, Bowman PD, Goldstein GW (1983): Glucose transport in microvascular endothelial cells cultured from bovine retina. *Exp. Eye Res.*, *36*, 269.
177. Tripathi BJ, Tripathi RC (1982): Human retinal vessels in tissue culture. A preliminary report of the effect of acute glucose poisoning on cultured vascular cells. *Ophthalmology*, *89*, 858.
178. Palmer GC, Wilson GL, Chronister RB (1983): Streptozotocin induced diabetes produces alterations in adenylate cyclase in rat cerebrum, cerebral microvessels and retina. *Life Sci.*, *32*, 365.
179. Paton RC, Guillot R, Passa P, Canivet J (1982): Prostacyclin production by human endothelial cells cultured in diabetic serum. *Diabète Métab.*, *8*, 323.
180. Buzney SM, Masicotte SJ, Hety N, Zetter BR (1983): Retinal vascular endothelial cells and pericytes. Different growth characteristics in vitro. *Invest. Ophthalmol. Vis. Sci.*, *24*, 470.
181. Blair NP, Tso MOM, Dodge JT (1984): Studies of the blood retinal barrier in the spontaneously diabetic BB rat. *Invest. Ophthalmol. Vis. Sci.*, *25*, 302.

182. Tso MOM (1982): Pathology of cystoid macular oedema. *Ophthalmology, 89*, 902.
183. Marshall J, Clover G, Rothely S (1984): Some new findings on retinal irradiation by krypton and argon lasers. In: *Documenta Ophthalmologica Proceedings Series 36*, p. 21. Editors: R. Bringruber, V.P. Gabel. Dr W. Junk, The Hague.
184. Gregerson DS, Abrahams IW, Puklin JE (1982): Serum antibody responses to bovine retinal S-antigen and rod outer segments in proliferative diabetic retinopathy before and after argon laser photocoagulation. *Ophthalmology, 89*, 767.
185. Eagerman RL, Kern TS (1984): Experimental galactosemia produces a diabetic-like retinopathy. *Diabetes, 33*, 92.
186. Russell P, Merola LO, Yajima Y, Kinoshita JM (1982): Aldose reductase activity in cultured human retinal cell line. *Exp. Eye Res., 35*, 331.
187. Robinson WG, Kador PF, Kinoshita JH (1983): Retinal capillaries: basement membrane thickening by galactosaemia prevented with aldose reductase inhibitor. *Science, 221*, 1177.
188. Kennedy A, Frank RN, Varma S (1983): Aldose reductase activity in retinal and cerebral microvessels and cultured vascular cells. *Invest. Ophthalmol. Vis. Sci., 24*, 125c.
189. Poulsom R, Boot-Handford RP, Heath H (1983): The effect of long term treatment of streptozotocal diabetic rats with aldose reductase inhibitor. *Exp. Eye Res., 37*, 507.
190. Poulsom R, Mirrless DJ, Earl DCN, Heath H (1983): The effect of an aldose reductase inhibitor upon the sorbitol pathway, fructose-1-phosphate and lactate in the retina and nerve of streptozotocin diabetic rats. *Exp. Eye Res., 36*, 751.
191. Poulsom R, Heath H (1983): Inhibitor of aldose reductase in five tissues of the streptozotocin diabetic rat. *Biochem. Pharmacol., 32*, 1495.

The Diabetes Annual/1
K.G.M.M. Alberti and L.P. Krall, editors

ISBN 0444 90 343 7
$0.85 per article per page (transactional system)
$0.20 per article per page (licensing system)

16 Diabetic neuropathy

J.D. WARD

Progress in the understanding of nerve damage in diabetes is bedevilled by our inability to carry out meaningful studies directly on human tissue although clinical observation continues to increase our knowledge of the widespread effects of such damage.

Histopathological studies are almost all carried out on nerves from animal models. Are these the changes caused by the same factors that afflict human nerve within weeks of developing diabetes or after thirty years of the disease?

Electrophysiological measurement can be made with increasing degrees of sophistication but still we are uncertain what they tell us – indeed very little about basic etiology.

Sorbitol and myo-inositol pathways are deranged and at the moment provide the only active reasonable biochemical hypothesis to explain nerve damage. At the same time *vascular* factors continue to be ignored despite the obvious occurrence of severe neuropathic syndromes in those whose glucose (sorbitol) status is not particularly abnormal.

Clinical observations help to identify likely etiological factors in a very general way and are certainly necessary to define the natural history of the many differing syndromes of the *'diabetic neuropathies'* and hence to allow attempts at therapeutic intervention.

Autonomic dysfunction continues to be studied in very great depth and despite its relative rarity as a clinical problem may yet prove to have unidentified harmful effects on many bodily functions.

Impotence remains the meeting point of all the complexities of a human disease resulting from a variable combination of neurological, chemical, vascular and psychological factors, and not only remaining essentially incurable, but the problem most disturbing to the patient and most likely shunted about by the physician!

Histopathological changes

Descriptive histopathology of diabetic nerve is usually from animal tissues and there is a constant worry that this may not reflect the situation in the human subject. Recent studies have involved the dog (1), inbred spontaneously diabetic rat (2), streptozotocin-induced diabetes in rats (3), the Chinese hamster (4) and the diabetic mutant mouse (5). Unfortunately, the pathological changes described in these animals are not identical, further raising the fear that the human will also be different. The dog has axon and myelin changes in distal but not proximal nerves. The inbred rats did not show morphometric structural differences in unmyelinated axons at 2 months whereas at 6 months there was a reduction in nerve fiber size and axonal size. Conduction velocities, however, were abnormal within the first 2 months. In the streptozotocin rat at 6 months there was splitting and notching of myelin sheaths, decrease in the ratio of internodal length and diameter, and widening of the nodal gaps. By contrast the Chinese hamster, although showing delayed conduction velocity, showed very little in the way of abnormal morphology. In the diabetic mutant mouse myelinated fiber size was less while unmyelinated axons were unaffected. Axonal material in this animal was not particularly abnormal, arguing against a primary axonopathy.

In an important review (6) it is recommended that in view of such widely varying histopathological changes, if animal models are to be studied, a careful characterization of the type of 'neuropathy' be attempted with long-term evaluation of many aspects of the animal. By such careful characterization similarities of morphology, biochemistry, function and physical behavior may be identified to allow justification of extrapolation to the human subject. In many respects continuing studies on the spontaneously diabetic BB-Wistar rat give some encouragement that this animal model is a useful indicator of the state in man (7). This rat has an acute onset of ketosis-prone insulin-dependent diabetes (although very unlike the human with non-insulin-dependent 'mild' diabetes who suffers from severe neuropathic syndromes). Neurophysiological abnormalities occur early in the course of hyperglycemia and ultrastructural examination indicates axonal change of a dying back neuropathy. Myelinated fiber atrophy occurs earlier in sensory than in motor nerves progressing with continued duration of diabetes. Axon shrinkage occurs earlier in sural nerve than in peroneal nerve (4 and 8 months respectively). It is assumed that the early appearance of the conduction defect is due to conduction blockage of large myelinated fibers relating to inactivation of sodium ions.

In relation to human neuropathy even more important observations have been made on the BB-Wistar rat (8). By maintaining a state of rather poor metabolic control animals with weakness could be identified in which conduction velocity was only impaired in proximal nerves – the assumption being that this state was similar to the proximal motor neuropathy of human diabetes. A striking finding in the ventral roots was multiple infarcted areas, recent and old, with the demonstration of occluded vessels near such infarcts. One vessel was identified in which total occlusion of the vessel was due to a plug of degranulated platelets. The finding of diseased neural vessels has been described in human neuropathy (9). A further group of 11 patients with severe neuropathy and good metabolic control have recently been studied by the same team and all of them, on sural nerve biopsy, showed severe endothelial disease with occlusion of small vessels and in 1 subject there was a similar plug of degranulated platelets (116). These findings indicate the need to re-examine the vascular hypothesis as a cause of nerve damage in human diabetes, although human tissue is obviously more difficult to acquire in suitable quantities.

An autopsy examination has been reported from patients with a symmetrical sensory distal neuropathy (10). Severe diffuse fiber loss was seen in peripheral nerves, while nerve roots appeared unaffected, and the general appearance suggested a patchy interstitial process rather than a metabolic cause.

Another area requiring further evaluation concerns the non-enzymatic glycosylation of nervous tissue (11). Nerve myelin in diabetic rats seems to be the major component undergoing glycosylation, and in brain excess glycosylation was observed. It would seem likely that this abnormality must play a part in nerve dysfunction.

Two studies (12, 13) raise a number of fundamental problems. Essentially it was shown that when compared with control non-diabetic rats or untreated alloxan diabetic rats, animals treated with insulin showed a greater degree of nerve damage. The changes consisted of altered axon:myelin ratios, teased fiber preparations with ovoids consistent with wallerian-type degeneration and decreased fucose and leucine incorporation into nerves. Abnormal findings were particularly marked in animals receiving protamine zinc insulin (PZI), being less prominent when Ultralente insulin was used and least in the minipump insulin infusion group. It is suggested that insulin in some way precipitates nerve damage, although this denies that in human diabetes some of the worst neuropathic syndromes are seen in those who have never received insulin. An unusual interaction of PZI and alloxan-induced diabetes would seem to be the more likely explanation.

Axons and axonal transport

Experimental diabetes results in an early decrease in the delivery of structural proteins to axons probably leading to a decrease in axonal volume. This extensive area of study is well reviewed by Sidenius (14). Since that time work has focused on axonal transport of other compounds and on the relation to nerve myoinositol. Axonal transport of cholinergic transmitting enzymes (acetyl cholinesterase and choline acetyltransferase) is defective in diabetic animals as it is prevented by use of insulin (15). Results of noradrenaline transmission are conflicting in that this compound was found not to be altered in diabetic animals (16). However, these animals had undoubted histological evidence of abnormal nerve terminals to the vas deferens and impaired responses to stimulation, but no impairment of axonal transport. Further evidence was provided for lack of noradrenaline axon transport while at the same time a reduction in accumulation of fucose and leucine relating to high glucose in the incubating medium was demonstrated (17). With regard to myelin, fucose and leucine show increased incorporation (18).

Recent studies of nerve growth factor (NGF) could well be of great importance for future research (19). Decreased retrograde transport of NGF occurred in ganglia of nerves which are known to develop a distal axonopathy but not in ganglia whose nerves do not develop such lesions. NGF has also been localized in salivary glands of mice (20). In diabetic animals the pattern of catecholamine fluorescence was less marked than in normals, and this correlated with immunocytochemical staining for NGF suggesting a trophic influence of the NGF-containing duct cells on their sympathetic innervation.

Electrophysiology

The most important recent advance in electrophysiological technique has been the development of microneurography, in which microelectrodes are inserted intraneurally, allowing the recording of naturally occurring nerve discharges (21). Muscle and skin fibers may be studied and sympathetic activity in C fibers can be recorded, so that a full range of functions may be tested – vasoconstriction, thermoregulation, muscular activity. Fagius (22) has applied this technique to the study of sympathetic function in diabetic peripheral neuropathy, demonstrating that in neuropathy sensory-afferent impulses were always normal while muscular-afferent activity is often absent. Sympathetic activity could not be detected in more than half the subjects studied, correlating well with reduction in motor conduction velocity (MCV), whereas in non-diabetic neuropathy extremely low values of MCV may be observed in the presence of normal sympathetic activity. Impairment of sympathetic outflow obviously occurs much more commonly in diabetic neuropathy than had previously been assumed. Moreover this technique allows the indirect measurement of conduction velocity (CV) in the unmyelinated post-ganglionic C-fibers by recording reflex latency following various stimuli. Application of this technique will be useful in all types of study involving therapy in diabetic neuropathy.

Attempts continue to use CV in a more specific manner so that distinct groupings of fibers may be studied. By plotting the distributions of nerve fiber CV it is possible to define 2 groups of patients showing different degrees of selective dysfunction of 'fast-large' fibers, the abnormality always appearing to be greater than that indicated by the conventional CV

(23). It will be important in the future to adapt such selective electrophysiological measures to specific clinical syndromes.

With all electrophysiological techniques there is the major problem of understanding what an abnormality means in structural terms in the nerve. It is widely accepted that slowing of CV is related to reduction of fiber size, the presence of a myelin sheath and its thickness and the ratio between axon and myelinated nerve fiber diameter (22). However, in diabetes CV reduction may be present in the absence of measurable morphological change with rapid reversal following metabolic control – too rapid to reflect structural change. At no time when performing electrophysiological measurements in diabetes can we be certain of the exact metabolic state of the nerve at the time of the test. However, these techniques form a major part of the few measurements that can be applied to peripheral nerve – they should be used but interpreted with care. Simple conduction velocities have recently been performed in much younger people than in the past, showing 30% of significant abnormalities correlating positively with quality of glucose control (glycosylated hemoglobin and glycosuria) (24). Young et al. (25) report 72% of abnormalities in peripheral nerve function in diabetic teenagers between ages 16–19 years; 31% had abnormal cardiac parasympathetic tests. In another study 20% of juvenile diabetics within 5 years of diagnosis had delayed CV (26). Obviously these nerves do not function properly when stimulated – but does this necessarily mean structural change? Certainly for the future the subsequent clinical (and electrophysiological) fate of these subjects with regard to the development of 'neuropathic disease' will provide us with vital information concerning the usefulness of these techniques.

Unfortunately, the use of electrophysiology continues to be obsessed with the need to demonstrate that a particular test improves when blood glucose control is improved, usually in short-term studies. For years there has been no doubt that conduction velocities (motor more readily than sensory), latencies and H-reflexes all improve following improved metabolic control. Perhaps all that recent studies have achieved is to underline the correlation of reduction of CV to glycosylated hemoglobin providing further evidence of the relationship of metabolic factors to nerve damage (27–29). However, the argument that diffuse electrophysiological abnormalities in diabetic nerve are closely related to measures of poor glycemic control, although strongly in favor of the metabolic theory of etiology, should not eliminate thought as to other possible factors.

Polyols: sorbitol and myo-inositol

Abnormalities of sorbitol and myo-inositol remain the single most interesting and important area in the understanding of the pathogenesis of nerve damage in diabetes, especially to those who look only for a metabolic explanation. From the knowledge gained so far clinical intervention is being attempted. The background to the 'Polyol Story' is well reviewed by Clements (30) and since that time there has been ample confirmation of the presence of elevated levels of sorbitol and fructose in animal diabetic nerve. However, attention is now focused much more on myo-inositol, concentrations of which are undoubtedly reduced in both animal and human nerve (31–32). Nerve utilizes myo-inositol and its phospholipid derivatives and recent work stresses the importance of this pathway in leading to both nerve dysfunction and axonal damage.

Sorbitol and fructose accumulation in nerve, relating directly to the extracellular glucose concentration, influences the uptake of myo-inositol (33). There is now clear evidence that aldose reductase inhibitors (ARI) prevent the accumulation of sorbitol and fructose but also prevent the reduction of myo-inositol in diabetic nerve independent of the ambient blood glucose (34). However, whereas myo-inositol supplementation of diabetic animals leads to normalization of nerve concentrations of this polyol, it has no effect whatsoever on sorbitol concentrations (35). A further result of the use of ARI agents is improvement in nerve conduction velocities (31, 36, 37) as does myo-inositol supplementation (31). Thus improvement in nerve myo-inositol content by whatever means results in improved nerve function underlining the central position of myo-inositol and the peripheral position of sorbitol. Greene et al. (38), while demonstrating this improvement in CV with myo-inositol feeding, assessed such measurements in 2 populations of motor nerve fibers (large myelinated fibers) which were affected by growth, diabetes and dietary myo-inositol at rather different rates. Supplementation improved conduction at different rates depending on these factors, which could lead to a discrepancy in reported results if they are not standardized. The state of growth and development of the animal itself is an important factor, for functional benefits of myo-inositol feeding are not so readily apparent once growth has ceased (39).

A defect in sodium-potassium adenosine triphosphatase (Na/K ATPase) function may be a result of altered myo-inositol metabolism and this defect is prevented by myo-inositol administration (40). The link could well be in the altered activity of phosphatidylinositol for the water soluble myo-inositol influences nerve inositol phospholipid metabolism (41); hence this derangement could affect Na/K APTase. Moreover, it is argued that while myo-inositol supplementation corrects the reduced Na/K APTase activity, the uptake of myo-inositol itself may be regulated by Na/K APTase allowing the development of a vicious circle (42, 43). Indeed Greene and Lattimer (44) have demonstrated that the reduction in APTase activity seen in diabetic animals was prevented by myo-inositol feeding.

A further possibly important link is to relate myo-inositol abnormalities to defects in axonal transport which are marked in diabetic nerve (35), and Mayer and Tomlinson (31) have recently reported a significant effect of myo-inositol feeding and ARI on such transport. If constriction for 24 hours is applied to the sciatic nerve measurement of the accumulation of choline acetyltransferase (CA) activity proximal to the constriction serves as a measure of orthograde axonal transport of that enzyme. In untreated diabetic animals there is a reduction in CA along with a fall in nerve conduction velocity which is prevented either by the use of ARI or myo-inositol feeding. Again the common pathway would seem to be through myo-inositol in keeping with the observation that reduction of this polyol arises as a result of competitive inhibition of uptake by high levels of extracellular glucose (45).

All the work described above has been carried out on animals. It is obviously important to apply these principles to man. It has been shown that nerve conduction velocity improves significantly following treatment with an ARI (sorbinil) in patients with diabetes but without overt neuropathy (46). It must be stressed that the improvements were extremely small (0.70 m/sec for motor velocity and 1.16 for sensory velocity). Two studies involved themselves with symptomatic neuropathy. In a double-blind placebo-controlled crossover trial of sorbinil there was improvement in only 3 of many measurements – pain, tendon reflexes and sural sensory potential amplitude – while clinical sensory testing deteriorated (47). In a more open-ended anecdotal study, marked improvement in severe symptoms and conduction velocities, with deterioration on withdrawal of the drug is reported following treatment with sorbinil (48). Some subjects improved within days of treatment – in a way difficult to equate with known chemical and structural abnormalities.

Evidence as to the benefits to man of myo-inositol supplementation is not yet available. Studies have been inconclusive, the most recent claiming lack of improvement of all measurements (49).

For the future basic animal biochemical work into sorbitol, myo-inositol and axonal interrelationships should lead to a greater understanding of pathogenetic processes in diabetic nerve. Unfortunately the situation in man is likely to be far more complex, for most animal studies apply themselves to relatively acute and early changes whereas in man the nerves have been abused for years. Some encouragement should be taken from the suggestion of functional and symptomatic improvement in ARI drug trials so far reported.

Clinical observations

Physicians deal with people with diabetes, not with animals. While accepting that animal work will lead to an understanding of fundamental biochemistry, pathology and function of diabetic peripheral nerve, it is to the human subject that the physician must turn. In doing this the clinician can contribute to the understanding of etiology, natural history, presentation and treatment. These are the areas to be covered in this section.

Etiology

Because most cases of diabetic neuropathy are diffuse and symmetrical both clinically and electrophysiologically, it is assumed that the basic cause must be metabolic – a dangerous assumption. Metabolic factors, particularly polyol pathways, are reviewed earlier in this Chapter and comment is made about the role of small vessel disease in pathogenesis. In the clinical field attempts are still being made to relate the development of neuropathy to the quality of blood glucose control. In a recent extensive review of diabetic neuropathy, Brown and Asbury (50) reiterate the view that hyperglycemia is the major factor involved. Glycosylated hemoglobin, an index of glycemic control for a period of a month or so was shown to be elevated in a group of 36 subjects with a variety of clinical syndromes of diabetic neuropathy (51), lending further support to this metabolic-glycemic hypothesis. A number of studies have shown a distinct correlation between elevated glycosylated hemoglobin and electrophysiological measurements (see Electrophysiology, above). Improvement in electrophysiological function in nerve has always been quoted as evidence of the importance of glucose-related metabolic factors, but we are uncertain of the exact significance of such changes which rarely specify the actual pathological change in the nerve.

Beneficial clinical response to blood glucose control may be taken as an indication that nerve function (and hopefully structure) has improved and it seems reasonable to assume that in many instances more adequate glycemic control from an earlier period would have prevented the development of such clinical states. Continuous subcutaneous insulin infusion (CSII) as a method of producing normoglycemia has been shown to produce considerable improvement in 9 patients with severe unremitting painful neuropathy (present for more than 1 year) associated with improvement in motor but not sensory conduction velocities and improved vibration perception threshold (52). It must be noted that this was an uncontrolled open-ended study, but the results have been confirmed by other workers (53, 54). In a much larger study, vibration perception was measured in 74 insulin-requiring diabetic subjects who were randomized to more intensive treatment or usual clinical attendance. After 2 years glycosylated hemoglobin was significantly better in the intensive treatment group as was the vibration perception threshold (55).

Returning to electrophysiological measurements, it has been shown that over 3 years of a study in which treatment was aimed at achieving glucose values between 8.3 mmol/l and 11.1 mmol/l no improvement could be demonstrated in such function (56). Clearly the aim of physicians must be to achieve the best levels of blood glucose control possible, especially when faced with a neuropathic problem. Realism forces one to question how feasible this is in the average large diabetic clinic or practice.

Attempts have also been made to identify other factors relating to the development of nerve damage. Genetic factors as indicated by HLA status or the chlorpropamide alcohol flush do not seem to be important (51). Acetylator status which had been suggested as a factor does not seem to be implicated (51, 57). With the increasing understanding of the role of auto-immune factors involved in the pathogenesis of Type 1 diabetes there is a need to consider this area in relation to the development of nerve damage. One study so far suggests a possible link with 62% of neuropathic patients showing lymphocyte sensitization to central and peripheral nerve antigens (58).

Treatment

There is an enormous need for more accurate detailed classification of the 'diabetic neuropathies', for it seems likely that each syndrome could have a different etiological background. Brown and Asbury (50) suggest a simple classification but more prospective studies are needed to study subjects with as many of the techniques that are used in animals as possible (a difficult proposition). The natural history of syndromes is very different. Nine patients with severe acute painful neuropathy accompanied by depression, weight loss and impotence were shown to have improved within 10 months (59), while 39 patients with less severe sensory symptoms of a 'chronic' nature were seen to improve very little over nearly 5 years (60), and 9 other patients with very painful neuropathy treated with CSII described symptoms of 1–4 years (52). Motor neuropathy from personal experience may develop suddenly with accompanying high glucose levels or more slowly with apparent good control. Extensive wasting of the small muscles of the hand was noted by routinely examining a large number of diabetic subjects. This sign of severe nerve damage, in conjunction with weakness and abnormal electrophysiological measurements had obviously gone unnoticed by the patients themselves (61).

Accurate clinical classification is vital in any treatment trial. It is still all too common to read of a drug trial for diabetic neuropathy of any type – which may well result in a negative result as the treatment might well be inappropriate to some of the etiologies. More careful assessment of symptoms, signs and electrophysiology, temperature and vibration sense, and exclusion of vascular disease are suggested (62). The very detailed methods of clinical and electrophysiological evaluation suggested by Dyck et al. (63, 64) must remain the council of perfection but unfortunately are extremely time consuming and expensive. Treatment with drugs, however, along with blood glucose control, will remain an aim for those with diabetic nerve damage. The use of sorbitol blockers is mentioned elsewhere in this chapter (p. 294). Other drugs have been tried on rather empirical grounds with some indications of success – at least enough to warrant occasional use by physicians when faced with intractable problems – namely gangliosides (65, 66), isaxonine (67), amitryptilene and fluphenazine (68).

There are other clinically interesting studies to report: (1) the occurrence of keratopathy in those with neuropathy, the vibration perception threshold being a predictor of this problem (69); (2) the use of ultrasound to detect the presence of residual urine in those with neuropathy (70); (3) the further use of von Frey hairs for sensory testing on the fingers showing rather small abnormalities not associated with reported symptoms of neuropathy (71).

The diabetic leg

The major clinical manifestation of nerve damage in diabetes are problems of the neuropathic foot. The publication by Levin and O'Neal (72) remains the most extensive and authoritative review of this subject. At the simplest level it can be shown that a foot-care collaborative clinic of physician, nurse, chiropodist, shoe-designer and surgeon can radically reduce the incidence of significant foot ulceration (73). Extremely high pressures are exerted through points in neuropathic feet and this can be quantitated accurately by a microprocessor-controlled optical system (74). Such a system should allow its use in identifying dangerous pressure points and studying the benefits of shoe design or pressure-relieving materials. A visco-elastic polymer material (Sorbothane) has been shown to lower pressure at points in the feet (75) and materials of this nature should have a place in prevention of ulceration. In these studies vibration perception has been shown to correlate very significantly with the presence of high pressure, thus in screening for patients at risk impairment of vibration sense should be sought.

There is a need for careful description of types of diabetic foot problem for many such problems are clearly related to degenerative vascular ischemic disease in proximal vessels. This would then prevent statements that neuropathy was not important in the development of foot lesions when vascular disease was the prominent etiological factor (76).

Arteriovenous shunting

We have now a completely different concept of blood flow in the diabetic neuropathic leg and foot from that of arteriosclerotic obstructive disease or distal small vessel disease. It has been established that in many, especially those with foot ulcers past or present, arteriovenous shunting is occurring. In a typically warm neuropathic foot a bounding visible dorsalis pedis pulse may be observed close to gangrene and ulceration. The veins on the foot are grossly distended (77) and in the supine position they do not collapse until the leg is elevated. The temperature of the foot is well above room temperature and the oxygen concentration of the blood from these veins approaches arterial levels (78). Doppler studies of blood flow indicate increased forward flow (i.e. fast flow) (79) and an increase in transit time suggests rigidity of vessels (62). The presence of medial arterial calcification has been demonstrated in such problems of diabetic neuropathy and it is suggested that sympathetic nerve damage is a potent cause of the described abnormalities (80).

The Charcot foot is the most destructive manifestation of peripheral and autonomic nerve damage and it is likely that the destruction of joints seen in this condition is due to increased blood flow for there is increased uptake of isotope in the bone of joints (81). In the unusual condition of neuropathic edema this abnormal pattern of blood flow is present and may be returned to normal, with resolution of the edema by the use of ephedrine as a sympathetic stimulant (82). It is suggested that abnormal blood flow may be a cause of pain in the diabetic leg rather than neuropathy itself (83). Muscle blood flow estimated by a clearance method has been shown to be reduced in neuropathy but it seems likely that these were not similar subjects to those described above (84).

Autonomic neuropathy

The various tests to assess autonomic function are now well established. Parasympathetic function is tested by measuring heart rate change during the Valsalva maneuver, deep breathing or on standing up, and sympathetic function by assessing blood pressure response to standing up or sustained hand grip (25). Abnormalities of parasympathetic function have been extensively studied in the past decade and it has been assumed that changes in sympathetic function occur much later in the natural history of the condition. A recent review by Watkins (83) stresses the wide-spread effects of sympathetic dysfunction – cardiac denervation, postural hypotension, vascular calcification and arteriovenous shunting in the diabetic leg. Abnormalities of sympathetic function as measured by microneurography occur early on even in patients with 'simple' peripheral neuropathy (see Electrophysiology, p. 291). Involvement of the sympathetic system is suggested by the demonstration of impaired noradrenaline secretion and lack of increase in heart rate following an oral glucose load (85).

Change in heart rate continues to be the single most common measurement performed, being relatively simple to monitor in response to various maneuvers (86). Recent studies describe simplification of many of these tests but also underline how common these abnormalities are, which presumably has prognostic importance to those with longstanding diabetes (87). Heart rate response to deep breathing comparing the longest R–R interval in expiration with the shortest in inspiration seems to be a simple bedside test (88) and Wieling et al. (89) also describe similar responses to forced breathing and standing, pointing out that there was no correlation between the response to both maneuvers. In both these studies increasing age blunted the response. Standing and hand grip are claimed to be superior to head up tilt as a test of vagal heart rate control (90), an abrupt and large increase in heart rate after standing excluding parasympathetic damage. The use of beta-blocking drugs adds a new dimension to the study of the autonomic nervous system allowing analysis of parasympathetic function independent of any sympathetic activity (91). Beta-blockade results in less R–R variation in diabetics with or without autonomic neuropathy when compared to normals.

Abnormalities of heart rate have also been shown in children and adolescents indicating the very early stage at which alteration occurs. In an attempt to overcome the inherent variability of heart rate (sinus arrhythmia) in children the ratio of maximum R–R interval to minimum was used and shown to be abnormal in 15% of children on standing (92). Using heart rate response to standing single deep breath and the Valsalva maneuver in younger people, no abnormalities were found but the resting heart rate was indeed faster in the diabetic (93). Certainly gross abnormalities of the autonomic system have not been described.

In a 24-hour continuous ECG monitoring study of adults with degrees of autonomic dysfunction no arrhythmias were detected but a higher mean hourly heart rate was noted with the minimum heart rate being much higher in those with severe degrees of autonomic damage (94). With increasing damage there was a reduction in diurnal heart rate variation, and it is suggested that at night, when the vagus should still be operative, if there is vagal damage then some sympathetic stimulation is all that is required to cause an increased heart rate. One would tend to assume that an increased heart rate was in some way harmful. However, diabetic subjects with autonomic neuropathy have been found to have a reasonably normal fibrinolytic response when compared to those without neuropathy (95), suggesting the intriguing possibility that heart rate increase is similar to exercise in improving coagulation factors and thus, coupled with dilated vascular channels in denervated vessels, protects against degenerative atheromatous change. However, the known decreased life expectancy of those with autonomic damage denies this as a serious protective factor. Cardiac stroke volume is however lower in those with autonomic neuropathy with a decreased response to exercise, and indeed there was a degree of impairment in diabetics generally (96).

Unexplained cardiorespiratory arrest is now well recognized in autonomic neuropathy (97) but peripheral chemoreceptors are intact in this condition (98), there being no difference between the ventilatory response to transient hypoxia.

The pupil is a fruitful area in which to study autonomic function where the light reflex response is impaired and relates to the presence of autonomic neuropathy (99). Both parasympathetic and sympathetic systems are equally affected in the eye. Each system may be studied separately by the instillation of specific blocking agents (100). Dark adapted pupil size is an index of sympathetic activity when parasympathetic blockade is present and the time from light stimulation to pupil response a measure of parasympathetic activity.

Hormonal secretion is frequently seen to be abnormal when autonomic dysfunction is present. The most obvious hormones to study are adrenaline and noradrenaline seeming to be a direct measure of an intact system. Basal noradrenaline levels are lower in autonomic neuropathy with a poor response to standing although during exercise there is a normal response (101). Norepinephrine levels rise less after insulin administration in autonomic neuropathy with an increase in renin suggesting impaired conversion of inactive renin (102). Gross derangements of gut hormone secretion have now been described and completely reviewed by Vinik and Glownia (103). Since these hormones influence motility, digestion and absorption, they should be regarded not only as an effect of nerve damage but a cause of problems in control of the blood glucose in many subjects. For example, no increase in glucagon pancreatic polypeptide and somatostatin was found after insulin-induced hypoglycemia in autonomic neuropathy (104) and it will be important in the future to relate such abnormalities to clinical situations especially where erratic control is present.

Very little information is available concerning pathological change in autonomic tissue in man and there is no direct evidence of any improvement in various measures of autonomic function relating to quality of metabolic control. Streptozotocin-diabetic rats develop gut dilatation and damage to unmyelinated axons supplying the bowel wall with dilatation of the axon by subcellular organelles (105). When these animals received transplantation of pancreatic islets at a time when this axonopathy was known to be present, subsequent histological examination revealed absence of axon degeneration and bowel function returned to normal. In this animal model at least recovery of neurological function was possible. Degenerative axon changes were seen to be less severe in similar animals when a degree of glucose control was produced with insulin (106). In man autonomic nerve fibers showed beading, spindle-shaped thickening and fragmentation in regions adjacent to sweat glands in skin biopsies from subjects with autonomic neuropathy and anhydrotic skin (107).

Impotence

The commonest most distressing result of nerve damage in diabetes is to interfere with sexual function. It is assumed that autonomic dysfunction is a major etiological factor along with somatic nerve damage and blood flow abnormalities. Psychological factors also play a very large part both in the development of the problem and in its treatment. This important subject requires a major review in itself. Animal studies can surely have very little to offer in the understanding of this most complex of human functions other than in the demonstration of biochemical or anatomical changes. In diabetic rats changes in autonomic fibers were observed similar to those seen in man (108) and perhaps this could allow an understanding of the relationship between noradrenergic innervation of the penis and erectile tissue. Vasoactive intestinal polypeptide is reduced in diabetic rat penile tissue (109).

All human studies should attempt to look at every aspect known to contribute to the eventual development of impotence so that ultimately it should be possible to identify the most important factor in an individual rather than simply record the incidence in a large number of subjects (110). A detailed study of 27 impotent diabetic men demonstrates the need for this in-depth approach (111). Half those with impotence reported morning erections but reduced sexual interest, one third had spontaneous erections and many had disorders of ejaculation. In this study, however, no relationship was found between impotence and autonomic neuropathy, retinopathy or obvious psychological factors – perhaps against the likely view of many physicians. The importance of vascular abnormalities has been stressed (112), for 68% of impotent diabetics studied had evidence of vascular occlusion, while only 26% had electrophysiological abnormalities. In this group 19% had low plasma testosterone levels and although 38% had psychological problems, in only 19% these were regarded as relevant. The exact role of psychological factors in etiology remains to bc determined. However, psychological techniques are of great importance in treatment either aiming at a 'cure' of the physical inability or helping in coping with an insoluble problem. The great need for psychological support and counselling is well reviewed by Smith (113). Proven benefits from such techniques must be put to the test of properly constructed trials.

In the totally incurable situation attempts may be made to provide the patient with an artificial erection by the implantation of rigid or inflatable penile prosthesis, perhaps with some psychological benefit to the man or his partner. Studies tend to indicate an acceptable degree of satisfaction with these implants for those who want the procedure (114, 115).

References

1. Braund KG, Steiss JE (1982): Distal neuropathy in spontaneous diabetes mellitus in the dog. *Acta Neuropathol.*, *57*, 263.
2. Yagihashi S, Tonosaki A, Yamada K (1982): Peripheral neuropathy in selectively inbred spontaneously diabetic rats. *Tohoku J. Exp. Med.*, *138*, 39.
3. Mattingly GE, Fischer VW (1983): Peripheral neuropathy following prolonged exposure to streptozotocin induced diabetes in rats: a teased nerve fiber study. *Acta Neuropathol.*, *59*, 133.
4. Kennedy WR, Quick DC, Miyoshi T, Gerritsen GC (1982): Peripheral neurology of the diabetic Chinese hamster. *Diabetologia*, *23*, 445.
5. Sharma AK, Thomas PK, Gabriel G, Stolinski C, Dockery P, Hollins GW (1983): Peripheral nerve abnormalities in the diabetic mutant mouse. *Diabetes*, *32*, 1152.
6. Brown MR, Dyck PJ, McClearn GE, Sima AAF, Powell HC, Porte D Jr (1982): Central and peripheral nervous system complications. *Diabetes*, *31*, *Suppl. 1*, 65.
7. Sima AAF, Bouchier M, Christensen H (1983): Axonal atrophy in sensory nerves of the diabetic BB-Wistar rat: a possible early correlate of human diabetic neuropathy. *Ann. Neurol.*, *13*, 264.
8. Sima AAF, Thibert P (1982): Proximal motor neuropathy in the BB-Wistar rat. *Diabetes*, *31*, 784.
9. Williams E, Timperley WR, Ward JD, Duckworth T (1980): Electron microscopical studies of vessels in diabetic peripheral neuropathy. *J. Clin. Pathol.*, *33*, 462.
10. Sugimura K, Dyck PJ (1982): Multifocal fiber loss in proximal sciatic nerve in symmetric distal diabetic neuropathy. *J. Neurol. Sci.*, *53*, 501.
11. Vlassara H, Brownlee M, Cerami A (1983): Excessive nonenzymatic glycosylation of peripheral and central nervous system myelin components in diabetic rats. *Diabetes*, *37*, 670.
12. Westfall SG, Felten DL, Mandelbaum JA, Moore SA, Petersen RG (1983): Degenerative neuropathy in insulin-treated rats. *J. Neurol. Sci.*, *61*, 93.
13. Mandelbaum JA, Felten DL, Westfall SG, Newlin GE, Petersen RG (1983): Neuropathic changes associated with insulin treatment of diabetic rats: electron microscopic and morphometric analysis. *Brain Res. Bull.*, *10*, 377.
14. Sidenius P (1982): The axonopathy of diabetic neuropathy. *Diabetes*, *31*, 356.
15. Mayer JH, Tomlinson DR (1983): Axonal transport of cholinergic transmitter enzymes in vagus and sciatic nerves of rats with acute experimental diabetes mellitus: correlation with motor nerve conduction velocity and effects of insulin. *Neuroscience*, *9*, 951.
16. Tomlinson DR, Gillon KRW, Smith MG (1982): Axonal transport of noradrenaline and noradrenergic transmission in rats with streptozotocin-induced diabetes. *Diabetologia*, *22*, 199.
17. Tomlinson DR (1983): Axonal transport of noradrenaline, protein and glycoprotein in cat hypogastric nerves in vitro under conditions of high extracellular glucose. *Diabetologia*, *24*, 172.
18. Chez MG, Peterson RG (1983): Altered metabolic incorporation of fucose

and leucine into PNS myelin of 25 week old diabetic (C57BL/Ks (DB/DB)) mice: effects of untreated diabetes on nerve metabolism. *Neurochem. Res.*, *8*, 465.
19. Schmidt RE, Modert CW, Yip HK, Johnson EM Jr (1983): Retrograde axonal transport of intravenously administered nerve growth factor in rats with streptozocin induced diabetes. *Diabetes*, *37*, 654.
20. Carson KA, Sar M, Hanker JS (1982): Immunocytochemical demonstration of nerve growth factor and histofluorescence of catecholaminergic nerves in the salivary glands of diabetic mice. *Histochem. J.*, *14*, 35.
21. Wallin BG (1981): New aspects of sympathetic function in man. In: E. Stalberg and R Young (Eds), *Neurology I, Clinical Neurophysiology*, p. 145. Butterworths, London-Boston.
22. Fagius J (1982): Microneurographic findings in diabetic polyneuropathy with special reference to sympathetic nerve activity. *Diabetologia*, *23*, 415.
23. Dorfman LJ, Cummins KL, Reaven GM (1983): Studies of diabetic polyneuropathy using conduction velocity distribution (DCV) analysis. *Neurology*, *33*, 773.
24. Kaar ML, Saukkonen AL, Pitkanen M, Akerblom HK (1983): Peripheral neuropathy in diabetic children and adolescents. A cross-sectional study. *Acta Paediatr. Scand.*, *72*, 373.
25. Young RJ, Ewing DJ, Clarke BF (1983): Nerve function and metabolic control in teenage diabetics. *Diabetes*, *32*, 142.
26. Hoffman WH, Hart ZH, Frank RN (1983): Correlates of delayed motor nerve conduction and retinopathy in juvenile-onset diabetes mellitus. *J. Pediatr.*, *102*, 351.
27. Mabin D, Darragon T, Menez JF (1982): Influence of glycaemic control on peripheral nerve conduction in insulin-dependent diabetic subjects. *Rev. Electroencephalogr. Neurophysiol. Clin.*, *12*, 72.
28. Halar EM, Graf RJ, Halter JB (1982): Diabetic neuropathy: a clinical, laboratory and electrodiagnostic study. *Arch. Phys. Med. Rehabil.*, *63*, 298.
29. Agardh CD, Rosen I, Schersten B (1983): Improvement of peripheral nerve function after institution of insulin treatment in diabetes mellitus. A case control study. *Acta Med. Scand.*, *213*, 283.
30. Clements RS Jr (1979): Diabetic neuropathy: new concepts of its etiology. *Diabetes*, *28*, 604.
31. Mayer JH, Tomlinson DR (1983): Prevention of defects of axonal transport and nerve conduction velocity by oral administration of myo-inositol or an aldose reductase inhibitor in streptozotocin-diabetic rats. *Diabetologia*, *25*, 433.
32. Mayhew JA, Gillon KRW, Hawthorne JN (1983): Free and lipid inositol, sorbitol and sugars in sciatic nerve obtained post-mortem from diabetic patients and control subjects. *Diabetologia*, *24*, 13.
33. Simmonds DA, Winegrad AI, Martin DB (1982): Significance of tissue myo-inositol concentrations in metabolic regulation in nerve. *Science*, *217*, 848.
34. Finegold D, Lattimer SA, Nolle S, Bernstein M, Greene DA (1983): Polyol pathway activity and myo-inositol metabolism. A suggested relationship in the pathogenesis of diabetic neuropathy. *Diabetes*, *32*, 988.
35. Gillon KRW, Hawthorne JN, Tomlinson DR (1983): Myo-inositol and sor-

bitol metabolism in relation to peripheral nerve function in experimental diabetes in the rat: the effect of aldose reductase inhibition. *Diabetologia*, *25*, 365.

36. Yue DK, Hanwell MA, Satchell PM, Turtle JR (1982): The effect of aldose reductase inhibition on motor nerve conduction velocity in diabetic rats. *Diabetes*, *31*, 789.
37. Kikkawa R, Hatanaka I, Yasuda H, Kobayashi N, Shigeta Y, Terashima H, Morimura T, Tsuboshima M (1983): Effect of a new aldose reductase inhibitor on peripheral nerve disorders in streptozotocin diabetic rats. *Diabetologia*, *24*, 290.
38. Greene DA, Lewis RA, Lattimer SA, Brown MJ (1982): Selective effects of myo-inositol administration on sciatic and tibial motor nerve conduction parameters in the streptozocin-diabetic rat. *Diabetes*, *31*, 573.
39. Thomas PK, Jefferys JGR, Sharma AK, Bajada S (1981): Nerve conduction velocity in experimental diabetes in the rat and rabbit. *J. Neurol. Neurosurg. Psychiatry*, *44*, 233.
40. Greene DA, Lattimer SA (1983): Na/K AtPase defect in diabetic rat peripheral nerve: correction by myo-inositol administration. *J. Clin. Invest.*, *72*, 1058–1063.
41. Simmons DA, Winegrad AI, Martin DB (1982): Significance of tissue myo-inositol concentrations in metabolic regulation in nerve. *Science*, *217*, 848.
42. Greene DA (1983) Metabolic abnormalities in diabetic peripheral nerve: relation to impaired function. *Metabolism*, *32*, *Suppl. 1*, 118.
43. Greene DA, Lattimer SA (1982): Sodium and energy dependent uptake of myo-inositol by rabbit peripheral nerve: competitive inhibition by glucose and lack of an insulin effect. *J. Clin. Invest.*, *70*, 1009.
44. Greene DA, Lattimer SA (1983): Impaired rat sciatic nerve sodium-potassium adenosine triphosphatase in acute streptozotocin diabetes and its correction by dietary myo-inositol supplementation. *J. Clin. Invest.*, *72*, 1058.
45. Gillon KRW, Hawthorne JN (1983): Transport of myo-inositol into endoneurial preparations of sciatic nerve from normal and streptozotocin-diabetic rats. *Biochem. J.*, *210*, 775.
46. Judzewitsch RG, Jaspan JB, Polonsky KS, Weinberg CR, Halter JB, Halar E, Pfeifer MA, Vukadinovic C, Bernstein L, Schneider M, Liang KY, Gabbay KH, Rubenstein AH, Porte D (1983): Aldose reductase inhibition improves nerve conduction velocity in diabetic patients. *N. Engl. J. Med.*, *308*, 119.
47. Young RJ, Ewing DJ, Clarke BF (1983): A controlled trial of sorbinil, an aldose reductase inhibitor, in chronic painful diabetic neuropathy. *Diabetes*, *32*, 938.
48. Jaspan J, Herold K, Maselli R, Bartkus C (1983): Treatment of severely painful diabetic neuropathy with an aldose reductase inhibitor: relief on pain and improved somatic and autonomic nerve function. *Lancet*, *2*, 758.
49. Gregerson G, Bertelsen B, Harbo H, Larsen E, Anderson JR, Helles A, Schmiegelow M, Christensen JE (1982): No effect of myo-inositol on function of peripheral nerves in diabetics. *Acta Endocrinol. (Copenhagen)*, *247*, *Suppl. 100*, 23.

50. Brown MJ, Asbury AK (1984): Diabetic Neuropathy. *Ann. Neurol.*, *15*, 2.
51. Boulton AJM, Worth RG, Drury J, Hardisty CA, Wolf E, Cudworth AG, Ward JD (1984): Genetic and metabolic studies in diabetic neuropathy. *Diabetologia*, *26*, 15.
52. Boulton AJM, Drury J, Clarke B, Ward JD (1982): Continuous subcutaneous insulin infusion in the management of painful diabetic neuropathy. *Diabetes Care*, *5*, 386.
53. White NH, Skor D, Santiago JV (1982): Long term effect of intensive insulin therapy on peripheral and autonomic neuropathy in insulin dependent diabetes. *Diabetes*, *31*, *Suppl. 2*, 66A.
54. Tolaymat A, Roque JL, Russo LS Jr (1982): Improvement of diabetic peripheral neuropathy with the portable insulin infusion pump. *South. Med. J.*, *75*, 185.
55. Holman RR, Dornan TL, Mayon-White V, Williams JH, Peckar CO, Jenkins L, Steemson J, Rolfe R, Smith B, Barbour D, McPherson K, Poon P, Rizza C, Mann JI, Knight AH, Bron AJ, Turner RC (1983): Prevention of deterioration of renal and sensory nerve function by more intensive management of insulin-dependent diabetic patients. A two-year randomised prospective study. *Lancet*, *1*, 204.
56. Service FJ, Daube JR, O'Brien PG, Zimmerman BR, Brennan MD, Swanson CJ, Dyck PJ (1983): Effect of blood glucose control on peripheral nerve function in diabetic patients. *Mayo Clin. Proc.*, *58*, 283.
57. Shenfield GM, McCann VJ, Tjokresetio R (1982): Acetylator status and diabetic neuropathy. *Diabetologia*, *22*, 441.
58. Segal P, Teitelbaum D, Ohry A (1983): Cell-mediated immunity to nervous system antigens in diabetic patients with neuropathy. *Isr. J. Med. Sci.*, *19*, 7.
59. Archer AG, Watkins PJ, Thomas PK, Sharma AK, Payan J (1983): The natural history of acute painful neuropathy in diabetes mellitus. *J. Neurol. Neurosurg. Psychiatry*, *46*, 491.
60. Boulton AJM, Armstrong WD, Scarpello JHB, Ward JD (1983): The natural history of painful diabetic neuropathy – a 4 year study. *Postgrad. Med. J.*, *59*, 556.
61. Borsey DQ, Cull RE, Fraser DM, Ewing DJ, Campbell IW, Clarke BW (1983): Small muscle wasting of the hands in diabetes mellitus. *Diabetes Care*, *6*, 10.
62. Ward JD (1982): The diabetic leg. *Diabetologia*, *22*, 141.
63. Dyck PJ, Sherman WR, Hallcher LM, Service FJ, O'Brien PC, Grina LA, Palumbo PJ, Swanson CJ (1980): Human diabetic endoneurial sorbitol, fructose and myo-inositol related to sural nerve morphometry. *Ann. Neurol.*, *8*, 590.
64. Dyck PJ, Zimmerman IR, O'Brien PC, Ness A, Caskey PE, Karnes J, Bushek W (1978): Introduction of automated systems to evaluate touch pressure, vibration and thermal cutaneous sensation in man. *Ann. Neurol.*, *4*, 502.
65. Montenero P, Marozzi G, Chiaramonte F (1983): Possibilities of using brain gangliosides in treatment of peripheral diabetic neuropathy. *Clin. Ter. (Roma)*, *106*, 169.

66. Bassi S, Albizzati MG, Frattola L (1982): Electromyographic study of diabetic and alcoholic polyneuropathic patients treated with gangliosides. *Muscle Nerve*, *5*, 351.
67. Augustin P, Rathery M (1982): Clinical trial of isaxonine in diabetic neuropathies. *Nouv. Presse Méd. (Paris)*, *11*, 1265.
68. Mitas JA II, Mosley CA Jr, Drager AM (1983): Diabetic neuropathic pain: control by amitriptyline and fluphenazine in renal insufficiency. *South. Med. J.*, *76*, 462.
69. Schultz RO, Peters MA, Sobocinski K (1983): Diabetic keratopathy as a manifestation of peripheral neuropathy. *Am. J. Ophthalmol.*, *96*, 368.
70. Beylot M, Marion D, Noel G (1982): Ultrasonographic determination of residual urine in diabetic subjects: relationship to neuropathy and urinary tract infection. *Diabetes Care*, *5*, 501.
71. Magelende R, McBride P, Mistretta CM (1982): Light touch thresholds in diabetic patients. *Diabetes Care*, *5*, 311.
72. Levin ME, O'Neal LW (Eds) (1983): *The Diabetic Foot, 3rd Edition*. The CV Mosby Company, St. Louis-Toronto-London.
73. Edmonds ME, Blundell MP, Morris M, Thomas EM, Williamson M, Watkins PJ (1982): The 'Combined Diabetic Foot Clinic'. A major development in diabetic foot care. *Diabetologia*, *23*, 468A.
74. Boulton AJM, Hardisty CA, Betts RP, Franks CI, Worth RC, Ward JD, Duckworth T (1983): Dynamic foot pressure and other studies as diagnostic and management aids in diabetic neuropathy. *Diabetes Care*, *6*, 26.
75. Boulton AJM, Franks CI, Betts RP, Duckworth T, Ward JD (1984): Reduction of abnormal foot pressures in diabetic neuropathy using a new Polymer insole material. *Diabetes Care*, *7*, 42.
76. Delbridge L, Appelberg M, Reeve TS (1983): Factors associated with development of foot lesions in the diabetic. *Surgery*, *93*, 78.
77. Ward JD, Simms JM, Knight G, Boulton AJM, Sandler DA (1983): Venous distension in the diabetic neuropathic foot (physical sign of arteriovenous shunting). *J. R. Soc. Med.*, *76*, 1011.
78. Boulton AJM, Scarpello JHB, Ward JD (1982): Venous oxygenation in the diabetic neuropathic foot: evidence of arteriovenous shunting? *Diabetologia*, *22*, 6.
79. Edmonds ME, Roberts VC, Watkins PJ (1982): Blood flow in the diabetic neuropathic foot. *Diabetologia*, *22*, 9.
80. Edmonds ME, Morrison N, Laws JW, Watkins PJ (1982): Medial arterial calcification and diabetic neuropathy. *Br. Med. J.*, *284*, 928.
81. Watkins PJ, Edmonds ME (1982): Autonomic neuropathy: blood flow in the diabetic foot. In: Bostrom and H. Ljungstedt (Eds), *Recent Trends in Diabetic Research*, p. 211. Almqvist & Wiksell International, Stockholm.
82. Edmonds ME, Archer AG, Watkins PJ (1983): Ephedrine: a new treatment for diabetic neuropathic oedema. *Lancet*, *1*, 548.
83. Watkins PJ, Edmonds ME (1983): Sympathetic nerve failure in diabetes. *Diabetologia*, *25*, 73.
84. Matikainen E, Leinonen H, Juntunen J (1982): Capillary morphology and muscle blood flow in diabetic neuropathy. *Eur. Neurol.*, *21*, 22.

85. Hegedus L, Christensen NJ, Sestoft L (1983): Abnormal regulation of sympathetic nervous activity and heart rate after oral glucose in Type 1 (insulin-dependent) diabetic patients. *Diabetologia, 25*, 242.
86. Ewing DJ, Campbell IW, Clarke BF (1981): Heart rate changes in diabetes mellitus. *Lancet, 1*, 183.
87. Ewing DJ, Campbell IW, Clarke BF (1980): Assessment of cardiovascular effects in diabetic autonomic neuropathy. *Ann. Intern. Med., 92*, 308.
88. Smith SA (1982): Reduced sinus arrhythmia in diabetic autonomic neuropathy: diagnostic value of an age-related normal range. *Br. Med. J., 285*, 1599.
89. Wieling W, Van Brederode JF, De Rijk LG, Borst C, Dunning AJ (1982): Reflex control of heart rate in normal subjects in relation to age: a data base for cardiac vagal neuropathy. *Diabetologia, 22*, 163.
90. Wieling W, Borst C, Van Brederode JFM, Van Dongen Torman MA, Van Montfrans GA, Dunning AJ (1983): Testing for autonomic neuropathy: heart rate changes after orthostatic manoeuvres and static muscle contractions. *Clin. Sci., 64*, 581.
91. Pfeifer MA, Cook D, Brodsky J, Tice D, Reenan A, Swedine S, Halter JB, Porte D Jr (1982): Quantitative evaluation of cardiac parasympathetic activity in normal and diabetic man. *Diabetes, 31*, 339.
92. Mitchell EA, Wealthall SR, Elliott RB (1983): Diabetic autonomic neuropathy in children: immediate heart-rate response to standing. *Aust. Paediatr. J., 19*, 175.
93. Koepp P, Hamm H (1983): Testing for autonomous nervous function in children and adolescents with insulin-dependent diabetes mellitus. *Monatsschr. Kinderheilkd., 131*, 273.
94. Ewing DJ, Borsey DQ, Travis P, Bellauere F, Neilson JMM, Clarke BF (1983): Abnormalities of ambulatory 24-hour heart rate in diabetes mellitus. *Diabetes, 32*, 101.
95. Almer LO, Sundqvist G, Lilja B (1983): Fibrinolytic activity, autonomic neuropathy, and circulation in diabetes mellitus. *Diabetes, 32, Suppl.*, 4.
96. Hilsted J, Galbo H, Christensen NJ, Parving HH, Benn J (1982): Haemodynamic changes during graded exercise in patients with diabetic autonomic neuropathy. *Diabetologia, 22*, 318.
97. Lloyd-Mostyn RH, Watkins PJ (1976): Total cardiac denervation in diabetic autonomic neuropathy. *Diabetes, 25*, 748.
98. Calverley PMA, Ewing DJ, Campbell IW, Wraith PK, Brash HM, Clarke BF, Flenley DC (1982): Preservation of the hypoxic drive to breathing in diabetic autonomic neuropathy. *Clin. Sci., 63*, 17.
99. Smith SA, Smith SE (1983): Reduced pupillary light reflexes in diabetic autonomic neuropathy. *Diabetologia, 24*, 330.
100. Pfeifer MA, Cook D, Brodsky J, Tice D, Parrish D, Reenen A, Halter JB, Porte D (1982): Quantitative evaluation of sympathetic and parasympathetic control of iris function. *Diabetes Care, 5*, 518.
101. Caviezel F, Picotti GB, Margonato A, Slaviero G, Galva MD, Camagna P, Bondiolotti GP, Carruba MO, Pozza G (1982): Plasma adrenaline and noradrenaline concentrations in diabetic patients with and without autonomic neuropathy at rest and during sympathetic stimulation. *Diabetologia, 23*, 19.

102. Nakamaru M, Ogihara T, Higaki J (1983): Plasma inactive renin in diabetic patients with neuropathy: a role for the sympathetic nervous system in the conversion in vivo of inactive renin. *Acta Endocrinol.*, *104*, 216.
103. Vinik AI, Glownia KJV (1982): Hormonal secretion in diabetic autonomic neuropathy. *NY State J. Med.*, *82*, 871.
104. Hilstead J, Madsbad S, Krarup T (1982): No response of pancreatic hormones to hypoglycaemia in diabetic autonomic neuropathy. *J. Clin. Endocrinol. Metab.*, *54*, 815.
105. Schmidt RE, Plurad SB, Olack BJ, Scharp DW (1983): The effect of pancreatic islet transplantation and insulin therapy on experimental diabetic autonomic neuropathy. *Diabetes*, *32*, 532.
106. Monckton G, Pehowich E (1982): The effects of intermittent insulin therapy on the autonomic neuropathy in the streptozotocin diabetic rat. *Can. J. Neurol. Sci.*, *9*, 79.
107. Faerman I, Faccio E, Calb I, Razumny J, Franco N, Dominguez A, Podesta P (1982): Autonomic neuropathy in the skin: a histological study of the sympathetic nerve fibres in diabetic anhydrosis. *Diabetologia*, *22*, 96.
108. Felten DL, Felten SY, Melman A (1983): Noradrenergic innervation of the penis in control and streptozotocin diabetic rats: evidence of autonomic neuropathy. *Anat. Rec.*, *206*, 49.
109. Crowe R, Lincoln J, Blacklay PF (1983): Vasoactive intestinal polypeptide-like immunoreactive nerves in diabetic penis. A comparison between streptozotocin-treated rats and man. *Diabetes*, *32*, 1075.
110. McCulloch DK, Campbell IW, Wu FC, Prescott RJ, Clarke BF (1980): The prevalence of diabetic impotence. *Diabetologia*, *18*, 279.
111. Fairburn CG, Wu FC, McCulloch DK, Borsey DQ, Ewing DJ, Clarke BF, Bancroft JHJ (1982): The clinical features of diabetic impotence: a preliminary study. *Br. J. Psychiatry*, *140*, 453.
112. Lehman TP, Jacobs JA (1983): Aetiology of diabetic impotence. *J. Urol.*, *129*, 291.
113. Smith BC (1983): Sexual counselling of diabetic impotence. *Patient Couns. Health Educ.*, *4*, 10.
114. Segraves RT, Schoenberg HW, Zarins CK (1982): Psychosexual adjustment after penile prosthesis surgery. *Sex. Disability*, *5*, 222.
115. Pfeifer M, Reenan A, Berger R, Best J (1983): Penile prosthesis and quality of life. *Diabetes*, *32*, 77A.
116. Timperley WR, Boulton AJM, Davies-Jones GAB, Jarratt J, Ward JD (1984): Small vessel disease in progressive diabetic neuropathy with good metabolic control. *Diabetologia, 27*, 339A.

The Diabetes Annual/1
K.G.M.M. Alberti and L.P. Krall, editors

ISBN 0444 90 343 7
$0.85 per article per page (transactional system)
$0.20 per article per page (licensing system)

17 Diabetic nephropathy

EILEEN N. ELLIS AND S. MICHAEL MAUER

Diabetic nephropathy and its end result, renal failure, is a vast problem both for diabetic patients and those health care teams who care for them. Nearly 40% of insulin-dependent diabetic (Type 1 – IDDM) patients will develop renal failure on average about 20 years after onset of diabetes (1–3). Although the incidence of renal failure is much lower, Type 2 diabetes is so common that it contributes almost equally to the renal failure population (4). Together, diabetes-related kidney failure accounts for approximately 25% of new end-stage renal disease patients in the United States (5). In the United Kingdom in 1979, 33% of diabetic patients under the age of 50 years either died of uremia or of other causes but with evidence of nephropathy (6). Herein, with special emphasis on recent advances, we review aspects of the pathogenesis and treatment of diabetic renal lesions.

Pathology of the diabetic kidney: relationship of structure and function

Renal structural and functional changes have been recognized to occur soon after onset of IDDM. Renal hypertrophy occurs in early diabetes mellitus (7–13) and in animals with experimental diabetes (14–22). In both patients and animals, kidney enlargement is noted shortly after the onset of hyperglycemia (8, 9, 16). Both glomerular and tubular size are significantly increased with a 30% increase in total glomerular volume (16), an increase in glomerular filtration surface area (17, 18), podocyte hypercellularity (19), and proximal and distal tubular cellular hypertrophy and hyperplasia (21). Precise glycemic control by insulin administration can prevent these structural changes in animals (23) and return these early structural alterations toward normal in diabetic patients (8).

Hyperfunction of the kidney is well documented early in IDDM (7–11) and is the subject of an extensive recent review (24). Glomular filtration rate (GFR), renal plasma flow (RPF), and filtration fraction (FF) are increased in newly diagnosed patients prior to insulin treatment (8, 11), while micropuncture studies of diabetic rats have demonstrated an increase in single nephron GFR and RPF with no change in FF (25). In newly diagnosed IDDM patients, GFR is elevated nearly 50% over normal prior to insulin treatment and remains 20% higher than normal after 8 days of insulin treatment achieving near-normal blood glucose values (9). Patients with good metabolic control appear to have lower GFR than patients with poor metabolic control (24), but GFR remains elevated by 20–30% in diabetics on standard insulin treatment, unless the patient develops clinical nephropathy (26). This increased GFR is closely correlated with the enlarged kidney size in both newly diagnosed diabetics (7, 8) and in those with longer duration without evidence of nephropathy (12, 13). However, renal size measured röntgenographically and GFR in the normal range in patients with long-standing IDDM do not indicate the severity of diabetic renal size measured roentgenographically and GFR in the normal range in have been conflicting most likely because of differences in study design, patient selection, and degree of metabolic control, but an increase of at least 10% in patients in usual metabolic control is probably accurate (24). A linear relationship has been found between GFR and RPF (24).

The mechanism of renal hyperfunction in diabetes is unclear; however, vascular volume expansion has been excluded as a possibility (27). Glucose infusion alone has been shown to increase GFR by 6% in normal man (28). In diabetics, a rise in blood glucose from normoglycemic levels to moderately hyperglycemic levels also results in a 5% increase in GFR (28). Micropuncture studies in rats have shown that increased GFR is secondary to increased glomerular plasma flow and transcapillary hydraulic pressure, the latter apparently secondary to alterations in the balance of afferent and efferent glomerular arteriolar resistances (25). Ditzel and Brochner-Mortensen have proposed that these functional changes result from altered tubulo-glomerular feedback mechanisms (29). They based this argument on the accompaniment of increased GFR by demonstrably increased tubular reabsorption rates for sodium, glucose, and calcium (29, 30). They proposed that elevated plasma and ultrafiltrate glucose stimulates tubular reabsorption of sodium by the sodium-glucose co-transport mechanism, thus producing increased solute-linked water reabsorption and a net increase in GFR and FF (29). Others have proposed additional factors which may influence the hyperfunction in IDDM. Although glucagon administration has been shown to increase GFR in animals (31), normal man (32) and well-controlled diabetics (33), the mechanism of this rise in GFR is unclear. It has been proposed that growth hormone may also play a role in the hyperfunction of diabetes, based on the finding that administration of growth hormone to diabetics while maintaining usual glycemic control results in an elevation of GFR and RPF over baseline values (34). Thus, the growth hormone elevation usually found in Type 1 diabetics under usual metabolic control may contribute to the enhanced GFR and RPF.

Overt *proteinuria* has long been recognized as one of the hallmarks of clinically apparent diabetic nephropathy. Recent work has focused on the *microalbuminuria* which can be detected earlier in the disease process. Microalbuminuria can be defined as an increase in urinary albumin excretion (UAE) not detectable by Albustix®. UAE is increased both at rest and during exercise in newly diagnosed diabetics prior to insulin treatment; a decrease in microalbuminuria occurs after a few days of insulin treatment (35). Further, diabetics with longer duration of diabetes demonstrate an abnormal elevation in UAE with less exercise when compared to normals (35). In diabetic animals, albuminuria normalizes with effective insulin treatment or pancreatic islet transplantation (36, 37). Importantly, microalbuminuria reflects glycemic control as estimated by glucosylated hemoglobin (38).

Attempts have been made to relate microalbuminuria to later development of clinical nephropathy. In a 14-year follow-up of 87 IDDM patients, Viberti suggested that patients with 30 to 140 μg/min UAE at initial study were 24 times more likely to develop overt proteinuria than those subjects with less than 30 μg/min UAE (39). Similarly, 5 of 8 diabetics with a mean UAE of 115 mg/24 hours developed proteinuria, hypertension and rising serum creatinine within 6 years follow-up while only 2 of 15 diabetics with mean UAE of 17 mg/24 hours developed intermittent or persistent albuminuria and none developed overt proteinuria, hypertension, or increased serum creatinine during this same time period (40). In Type 2 diabetics, Mogensen has shown that UAE of 30 to 140 μg/min is more often associated with increased proteinuria on follow-up 10 years later (41). We have not found a clear relationship between UAE and GBM thickness or mesangial expansion on renal biopsy (42). Taken together, one possible interpretation of these studies is that microalbuminuria serves as a marker of nephropathy risk by reflecting glycemic control rather than indicating the severity of underlying glomerular lesions. However, when UAE exceeds 300 μg/min or 400 mg/24 hr, this regularly indicates severe glomerulopathy (42).

Other urinary proteins have been measured in diabetes. Beta-2-microglobulin excretion, a measure of tubular protein reabsorption, is normal at rest and with exercise in newly diagnosed and in longer duration IDDM patients (35, 38). Urinary IgG excretion rates are increased in diabetics with microalbuminuria and in clinically proteinuric diabetics (38). Improved glycemic control with continuous subcutaneous insulin infusion corrects the elevated IgG excretion in IDDM patients with microalbuminuria. In clinically proteinuric subjects, improved glycemic control does not correct urinary albumin or IgG excretion (38).

Myers and co-workers have used the clearances of neutral dextran to study the permselectivity properties of diabetics with proteinuria greater than 1 g/24 hours (43–45). The data from these investigations, subjected to mathematical modeling, suggested that 2 populations of 'pores' are distributed in the glomerular filtration 'barrier'. In IDDM patients with mildly increased urinary IgG excretion the fractional clearance of smaller molecular weight dextrans was diminished compared to normals (43–45). In contrast, the fractional clearance of large molecular weight dextrans (corresponding to the large 'pore' component of the 'membrane') was increased, presumably reflecting the defect resulting in increased urinary IgG excretion. These abnormalities were even greater in those diabetics with more marked urinary IgG excretion. The modeling suggested that the fraction of glomerular filtrate passing through the large 'pores' is greater in the diabetic group with marked proteinuria (45). These studies suggested that, in part, UAE in diabetic patients with overt nephropathy is due to partial loss of the charge selective properties of the glomerular filtration barrier. Viberti has focused attention on the protein selectivity of 3 stages of diabetic proteinuria: (1) diabetics with microalbuminuria less than 60 μg/min where there is increased excretion of both albumin and IgG; (2) diabetics with more than 60 μg/min UAE and normal GFR where there is a selective proteinuria with disproportionate increase in albumin excretion over IgG excretion; and (3) diabetics with declining GFR where selectivity is lost and the heavy proteinuria consists of both massive albumin and IgG excretion (46). The selective proteinuria of the Stage 2 group was interpreted as a charge defect in the glomerular permselectivity barrier while pore size defects were mainly responsible for the marked proteinuria of clinical diabetic nephropathy. Although studies of diabetic rats have not demonstrated a charge selective defect, these animals have only mild proteinuria (47). Three-month untreated and insulin-treated diabetic rats have, in fact, increased restriction to the passage of anionic macromolecules despite increased albumin excretion (47). Thus, the factors responsible for microalbuminuria remain enigmatic. Perhaps, the discrepancies can in part be explained by the recent demonstration of glycosylation of serum albumin in diabetics. This glycosylation results in the formation of cationic albumin subunits which undergo enhanced renal excretion compared to anionic albumin (48).

The structural lesions of diabetic nephropathy are well described and include the Kimmelsteil-Wilson nodular lesion, diffuse mesangial expansion, glomerular (GBM) and tubular (TBM) basement membrane thickening, afferent and efferent glomerular arteriolar hyalinosis, capsular drops, hyaline caps and increased GBM, TBM, and Bowman's capsular localization of albumin and other plasma proteins as detected by immunofluorescence microscopy. The etiology of the abnormal immunofluorescent binding of plasma proteins is unknown, but glycosylation, for example, of albumin or renal basement membranes does not appear to play a role (49). Melvin and co-workers have shown that increased localization of individual plasma proteins to renal extracellular basement membranes is highly dependent on a given protein molecule's inherent electrical charge, hence, the highly negatively charged albumin is heavily localized (50). Although IgG4 is of relatively low concentration in plasma, it is the dominant IgG in renal extracellular membranes in diabetes since this form of IgG is the only one which is negatively charged (50). Thus, one hypothesis which would explain this phenomenon is that there are increased binding sites for negatively charged molecules within renal and other basement membranes in diabetics. Since the binding is firm, releasable only with collagenase or a drastically acidic environment, it is highly unlikely that this feature of human diabetic pathology is an epiphenomenon to increased capillary permeability to protein. It is known from studies of normal kidneys transplanted into diabetic patients that this is an early phenomenon, not necessarily associated with significant glomerular pathology. Further, rodents with diabetes develop GBM thickening and mesangial expansion but do not manifest increased linear renal extracellular basement membrane plasma protein localization. Therefore, it may be that the extracellular protein binding is not an essential contributor to the development of the important lesions of diabetic nephropathy.

The elegant ultrastructural work of Østerby showed that GBM thickening and glomerular mesangial expansion are hallmarks of early diabetic glomerular pathology (51). She demonstrated that both GBM thickness and mesangial area are normal at the onset of Type 1 diabetes but by 2½ years after onset, glomerular changes were discernible and within 5 years after onset these changes were clear cut (51). Soon after induction of diabetes in animals, there is a rapid increase in substrates utilized in the synthesis of glycoprotein and glycosaminoglycans necessary for increase in basement membrane material (52). In-vivo studies of hydroxylation of proline in GBM of diabetic rats have shown a synthesis rate twice normal as early as 9 days after onset of hyperglycemia (53). Glycosyl transferase, which is involved in the synthesis of GBM, is increased in diabetic rats, and this abnormality can be reversed with insulin treatment (54). Further, GBM collagen turnover may be decreased since the calculated turnover rate for labeled hydroxyproline in GBM was 20% less in diabetic rats than in controls (55). Decreased activity of glucosyl-galactosyl-hydroxylysine glucohydrolase, an enzyme involved in basement membrane collagen catabolism, is seen in rats at a glucose concentration seen in diabetics (56). Thus, increased synthesis and decreased degradation are probably both involved in the GBM thickening characteristic of diabetes.

Abnormalities in the constituents of the GBM have been studied. In human diabetes, immunohistopathologic studies have shown a polyantigenic expansion of all of the examined intrinsic components of GBM, TBM, and mesangium in early and moderate stages of nephropathy (57). In late stages there was a decrease in the normal antigenic components in the mesangium and GBM and the presence in these sites of fetal antigens not normally found in adult kidneys (57). Thus, complex polyantigenic alterations accompany the development of nephropathy. In this regard it should be clear that little is likely to be gained from biochemical studies which, for example, examine the amino acid content of diabetic GBM since changes in protein constituents are so complex. In diabetic animals, the metabolism of glycosaminoglycans has been extensively studied. Reduced levels of dermatan sulfate, heparan sulfate, and hyaluronic acid have been found in the renal cortex of diabetic rats (58). Incorporation of $^{35}SO_4$ into glycosaminoglycans in diabetic glomeruli in vivo and in vitro, into diabetic GBM fractions, and into basement membrane producing tumor in diabetic mice is decreased (59–61). It has been speculated that these abnormalities of renal glycosaminoglycan metabolism may alter the negative charge of diabetic nephropathy. However, results of studies of the charge selective properties of the glomerulus in diabetic rats are not consistent with a loss of fixed anionic sites. Less direct human studies confirm this view in that charge related functional defects in the glomerular filter system appear to be a manifestation of far advanced nephropathy and cannot explain the initial proteinuria.

Many compositional studies have emphasized GBM thickening as the central renal lesion in diabetes. In part, this emphasis may be related to the ease of measurement and small interindividual variation of the GBM width and in isolation of GBM for biochemical studies. Parenthetically GBM preparations are now known to be markedly contaminated by mesangial material. We have been unable to demonstrate that the GBM plays a critical role in renal dysfunction in diabetes. In 48 patients with Type 1 diabetes with a mean duration of diabetes of 18.5 ± 6.2 years the width of the GBM was not related to the clinical manifestations of nephropathy, proteinuria, hypertension or reduced creatinine clearance (42). Further GBM width also did not correlate with other glomerular structural measurements including fractional mesangial volume, capillary luminal volume, and relative peripheral capillary filtering surface area (42). Rather, mesangial expansion probably plays an important role in the functional deterioration of glomerulus, since fractional mesangial volume is related to the clinical parameters of nephropathy and is very closely related to the structural parameters of fractional capillary lumenal volume and relative peripheral capillary filtering surface area (42). Thus, we support the observations of Gellman et al. made in 1959 that hypertension, proteinuria, and renal failure correlate with the severity of diffuse glomerulosclerosis (62). It is difficult to understand how expansion of the mesangium could play such a vital role in glomerular functional deterioration unless it is hypothesized that it does so as a consequence of a process of impingement on contiguous structures including the glomerular capillary luminal space and the peripheral capillary filtration surface. It may be that reduction in the functional potential of these latter structures results in compensatory processes which resemble those seen in the remnant kidney model in rats. If this is true, then once significant clinical nephropathy is present, the continued deterioration of renal structure and function may become independent of the diabetic state.

Numerous animal models including rodents, dogs, and primates with both induced and spontaneous diabetes have been used to elucidate the structural renal changes occurring in diabetes (22, 63–67) although differences between animal and human pathology are well known (65). The reversibility of diabetic renal lesions has been extensively studied in animals. When kidneys from highly inbred Lewis rats which were made diabetic 6 months previously were transplanted to non-diabetic rats, the mesangial thickening and immunoglobulin deposition which had been present was markedly improved after 2 months in a normal metabolic environment (68). Similarly, mesangial thickening and immunoglobulin deposition decreased after normoglycemia was established in diabetic rats with pancreatic islet transplantation (69, 70). In addition, pancreatic islet transplantation results in a normalization of glomerular capillary parameters such as the peripheral capillary filtering surface area (69). On the other hand, GBM thickness, which is increased at the time of establishment of normoglycemia, is unaffected by pancreatic islet transplantation (71). Again, urinary albumin excretion which is elevated in the diabetic animals, returns to normal in the animals receiving pancreatic transplantation (37) while GBM thickness is unchanged, which emphasizes the fact that GBM thickening alone cannot explain the abnormal permeability to albumin. More recent studies have shown uninephrectomy which accelerates diabetic lesions (67) prevents the return of mesangial volume to normal with establishment of normoglycemia by pancreatic islet transplantation (64). This supports the idea that the hemodynamic state of the glomerulus affects the rate of development of glomerular lesions and that with advanced glomerulopathy, establishment of normoglycemia may not be able to reverse the structural changes (64). In man, 2 cadaver kidneys showing typical diabetic diffuse nephrosclerosis were transplanted into 2 non-diabetic patients (72). At 7 months post-transplantation, renal biopsy showed reversal of mesangial and basement membrane lesions in 75% of glomeruli studied and the remainder showed minimal residual lesions (72, 73). The report that improved diabetic control normalizes urinary albumin excretion in patients without clinical nephropathy but fails to do so in patients with clinical nephropathy (38) suggests that the functional manifestations of diabetic nephropathy can be influenced only prior to the development of advanced lesions. This supports the concept that the proteinuria of advanced diabetic nephropathology may be independent of the diabetic state and may represent the establishment of new intraglomerular forces analogous to those of the remnant kidney. It is wholly unknown whether glycemic control sufficient to reduce microalbuminuria into the normal range is sufficient to significantly reduce the rate at which diabetic lesions develop.

Management of the diabetic patient with nephropathy

Early treatment

At the present time, clearly established treatment effective in preventing diabetic nephropathy has not been delineated. Meticulous metabolic control of the diabetic state is currently being offered to many patients in the hope that complications, including nephropathy, will be delayed or prevented. Indeed, in animal studies, correction of the diabetic state can reverse renal structural lesions and albuminuria. Whether this is possible in diabetic patients remains uncertain. However, the experience referred to above (17) suggests that this is possible. In patients treated with one year of continuous subcutaneous insulin infusion, despite improved metabolic control retinal findings appeared to deteriorate particularly in those patients with the best glycemic control (74). In two adolescent diabetics the development of overt proteinuria occurred during rapid improvement in glycemic control (75). The long-term meaning of these very preliminary observations is entirely unclear. The degree of renal pathology present at the institution of strict metabolic control may determine the response. In diabetics without overt nephropathy, strict metabolic control with continuous subcutaneous insulin infusion of Ultralente® insulin plus regular insulin resulted in a more normal GFR and decreased urinary albumin excretion (76, 77). On the other hand, in diabetics with overt proteinuria long-term improved metabolic control did not change the rate of decline of renal function (78). Thus, early in the course of the disease before significant deterioration has taken place improvement in glycemic control may potentially delay or reverse the renal lesions. But when overt clinical proteinuria is present, as discussed earlier, no change in rate of deterioration has been demonstrated. At this stage, progression to renal insufficiency appears independent of the diabetic state.

Hypertension, one of the hallmarks of diabetic nephropathy, is usually seen at or shortly after the development of overt persistent proteinuria (79). Essential hypertension may be relatively uncommon in patients without overt nephropathy (79). The management of hypertension in the nephropathic diabetic clearly has a beneficial effect on the progression of renal insufficiency. Effective antihypertensive treatment decreases the rate of decline of GFR (80, 81) and is the most important factor in the management of the overtly proteinuric diabetic.

Recently, two groups have reported a return toward normal of muscle capillary basement membrane width with continuous subcutaneous insulin infusion in insulin dependent diabetics (82) and with glipizide treatment in chemical diabetics (83). Since the relationship between muscle capillary basement membrane width and the important renal structural changes in diabetes – the mesangium and its related parameters, has not been demonstrated, to assume that a decrease in muscle capillary basement membrane width reflects an improvement in other manifestations of microvascular disease in diabetes is premature.

Management of end-stage renal disease in the diabetic

In the past, uremic diabetic patients were considered at high risk for the advanced technologies of dialysis and transplantation, primarily due to multiple organ system involvement and because initial results with dialysis and transplantation were disappointing. Recently, significant improvements in the survival and rehabilitation of diabetic patients undergoing hemodialysis make this a reasonable therapy in end-stage renal disease (84–86). Continuous ambulatory peritoneal dialysis with intraperitoneal administration of insulin provides another realistic option for the treatment of end stage renal disease even in the blind diabetic (87). Despite these good results with dialysis, a functioning renal transplant offers a degree of rehabilitation not easily obtainable with dialysis. Further, renal transplantation in diabetics need not be of higher risk than in non-diabetics with patient and graft survival reported as high as 88 and 82%, respectively, at 2 years, including all donor sources (88–91) and 100% 2-year patient and graft survival in HLA-identical sibling transplants (88). Thus, tremendous strides have been made in therapy for the uremic diabetic, and dialysis and transplantation should be considered as realistic options.

References

1. Knowles HC Jr, Guest GM, Lampe J, Kessler M, Skillman TG (1965): The course of juvenile diabetes treated with unmeasured diet. *Diabetes, 14*, 239.
2. Deckert T, Poulsen J, Larsen M (1976): Prognosis in juvenile diabetes mellitus. *Acta Endocrinol. (Copenhagen), 203, Suppl. 82*, 15.
3. Andersen AF, Sandahl-Christiansen J, Anderson JK, Kreiner S, Deckert T (1983): Diabetic nephropathy in type I (insulin-dependent) diabetes: An epidemiological study. *Diabetologia, 25*, 496.
4. Fabre J, Balant LP, Dayer PG, Fox HM, Vernet AT (1982): The kidney in maturity onset diabetes mellitus: A clinical study of 510 patients. *Kidney Int., 21*, 730.
5. Rao TKS, Hirsch S, Avram MM, Friedman EA (1980): Prevalence of diabetic nephropathy in Brooklyn. In: *Diabetic Renal-Retinal Syndrome*, p 205. Editors: E.A. Friedman and F.A. L'Esperance Jr. Grune and Stratton, New York.
6. Moloney A, Tunbridge WMG, Ireland JT, Watkins PJ (1983): Mortality from diabetic nephropathy in the United Kingdom. *Diabetologia, 25*, 26.
7. Mogensen CE, Andersen MJF (1973): Increased kidney size and glomerular filtration rate in early juvenile diabetes. *Diabetes, 22*, 706.

8. Mogensen CE, Andersen MJF (1975): Increased kidney size and glomerular filtration rate in untreated juvenile diabetes: Normalization by insulin-treatment. *Diabetologia, 11*, 221.
9. Christiansen JS, Gammelgaard J, Tronier B, Svendsen PA, Parving HH (1982): Kidney function and size in diabetics before and during initial insulin treatment. *Kidney Int., 21*, 683.
10. Puig JG, Anton FM, Grande C, Pallardo LF, Arnalich F, Gil A, Vazquez JJ, Garcia AM (1981): Relation of kidney size to kidney function in early insulin-dependent diabetes. *Diabetologia, 21*, 363.
11. Christiansen JS, Gammelgaard J, Frandsen M, Parving HH (1981): Increased kidney size, glomerular filtration rate and renal plasma flow in short-term insulin-dependent diabetes. *Diabetologia, 20*, 451.
12. Wiseman M, Viberti GC (1983): Kidney size and glomerular filtration rate in type I (insulin-dependent) diabetes mellitus revisited. *Diabetologia, 25*, 530.
13. Ellis EN, Steffes MW, Goetz FC, Sutherland DER, Mauer SM (1984): Relationship of renal size to nephropathy in insulin dependent diabetes mellitus. Submitted for publication.
14. Seyer-Hansen K (1976): Renal hypertrophy in streptozotocin diabetic rats. *Clin. Sci. Mol. Med., 51*, 551.
15. Seyer-Hansen K, Hansen J, Gundersen HJG (1980): Renal hypertrophy in experimental diabetes. *Diabetologia, 18*, 501.
16. Seyer-Hansen K (1983): Renal hypertrophy in experimental diabetes mellitus. *Kidney Int., 23*, 643.
17. Kroustrup JP, Gundersen HJG, Osterby R (1977): Glomerular size and structure in diabetes mellitus. III. Early enlargement of the capillary surface. *Diabetologia, 13*, 207.
18. Mogensen CE, Osterby R, Gundersen HJG (1979): Early functional and morphologic vascular renal consequences of the diabetic state. *Diabetologia, 17*, 71.
19. Romen W, Takahashi A (1982): Autoradiographic studies on the proliferation of glomerular and tubular cells of the rat kidney in early diabetes. *Virchows Arch. B, 40*, 339.
20. Rasch R, Rytter Norgaard JO (1983): Renal enlargement: Comparative autoradiographic studies of ^{3}H-thymidine uptake in diabetic and uninephrectomized rats. *Diabetologia, 25*, 280.
21. Broulik PD, Schreiber J (1982): Effect of alloxan diabetes on kidney grown in intact and castrated mice. *Acta Endocrinol. (Copenhagen), 99*, 109.
22. Brown DM, Steffes MW, Thibert P, Azar SM, Mauer SM (1983): Glomerular manifestations of diabetes in the BB rat. *Metabolism, 32*, 131.
23. Rasch R (1979): Prevention of diabetic glomerulopathy in streptozotocin diabetic rats by insulin treatment. Kidney size and glomerular volume. *Diabetologia, 16*, 125.
24. Christiansen JS (1984): *On the Pathogenesis of the Increased Glomerular Filtration Rate in Short-Term Insulin-Dependent Diabetes*. Thesis, University of Copenhagen.
25. Hostetter TH, Troy JL, Brenner BM (1981): Glomerular hemodynamics in experimental diabetes mellitus. *Kidney Int., 19*, 410.

26. Mogensen CE, Christensen CK, Vittinghus E (1983): The stages of diabetic renal disease with emphasis on the stage of incipient diabetic nephropathy. *Diabetes*, *32*, *Suppl. 2*, 64.
27. Brochner-Mortensen J, Ditzel J (1982): Glomerular filtration rate and extracellular fluid volume in insulin-dependent patients with diabetes mellitus. *Kidney Int.*, *21*, 696.
28. Christiansen JS, Frandsen M, Parving HH (1981): Effects of intravenous glucose infusion on renal function in normal man and in insulin-dependent diabetics. *Diabetologia*, *21*, 368.
29. Ditzel J, Brochner-Mortensen J (1983): Tubular reabsorption rates as related to elevated glomerular filtration in diabetic children. *Diabetes, 32, Suppl. 2*, 28.
30. Ditzel J, Brochner-Mortensen J (1983): Renal glomerular and tubular dysfunction in short-term insulin-dependent diabetic subjects. *Aktuel. Endokrinol. Stoffwechsel*, *4*, 16.
31. Levy M (1975): The effect of glucagon on glomerular filtration rate in dogs during reduction of renal blood flow. *Can. J. Physiol. Pharmacol.*, *53*, 660.
32. Parving HH, Noer I, Kehlet H, Mogensen CE, Svendsen PA, Heding LG (1977): The effects of short-term glucagon on kidney function in normal man. *Diabetologia*, *13*, 323.
33. Parving HH, Christiansen JS, Noer I, Tronier B, Mogensen CE (1980): The effects of glucagon infusion on kidney function in short-term insulin-dependent juvenile diabetics. *Diabetologia*, *19*, 350.
34. Christiansen JS, Gammelgaard J, Frandsen M, Orskov H, Parving HH (1982): Kidney function and size in type I (insulin-dependent) diabetic patients before and during growth hormone administration for one week. *Diabetologia*, *22*, 333.
35. Vittinghus E, Mogensen CE (1982): Graded exercise and protein excretion in diabetic man and the effect of insulin treatment. *Kidney Int.*, *21*, 725.
36. Pennell JP, Meinking TL (1982): Pattern of urinary proteins in experimental diabetes. *Kidney Int.*, *21*, 709.
37. Mauer SM, Brown DM, Matas AJ, Steffes MW (1978): Effects of pancreatic islet transplantation in the increased urinary albumin excretion rates in intact and uninephrectomized rats with diabetes mellitus. *Diabetes*, *27*, 959.
38. Viberti GC, Mackintosh D, Bilous RW, Pickup JC, Keen H (1982): Proteinuria in diabetes mellitus: Role of spontaneous and experimental variation in glycemia. *Kidney Int.*, *21*, 714.
39. Viberti GC, Jarrett RJ, Mahmud U, Hill RD, Argyropoulos A, Keen H (1982): Microalbuminuria as a predictor of clinical nephropathy in insulin-dependent diabetes mellitus. *Lancet*, *1*, 1430.
40. Parving HH, Oxenboll B, Svendsen PA, Christiansen JS, Andersen AR (1982): Early detection of patients at risk of developing diabetic nephropathy. A longitudinal study of urinary albumin excretion. *Acta Endocrinol. (Copenhagen)*, *100*, 550.
41. Mogensen CE (1984): Microalbuminuria predicts clinical proteinuria and early mortality in maturity-onset diabetes. *N. Engl. J. Med.*, *310*, 356.
42. Mauer SM, Steffes MW, Ellis EN, Sutherland DER, Brown DM, Goetz FC

(1984): Structural-functional relationships in diabetic nephropathy. *J. Clin. Invest., 74*, 1143.
43. Myers BD, Winetz JA, Chui F, Michaels AS (1982): Mechanisms of proteinuria in diabetic nephropathy: A study of glomerular barrier function. *Kidney Int., 21*, 633.
44. Winetz JA, Golbetz HV, Spencer RJ, Lee JA, Myers BD (1982): Glomerular function in advanced human diabetic nephropathy. *Kidney Int., 21*, 750.
45. Friedman S, Jones HW, Golbetz HV, Lee JA, Little HL, Myers BD (1983): Mechanisms of proteinuria in diabetic nephropathy II: A study of size selective glomerular filtration barrier. *Diabetes, 32, Suppl. 2*, 40.
46. Viberti GC, Mackintosh D, Keen H (1983): Determinants of the penetration of proteins through the glomerular barrier in insulin-dependent diabetes mellitus. *Diabetes, 32, Suppl. 2*, 92.
47. Michaels LD, Davidman M, Keane WF (1982): Glomerular permeability to neutral and anionic dextrans in experimental diabetes. *Kidney Int., 21*, 699.
48. Ghiggeri GM, Candiano G, Delfino G, Bianchini F, Queirolo C (1984): Glycosyl albumin and diabetic microalbuminuria: Demonstration of an altered renal handling. *Kidney Int., 25*, 565.
49. Jeraj KP, Michael AF, Mauer SM, Brown DM (1983): Glucosylated and normal human or rat albumin do not bind to renal basement membranes of diabetic and control rats. *Diabetes, 32*, 380.
50. Melvin T, Kim Y, Michael AF (1984): Selective binding of IgG4 and other negatively charged plasma proteins in normal and diabetic human kidneys. *Am. J. Pathol., 115*, 143.
51. Østerby R (1975): Early phases in the development of diabetic glomerulopathy. *Acta Med. Scand., Suppl., 574*, 14.
52. Cortes P, Dumler F, Sastry KSS, Verghese CP, Levin NW (1982): Effects of early diabetes on uridine diphosphosugar synthesis in the rat renal cortex. *Kidney Int., 21*, 676.
53. Brownlee M, Spiro RG (1979): Glomerular basement membrane metabolism in the diabetic rat. *Diabetes, 28*, 121.
54. Spiro RG, Spiro MJ (1971): Effect of diabetes of the biosynthesis of the renal glomerular basement membrane. Studies on the glucosyltransferase. *Diabetes, 20*, 641.
55. Romen W, Lange HW, Hempel K, Heck TH (1981): Studies on collagen metabolism in rats. II. Turnover and amino acid composition of the collagen of glomerular basement membrane in diabetes mellitus. *Virchows Arch. B, 36*, 313.
56. Sternberg M, Andre J, Peyroux J (1983): Inhibition of the alpha-glucosidase specific for collagen disaccharide units in diabetic rat kidney by in vivo glucose levels: Possible contribution to basement membrane thickening. *Diabetologia, 24*, 286.
57. Falk RJ, Scheinman JI, Mauer SM, Michael AF (1983): Polyantigenic expansion of basement membrane constituents in diabetic nephropathy. *Diabetes, 32*, 34.
58. Saraswathi S, Vasan NS (1983): Alterations in the rat renal glycosaminoglycans in streptozotocin-induced diabetes. *Biochim. Biophys. Acta, 755*, 237.

59. Brown DM, Klein DJ, Michael AF, Oegema TR (1982): 35S-glycosaminoglycan and 35S-glycopeptide metabolism by diabetic glomeruli and aorta. *Diabetes*, *31*, 418.
60. Cohen MP, Surma ML (1984): Effect of diabetes on in vivo metabolism of (35S)-labeled glomerular basement membrane. *Diabetes*, *33*, 8.
61. Rohrbach DH, Hassell JR, Kleinman HK, Martin GR (1982): Alterations in the basement membrane (heparan sulfate) proteoglycan in diabetic mice. *Diabetes*, *31*, 185.
62. Gellman DD, Pirani CL, Soothill JF, Muehrcke RF, Maduros W, Kark RM (1959): Structure and function in diabetic nephropathy. The importance of diffuse glomerulosclerosis. *Diabetes*, *8*, 251.
63. Rodrigues M, Currier C, Yoon J (1983): Electron microscopy of renal and ocular changes in virus-induced diabetes mellitus in mice. *Diabetologia*, *24*, 293.
64. Steffes MW, Vernier RL, Brown DM, Basgen JM, Mauer SM (1982): Diabetic glomerulopathy in the uninephrectomized rat resists amelioration following islet transplantation. *Diabetologia*, *23*, 347.
65. Hirose K, Osterby R, Nozawa M, Gundersen HJ (1982): Development of glomerular lesions in experimental long-term diabetes in the rat. *Kidney Int.*, *21*, 689.
66. Steffes MW, Buchwald H, Wigness BD, Groppoli TJ, Rupp WM, Rohde TD, Blackshear PJ, Mauer SM (1982): Diabetic nephropathy in the uninephrectomized dog: Microscopic lesions after one year. *Kidney Int.*, *21*, 721.
67. Steffes MW, Brown DM, Mauer SM (1978): Diabetic glomerulopathy following unilateral nephrectomy in the rat. *Diabetes*, *27*, 35.
68. Lee CS, Mauer SM, Brown DM, Sutherland DER, Michael AF, Najarian JS (1974): Renal transplantation in diabetes mellitus in rats. *J. Exp. Med.*, *139*, 793.
69. Steffes MW, Brown DM, Basgen JM, Mauer SM (1980): Amelioration of mesangial volume and surface alterations following islet transplantation in diabetic rats. *Diabetes*, *29*, 509.
70. Mauer SM, Sutherland DER, Steffes MW, Leonard RJ, Najarian JS, Michael AF, Brown DM (1974): Pancreatic islet transplantation: Effects on the glomerular lesions of experimental diabetes in the rat. *Diabetes*, *23*, 748.
71. Steffes MW, Brown DM, Basgen JM, Matas AJ, Mauer SM (1979): Glomerular basement membrane thickness following islet transplantation in the rat. *Lab. Invest.*, *41*, 116.
72. Abouna GM, Al-Advani MS (1983): Reversibility of diabetic nephropathy after transplantation of affected kidney. *Lancet*, *2*, 1274.
73. Pyke DA, Watkins PJ (1984): Reversibility of diabetic nephropathy after transplantation of affected kidney. *Lancet*, *1*, 163.
74. Lauritzen T, Larsen HW, Frost-Larsen K, Deckert T (1983): Effect of 1 year of near-normal blood glucose levels on retinopathy in insulin-dependent diabetics. *Lancet*, *1*, 200.
75. Ellis D, Avner ED, Transue D, Yunis EJ, Drash AL, Becker DJ (1983): Diabetic nephropathy in adolescence: Appearance during improved glycemic control. *Pediatrics*, *71*, 824.

76. Steno Study Group (1982): Effect of 6 months of strict metabolic control on eye and kidney function in insulin-dependent diabetics with background retinopathy. *Lancet*, *1*, 121.
77. Holman RR, Mayon-White V, Orde-Peckar C, Steemson J, Smith B, McPherson K, Rizza C, Knight AH, Dornan TL, Howard-Williams J, Jenkins L, Rolfe R, Barbour D, Poon P, Mann JI, Bron AJ, Turner RC (1983): Prevention of deterioration of renal and sensory-nerve function by more intensive management of insulin-dependent diabetic patients. *Lancet*, *1*, 204.
78. Viberti GC, Bilous RW, Mackintosh D, Bending JJ, Keen H (1983): Long-term correction of hyperglycaemia and progression of renal failure in insulin dependent diabetes. *Br. Med. J.*, *286*, 598.
79. Parving HH, Andersen AR, Smidt UM, Oxenboll B, Edsberg B, Christiansen JS (1983): Diabetic nephropathy and arterial hypertension. *Diabetologia*, *24*, 10.
80. Parving HH, Smidt, UM, Andersen AR, Svendsen PA (1983): Early agressive antihypertensive treatment reduces rate of decline in kidney function in diabetic nephropathy. *Lancet*, *1*, 1175.
81. Mogensen CE (1982): Long-term antihypertensive treatment inhibiting progression of diabetic nephropathy. *Br. Med. J.*, *285*, 685.
82. Raskin P, Pietri AO, Unger R, Shannon WA Jr (1983): The effect of diabetic control on the width of skeletal-muscle capillary basement membrane in patients with type I diabetes mellitus. *N. Engl. J. Med.*, *309*, 1546.
83. Camerini-Davalos RA, Velasco C, Glasser M, Bloodworth JMB (1983): Drug-induced reversal of early diabetic microangiopathy. *N. Engl. J. Med.*, *309*, 1551.
84. Comty C, Kjellsen D, Shapiro F (1976): A reassessment of the prognosis of diabetic patients treated by chronic hemodialysis. *Trans. Am. Soc. Artif. Intern. Organs*, *22*, 404.
85. Ma K, Masler D, Brown D (1975): Hemodialysis in diabetic patients with chronic renal failure. *Ann. Intern. Med.*, *83*, 215.
86. Totten M, Izenstein B, Gleason R, Takacs F, Libertino J, D'elia J (1978): Chronic renal failure in diabetes: Survival with hemodialysis vs. transplantation. *J. Dialysis*, *2*, 17.
87. Amair P, Khanna R, Leibel B, Pierratos A, Vas S, Meema E, Blair G, Chisolm L, Vas M, Zingg W, Digenis G, Oreopoulos D (1982): Continuous ambulatory peritoneal dialysis in diabetics with end-stage renal disease. *N. Engl. J. Med.*, *306*, 625.
88. Sutherland DER, Morrow CE, Fryd DS, Ferguson R, Simmons RL, Najarian JS (1982): Improved patient and primary renal allograft survival in uremic diabetic recipients. *Transplantation*, *34*, 319.
89. Khauli RB, Novick AC, Braun WE, Steinmuller D, Buezta C, Goormastic M (1983): Improved results of cadaver renal transplantation in the diabetic patient. *J. Urol.*, *130*, 867.
90. Oktye SE, Engen DE, Sterioff SS, Frohnect PP, Johnson WJ, Offord KP, Zincke H (1983): Primary and secondary renal transplantation in diabetic patients. *J. Am. Med. Assoc.*, *249*, 492.
91. Larsson O, Attman PO, Blohme I, Bryngerlt (1982): Transplantation in patients with diabetic nephropathy: A 10-year experience. *Trans. Proc.*, *14*, 30.

The Diabetes Annual/1
K.G.M.M. Alberti and L.P. Krall, editors

ISBN 0444 90 343 7
$0.85 per article per page (transactional system)
$0.20 per article per page (licensing system)

18 Diabetic macroangiopathy

ALAN CHAIT, EDWIN L. BIERMAN AND JOHN D. BRUNZELL

Macrovascular complications of diabetes mellitus remain the major cause of morbidity and mortality in diabetes today. Because of the alarming frequency of macrovascular complications in all types of diabetics in most industrialized populations throughout the world, and the high likelihood of an individual diabetic succumbing to the consequences of arterial disease, recent attention has focused on the pathogenetic mechanisms of atherosclerosis in the diabetic.

The focus of research over the past several years appears to be shifting from epidemiological studies to basic investigation of the cell biology of atherosclerosis. Population studies have provided important insights and clues as to potential pathogenetic mechanisms. This has resulted in studies that have evaluated the interaction between circulating humoral and cellular elements with cells of the arterial wall. An understanding of the interaction of extrinsic factors, such as lipoproteins and platelets, with intrinsic factors such as smooth muscle cells and macrophages in the artery wall, is likely to provide important insights into the pathogenesis and prevention of atherosclerosis in the diabetic.

Progress in understanding the relationship between diabetes and its macrovascular complications has been impeded for several reasons. First, conclusions from epidemiological studies have in some instances been unclear: the several types of diabetics have often been studied as a single group and relatively little attention has been given to the mode of therapy. Second, the inability to detect subclinical atherosclerosis compounds the issue. Third, certain key measurements, such as of plasma lipoproteins and platelet function, are difficult to perform in large epidemiological studies. Fourth, even careful evaluation of such measurements in small groups of well characterized diabetics also can be limited, since these studies must be restricted to blood and a few other accessible tissues. The arterial wall obviously is inaccessible for routine study. Thus, studies in human diabetes have tended to focus on circulating factors that may be important in atherogenesis, but which often are indirect, e.g. endothelial cell products, platelet release products and lipoproteins. Most studies neglect the interaction of these circulating factors with the arterial wall. Fifth, the tissue culture studies that evaluate these interactions suffer from the difficulty of extrapolation of findings to the patient. Finally, animal studies have their problems as well, since a major difficulty is the lack of ideal models of either human diabetes or atherosclerosis.

Despite these difficulties, information gained from all these approaches appears to be culminating in greater understanding of atherogenesis in general and in the diabetic in particular. Epidemiological studies published during the past several years have provided powerful confirmatory evidence of the importance of certain atherosclerotic risk factors in diabetes. Advances in the prevention of atherosclerosis in non-diabetics provide encouragement that similar results can be achieved in diabetics as well. Perhaps most encouraging is the emergence of consensus about multiple potentially important pathogenetic mechanisms related to the diabetes–atherosclerosis connection.

This chapter will outline some of the recent epidemiological findings. It will discuss the emerging knowledge of the understanding of the cell biology of atherosclerosis and will summarize some of the recent studies regarding several of these pathogenetic mechanisms of atherosclerosis in the diabetic.

EPIDEMIOLOGICAL STUDIES

Perhaps the most important recent information derives from the publication of a number of previously unexplored relationships between cardiovascular risk factors and vascular disease in diabetes from the 14-nation WHO study (1), which evaluated coronary artery disease (CAD), peripheral vascular disease (PVD) and cerebrovascular disease in diverse populations of diabetics of different ethnic origin living in a variety of environments.

Macrovascular disease is not inevitable in diabetes

The very marked differences in frequency of vascular complications in the WHO study strongly implies that macrovascular disease need not inevitably accompany diabetes, a conclusion already reached from studies of Asian diabetic subjects. When Asian diabetics change their environment (e.g. from Japan to Hawaii) (2), their low CAD incidence increases in conjunction with change in diet and lifestyle, emphasizing the important interaction of diabetes with genetic and environmental factors in the pathogenesis of atherosclerosis. These observations provide a ray of hope that atherosclerosis in the diabetic may be prevented by definition and correction of atherogenic environmental factors.

Plasma lipids and lipoproteins

The WHO multinational study strongly confirmed that plasma lipids are important risk factors for atherosclerosis in the diabetic. Hypertriglyceridemia, which is due to increased plasma levels of very low-density lipoprotein (VLDL), occurs frequently amongst diabetics of all types (see Chapter 26). Two earlier studies strongly suggest that hypertriglyceridemic diabetics have more CAD than do normotriglyceridemic diabetics (3, 4). In the WHO study, plasma triglycerides showed a strong correlation with CAD independent of other risk factors. Further, the ranking of mean triglyceride values in the populations studied coincided with the ranking of CAD rates. Elevated plasma triglyceride levels did not appear to increase the risk of either PVD or cerebrovascular disease.

Plasma cholesterol levels in the WHO study were associated with CAD, but less strongly than were plasma triglycerides. Inclusion of triglycerides in the multivariate analysis rendered the apparent correlation between cholesterol and CAD insignificant in patients with non-insulin-dependent diabetes mellitus (NIDDM). It is possible that the correlation of cholesterol and CAD in diabetics, especially those with NIDDM, reflects elevated plasma levels of VLDL, since the cholesterol component of VLDL can influence the total plasma cholesterol level. Reduced high density lipoprotein (HDL) cholesterol has been shown to be a powerful predictor of atherosclerosis in the diabetic (5), but no recent studies have expanded upon this relationship. The more detailed relationship between plasma lipids, lipoproteins and diabetes and the potentially beneficial role of improved glycemic control and dietary factors on plasma lipids and lipoproteins is more fully discussed in Chapter 26.

Hyperinsulinemia

Three recent prospective studies have shown an independent predictive relationship between plasma insulin levels, both fasting and after stimulation, and the development of CAD in the general population (6–8). These results support the hypothesis that hyperinsulinemia promotes atherogenesis (9). In the Helsinki study, the effect of insulin clearly was independent of either glucose levels or obesity (6). Since both NIDDM, by virtue of peripheral insulin resistance, and IDDM, by virtue of intermittent high peripheral insulin levels following absorption of injected insulin, are characterized by at least intermittent hyperinsulinemia, potential mechanisms by which insulin can promote atherogenesis should be elucidated.

Other risk factors

Risk factors associated with atherosclerosis in the non-diabetic subject appear to have a similar relation to CAD among diabetics (10). In a recent population-based study, both diabetics and non-diabetics with a single cardiovascular risk factor (high serum cholesterol, high serum triglycerides, hypertension, obesity or cigarette smoking) were likely to have other risk factors in addition (11). Clustering of risk factors was more marked in diabetics than in non-diabetics, and was more marked in females than males. These observations may help explain the increased cardiovascular risk of diabetics over non-diabetics and also the relative lack of protection in females with diabetes.

Site of the macrovascular disease

Although the pathology of CAD, PVD and cerebrovascular disease appears to be the same, marked differences in risk factor associations occur at these different sites. This was again clearly demonstrated by the WHO multinational study (1) in which CAD was most strongly related to plasma lipid levels and was unrelated to the duration of diabetes or to fasting plasma glucose levels. Conversely, both PVD and cerebrovascular disease were strongly related to duration of diabetes and to the plasma glucose levels, but not to plasma triglycerides. A smaller study also demonstrated an association between PVD and diabetes duration, but smoking appeared to be the major determinant of PVD in this study (12). Hypertriglyceridemia and reduced levels of HDL also were associated with PVD (13). In the WHO study, amputation was more common in insulin-treated cases, but the duration of diabetes also was longer in this group of patients. Since other recent studies concerning the relationship between insulin treatment and PVD in diabetes were retrospective (12, 14), no firm conclusions can be drawn.

In the WHO study (1), hypertension was associated with both CAD and cerebrovascular disease. A relationship between cerebrovascular disease and serum cholesterol also was observed. This observation is supported by a smaller study in the USA, in which serum cholesterol was associated with occlusive carotid artery disease (15).

Insulin dependent vs non-insulin dependent diabetes mellitus

Interpretation of many epidemiological studies is hampered by inadequate separation of insulin dependent diabetes mellitus (IDDM) from NIDDM and lack of standardization of diagnostic criteria. While the final report of the University Group Diabetes Program (16) emphasizes the low morbidity and mortality from CAD in NIDDM, many of the subjects studied would not be classified as diabetic by today's criteria. Another study suggests that the type of diabetes is of little importance in relation to the frequency of occlusive carotid artery disease (15). Thus far there is little evidence that the frequency of atherosclerotic sequela differs between IDDM and NIDDM.

Sex differences in atherosclerotic complications

The WHO trial also re-emphasized the well-documented observation that despite major variations in arterial disease between different populations, the cardiovascular disease risk for diabetic women equalled that for diabetic men (1). This loss of protection against CAD in diabetic women pertains to all age groups and occurs with both IDDM and NIDDM. It also was seen in the Pittsburgh IDDM prospective morbidity and mortality study (17), in which cardiovascular mortality was a significant cause of death among older diabetic patients in this study. Mortality rates for male and female diabetics were 11 and 16 times greater than for non-diabetics.

Age vs duration of diabetes

Since development of arteriosclerotic lesions precedes the first clinical episode by many years, macrovascular complication rates might be expected to relate to the duration of diabetes. Yet several recent studies again have failed to demonstrate a relationship between CAD mortality and diabetes duration (1, 17, 18). Despite the lack of association between CAD mortality and diabetes duration in the WHO study, it is of interest that both stroke and amputation did relate to diabetes duration. This lack of correlation between CAD and diabetes duration appears to pertain mainly to NIDDM. Jarrett (19) recently has used this lack of correlation in suggesting that predisposition towards CAD might be a risk factor for the development of diabetes, rather than the converse as is usually assumed. However, he neglects the fact that it is impossible to determine the onset of NIDDM with any degree of certainty. Also, since onset and the gradual development of atherosclerosis may have antedated the onset of NIDDM by many years, lack of a relationship between diabetes duration and atherosclerosis is perhaps not surprising in NIDDM. Jarrett also points out that subjects with impaired glucose tolerance but not diabetes have an increased risk of cardiovascular disease relative to non-diabetics. Thus, he claims that it is conceivable that NIDDM and atherosclerosis share a number of antecedent metabolic risk factors, possibly on a genetic basis (20), which predisposes the individual to either diabetes, atherosclerosis or both of these clinical outcomes. This is supported by the recent finding that specific DNA fragments that flank the insulin gene occur with increased frequency both in NIDDM and in non-diabetics with atherosclerotic complications (21). While Jarrett provides no direct evidence to support his hypothesis, this intriguing concept emphasizes some of the as yet unexplained inconsistencies in the epidemiology of atherosclerosis in the non-insulin dependent diabetic.

BASIC MECHANISMS OF ATHEROGENESIS

Before consideration of the several areas in which diabetes and factors associated with the diabetic state could potentially play a role in atherogenesis, recent developments in the understanding of the cell biology of atherosclerosis will be reviewed. The three major features of atherosclerosis, i.e. (a) lipid accumulation, (b) cellular accumulation within the arterial intima (smooth muscle cell proliferation and macrophage recruitment), and (b) connective tissue deposition, all may be influenced by the interaction of circulating cellular and humoral factors with the cells of the artery wall. Although morphological and biochemical studies of lesions have provided insight into the cellular pathology of atherosclerosis, the recent use of careful longitudinal studies of the artery wall in suitable animal models has provided important new information about the time sequence of events (22, 23). In-vitro studies using cultured endothelial cells, macrophages and arterial smooth muscle cells have provided new and important insight into the cell biology of the artery wall and potential mechanisms of atherosclerosis. The subject has been reviewed recently (24) and is an extension of the reaction to injury hypothesis expounded by Ross and Glomset (25) nearly a decade ago.

Endothelial injury, whether initiated by hyperlipidemia, hypertension, diabetes mellitus or other injurious agents, is now believed to be associated with adherence of circulating monocytes to the endothelial surface. These monocytes then migrate across an intact endothelial barrier, possibly in response to chemotactic factors. The monocytes in the artery wall accumulate lipid and become lipid laden foam cells in the subendothelial space. Smooth muscle cells then migrate from the media to the intima, where they begin to proliferate, possibly in response to mitogens secreted by the macrophages. Loss of endothelial integrity might then occur, followed by the adherence of platelets to the exposed subendothelial connective tissue and macrophages. This is accompanied by the release of a powerful mitogen from platelets, the platelet-derived growth factor (PDGF). PDGF is a smooth muscle cell chemotactin, which stimulates further migration of smooth muscle cells into the arterial intima. PDGF also stimulates smooth muscle cell proliferation leading to intimal thickening. Uptake of low density lipoprotein (LDL) by smooth muscle cells via both receptor and non-receptor mediated pathways also is stimulated by PDGF and by secretory products of the macrophages themselves. Accumulation of lipid by macrophages probably occurs by a different mechanism. LDL that has been modified chemically or biologically can be taken up by distinct 'scavenger' receptors on macrophages and results in cholesteryl ester accumulation. Both endothelial cells and arterial smooth muscle cells can modify LDL such that they are taken up by the macrophage 'scavenger' receptors. In addition, interaction of lipoproteins with connective tissue elements in the interstitial space could lead to enhanced lipoprotein uptake by macrophages. Smooth muscle cells can secrete collagen, proteoglycans and other connective tissue elements, which may play a role in the fibrosis seen in atherosclerotic plaques.

Many of these events are reversible. They probably all represent normal defense mechanisms by the host against arterial injury. Thus it is entirely conceivable that repair can occur; for example, endothelial breaks can be repaired, lipid that has accumulated can be removed and cell proliferation can cease and regress. The net result may be some residual arterial thickening or scarring. However, if the injurious insult is of a repetitive or constant nature, the process becomes progressive, until occlusion, thrombosis or embolism result in clinical manifestations of the atherosclerosis.

Several of the metabolic disturbances and cellular dysfunctions that occur in the diabetic state have now been studied with particular relevance to their interaction with the arterial cellular elements that are important in atherosclerosis. The circulating humoral and cellular factors that have been most extensively studied include platelets, monocytes, lipoproteins, glucose and insulin. The main arterial wall cells that are receiving attention are endothelial cells, arterial smooth muscle cells and macrophages. Despite the use of widely different in vivo and in vitro techniques, the study of different forms of human diabetes and the use of different models of experimental diabetes, consensus appears to be emerging on a number of fronts. Several of these will now be evaluated in turn, with particular relevance to studies published during the past 2 years.

MECHANISMS OF ATHEROSCLEROSIS IN DIABETES MELLITUS

Monocytes

The adherence of monocytes to the intact arterial endothelium is an early and important event in atherosclerosis. Monocyte adherence would likely precede the attraction of monocytes into the arterial intima, presumably in response to a chemotactic gradient. Yet very little is known about the processes of monocyte adherence and chemotaxis in diabetes.

Monocyte adherence

A major deficiency in our knowledge of monocyte function in general and in diabetes in particular relates to the adhesive properties of this important cell. Recent studies in patients who are unable to form pus in response to infections have revealed that a specific protein on the cell surface of neutrophils and monocytes is responsible for their adhesion and spreading both to foreign surfaces and to endothelial monolayers (26). Unfortunately, no studies to date have reported on the effect of diabetes on monocyte adherence. It is entirely conceivable that this process could be deranged in diabetes, either due to alteration of monocyte function or to changes in the endothelium which cause it to be a better surface for adherence than is normal endothelium. A recent study demonstrated increased adherence of erythrocytes from diabetic patients to cultured human umbilical vein endothelial cells (27). When surfaces other than endothelial cells were tested, diabetic erythrocyte still exhibited greater adherence than did non-diabetic cells, thus suggesting an intrinsic abnormality in diabetic cells that resulted in increased cell adherence. Although the proteins responsible for adherence of neutrophils and monocytes do not appear to be present on the surface of red blood cells, it is conceivable that the adhesive properties of monocytes could be altered in diabetes in a manner similar to that reported for erythrocytes. This potentially important area of monocyte/endothelial cell interaction clearly requires additional attention.

Monocyte chemotaxis

After adherence of monocytes to the arterial endothelium, directed migration into the arterial wall intima is believed to occur along a chemical gradient created by chemotactic factors. Both cultured human monocyte-derived macrophages and arterial smooth muscle cells can secrete factors that are chemotactic for human monocytes (28).

Several early studies showed that polymorphonuclear leukocyte chemotaxis was reduced in diabetics (29–32), whether insulin- or non insulin-dependent. Incubation in vitro of leukocytes from insulin-dependent diabetics with insulin resulted in correction of the impaired chemotactic responsiveness (31).

Of two more recent studies of monocyte chemotaxis in diabetes, one appears to support the findings observed in neutrophils, while the other does not. Hill et al. (33) found that both directed and random mobility of monocytes from a mixed group of insulin- and non-insulin-dependent diabetics were lower in the diabetics than in a control group. Unlike their earlier studies using polymorphonuclear leukocytes (31) insulin added to diabetic cells failed to correct the defect in chemotaxis. However, it was corrected by the use of antioxidants both in vitro and in vivo. The in vitro addition of scavengers of superoxide anion and of hydrogen peroxide, or the administration of the antioxidant, vitamin E, to diabetic patients, reversed these defects in monocyte chemotaxis. These findings raise the interesting speculation that these defects in cellular function might have resulted from autooxidative membrane damage consequent to the diabetes. Thus, consideration of lipid peroxidation in diabetes is important (see the section on oxidative metabolism).

In contrast, in a smaller group of mixed insulin-dependent and non-insulin-dependent subjects, Geisler et al. (34) demonstrated that the chemotaxis of monocytes towards casein was increased in diabetics relative to controls. They were unable to find differences in the chemotactic activity of sera from their diabetics and controls, and concluded that an intrinsic abnormality of the diabetic monocytes was responsible for the enhanced chemotaxis observed. The reason for the difference between these two studies is not apparent, and clearly, further studies of monocyte chemotaxis in diabetes are warranted.

Oxidative metabolism

Neutrophil or monocyte activation is accompanied by a burst of oxidative metabolism, which generates several highly reactive metabolites of oxygen. Since these may be important in monocyte chemotaxis and in modification of lipoproteins (see sections on monocyte chemotaxis and low-density lipoprotein), examination of recent observations of cellular oxidative metabolism in diabetes is in order. Two groups of investigators have reported conflicting data on oxidative metabolism by leukocytes in diabetes. Stimulated polymorphonuclear leukocytes from diabetics demonstrated reduced superoxide production and chemoluminescence, a measure of oxidative metabolism (35). In a similar group of diabetic subjects, although with somewhat worse glycemic control, diabetic monocytes rather than neutrophils showed increased rather than reduced chemiluminescence and superoxide production than did monocytes from non-diabetics (36).

A potentially important role for glucose in determining the production of reactive oxygen metabolites is suggested by several lines of evidence (36). First, the extent of chemoluminescence correlated with the blood glucose level. Second, insulin treatment resulted in reduced oxygen metabolism, and third, addition of glucose directly to monocytes from normal or diabetic subjects led to enhanced chemoluminescence. Generation of these potentially toxic reactive oxygen species appears to result from increased glucose metabolism via the hexose monophosphate shunt pathway. Thus it was suggested that enhanced cellular hexose monophosphate shunt activity, whether a result of increased glucose concentrations or hypoinsulinism, could stimulate oxidative metabolism, with potential effects on some of the events that are important in atherosclerosis.

Platelets

Platelets are believed to play an important role in atherosclerosis. They adhere to areas of denuded endothelium and exposed subendothelial macrophages and connective tissue. There they are capable of releasing PDGF, the powerful mitogen and chemotactic agent for arterial smooth muscle cells. They also release arachidonate metabolites such as thromboxanes, leukotrienes and lipid peroxides which are likely to be important in atherogenesis.

Platelet function, as measured by a variety of in vitro techniques, has been widely studied in diabetes during the past several years and is the subject of several extensive reviews (see also Chapter 19). In addition, an update on alteration of platelet function in diabetes is included in an excellent recent review on the pathogenesis of atherosclerosis in diabetes mellitus (37).

Platelet adherence and aggregation in vitro

Although not all studies are in agreement, platelet adherence and aggregation in vitro appear to be increased in all forms of human and experimental diabetes (37). However, most of the studies of platelet adherence unfortunately have used foreign surfaces rather than endothelial cells. Further, there is general agreement that platelets from diabetics studied in vitro demonstrate a hypersensitivity to aggregating agents, even before clinical evidence of angiopathy. Thus factors associated with the diabetic state, rather than primary vascular damage, might produce the observed abnormalities of platelet function.

Platelet aggregation in vivo

To evaluate the relationship between platelet aggregation and endothelial integrity in vivo, indirect measurements of platelet aggregation (e.g. circulating β-thromboglobulin and platelet factor 4 or platelet survival studies) and endothelial damage (e.g. Factor VIII related antigen) have been performed. Since platelet aggregation and endothelial damage can be focal and limited, these in vivo measures are indirect and potentially insensitive. Nevertheless, there is a surprising consensus of findings; i.e. increased platelet consumption and decreased platelet survival occur commonly in diabetes, even in the young insulin-dependent patient without evidence of overt micro- or macrovascular disease.

Two recent studies have evaluated whether abnormalities of platelet aggregation precede vascular complications by the concurrent measurement of β-thromboglobulin and Factor VIII related antigen (as indices of platelet consumption and endothelial damage, respectively) in a wide spectrum of diabetics. In one study (38), plasma levels of both proteins were found to be elevated in diabetics of all age groups and in non-diabetic atherosclerosis patients. Higher levels were observed in subjects with atherosclerosis independent of diabetes. Diabetic children also showed evidence of increased platelet consumption, but since they also had increased plasma levels of Factor VIII related antigen, it is difficult to decide whether platelet aggregation preceded endothelial damage or vice versa. Further, since an interaction between platelets and endothelial cells is likely to play a role in the pathogenesis of diabetic microangiopathy as well as macroangiopathy, the relationship of these observations to atherogenesis is difficult to evaluate. The other recently reported study also evaluated platelet aggregation and endothelial injury in a large group of diabetics (39). An increase in Factor VIII related antigen was observed in all groups of diabetics, while plasma β-thromboglobulin levels were only elevated in those with retinal disease, suggesting that endothelial damage precedes platelet aggregation. Even though the insensitivity of these indirect measurements makes such studies difficult to interpret, endothelial injury appears to occur early in diabetics of all types, and in conformity with studies in non-diabetic animals (22, 23), could be an important stimulus to platelet aggregation.

Platelet arachidonate metabolism

Consensus also exists that platelet prostaglandin and thromboxane synthesis is increased in human and experimental diabetes (37), although the precise enzymes affected are not known with certainty. In one recent study, platelet production of thromboxane was measured in insulin-dependent diabetics, with and without angiographically proven CAD, and in non-diabetic patients with CAD (40). Although no evidence was provided that the uncomplicated diabetic patients were free of CAD, platelets from diabetics with and without CAD nonetheless produce more thromboxane than did platelets from normal controls. Furthermore, thromboxane production was greater in platelets from diabetics with CAD than in platelets from those without. Platelets from non-diabetic CAD patients also produced high levels of thromboxane. A further interesting and potentially important finding was that thromboxane production by platelets correlated with plasma cholesterol and triglyceride levels, independent of the presence of diabetes. Thus, part of the increased cardiovascular risk of hyperlipidemia might relate to abnormalities of platelet aggregation and thromboxane synthesis through as yet undetermined mechanisms.

Platelet thromboxane synthesis might be related to diabetic control (41).

In a recent study, one small group of IDDM subjects was treated with conventional insulin therapy, while a second group received intensive therapy with continuous subcutaneous insulin infusion. Excellent glycemic control was achieved in the intensively treated group, whose platelet thromboxane production was normal. Platelets from diabetics receiving conventional therapy produced more thromboxane than did platelets from either the control group or the intensively treated diabetics. There are several potential problems with this study, including the small number of patients studied and the failure to reach statistical significance between groups for some of their measurements. Also, it is not clear that the duration of diabetes was equal in the two groups. Despite these shortcomings, this study raises the intriguing possibility that changes in platelet function in diabetes may be preventable by adequate glycemic (and lipidemic) control. An attempt to correct platelet abnormalities by intensive therapy in diabetics in whom abnormalities were observed previously, would be a logical next step.

Platelet derived growth factor (PDGF) and other mitogens

A major effect of platelets in atherogenesis is likely to be mediated by PDGF. Assays of circulating levels of PDGF recently have become available, but they suffer from the same disadvantages as other indirect measures of platelet aggregation and degranulation. Nonetheless, measurement of the level of this mitogen in the plasma of diabetics is awaited with interest, especially since PDGF is more likely to be directly involved in atherogenesis than are β-thromboglobulin and platelet factor 4.

Other potential circulating mitogens such as low molecular weight mitogens (42), growth hormone (43) or insulin-like growth factors may exist in the diabetic state. Clearly, smooth muscle cell mitogens that are active in vivo could be of major importance in atherogenesis in the diabetic. However, in view of their likely local action in the arterial wall, measurement of circulating levels of mitogenic activity in diabetes may be of limited value.

Arterial wall cells

The three major arterial wall cells that play a role in atherogenesis are the endothelial cells, the arterial smooth muscle cell and the monocyte-derived macrophage. Of these three cells, most is known about endothelial cell function in diabetes, which recently has been discussed in detail in the review by Colwell et al. (37). Much less is known about arterial smooth muscle cells and macrophage metabolism and function in diabetes, but these two cells are likely to receive increased attention in the near future.

Endothelial cells

Abnormalities of endothelial cell function as evaluated by circulating Factor VIII related antigen are common even in young diabetic children shortly after the onset of their disease (44). Prostacyclin, which can be synthesized by vascular endothelial cells and which can inhibit platelet adhesion and aggregation, is a potentially important inhibitor of platelet aggregation in atherosclerosis. Therefore it is of interest that prostacyclin production by arteries from animals with experimental diabetes is reduced and can be restored towards normal by treatment of the diabetes. Studies of human endothelial tissue cells and measurement of prostacyclin metabolites in the plasma of human diabetics are in general consistent with this notion. Two recent studies using endothelial cells in culture provide evidence that serum from diabetic subjects contain factors which inhibit prostacyclin production relative to non-diabetic control (45, 46). The nature of the inhibitory factors is unknown, but is has been suggested that lipid peroxides, which are inhibitors of prostacyclin synthesis and which can be elevated in the plasma of diabetics (see later) might play a role in this respect. This interesting possibility awaits further testing.

Increased endothelial permeability has been suggested to be an early event in atherosclerosis and is associated with increased arterial wall histamine synthesis and histamine content in non-diabetic animal models of atherosclerosis (47). Therefore it is of interest that increases in arterial histamine levels in association with increased levels of enzymes important in histamine synthesis and decreased levels of enzymes important in its catabolism also have been shown to occur in rats made diabetic by the administration of streptozotocin. These changes could be reversed by insulin therapy and normalization of glycemic control (48). Although there is no evidence that similar changes occur in human arteries, these findings nonetheless provide a mechanism by which diabetes could lead to endothelial injury, thereby initiating the chain of events that result in the development of atherosclerotic lesions.

Repair of endothelial cell injury could be impaired in diabetes, since proliferation of mesenchymal cells is known to be slow in wound healing in diabetes (9).

Arterial smooth muscle cells and macrophages

Very little is known about the function of these two cell types in diabetes. Studies on arterial smooth muscle cells will need to be performed using cells from animals with experimental diabetes. Studies with macrophages will need to be performed using macrophages from other sites. In humans, cultured macrophages can be derived from blood monocytes; also pulmonary alveolar macrophages are accessible for study. No major findings have been published during the past two years which enhance our understanding of the role of these two arterial wall cells in diabetes, and further studies in this area clearly would be of value.

Plasma lipids and lipoproteins

Plasma lipid and lipoprotein abnormalities in human diabetes are extensively discussed in Chapter 26. Information regarding circulating levels of lipoproteins in diabetes has been available for many years. More recently, attention has focused on qualitative changes in plasma lipoproteins in diabetes, e.g. that due to glucosylation. Another lipoprotein modification which may be important in diabetes is that due to oxidation. Because of the potential pathogenetic importance of lipoproteins that have been modified by oxidation, it is of interest that two recent studies, one in diabetic animals (50), and the other in human diabetic subjects (51), have actually demonstrated increased circulating levels of oxidized lipoproteins. In a group of elderly diabetics with angiopathy, an increased proportion of lipid peroxides was observed in both LDL and HDL. Unfortunately, no non-diabetic control group with angiopathy of an equal degree was studied (51). The significance of these findings is not clear. However, it has been known for many years that an association exists between circulating and arterial wall lipid peroxides and atherosclerosis. Hopefully, future studies will allow the nature of this association to be determined, particularly with respect to diabetes mellitus.

Lipoprotein–cell interactions

Recent attention has focused on the interaction of lipoproteins with arterial wall cells, which occur at two distinct levels. First, arterial endothelial cells are in direct contact with circulating lipoproteins, which are potentially cytotoxic. Second, lipoproteins in the interstitial space or the artery wall can interact with both arterial smooth muscle cells and macrophages and induce cellular lipid accumulation. Also, lipoproteins can interact with extracellular connective tissue elements.

Very low-density lipoprotein

Cytotoxicity. Since VLDL levels frequently are elevated in both types of human diabetes and in experimental diabetes, the recent demonstration that VLDL isolated from diabetic rats is toxic to endothelial cells (52), illustrates a possible mechanism of endothelial injury in diabetes. VLDL isolated from plasma or serum of streptozotocin diabetic rats were toxic to cultured porcine endothelial cells by an unknown mechanism. However, recent studies suggest that oxidation of lipoproteins may occur either during their in vitro preparation in the absence of sufficient antioxidants or EDTA (53) or by cell-mediated mechanisms (54, 55). Oxidized LDL is markedly cytotoxic due to substances in the lipid moiety (56), presumably lipid peroxides. VLDL from diabetic animals were more cytotoxic than VLDL from control animals even when isolated in the presence of EDTA. This effect could be reversed by insulin treatment (52). Thus, it is possible that some lipid peroxides were being formed in vivo in the diabetic animals or that VLDL from diabetic animals was more susceptible to oxidation during its isolation. These potentially important findings clearly need to be pursued and extended to other lipoproteins in both experimental and human diabetes. Oxidant damage to lipoproteins certainly is a potential mechanism for arterial cell injury which initiate the events leading to atherosclerosis.

Lipid accumulation. VLDL also could play an important role in atherogenesis by delivery of lipid to arterial wall cells. Fibroblasts, as an arterial cell model, do not appear to recognize normal VLDL by the classical LDL receptor pathway. However, VLDL isolated from subjects with a primary form of hypertriglyceridemia can be recognized and taken up by the LDL receptor (57). Uptake is related to the apoprotein E component of VLDL. 'Hypertriglyceridemic' VLDL also was taken up by resident mouse peritoneal macrophages (58), while 'normotriglyceridemic' VLDL was not. The uptake of 'hypertriglyceridemic' VLDL by macrophages is believed to be via the β-VLDL receptor, which is distinct from both the acetyl LDL receptor, and the tightly regulated LDL receptor. VLDL from hypertriglyceridemic subjects thus can lead to massive lipid accumulation, with the macrophages developing the appearance of foam cells in vitro. Recently, Kraemer et al. (59) have demonstrated that normal human VLDL also can be taken up by these receptors on cultured macrophages. The reason for differences between this and the previous study is unclear. Recent preliminary evidence indicates that VLDL from non-insulin dependent diabetic donors actually is taken up to a greater extent and results in more lipid accumulation in macrophages than does normal VLDL (60).

Remnants of triglyceride-rich lipoprotein catabolism

Catabolism of VLDL and chylomicrons to their remnants is mediated by lipoprotein lipase. Remnant accumulation in plasma can result from decreased cellular uptake and may lead to increased levels of intermediate density lipoprotein (IDL), the remnant-rich lipoprotein fraction, seen in diabetes (see Chapter 26). Remnant formation is an important factor in the uptake of triglyceride-rich lipoproteins by macrophages (61, 62) and arterial smooth muscle cells (63).

Low-density lipoprotein

LDL can be taken up by arterial cells other than macrophages via the classical LDL receptor pathway (64). LDL receptor activity does not appear to be altered in cells cultured from subjects with either insulin-dependent or non-insulin dependent diabetes (65). Macrophages possess few LDL receptors, and uptake of LDL by both human and rodent macrophages results in little lipid accumulation. Massive cholesterol ester deposition occurs when macrophages are exposed to LDL that has been modified chemically (64, 66) or biologically (54, 55, 66, 67). Since LDL composition can be altered in diabetes (see Chapter 26), the effect of these compositional changes on LDL cellular interaction in diabetes is of obvious import.

LDL isolated from subjects with mild to moderate non-insulin dependent diabetes are bound and degraded by skin fibroblasts and mouse peritoneal macrophages identically to normal LDL (68), despite diabetic LDL having a more heterogeneous hydrated density and triglyceride enrichment compared to normal LDL. By contrast, LDL isolated from poorly controlled subjects with insulin-dependent diabetes was taken up and degraded to a lesser extent than LDL from normal subjects or from the same diabetic subjects after a period of metabolic control (69). It was suggested that triglyceride enrichment of the LDL particles that occurred in these poorly controlled diabetic subjects might interfere with cellular LDL metabolism. Elucidation of the potential role of triglyceride enrichment (and reciprocal cholesterol depletion) of LDL derives from the recent observation that LDL, modified by in-vitro incubation with VLDL and lipid transfer protein, also resulted in decreased uptake and degradation by fibroblasts (70). Also, LDL from severely hypertriglyceridemic diabetics, which resulted in more marked triglyceride enrichment of the lipoprotein, was catabolized slowly by fibroblasts and was associated with altered regulation of cellular cholesterol synthesis and LDL receptor activity (71). Thus, the extent of modification of LDL, by triglyceride enrichment, cholesterol depletion or possibly other changes including apoprotein alterations, can inhibit uptake and catabolism via the LDL receptor pathway.

Another modification pertinent to the diabetic state that alters the interaction of LDL with its receptor is non-enzymatic glucosylation of lysine residues on the apoprotein (72, 75). Glucosylated LDL exists in the plasma of normal individuals and diabetics (72, 73), with higher levels in the serum of diabetics (72, 75). Non-enzymatic glucosylation also alters the biological reactivity of LDL, resulting in reduced uptake and degradation by cells (74, 75). Inhibition of degradation was observed when as few as 6–15% of LDL lysine residues were glucosylated and was completely lost when one-third of the lysine residues were blocked (75). Further, in vivo catabolism of glucosylated LDL in guinea pigs was delayed (75), consistent with delayed clearance by the cellular LDL receptor pathway in vivo. Glucosylation failed to stimulate LDL uptake by macrophages (74, 75). The extent of LDL glucosylation that is likely to occur in vivo may be of sufficient magnitude to alter its catabolism, since the degree of modification observed in the circulating LDL from some diabetic patients was shown to be sufficient to inhibit catabolism of this lipoprotein (76). Another potential modification of LDL that could be of importance in the diabetic, especially with renal complications, is carbamylation. Modification of lysine residues on LDL by carbamylation results in reduced catabolism by fibroblasts in a fashion similar to that observed with glucosylated LDL (77).

The potential mechanisms by which LDL with chemically altered lysine residues is atherogenic remains speculative. However, markedly accelerated atherosclerosis occurs in homozygous familial hypercholesterolemia and in the Watanabe Heritable Hyperlipidemic (WHHL) rabbit, both of whom have no functional LDL receptors. Thus, uptake of lipid into the cells of the artery wall which lead to atherosclerosis must occur via non-LDL receptor-mediated mechanisms. Non-LDL receptor-mediated uptake is likely to be enhanced when the interaction of LDL with its receptor is blocked, e.g., non-enzymatic glucosylation or by carbamylation, both of which thereby might play important roles in the atherogenesis of diabetes. Another potentially atherogenic mechanism relates to arterial uptake of immune-complexes in diabetes. It has been shown recently that non-enzymatically glucosylated LDL is immunogenic when injected into guinea pigs (78). Similar immunogenicity also probably occurs in human diabetics as evidenced by anomalously rapid clearance of glucosylated LDL when injected into diabetic subjects (79). Thus it is conceivable that immune complexes of modified LDL and antibody could damage arterial endothelium or be ingested by macrophages, thus resulting in foam cell formation.

High-density lipoproteins

HDL may play an important role in reverse cholesterol transport, i.e. the transport of cholesterol from extrahepatic cells to the liver for excretion. Transport of HDL from extrahepatic cells is facilitated by the interaction of HDL particles with specific receptors on these cells (80). The protective role of HDL against atherosclerosis is believed to be by this mechanism applied to arterial wall cells. The precise mechanism by which HDL removes cholesterol from cells is not known with certainty, nor is much known about the functional significance of the several HDL subclasses and subspecies that are found in plasma. HDL levels and composition can be profoundly affected by diabetes and these changes appear to differ between IDDM and NIDDM (see Chapter 26).

At a cellular level, a recent provocative study by Fielding et al. (81) raises some interesting questions regarding HDL and its potential role in atherogenesis. These investigators incubated low concentrations of plasma from individual subjects with cultured normal skin fibroblasts and evaluated the net transport of cholesterol between cells and plasma compared to control incubations without cells. Plasma from a small group of subjects with poorly controlled diabetes exhibited inhibition of net transport of cholesterol from cells to medium relative to non-diabetic controls. This abnormality reverted to normal with improved glycemic control by insulin and also was improved by adsorption of the high levels of plasma apoprotein E that was found in these diabetics. An abnormality in the esterification of cholesterol and transfer of the cholesteryl ester to lipoproteins of lower density, i.e. subsequent events in the chain of reverse cholesterol transport, also was inhibited in NIDDM. These alterations were corrected by insulin therapy, but not by removal of apoprotein E. Thus, NIDDM appears to be associated with a reduction in the metabolic events that result in the transfer of cholesterol from cells to plasma, i.e. reverse cholesterol transport. The potential role of apoprotein E in these events is supported by a study in which lipoproteins from cholesterol-fed alloxan diabetic rabbits contained less of this apoprotein than did lipoproteins from cholesterol-fed controls (82). Although it has long been appreciated that atheroscleroris is actually reduced in cholesterol-fed animals when they are made diabetic (83), perhaps in part attributable to insulin lack, the finding that their lipoproteins were apoprotein E deficient, provides a fresh view of this phenomenon.

In an extension of their earlier findings, Fielding et al. (84) now suggest that changes in VLDL and LDL composition are responsible for the defect in cholesterol transport from cells observed in diabetics, since their free cholesterol to phospholipid ratio was increased. Spontaneous transfer of free cholesterol from these lipoproteins to HDL occurred, in turn leading to reduced uptake of cellular cholesterol by HDL. These findings using plasma from a small group of subjects with NIDDM could be of importance for atherogenesis in the diabetic, by inhibition of reverse cholesterol transport from artery wall cells.

HDL can also undergo non-enzymatic glucosylation (85). Unlike glucosylated LDL, which is more slowly catabolized than normal LDL, glucosylated HDL appears to be cleared at an increased rate in guinea pigs. The reason remains unknown, especially since a macrophage cell line failed to show enhanced uptake of this modified lipoprotein. The significance of these findings is not clear, but could provide another mechanism by which HDL levels could be reduced in diabetes. However, one would predict glucosylation of HDL also to occur in IDDM, in which HDL levels tend to be elevated. Nevertheless, it is conceivable that glucosylation of HDL affects HDL levels and cholesterol efflux in some diabetic individuals. Also, it is possible that glucosylated HDL can be taken up by arterial wall macrophages.

HDL also may potentially influence atherogenesis in other ways. HDL appears to protect cells against cytotoxic damage that results from other oxidized lipoproteins (53). The mechanism of this protection is unknown at present, as is the role of HDL in preventing lipid accumulation in macrophages exposed to modified lipoproteins. Another recent report indicated that HDL can be a substrate for prostacyclin synthesis by endothelial cells (86). In view of the changes in HDL composition that are known to accompany diabetes, further evaluation of the detailed mechanism by which HDL can function in this respect is likely to yield meaningful information. In addition, the effect of diabetes on the newly described HDL receptor in arterial wall cells, which functions to promote cholesterol efflux (87), needs to be determined.

Connective tissue

Connective tissue accumulation in the artery wall is also a feature of the atherosclerotic plaque. Elastin and collagen are normal components of the arterial wall that provide for the elastic properties and tensile strength. Proteoglycans probably function in arteries as in other tissues to resist compression, and act as a medium for the diffusion of nutrients to arterial wall cells. Atherosclerotic lesions appear to be associated with an increase in collagen content due to increased biosynthesis, but knowledge of the precise changes in the nature of the collagen is incomplete. Changes in glycosaminoglycans have been documented in arteriosclerosis, but little is known about the proteoglycans to which they are attached. However, formation of proteoglycan–lipoprotein complexes in the interstitial tissue of the artery wall probably is an important component of the extracellular trapping of lipoproteins in atherosclerosis.

Little is known about the effect of diabetes on the modulation of connective tissue metabolism. However, since non-enzymatic glucosylation of other slowly turning over proteins is increased in diabetes mellitus, it is not surprising that several recent studies have demonstrated that glucosylation of collagen also is increased in diabetes. Increased glucosylation of human tendon and skin collagen is a normal accompaniment of the aging process. Collagen isolated from these sites from diabetics showed a marked increase in glycosylation, which was associated with a decreased susceptibility to collagenase digestion (88). This appears to result from glucosylation-induced cross-linking, which might be associated with increased stiffening and premature aging of collagen, including that of the aorta. Another recent study also points out that collagen isolated from the dura mater of a small number of young Type 1 and Type 2 subjects was glucosylated in the same manner as collagen non-enzymatically glucosylated in vitro (89). The amount of the altered collagen corresponded to that found in non-diabetics twice their age. Apart from altered stiffening, glucosylated collagen could have another potentially important role in atherogenesis. Collagen that was glucosylated either in vitro or in vivo in diabetic rats has recently been shown to be a better stimulus for platelet aggregation than non-glucosylated collagen (90). If increased amounts of glucosylated collagen are present in the subendothelial space in diabetics, increased platelet aggregation and all its consequences may be stimulated, thereby providing another link between diabetes and accelerated atherogenesis.

Even less is known about alteration of arterial wall glycosaminoglycans and proteoglycans in diabetes. However, changes in the proteoglycan (91) and glycosaminoglycan (92) content of tissue from animals with experimental diabetes have been documented. Of particular interest was the observation that changes in glycosaminoglycan content and composition might be related to hyperinsulinism, since non-diabetic hypophysectomized animals infused with insulin demonstrated similar changes in arterial glycosaminoglycans (92). Thus, changes in these connective tissue components could play a role in altered arterial permeability or ability to interact with and bind to lipoproteins in diabetes. Clearly, these issues need to be further examined in the future.

CONCLUSIONS

Much has been learned about the relationship of diabetes mellitus to atherosclerosis. The recent increase in interest in the cell biology of atherosclerosis and the interaction of extrinsic humoral and cellular factors with the cells of the arterial wall is likely to provide important insights into mechanisms of atherogenesis in diabetes. It is particularly encouraging to see the number of instances in which multiple experimental approaches have yielded similar conclusions as to the role of diabetes at specific sites of potential defects. Also, it is encouraging to witness the parallel yet intertwining advances being made in the areas of epidemiology, experimental medicine and cell biology. Nonetheless, as alluded to throughout this chapter, several areas exist in which there are huge hiatuses in our knowledge. These include the role of monocyte adhesion and chemotaxis in the initiation of the atherosclerotic process, the role of mitogens in atherogenesis, the intraarterial metabolic abnormalities that result in lipid accumulation in arterial smooth muscle cells and macrophages, and the role of connective tissue abnormalities in atherogenesis.

It is clear that factors associated with diabetes mellitus can interact adversely at multiple levels in this clearly multifaceted disorder. Perhaps this is why atherosclerosis is so common and so rampant in diabetes mellitus. However, it is only by a further understanding of these relationships and pathogenetic mechanisms that it will be possible for interventions aimed at the prevention of atherosclerosis to be undertaken rationally.

References

1. West KM, Ahuja MM, Bennett PH, Czyzyk A, Matco de Acosta O, Fuller JH, Grab B, Grabauskas V, Jarrett RJ, Kosaka K, Keen H, Krolewski AS, Miki E, Schliack V, Teuscher A, Watkins PJ, Stober JA (1983): The role of circulating glucose and triglyceride concentrations and their interactions with other 'risk factors' as determinants of arterial disease in nine diabetic population samples from the WHO multinational study. *Diabetes Care, 6*, 361.
2. Kawate R, Miyanishi M, Yamakido M, Nishimoto Y (1978): Preliminary studies of the prevalence and mortality of diabetes mellitus in Japanese in Japan and on the island of Hawaii. *Adv. Metab. Dis., 9*, 201.
3. Santen RJ, Willis PW, Fajans SJ (1972): Atherosclerosis in diabetes mellitus. *Arch. Intern. Med., 130*, 833.
4. Kudo H (1969): Serum triglyceride levels of untreated diabetes in relation to vascular lesions and obesity. *Tohoku J. Exp. Med., 97*, 47.
5. Gordon T, Castelli WP, Hjortland MC, Kannel WB, Dawber TR (1977): Diabetes, blood lipids and the role of obesity in coronary heart disease risk for woman. The Framingham study. *Ann. Intern. Med., 87*, 393.
6. Pyorala K (1979): Relationship of glucose tolerance and plasma insulin to the incidence of coronary heart disease: results from two population studies in Finland. *Diabetes Care, 2*, 131.
7. Welborn TA, Wearne K (1979): Coronary heart disease incidence and cardiovascular mortality concentrations. *Diabetes Care, 2*, 154.
8. Ducimetiere P, Eschwege E, Papoz L, Richard JL, Clude JR, Rosselin G (1980): Relationship of plasma insulin levels to the increase of myocardial infarction and coronary heart lesion mortality in a middle-aged population. *Diabetologia, 19*, 205.
9. Stout RW (1981): Blood glucose and atherosclerosis. *Arteriosclerosis, 1*, 227.
10. Kannel WB, McGee DL (1979): Diabetes and cardiovascular risk factors: the Framingham study. *Circulation, 59*, 8.
11. Wingard DL, Barrett-Connor E, Criqui MH, Suarez L (1983): Clustering of heart disease risk factors in diabetic compared to nondiabetic adults. *Am. J. Epidemiol., 117*, 19.
12. Beach KW, Brunzell JD, Strandness DE (1982): Prevalence of severe arteriosclerosis obliterans in patients with diabetes mellitus: relation to smoking and form of therapy. *Arteriosclerosis, 2*, 275.
13. Beach KW, Brunzell JD, Conquest U, Strandness DE (1979): The correlation of arteriosclerosis obliterans with lipoproteins in insulin-dependent and non-insulin-dependent diabetes. *Diabetes, 28*, 836.
14. Vaccaro O, Rivellese A, Annuzzi G, Riccardi G, Furnari M, Rubba P, Mancini M (1982): Risk factors for peripheral atherosclerosis in non insulin dependent diabetes. *Artery, 10*, 341.
15. Kuebler TW, Bendick PJ, Finebers E, Markana ON, Norton JA, Vinicer FN, Clark CM (1983): Diabetes mellitus and cerebrovascular disease: prevalence of carotid artery occlusive disease and associated risk factors in 482 adult diabetic patients. *Diabetes Care, 6*, 274.
16. The University Group Diabetes Program (1982): Effects of hypoglycemic

agents on vascular complications in patients with adult-onset diabetes. VII. Evaluation of insulin therapy: Final report. *Diabetes*, *31*, *Suppl. 5*, 1.

17. Dorman JS, Laporte RE, Kuller LH, Cruickshanks KJ, Orchard TJ, Wagener DK, Becker DJ, Cavender DE, Drash AL (1984): The Pittsburgh insulin-dependent diabetes mellitus (IDDM) morbidity and mortality study. *Diabetes*, *33*, 271.
18. Tunbridge WM (1981): Factors contributing to deaths of diabetics under fifty years of age. *Lancet*, *2*, 569.
19. Jarrett RJ (1984): Type 2 (non-insulin-dependent) diabetes mellitus and coronary heart disease-chicken, egg or neither? *Diabetologia*, *26*, 99.
20. Brunzell JD (1984): Obesity and coronary heart disease: a targeted approach. *Arteriosclerosis*, *4*, 180.
21. Owerbach D, Johansen K, Billesbolle P (1982): Possible association between DNA sequences flanking the insulin gene and atherosclerosis. *Lancet*, *2*, 1291.
22. Faggiotto A, Ross R, Harker LA (1984): Studies of hypercholesterolemia in the non-human primate. I. Changes that lead to fatty streak formation. *Arteriosclerosis*, *4*, 323.
23. Faggiotto A, Ross R (1984): Studies of hypercholesterolemia in the non-human primate. II. Fatty streak conversion to fibrous plaque. *Arteriosclerosis*, *4*, 341.
24. Ross R (1981): Atherosclerosis: a problem of the biology of arterial wall cells and their interactions with blood components. *Arteriosclerosis*, *1*, 293.
25. Ross R, Glomset J (1976): The pathogenesis of atherosclerosis. *N. Engl. J. Med.*, *295*, 369.
26. Beatty PG, Harlan JM, Rosen H, Hansen JA, Ochs HD, Price TH, Taylor RF, Klebanoff SJ (1984): Absence of monoclonal-antibody-defined protein complex in boy with abnormal leukocyte function. *Lancet*, *1*, 535.
27. Wautier J-L, Paton C, Wautier M-P, Pintigny D, Abadic E, Passa P, Caen JP (1981): Increased adhesion of erythrocytes to endothelial cells in diabetes mellitus and its relation to vascular complications. *N. Engl. J. Med.*, *305*, 237.
28. Mazzone T, Jensen M, Chait A (1983): Human arterial cells secrete factors that are chemotactic for monocytes. *Proc. Natl Acad. Sci. USA*, *80*, 5094.
29. Mowat AG, Baum J (1971): Chemotaxis of polymorphonuclear leukocytes from patients with diabetes mellitus. *N. Engl. J. Med.*, *284*, 621.
30. Miller ME, Baker L (1972): Leukocyte function in juvenile diabetes mellitus: humoral and cellular aspects. *J. Pediatr. (St. Louis)*, *81*, 979.
31. Hill HR, Sauls HS, Dettloff JL, Quie PG (1974): Impaired leukotactic responsiveness in patients with juvenile diabetes mellitus. *Clin. Immunol. Immunopathol.*, *2*, 395.
32. Molenaar DM, Palumbo PJ, Wilson WR, Ritts RE (1976): Leukocyte chemotaxis in diabetic patients and their nondiabetic firstdegree relatives. *Diabetes*, 25, *Suppl. 2*, 880.
33. Hill HR, Augustine NH, Rallison ML, Santos JI (1983): Defective monocyte chemotactic responses in diabetes mellitus. *J. Clin. Immunol.*, *3*, 70.
34. Geisler C, Almdal T, Bennedsen I, Rhodes JM, Kolendorf K (1982): Monocyte functions in diabetes mellitus. *Acta Pathol. Microbiol. Scand.*, *90*, 33.
35. Shah SV, Wallin JD, Eilen SD (1983): Chemiluminescence and superoxide

anion production by leukocytes from diabetic patients. *J. Clin. Endocrinol. Metab.*, *57*, 402.
36. Kitahara M, Eyre JH, Lynch RE, Rallison ML, Hill HR (1980): Metabolic activity of diabetic monocytes. *Diabetes*, *29*, 251.
37. Colwell JA, Winocour PD, Lopes-Virella M, Halushka PV (1983): New concepts about the pathogenesis of atherosclerosis in diabetes mellitus. *Am. J. Med.*, *74*, 67.
38. Rak K, Beck P, Udvardy M, Pfliegler G, Misz M, Boda Z (1983): Plasma levels of beta-thromboglobulin and factor VIII-related antigen in diabetic children and adults. *Thromb. Res.*, *29*, 155.
39. Janka HU, Standl E, Schramm W, Mehnert H (1983): Platelet enzyme activities in diabetes mellitus in relation to endothelial damage. *Diabetes*, *32*, *Suppl 2*, 47.
40. Butkus A, Shirey EK, Schumaker OP (1982): Thromboxane biosynthesis in platelets of diabetic and coronary artery diseased patients. *Artery*, *11*, 238.
41. McDonald JW, Dupré J, Rodger NW, Champion MC, Webb CD, Ali M (1982): Comparison of platelet thromboxane synthesis in diabetic patients on conventional insulin therapy and continuous insulin infusions. *Thromb. Res.*, *28*, 705.
42. Koschinsky T, Bunting CE, Schnippert B, Gries FA (1979): Increased growth of human fibroblasts and arterial smooth muscle cells from diabetic patients related to diabetic serum factors and cell origin. *Atherosclerosis*, *33*, 245.
43. Ledet T (1981): Diabetic macroangiopathy and growth hormone. *Diabetes*, *30*, *Suppl. 2*, 14.
44. Borkenstein MH, Muntean WE (1982): Elevated factor VIII activity and factor VIII-related antigen in diabetic children without vascular disease. *Diabetes, 31*, 1006.
45. Paton RC, Guillot R, Passa P, Canivet J (1982): Prostacyclin production by human endothelial cells cultured in diabetic serum. *Diabète Métab.*, *8*, 323.
46. Patel MK, McEvoy FA (1983): Stimulation of prostacyclin production in cultured human endothelial cells by sera from diabetics and matched controls. *Biochem. Soc. Trans.*, *11*, 309.
47. Hollis TM, Furniss JV (1980): Relationship between aortic histamine formation and aortic albumin permeability in atherogenesis. *Proc. Soc. Exp. Biol. Med.*, *165*, 271.
48. Orlidge A, Hollis TM (1982): Aortic endothelial and smooth muscle histamine metabolism in experimental diabetes. *Arteriosclerosis*, *2*, 142.
49. Rowe DW, Starman BJ, Fujimoto WY, Williams RH (1977): Abnormalities in proliferation and protein synthesis in skin fibroblast cultures from patients with diabetes mellitus. *Diabetes*, *26*, 284.
50. Higuchi Y (1982): Lipid peroxides and α-tocopherol in rat streptozotocin-induced diabetes mellitus. *Acta Med. Okayama*, *36*, 165.
51. Nishigaki I, Hagihara M, Tsunekawa H, Maseki M, Yagi K (1981): Lipid peroxide levels in serum lipoprotein fractions of diabetic patients. *Biochem. Med.*, *25*, 373.
52. Arbogast BW, Lee GM, Raymond TL (1982): *In vitro* injury of porcine aortic endothelial cells by very-low-density lipoproteins from diabetic rat serum. *Diabetes*, *31*, 593.

53. Hessler JR, Morel DW, Lewis LJ, Chisolm GM (1983): Lipoprotein oxidation and lipoprotein-induced cytotoxicity. *Arteriosclerosis*, *3*, 215.
54. Heinecke JW, Baker L, Rosen H, Chait A (1984): Superoxide generated by arterial smooth muscle cells mediates metal ion catalyzed low density lipoprotein modification. *Arteriosclerosis*, *4*, 551a.
55. Morel DW, Di Dorleto PE, Chisolm GM (1984): Endothelial and smooth muscle cells alter low density lipoprotein *in vitro* by free radical oxidation. *Arteriosclerosis*, *4*, 357.
56. Morel DW, Hessler JR, Chisolm GM (1983): Low density lipoprotein cytotoxicity induced by free radical peroxidation of lipid. *J. Lipid Res.*, *24*, 1070.
57. Gianturco SH, Gotto AM, Hwang S-LC, Karlin JB, Yin AH, Prasad SC, Bradle YWA (1983): Apolipoprotein E mediates uptake of S_f 100–400 hypertriglyceridemic very low density lipoproteins by the low density lipoprotein receptor pathway in normal human fibroblasts. *J. Biol. Chem.*, *258*, 4526.
58. Gianturco SH, Bradley WA, Gotto AM, Morrisett JD, Peavy DL (1982): Hypertriglyceridemic very low density lipoproteins induce triglyceride synthesis and accumulation in mouse peritoneal macrophages. *J. Clin. Invest.*, *70*, 168.
59. Kraemer FB, Chen Y-DI, Lopez RD, Reaven GM (1983): Characterization of the binding site on thioglycolate-stimulated mouse peritoneal macrophages that mediates the uptake of very low density lipoproteins. *J. Biol. Chem.*, *258*, 12190.
60. Kraemer FB, Chen Y-DI, Cheung RM, Reaven GM (1981): Binding and degradation of very low density lipoproteins (VLDL) from diabetics by mouse peritoneal macrophages. *Clin. Res.*, *29*, 411A.
61. Lindqvist P, Ostlund A-M, Witztum JL, Steinberg D, Little JA (1983): The role of lipoprotein lipase in the metabolism of triglyceride-rich lipoproteins by macrophages. *J. Biol. Chem.*, *258*, 9086.
62. Bates SR, Murphy PL, Feng Z, Kanazawa T, Getz GS (1984): Very low density lipoproteins promote triglyceride accumulation in macrophages. *Arteriosclerosis*, *4*, 103.
63. Floren CH, Albers JJ, Bierman EL (1981): Uptake of chylomicron remnants causes cholesterol accumulation in cultured human arterial smooth muscle cells. *Biochim. Biophys. Acta*, *663*, 336.
64. Goldstein TL, Brown MS (1982): The LDL receptor defect in familial hypercholesterolemia: implications for pathogenesis and therapy. *Med. Clin. North Am.*, *66*, 335.
65. Chait A, Albers JJ, Bierman EL (1979): Low density lipoprotein receptor activity in fibroblasts cultured from diabetic donors. *Diabetes*, *28*, 914.
66. Fogelman AM, Shechter I, Seager J, Hokom M, Child JS, Edwards PA (1980): Malondialdehyde alteration of low density lipoproteins leads to cholesteryl ester accumulation in human monocyte-macrophages. *Proc. Natl Acad. Sci. USA*, *77*, 2214.
67. Henricksen T, Mahoney EM, Steinberg D (1983): Enhanced macrophage degradation of biologically modified low density lipoprotein. *Arteriosclerosis*, *3*, 149.
68. Kraemer FB, Chen Y-DI, Cheung RM, Reaven GM (1982): Are the binding

and degradation of low density lipoprotein altered in type 2 (non-insulin-dependent) diabetes mellitus? *Diabetologia*, *23*, 28.
69. Lopes-Virella MF, Sherer GK, Lees AM, Wohltmann H, Mayfield R, Sagel J, LeRoy EC, Colwell JA (1982): Surface binding, internalization and degradation by cultured human fibroblasts of low density lipoproteins isolated from type I (insulin-dependent) diabetic patients: changes with metabolic control. *Diabetologia*, *22*, 430.
70. Chait A, Eisenberg S, Steinmetz A, Albers JJ, Bierman EL (1984): Low density lipoproteins modified by lipid transfer protein have altered biological activity. *Biochim. Biophys. Acta*, *795*, 314.
71. Hiramatsu K, Bierman EL, Chait A (1984): Metabolism of low density lipoprotein from patients with diabetic hypertriglyceridemia by cultured human skin fibroblasts. *Diabetes*, in press.
72. Schleicher E, Deufel T, Wieland OH (1981): Non-enzymatic glycosylation of human serum lipoproteins. *FEBS Lett.*, *129*, 1.
73. Kim H-J, Kurup IV (1982): Nonenzymatic glycosylation of human plasma low density lipoprotein: evidence for *in vitro* and *in vivo* glucosylation. *Metabolism*, *31*, 348.
74. Gonen B, Baenziger J, Schonfeld G, Jacobson D, Farrar P (1981): Nonenzymatic glycosylation of low density lipoproteins *in vitro*: effects on cell-interactive properties. *Diabetes*, *30*, 875.
75. Witztum JL, Mahoney EL, Branks MJ, Fisher M, Elan R, Steinberg D (1982): Nonenzymatic glucosylation of low-density lipoprotein alters its biologic activity. *Diabetes*, *31*, 283.
76. Steinbrecher UP, Witztum JL (1984): Glycosylation of low-density lipoproteins to an extent comparable to that seen in diabetes slows their catabolism. *Diabetes*, *33*, 130.
77. Gonen B, Cole T, Hahm KS (1983): The interaction of carbamylated low-density lipoprotein with cultured cells. *Biochim. Biophys. Acta*, *754*, 201.
78. Witztum JL, Steinbrecher UP, Fisher M, Kesaniemi A (1983): Nonenzymatic glucosylation of homologous low density lipoprotein and albumin renders them immunogenic in the guinea pig. *Proc. Natl Acad. Sci. USA*, *80*, 2757.
79. Kesaniemi YA, Witztum JL, Steinbrecher UP (1983): Receptor-mediated catabolism of low density lipoprotein in man: quantitation using glucosylated low density lipoprotein. *J. Clin. Invest.*, *71*, 950.
80. Biesbroeck R, Oram JF, Albers JJ, Bierman EL (1983): Specific high affinity binding of high density lipoproteins to cultured human skin fibroblasts and arterial smooth muscle cells. *J. Clin. Invest.*, *71*, 525.
81. Fielding CT, Reaven GM, Fielding PE (1982): Human noninsulin-dependent diabetes: identification of a defect in plasma cholesterol transport normalized in vivo by insulin and in vitro by selective immunoadsorption of apolipoprotein E. *Proc. Natl Acad. Sci. USA*, *79*, 6365.
82. Brecher P, Chobanian AV, Small DM, Van Sickle W, Tercyak A, Lazzari A, Baler J (1983): Relationship of an abnormal plasma lipoprotein to protection from atherosclerosis in the cholesterol-fed diabetic rabbit. *J. Clin. Invest.*, *72*, 1553.
83. Duff GL, McMillan GC (1949): The effect of alloxan diabetes on experimental atherosclerosis in the rabbit. I. The inhibition of experimental

atherosclerosis in alloxan diabetes. II. The effect of alloxan diabetes on the retrogression of experimental cholesterol atherosclerosis. *J. Exp. Med.*, *89*, 611.

84. Fielding DF, Reaven GM, Liu G, Fielding PE (1984): Increased free cholesterol in plasma low and very low density lipoproteins in non-insulin-dependent diabetes mellitus: its role in the inhibition of cholesteryl ester transfer. *Proc. Natl Acad. Sci. USA*, *81*, 2512.
85. Witztum JL, Fisher M, Pietro T, Steinbrecher U, Elam RL (1982): Nonenzymatic glucosylation of high-density lipoprotein accelerates its catabolism in guinea pigs. *Diabetes*, *31*, 1029.
86. Fleisher LN, Tall AR, Witte LD, Miller RW, Cannon PJ (1982): Stimulation of arterial endothelial cell prostacyclin synthesis by high density lipoproteins. *J. Biol. Chem.*, *257*, 6653.
87. Oram JF, Brinton EA, Bierman EL (1983): Regulation of high density lipoprotein receptor activity in cultured human skin fibroblasts and human arterial smooth muscle cells. *J. Clin. Invest.*, *72*, 1611.
88. Kohn RR, Schnider SL (1982): Glucosylation of human collagen. *Diabetes*, *31, Suppl. 3*, 47.
89. Monnier VM, Kohn RR, Cerami A (1984): Accelerated age-related browning of human collagen in diabetes mellitus. *Proc. Natl Acad. Sci. USA*, *81*, 583.
90. Le Pape A, Guitton JD, Gutman H, Legrand Y, Fauvel F, Muh JP (1983): Nonenzymatic glycosylation of collagen in diabetes: incidence or increased normal platelet aggregation. *Haemostasis*, *13*, 36.
91. Rohrbach DH, Hassel JR, Kleinman HY, Martin GR (1982): Alterations in the basement membrane (heparan sulphate) proteoglycan in diabetic mice. *Diabetes*, *31*, 185.
92. Sirek OV, Sirek A, Cukerman E (1981): Intermittent hyperinsulinemia and arterial glycosaminoglycans in dogs. *Diabetologia*, *21*, 154.

The Diabetes Annual/1
K.G.M.M. Alberti and L.P. Krall, editors

ISBN 0444 90 343 7
$0.85 per article per page (transactional system)
$0.20 per article per page (licensing system)

19 Hematologic changes in diabetes

DONALD E. McMILLAN

Diabetes mellitus is not normally considered to be a hematologic disorder. Our interest in blood in diabetic subjects is based, however, on the fact that many of the symptoms and complications of diabetes appear to be linked to alterations in blood. Attention will therefore be focussed on recent findings that appear to have the greatest linkage to diabetic symptoms and complications. For that purpose, it is useful first to review briefly the direct effects of hyperglycemia to help explain the link between hematologic changes and diabetic symptoms and complications.

Effects of hyperglycemia

Plasma from diabetics regularly contains excess glucose. The dynamic osmotic role of hyperglycemia on circulatory stability is not yet fully understood, but 1 milliosmole of a substance generates a water movement equivalent to a hydrostatic pressure of 19 mm Hg. Five excess milliosmoles of glucose, common in diabetes, can create an osmotic burden equal to the diabetic's blood pressure, generating fluid movements of considerable size. Erythrocytes, endothelial cells, and extravascular tissues would all become involved in this fluid movement. Rapid entry of glucose into human adult erythrocytes minimizes their role in this problem. In some mammals, notably pigs, rapid glucose entry and exit, a normal property of fetal erythrocytes, is lost by adult erythrocytes (1, 2). Changes in erythrocyte volume should occur as glucose level fluctuates in these animals. The effect of oscillating hyperglycemia on endothelial cell water content is less clear but may parallel erythrocyte behavior.

Protein changes

Proteins in the plasma of diabetic patients undergo subtle quantitative changes. The albumin level is depressed, and acute-phase proteins become elevated, as do certain other globulins. The degradation of albumin is slowed even though albumin synthesis is depressed, allowing relatively normal plasma albumin levels to be maintained by a reduced fractional catabolic rate secondary to diminished extravascular albumin concentration (3). Increased acute phase reactant levels have been associated with both increased platelet aggregation and serum lipid levels in diabetes with peripheral vascular disease (4).

Considerable interest has evolved in measuring glucose attached to red blood cell hemoglobin in diabetes (see also Peterson and Formby, Chapter 11). Glucose attachment occurs on amino groups located at the N-terminal valines or to lysine. Lysine-attached glucose usually fails to affect the charge on hemoglobin and is not normally detected by chromatography (5). Other proteins that come in contact with glucose in body areas affected by hyperglycemia, such as collagen (6), erythrocyte membranes, lens proteins, serum proteins and liver proteins become excessively glycosylated in diabetes. Gragnoli et al. (7) evaluated the potential value of glycosylated total serum proteins and liver proteins become excessively glycosylated in diabetes. Gragnoli et al. (7) evaluated the potential value of glycosylated total levels of glycosylated serum protein to glycohemoglobin in diabetes and found them to be similarly correlated with fasting plasma glucose. Kammerer et al. (9) found both glycosylated albumin and glycosylated hemoglobin elevated in patients with and without diabetic retinopathy. Manda et al. (10) studied glycosylated albumin, finding that it fell more rapidly than glycosylated hemoglobin following insulin therapy in Type 1 diabetes. While Jones et al. (11) found that glycosylated serum albumin falls in parallel with the fall in fasting glucose.

Glycosylated hemoglobin measurement has come into common use in the assessment of diabetic control. It is used in the management of both Type 1 (12, 13) and Type 2 (14, 15) diabetes, but has not proved useful as a replacement for glucose tolerance testing in detecting early Type 2 diabetes (16). Past studies assessing glycohemoglobin levels in diabetic retinopathy and neuropathy have usually shown only a non-significant trend to higher values, but some recent studies have shown a significant relation (17, 18). Special glycohemoglobin measurement applications include postmortem diagnosis (19), newborn evaluation using maternal glycohemoglobin (20) and an elevation with anxiety associated with diabetes (21). Glycosylated hemoglobin measurement has also been used in animals. The streptozotocin-diabetic and galactose-fed rat (22), the dog (23), the Celebes black ape (24), and the rodent *Mystromys* (25) show increases.

Chromatographically measured hemoglobin A_1 has been shown to fluctuate during the day (26) and a means of re-equilibrating erythrocytes to remove the labile component has been described (27). New chromatographic (28) and colorimetric techniques (29, 30) have been described, but the goal of a highly reproducible and a highly specific measurement of glycosylated proteins has probably not yet been reached.

Increased glycosylation of most proteins (6–13) in a high-glucose environment has led to a number of hypotheses linking increased glucose attachment with manifestations of diabetic complications. Both protein to protein cross-linking and impairment of enzymatic activity have been suggested as potential mechanisms for hyperglycemia-mediated tissue disruption. Because the average plasma glucose level is approximately twice normal in diabetes, glycosylation of long half-life proteins to about half the diabetic level occurs in the absence of diabetes. Aging and diabetes should therefore be additive for these proteins. Information about the turnover rate and glucose exposure of the protein studied must be used in interpreting experimental results. For erythrocytes, if the normal survival time of 120 days is decreased, glycosylated hemoglobin level will not fully reflect the metabolic abnormality. Following hemorrhage and in pregnancy, when the number of recently formed erythrocytes rises, glycosylated hemoglobin also underestimates the metabolic derangement.

Flow properties of erythrocytes

The flow properties of erythrocytes have regularly been found to be altered in diabetes. Five-μm polycarbonate (Nucleopore) filters, observations of capillary-sized micropipet flow, and formation of erythrocyte doublets in an artificial suspending fluid have been used to show reduced diabetic erythrocyte deformability (31). Insulin administered intravenously has been reported to reverse the diabetic erythrocyte deformability problem (32). In-vitro studies have suggested that non-diabetic erythrocyte filtration can be improved by incubation in 10^{-9} M insulin (32). Several studies have indicated that erythrocyte membrane lipid fluidity increases after exposure to insulin (31). Changes in proton transport also are seen when cells are incubated with insulin (33). The rapid reversal of reduced erythrocyte deformability by insulin argues against the hypothesis that increased glycosylation of erythrocyte plasma membrane proteins (29, 34) is responsible for their reduced deformability in diabetes.

Increased aggregability and sedimentation of diabetic erythrocytes has been observed regularly in the past. While this aberration has usually been attributed to elevated plasma levels of fibrinogen and other acute phase proteins, the possibility that diabetic erythrocytes could have an incomplete complement of negative charge has been suggested by observation of diminished sialic acid content of diabetic erythrocytes (35). The anticipated additional finding of reduced erythrocyte electrokinetic charge has not yet been reported. However, reduction in the negative charge of glycosaminoglycans in blood vessels in diabetes due to reduced sulfation has been described recently (36).

White blood cells

Leukocytes are also affected by the diabetic state. In order to accomplish their functions, polymorphonuclear leukocytes and monocytes utilize pseudopod-mediated movement and phagocytosis. They also generate free radicals and other active compounds from molecular oxygen. These substances are used to disrupt living substances engulfed by the phagocytic process. They include superoxide ions, hydroxyl radicals, and hydrogen peroxide. Leukocyte chemotactic motility (37), phagocytosis (38, 39), and the generation of these strong oxidants is impaired in poorly controlled diabetes (39, 40). Metabolic defects are also detectable in leukocytes in poorly controlled diabetes; glycolysis is diminished secondary to diminished phosphofructokinase activity (41), enzymatic oxidation of arachidonic acid to thromboxane is decreased (42), and lysosomal enzyme activities are depressed (43, 44). Satisfactory control of diabetes restores these functions, explaining why diabetics in adequate control are not unusually susceptible to most infectious disorders.

Altered function of lymphocytes is influenced by both type and duration of diabetes. Insulin plays a role in the response of lymphocytes to surface-reacting antigens. In both types of diabetes T-helper cell glycogen content rises (45). Serum from diabetic patients inhibits immunoglobulin production by B-lymphocytes (46). Mitogen-induced T-lymphocyte proliferation is affected by very low-density lipoproteins (47) and carnitine (48), while lymphocytes from infants of diabetic mothers respond excessively to mitogen exposure in vitro (49).

The immune competent cell is considered to be an agent in the generation of pancreatic damage in Type 1 diabetes (see also Chapter 2). Radioactive indium-labeled autologous human lymphocytes localize in the pancreatic area and remain detectable for several days (50). The helper component of the T-cell population is normal or increased and the suppressor component depressed in early Type 1 diabetes (51). In the BB Wistar rat, a useful Type 1 diabetes model, antibodies for pancreatic and lymphocyte antigens are detectable in diabetic but not in non-diabetic animals (52). In addition, a linkage has been made between control of immunocyte responses and individual plasma lipoproteins (47). The possibility that immune mechanisms play a role in diabetic complications has been reintroduced by recognition of an association of circulating immune complex levels with diabetic complications (53) and the finding of increased complement poly-C9 in vascular and nonvascular basement membranes of individual diabetic subjects (54).

Platelets

Blood platelets aggregate and fuse more easily in diabetes. This observation was made before the role of platelets in the pathogenesis of atherosclerosis was emphasized. Aggregability of platelets increases both with age and duration of diabetes. It also tends to be increased in individuals with advanced atherosclerosis. Several factors appear to be responsible for increased diabetic platelet aggregation. Aggregability is linked to platelet size and morphology, platelet biochemical propensities, and to substances in the plasma. Platelets are normally small, flat or lens-shaped discs. Their membranes become externally deformed after exposure to a number of agents or to most solid surfaces. This change, called pseudopod formation, favors platelet aggregation. Also favoring aggregation is the production of thromboxane from arachidonic acid by an oxygen-utilizing enzyme. This pathway is unusually active in the platelets of diabetics, an abnormality reversed by intravenous insulin therapy (55). The anti-aggregatory properties of prostacyclin are also reduced in diabetes (56), even though no change in binding of prostacyclin to platelets can be detected (57). Fasting has been found to reduce platelet thromboxane production in diabetic mice (58). Small-animal studies, however, provide a poor model of human platelet behavior. Although many of their responses are comparable, in some situations animal platelets manifest different responses than human platelets (59).

The oxygen-utilizing enzyme responsible for thromboxane and prostacyclin formation is inhibited by acetyl groups transferred from aspirin. Aspirin modifies platelet aggregation by this mechanism (60). Sulfonylureas also reduce platelet aggregation (61, 62) as does calcium dobesilate (63) but another mechanism appears to be involved.

Von Willebrand factor (VWF) is a plasma factor that influences platelet aggregation. VWF is a part of the Factor VIII complex. It is secreted into the plasma by endothelial cells and its absence is associated with the hemorrhagic diathesis of Von Willebrand's disease. It enhances the aggregability of platelets and is elevated in plasma from diabetic patients. It can be mobilized in increased amounts from endothelium in human diabetes by a vasopressin analogue (64). Increased VWF is not detectable until several days after increased platelet aggregation in streptozotocin-diabetic rats (65). This argument against VWF as the mediator of increased platelet aggregation in diabetes is further supported by a negative correlation between the two parameters in human diabetes (66).

Platelet volume, measured using electrical impedance is elevated both in human (67) and animal diabetes (68). Platelet aggregation is associated with release of β-thromboglobulin and platelet factor 4. The levels of both are elevated in blood from diabetic subjects (69). Platelets have been found to convert glucose to sorbitol but the increased sorbitol present is not linked to altered platelet structure or function (70).

Our inability to organize a hierarchy of responsibilities in the pathogenesis of diabetic complications has created a problem in interpreting platelet data. Do diabetic platelets become abnormal in response to developing complications or are they altered early in diabetes and then play a role in their development? Current observations suggest that platelet abnormalities are present early in diabetes (71), including VWF (ristocetin factor) elevation, but investigators appear to agree that platelet aggregation is further increased with duration of diabetes, in diabetic retinopathy, and in the presence of recognizable atherosclerosis. The injury hypothesis of atherogenesis requires a breakdown of the endothelial barrier and exposure of the underlying collagen for platelet adhesion to occur. Platelet accumulation is slowed by insulin (72). Platelets attached to blood vessel walls produce factors that favor the intimal migration and local proliferation of smooth muscle cells. The platelet hypothesis is now complicated by the fact that histiocytes, not smooth muscle cells, are the major storage site of lipids in atherosclerotic plaques. To support the hypothesis of platelet-mediated damage in diabetes, it would be particularly useful to demonstrate that platelets are present in increased amounts on the surface of anatomically healthy blood vessels in diabetes.

Oxygen transport

Glycosylation of hemoglobin affects tissue oxygen delivery. Glucose attachment at the β-chain N-terminal valine blocks the response of hemoglobin to 2,3-diphosphoglycerate (2,3-DPG). Madsen and Ditzel (73) studied red blood cell oxygen transport in diabetic pregnancy, finding that control of oxygen release by formation of 2,3-DPG is diminished in diabetes in such a way that it is possible to postulate that fetal hypoxia is occasionally present in fully regulated diabetic pregnancy. Dikker et al. (74) found that the circadian rhythm of oxygen balance was disturbed in diabetic patients with low oxygen tension seen in the evening. Reduced transcutaneous oxygen tension has been found in the diabetic foot, but this defect may be linked to occlusive arterial disease (75). Local tissue oxygen deficiency is postulated to cause an angiogenesis-promoting factor to be generated. This substance appears important in the pathogenesis of retrolental fibroplasia. It stimulates the growth of capillary microaneurysms and new microvessel proliferation in both neonatal and diabetic retinas. Work in identifying the angiogenesis factor has progressed to the point where its heparin-like conformation has been identified (76).

Viscosity

A substantial number of studies have been made of the viscosity of diabetic blood. They have commonly found a mild abnormality, more striking at low than at high shear rate. Blood viscosity is influenced principally by hematocrit, plasma viscosity (linked to plasma protein composition), erythrocyte aggregability, and erythrocyte deformability. The mild high shear rate blood viscosity elevation appears to be due principally to increased plasma viscosity. Direct measurement of the high shear rate viscosity of diabetic erythrocyte suspensions in artificial media has demonstrated little increase in flow resistance. Erythrocytes are known to undergo tank tread motion at high shear rate. They elongate into an elliptical shape and are sheared by adjacent plasma. Erythrocyte extensibility appears to be normal in diabetes. The greater viscosity at low shear rate (below 25 inverse seconds) is attributable to increased erythrocyte aggregation associated with diabetic plasma protein changes and reduced deformability of the now non-extended erythrocytes. At shear rates below 1 inverse second, a 20–30% elevation of diabetic blood viscosity is observed (77, 78). The elevation is more striking in diabetic proliferative retinopathy (79) and falls when either hyperglycemia is improved (80) or fibrinogen level is pharmacologically depressed (81). The viscosity of diabetic erythrocyte suspensions in this shear rate range is 5–10% greater than that of non-diabetic erythrocyte suspensions (77).

The elevated low shear rate blood viscosity is actually a transient process. It lasts until the disaggregation state becomes optimized for flow rate. After stable viscometric flow becomes established, diabetic blood viscosity is close to normal. The diabetic erythrocytes initially resist deformation more than normal erythrocytes but they can be placed into more streamlined configurations as flow is stabilized. The ability of blood and other materials to change in resistance after flow is initiated was described 50 years ago and designated by the word thixotropy – coined from Greek and meaning 'to change by touching'. Thixotropy is a property of a number of familiar materials including bread dough, mustard, soft tar, and an array of familiar emulsions. The additional burden produced by increased diabetic blood viscosity occurs in the brief period when blood flow is initiated or suddenly accelerated. These situations occur in arterial flow in early systole and as blood enters vessel branches. In the microcirculation it is seen when microaggregates are rapidly disrupted.

Vascular permeability

Control of permeability of the vascular system is central to the maintenance of the circulation. The system would not work without its ability to have oxygen diffuse rapidly outward while large molecules are retained in the vascular compartment. The rate of escape of plasma proteins from the vascular space can be assessed by using radioisotope-tagged proteins. O'Hare et al evaluated the effect of poor metabolic control, blood pressure elevation, and diabetic retinopathy on the plasma albumin escape rate in diabetes. They concluded that all three variables, blood pressure, metabolic status, and microvascular change, have separate effects that enhance the rate of albumin loss (82). Histamine-mediated accumulation of albumin in the aortic wall has been found to be increased in experimental diabetes (83). Urinary protein loss reflects increased permeability of the glomerular filtration surface. Poortmans et al. (84) studied urinary albumin and β_2-microglobulin excretion in diabetes, finding that elevations produced by exercise had no additional diagnostic value in comparison to urine collection at rest in evaluation for diabetic renal disease.

Vascular autoregulation

Microvascular flow is controlled by a process called autoregulation. Autoregulation matches local blood flow to need even when systemic blood pressure is made to fluctuate widely. The result is a stable local volume of flow over a wide arterial pressure range. Several studies have demonstrated impaired autoregulation in diabetes. Sinclair et al. (85) studied retinal vascular autoregulation using a blue-field entoptic technique, a novel self-testing process, finding impaired retinal autoregulation. Impaired retinal vasoconstriction due to oxygen administration is produced by acute hyperglycemia in non-diabetic animals (86). The coronary arteries become unusually sensitive to pharmacologic agents in the streptozotocin diabetic rat, apparently due to increased reactivity to arachidonic acid derivatives (87).

Conclusions

Hematologic changes associated with diabetes are linked to the vascular alterations characteristic of both acute hyperglycemia and chronic diabetes, but the exact nature of that linkage remains uncertain.

References

1. Jacquez JA (1984): Red blood cell as glucose carrier: significance for placental and cerebral glucose transfer. *Am. J. Physiol.*, *246*, R289.
2. Higgins PJ, Garlick RL, Bunn HF (1982): Glycosylated hemoglobin in humand and animal red cells. *Diabetes*, *31*, 743.
3. Murtiashaw MH, Baynes JW, Thorpe SR (1983): Albumin catabolism in diabetic rats. *Arch. Biochem. Biophys.*, *225*, 256.
4. Van Oost BA, Veldhuyzen BFE, Van Houwelingen HC, Timmermans APM, Sixma JJ (1982): Tests for platelet changes, acute phase reactants and serum

lipids in diabetes mellitus and peripheral vascular disease. *Thromb. Haemostasis*, *48*, 289.
5. Krishnamoorthy R, Cahour A, Elion J, Hartmann L, Labie D (1983): Monosaccharides bound to hemoglobins in normal and diabetic individuals: evidence for glucose, mannose and galactose as sugars released by methanolysis of the different hemoglobin components. *Eur. J. Biochem.*, *132*, 345.
6. Le Pape A, Gutman N, Guitton JD, Legrand Y, Muh JP (1983): Non enzymatic glycosylation increases platelet aggregating potency of collagen from placenta of diabetic human beings. *Biochem. Biophys. Res. Commun.*, *111*, 602.
7. Gragnoli G, Tanganelli I, Signorini AM, Tarli P, Paoli C (1982): Non-enzymatic glycosylation of serum proteins as an indicator of diabetic control. *Acta Diabetol. Lat.*, *19*, 161.
8. Mehl TD, Wenzel SE, Russell B, Gardner D, Merimee TJ (1983): Comparison of two indices of glycemic control in diabetic subjects: glycosylated serum protein and hemoglobin. *Diabetes Care*, *6*, 34.
9. Kammerer L, Jermendy G, Janosi L, Szelenyi J, Brosser G, Koltai M, Pogatsa G (1982): Investigation of glycosylized haemoglobin and albumin in diabetes mellitus with retinopathy. *Z. Gesamte Hyg. Ihre Grenzgeb.*, *37*, 474.
10. Manda N, Nakayama H, Aoki S, et al (1982): Determination of glucosylated albumin and its clinical significance in diabetes mellitus. *J. Jpn. Diabetes Soc.*, *25*, 691.
11. Jones IR, Owens DR, Williams S, Ryder REJ, Birtwell AJ, Jones MK, Gicheru K, Hayes TM (1983): Glycosylated serum albumin: an intermediate index of diabetic control. *Diabetes Care*, *6*, 501.
12. Mortensen HB, Vestermark S, Kastrup KW (1982): Metabolic control in children with insulin dependent diabetes mellitus assessed by hemoglobin A(lc). *Acta Paediatr. Scand.*, *71*, 217.
13. Richard L, Delaunay J, Dorleac E, Gillet P (1983): Apolipoprotéines et hémoglobine glycosylée chez le jeune diabétique insulino-dépendant. *Arch. Fr. Pédiatr.*, *40*, 11.
14. Ovalle BF, Rodrigues RE, Estrada A et al. (1982): Usefulness of hemoglobin A_1 determination in evaluation of efficacy chlorpropamide in the treatment of patients with diabetes type II. *Invest. Med. Int.*, *9*, 135.
15. Czech A, Taton J (1983): Glycosylated hemoglobin (Hb A_1) as an indicator of therapy effects in different clinical types of diabetes. *J. Chronic Dis.*, *36*, 803.
16. Orchard TJ, Daneman D, Becker DJ, Kuller LH, LaPorte RE, Drash AL, Wagener D (1982): Glycosylated hemoglobin: a screening test for diabetes mellitus? *Prev. Med.*, *11*, 595.
17. Hammerstein W, Berger M, Hennekes R (1983): The importance of an elevated hemoglobin A(IC) value for the pathogenesis of diabetic retinopathy. *Klin. Monatsbl. Augenheilkd.*, *182*, 298.
18. Boulton AJM, Hardisty CA, Worth RC, Drury J, Ward JD (1982): Elevated glycosylated hemoglobin in diabetic neuropathy. *Acta Diabetol. Lat.*, *19*, 345.
19. Chen C, Glagov S, Mako M, Rochman H, Rubenstein AH (1983): Post-mortem glycosylated hemoglobin (HBA(1C)): Evidence for a history of diabetes mellitus. *Ann. Clin. Lab. Sci.*, *13*, 407.

20. Zeller WP, Susa JB, Widness JA, Schwartz HC, Schwartz R (1983): Glycosylation of hemoglobin in normal and diabetic mothers and their fetuses. *Pediatr. Res.*, *17*, 200.
21. Turkat ID (1982): Glycosylated hemoglobin levels in anxious and nonanxious diabetic patients. *Psychosomatics*, *23*, 1056.
22. Powell HC, Ivor LP, Costello ML, Wolf PL (1982): Elevated hemoglobin A_1 in streptozotocin diabetic rats and in rats on sucrose and galactose-enriched diets. *Clin. Biochem.*, *15*, 133.
23. Mahaffey EA, Cornelius LM (1982): Glycosylated hemoglobin in diabetic and nondiabetic dogs. *J. Am. Vet. Med. Assoc.*, *180*, 635.
24. Howard CF (1982): Correlations of hemoglobin A(1C) and metabolic status in nondiabetic, borderline diabetic, and diabetic Macaca nigra. *Diabetes*, *31*, 1105.
25. Little RR, Parker KM, England JD, Goldstein DE (1982): Glycosylated hemoglobin in Mystromys albicaudatus: a diabetic animal model. *Lab. Anim. Sci.*, *32*, 44.
26. Daneman D, Luley N, Becker DJ (1982): Diurnal glucose-dependent fluctuations in glycosylated hemoglobin levels in insulin-dependent diabetes. *Metab. Clin. Exp.*, *31*, 989.
27. Huisman W, Kuijken JP, Tan-Tjiong HL, Duurkoop EP, Leijnse B (1982): Unstable glycosylated hemoglobin in patients with diabetes mellitus. *Clin. Chim. Acta*, *118*, 303.
28. Huisman THJ, Henson JB, Wilson JB (1983): A new high-performance liquid chromatographic procedure to quantitate hemoglobin A(1C) and other minor hemoglobins in blood of normal, diabetic, and alcoholic individuals. *J. Lab. Clin. Med.*, *102*, 163.
29. McMillan DE, Brooks SM (1982): Erythrocyte spectrin glucosylation in diabetes. *Diabetes*, *31*, 65.
30. Goldstein DE, Parker KM, England JD, England JE, Wiedmeyer HM, Rawlings SS, Hess R, Little RR, Simonds JF, Breyfogle RP (1982): Clinical application of glycosylated hemoglobin measurements. *Diabetes*, *31*, 70.
31. McMillan DE (1983): Insulin, diabetes, and the cell membrane: an hypothesis. *Diabetologia*, *24*, 308.
32. Juhan I, Vague P, Buonocore M, Moulin JP, Calas MF, Vialettes B, Verdot JJ (1981): Effects of insulin on erythrocyte deformability in diabetes-relationship between erythrocyte deformability in platelet aggregation. *Scand. J. Clin. Lab. Invest.*, *41*, 159.
33. Crane FL, Sun IL, Low H, Clark MG (1982): Insulin control of transplasma membrane NADH dehydrogenase. *Fed. Proc.*, *41*, 1339.
34. Miller JA, Gravallese E, Bunn HF (1980): Nonenzymatic glycosylation of erythrocyte membrane proteins. *J. Clin. Invest.*, *65*, 896.
35. Aminoff D, Jones TJ (1983): Erythrocyte sialoglycoconjugates in diabetes mellitus. *Fed. Proc.*, *42*, 507.
36. Rohrbach DH, Martin GR (1982): Structure of basement membrane in normal and diabetic tissue *Ann. NY Acad. Sci.*, *401*, 203.
37. Golub LM, Nicoll GA, Iacono VJ, Ramamurthy NS (1982): In vivo crevicular leukocyte response to a chemotactic challenge: inhibition by experimental diabetes. *Infect. Immun.*, *37*, 1013.

38. Katz S, Klein B, Elian I, Fishman P, Djaldetti M (1983): Phagocytotic activity of monocytes from diabetic patients. *Diabetes Care*, *6*, 479.
39. Gin H, Aubertin J, Ragnaud JM, Bonnal F (1982): Influence of normalisation of blood glucose levels on phagocytic and bactericidal properties of diabetic polynuclear leukocytes. *Rev. Med. Intern. Neurol. Psihiatr. Neurochir. Dermato-Venereol. Ser. Med. Intern.*, *3*, 321.
40. Shah SV, Wallin JD, Eilen SD (1983): Chemiluminescence and superoxide anion production by leukocytes from diabetic patients. *J. Clin. Endocrinol. Metab.*, *57*, 402.
41. Esmann V (1983): The polymorphonuclear leukocyte in diabetes mellitus. *J. Clin. Chem. Clin. Biochem.*, *21*, 561.
42. Qvist R, Larkins RG (1983): Diminished production of thromboxane B_2 and prostaglandin E by stimulated polymorphonuclear leukocytes from insulin-treated diabetic subjects. *Diabetes*, *37*, 622.
43. Finegold DN, Coates PM (1984): Effect of diabetes and insulin therapy on human mononuclear leukocyte lysosomal acid lipase activity. *Metab. Clin. Exp.*, *33*, 85.
44. Valerius NH, Eff C, Hansen NE, Karle H, Nerup J, Soeberg B, Sorensen SF (1982): Neutrophil and lymphocyte function in patients with diabetes mellitus. *Acta Med. Scand.*, *211*, 463.
45. Fuchs U, Dall E, Puschel W, Verlohren HJ, Marxhausen E, Shadow D, Mehner E, Wieniecki P (1982): Glycogen and acid alpha-naphthyl acetate esterase in lymphocytes of diabetic subjects. *Basic Appl. Histochem.*, *26*, 1.
46. Kaneshige H, Sakai H (1983): The inhibitory effects of diabetic sera on in vitro production of cytoplasmic immunoglobulins in normal lymphocytes. *J. Jpn. Diabetes Soc.*, *26*, 105.
47. Chi DS, Berry DL, Dillon KA, Arbogast BW (1982): Inhibition of in vitro lymphocyte response by streptozotocin-induced diabetic rat serum. A function of very-low-density lipoproteins. *Diabetes*, *31*, 1098.
48. Sensi M, Beales P, Zuccarini O, Spencer KM, Pozilli P (1982): Effect of carnitine on lymphocyte blastogenesis in patients with type 1 (insulin dependent diabetes). *IRCS J. Med. Sci.*, *10*, 305.
49. El Mohandes A, Touraine JL, Touraine F (1982): Lymphocyte populations and responses to mitogens in infants of diabetic mothers. *J. Clin. Lab. Immunol.*, *8*, 25.
50. Kaldany A, Hill T, Wentworth S, Brink SJ, D'Delia JA, Clouse M, Soeldner JS (1982): Trapping of peripheral blood lymphocytes in the pancreas of patients with acute-onset insulin-dependent diabetes mellitus. *Diabetes*, *31*, 463.
51. Pozzilli P, Zuccarini O, Iavicoli M, Andreani D, Sensi M, Spencer KM, Bottazzo GP, Beverley PCL, Kyner JL, Cudworth AG (1983): Monoclonal antibodies defined abnormalities of T-lymphocytes in type 1 (insulin-dependent) diabetes. *Diabetes*, *32*, 91.
52. Dyrberg T, Nakhooda AF, Baekkeskov S, Lernmark A, Poussier P, Marliss EB (1982): Islet cell surface antibodies and lymphocyte antibodies in the spontaneously diabetic BB Wistar rat. *Diabetes*, *31*, 278.
53. Dettori AG, Quintavalla R, Poli T (1983): Circulating platelet aggregates in diabetes mellitus. *Acta Haematol.*, *69*, 65.

54. Falk RJ, Scheinman JI, Mauer SM, Michael AF (1983): Polyantigenic expansion of basement membrane constituents in diabetic nephropathy. *Diabetes*, *32*, 34.
55. McDonald JWD, Dupré J, Rodger NW, Champion MC, Webb CD, Ali M (1982): Comparison of platelet thromboxane synthesis in diabetic patients on conventional insulin therapy and continuous insulin infusions. *Thromb. Res.*, *28*, 705.
56. Betteridge DJ, El Tahir KEH, Reckless JPD, Williams KI (1982): Platelets from diabetic subjects show diminished sensitivity to prostacyclin. *Eur. J. Clin. Invest.*, *12*, 395.
57. Shepherd GL, Lewis PJ, Blair IA, DeMey C, MacDermot J (1983): Epoprostenol (Prostacyclin, PGI_2) binding and activation of adenylate cyclase in platelets of diabetic and control subjects. *Br. J. Clin. Pharmacol.*, *15*, 77.
58. Rosenblum WI, Hirsh PD, Franson RC (1983): Overnight food deprivation in normal and diabetic mice markedly enhances thromboxane production by arachidonate stimulated platelet rich plasma and markedly increases platelet phospholipase A_2 activity. *Thromb. Res.*, *31*, 557.
59. Hamet P, Sugimoto H, Umeda F, Franks DJ (1983): Platelets and vascular smooth muscle: abnormalities of phosphodiesterase, aggregation, and cell growth in experimental and human diabetes. *Metab. Clin. Exp.*, *32*, 124.
60. Khosla PK, Seth V, Tiwari HK, Saraya AK (1982): Effect of aspirin on platelet aggregation in diabetes mellitus. *Diabetologia*, *23*, 104.
61. Valentovic MA, Lubawy WC (1983): Impact of insulin or tolbutamide treatment on ^{14}C-arachidonic acid conversion to prostacyclin and/or thromboxane in lungs, aortas, and platelets of streptozotocin-induced diabetic rats. *Diabetes*, *32*, 846.
62. Violi F, De Mattia GC, Alessandri C, Perrone A, Vezza E (1982): The effects of gliclazide on platelet function in patients with diabetes mellitus. *Curr. Med. Res. Opin.*, *8*, 200.
63. Youssef LO, Shalash BE, Afifi N, Hassanein A (1983): Calcium dobesilate in the treatment of diabetic retinopathy: Effect on platelet aggregation. *Acta Ther.*, *9*, 45.
64. Porta M (1982): Availability of endothelial von Willebrand factor and platelet function in diabetic patients infused with a vasopressin analogue. *Diabetologia*, *23*, 452.
65. Winocour PD, Lopes-Virella M, Laimins M, Colwell JA (1983): Time course of changes in in vitro platelet function and plasma von Willebrand factor activity (VIIIR:WF) and factor VIII-related antigen (VIIIR:AG) in the diabetic rat. *J. Lab. Clin. Med.*, *102*, 795.
66. Porta M, McCraw A, Kohner EM (1982): Inverse relationship between ristocetin co-factor levels and platelet aggregation in insulin dependent diabetes. *Thromb. Res.* *25*, 507.
67. Cagliero E, Porta M, Cousins S, Kohner EM (1982): Increased platelet volume in diabetic retinopathy. *Haemostasis*, *12*, 293.
68. Eriksson U, Ewald U, Tuvemo T (1983): Increased platelet volume in manifest diabetic rats. *Uppsala J. Med. Sci.*, *88*, 17.
69. Davi G, Rini GB, Averna M, Novo S, Di Fede G, Mattina A, Notarbartolo A, Strano A (1982): Enhanced platelet release reaction in insulin-dependent

and insulin-independent diabetic patients. *Haemostasis, 12*, 275.

70. O'Malley BC, Bidot-Lopez P, Lee EL, Robertson S (1982): Sorbitol accumulation in human normal and diabetic platelets. *J Fl Med. Assoc., 69*, 460.
71. Colwell JA, Winocour PD, Halushka PV (1983): Do platelets have anything to do with diabetic microvascular disease? *Diabetes, 32*, 14.
72. Rosenblum WI, El Sabban F (1983): Insulin delays platelet accumulation in injured cerebral microvessels of diabetic and normal mice. *Microvasc. Res., 26*, 254.
73. Madsen H, Ditzel J (1982): Changes in red blood cell oxygen transport in diabetic pregnancy. *Am. J. Obstet. Gynecol., 143*, 421.
74. Dikker VE, Galeniuk VA, Serykh IA, Kondiurina EG (1982): Circadian rhythms of tissue oxygen balance in diabetes mellitus. *Klin. Med. (Moscow), 60*, 64.
75. Railton R, Newman P, Hislop J, Harrower ADB (1983): Reduced transcutaneous oxygen tension and impaired vascular response in type 1 (insulin-dependent) diabetes. *Diabetologia, 25*, 340.
76. Shing Y, Folkman J, Sullivan R, Butterfield C, Murray J, Klagsbrun M (1984): Heparin affinity: purification of a tumor-derived capillary endothelial cell growth factor. *Science, 223*, 1296.
77. McMillan DE (1983): The effect of diabetes on blood flow properties. *Diabetes, 32*, 56.
78. Caimi G (1983): Blood viscosity and erythrocyte filterability: their evaluation in diabetes mellitus. *Horm. Metab. Res., 15*, 467.
79. Trope GE, Lowe GDO, Ghafour IM, Foulds WS, Forbes CD (1983): Blood viscosity in proliferative diabetic retinopathy and complicated retinal vein thrombosis. *Trans. Ophthalmol. Soc. UK, 103*, 108.
80. Poon PYW, Dornan TL, Orde-Peckar C, Mullins R, Bron AJ, Turner RC (1982): Blood viscosity, glycaemic control and retinopathy in insulin-dependent diabetes. *Clin. Sci., 63*, 211.
81. Itoh C, Ishii A, Iwafune Y, Yoshimoto H (1982): Fibrinolytic therapy and blood viscosity in simple diabetic retinopathy. *Nippon Ganka Kiyo (Fol. Ophthalmol. Jpn., 33*, 2469.
82. O'Hare JA, Ferriss JB, Twomey B, O'Sullivan DJ (1983): Poor metabolic control, hypertension and microangiopathy independently increase the transcapillary escape rate of albumin in diabetes. *Diabetologia, 25*, 260.
83. Hollis TM, Gallik SG (1982): Aortic histamine-mediated increased aortic albumin accumulation in experimental diabetes. *Fed. Proc., 41*, 1069.
84. Sinclair SH, Grunwald JE, Riva CE, Braunstein SN, Nichols CW, Schwartz SS (1982): Retinal vascular autoregulation in diabetes mellitus. *Ophthalmology, 89*, 748.
85. Poortmans J, Dorchy H, Toussaint D (1982): Urinary excretion of total proteins, albumin, and beta sub microglobulin during rest and exercise in diabetic adolescents with and without retinopathy. *Diabetes Care, 5*, 617.
86. Ernest JT, Goldstick TK, Engerman RL (1983): Hyperglycemia impairs retinal oxygen autoregulation in normal and diabetic dogs. *Invest. Ophthalmol. Vis. Sci., 24*, 985.

87. Reibel DK, Roth DM, Lefer BL, Lefer AM (1983): Hyperreactivity of coronary vasculature in platelet-perfused hearts from diabetic rats. *Am. J. Physiol.*, *14*, H640.

The Diabetes Annual/1
K.G.M.M. Alberti and L.P. Krall, editors

ISBN 0444 90 343 7
$0.85 per article per page (transactional system)
$0.20 per article per page (licensing system)

20 Organization of diabetic care

D.W. BEAVEN

Any organization in the field of diabetes care may be described as a framework of services provided for diabetes patients and designed to reduce morbidity and mortality. Mortality rates for diabetes mellitus can therefore be regarded as reflecting the efficacy of the organization of such services in a given community. Relevant data are cause-specific death rates from diabetic ketoacidosis (DKA) and from associated microvascular and accelerated macrovascular disease (myocardial infarction and strokes). A review of the United States DKA mortality figures (1) show these to be 8.4–10.6% of reported diabetic deaths each year from 1970 to 1978. Surprisingly, no changes were shown in comparison with figures for the period 1969–1973. Another paper from the US (2) shows diabetics under 45 years of age to have a minimal mortality rate 8 times that of a matched population group (408 per 100,000 versus 52 per 100,000).

TABLE 1 *Causes of mortality in diabetics as percentages of total deaths (2)*

Renal failure	34%
Myocardial infarction and strokes	29%
Diabetic ketoacidosis	18%
Infection	15%

In a survey conducted in Great Britain, 5971 British Diabetic Association members were followed 11–14 years for mortality rates (3). Diabetes as an underlying or first cause of death was excluded. Diabetes was found on only 60% of the remaining certificates! Standardized mortality ratios for cardiovascular disease were 11 times greater for both male and female diabetics. Equal mortality ratios for neoplasms and lower ratios for respiratory diseases support the accuracy of these figures.

If the present organization of delivery of diabetes care systems were better, technical developments could lower death rates from DKA and infection. The organization of and planning for delivery of services remain inadequate in most countries. Weinstein and Stason's review (4) on cost-effectiveness is an essential starting point if reorganization aims at a better distribution of restricted resources.

A more cost-efficient diabetes delivery service is based on the assumption that normalization of blood glucose levels, if achieved, can prevent disability and death. Studies by Raskin and colleagues and by Camerini Davalos and co-workers are critically reviewed by Siperstein (5). His summary 'to strive for the best possible control of blood glucose' sets the scene for the organizational methods by which this may be achieved.

Goals for the organization of diabetes services

Few critical reviews have emerged in the last two years on the effectiveness of diabetes services. Czyzyk (6) sets out the mechanism of the Polish two-tiered system for diabetes services. He states 'that health care for the diabetic will only be solved when there is better understanding of the relationship between primary health care services and specialized diabetic clinics'. The mortality of Memphis negro patients receiving oral hypoglycemic drugs and diet was compared with that of matched patients in Atlanta, USA (7), who had no oral drugs but aggressive diet therapy in a group program. After 9 years there were no significant differences in mortality figures.

Data from 6 USA states, covering the period 1976–1978, showed that 45% of all lower extremity amputations were performed on diabetics. Diabetics had a 15 times higher risk of amputation than non-diabetics (8). No detailed comparative data between states were presented on the degrees of hyperglycemia in toe, foot or leg amputations. The booklet *The Prevention and Treatment of Five Complications of Diabetes — A Guide for Primary Care Practitioners* (9) gives an excellent survey of the suggested organizational activities necessary to reduce morbidity and mortality.

The data of the Bedford study by Jarrett et al. (10) bear out the increased risks of hyperglycemia and impaired glucose tolerance. Age-corrected mortality rates from coronary heart disease were highest of all in the frankly diabetic Bedford patients. After statistical corrections for differences in age, blood pressure and obesity, increased coronary mortality remained in those with carbohydrate intolerance or diabetes. A 10-year mortality follow-up was undertaken on 18,000 male civil servants in London, UK (11). Coronary heart disease and stroke rates showed a non-linear relationship to blood glucose values (5.4 and 11 mmol/l). In glucose-intolerant and diabetic groups, other risk factors most strongly related to subsequent death from coronary heart disease were age and blood pressure. Any diabetes service should measure and control blood pressure in all glucose intolerant and diabetic people.

In 1983 the WHO Multinational Study Group (12) reported data from 9 of the 14 represented countries. A significant relationship was found between stroke, amputation and blood glucose concentration. Women and men had equal risks. Despite data variability between countries, the conclusion from this paper is that the variation in macrovascular disease was more related to the type of diabetes services provided, including dietary advice and its efficiency, rather than due to ethnicity. Microalbuminuria is a strong predictive index for increased mortality in non-insulin-dependent diabetics in the older age group from 50 to 75 (13), which again stresses the necessity for a yearly checklist to include microproteinuria.

Any organization needs to include goals for normalization of blood glucose levels and the control of raised blood pressure in carbohydrate-intolerant and diabetic persons. It is highly probable that daily multiple insulin injections pose less risk than once-daily injections, which sets another task for reorganization!

Organization at a national level

During the review period, few published reports give factual data on variations in the organization of diabetes care or compare efficiency. Thorn and Watkins (14) review teaching hospital out-reach programs in Wolverhampton but statistics are not given in this scheme, whereby 75% of patients seem to be seen in primary care practices, rather than in hospital clinic settings. Defaulting rates are said to be lower but no figures are given. They conclude 'effective diabetic care in general practice must be organized or it will not take place'.

The diabetes service is more organized in Croatia, Yugoslavia. Beaven (15) reported observations on the communications between primary care units, regional centers and a tertiary teaching institute in Zagreb, but again, without giving statistical data.

Organizational needs are different for various ethnic groups. The mortality and morbidity of diabetics in third-world countries such as Papua New Guinea is high (16). Half the surviving diabetic patients had microvascular complications and the average life expectancy of known diabetes was only 3.8 years. These figures compare unfavorably with the Japanese annual mortality rates of 2.5 for men and 1.4 for women (17). Premature death was seen with early age of onset, albuminuria, diabetic retinopathy and fasting glucose levels of over 11 mmol/l. Diabetes was observed in 5.9 per 1000 deliveries in South Carolina (18). The overall diabetic perinatal mortality rate was 102 per 1000 deliveries whereas non-diabetic perinatal mortality was 25 per 1000 deliveries. Fraser (19) reported a perinatal mortality in Kenya of 254 per 1000 population – 5 times the rate for non-diabetics.

Case finding: an integral part of diabetes services

The organization of diabetes care must be closely linked with case finding and with subsequent treatment programs. The 10-year follow-up in Bedford by Keen and colleagues (20) suggested hyperglycemia as a significant predictor of worsening tolerance in the second 5-year period. Surprisingly, obesity correlated weakly with a greater diabetes risk.

A more extensive review paper by Zimmet (21) presents a wealth of data on prevalence rates from 10 to 30% in a number of isolated communities over the last decade. As in communities with a high prevalence rate macrovascular disease is frequently associated with microvascular complications, often at diagnosis, detection drives should be an integral part of diabetes care services.

The *World Book of Diabetes in Practice* (22) offers no helpful studies regarding detection and subsequent organization of diabetes care. Detailed registers of all persons at risk in the community with marginal carbohydrate tolerance, with tissue typing of high-risk HLA subtypes, or close genetic linkage, require developing as part of a diabetes service, either on a regional or national organizational basis.

Diabetes organization

Special needs of a diabetes service

Cost-effectiveness depends upon incorporating the special needs of various groups into standard primary or secondary diabetes care services within the greater regional or national area. One critical period for the provision of diabetes care is when young diabetics are passed over to the responsibility of diabetes services for adults. Critical studies are urgently needed in this area. Adolescent diabetics referred to a tertiary center had emotional and psychological factors sorted out but the glycosylated hemoglobin levels remained high in this small patient group (23). A Danish report on a study in a population of 400 subjects aged 70 and over, showed an excess 10-year mortality if previously undiagnosed diabetes existed at the age of 70 or older (24). This well-documented prospective study showed impaired glucose tolerance tests in this age group to carry significant increase in cardiovascular mortality. This implies the need for diabetes organizations to survey and treat elderly populations regularly.

Should regular diabetes organizations meet intensive intervention needs?

This should be answered in the affirmative, but the high cost of such programs has prompted the US National Clinical Trial to assess critically the relationship between metabolic control and vascular complications in insulin-dependent diabetes (25).

Organization based on a philosophy of management

Most countries spend 6–9% of their gross domestic product on health. Selectively diverting resources into diabetes is slow, so that present economics demand reorganization of traditional diabetes delivery services. Muir Gray (26) speaks of 'two-box' health care and what he describes as the 'four-box system'. Adaptation to a full-circle model is set out in Figure 1. Secondary and tertiary care provisions are within one organizational structure. Increasingly, diabetes services are delivering 'shared-care' between patients and primary care provider and also between primary and secondary provider. Analyses of the financial cost for different combinations of self, primary, secondary and tertiary care are not available.

The health belief model

The Health Belief Model is 'an activity undertaken by a person who believes himself to be healthy for the purpose of preventing disease' (27). Provisions for improving positive health belief and health behavior will depend upon the general level of education, social and cultural beliefs of the community and the provision of health education within diabetes services. Lay diabetes societies serving as voluntary consumer groups to a regional or national organization need encouragement. Beaven and colleagues (28) descriptively report such a regional relationship in New Zealand, where an independent diabetes education and resource center was set

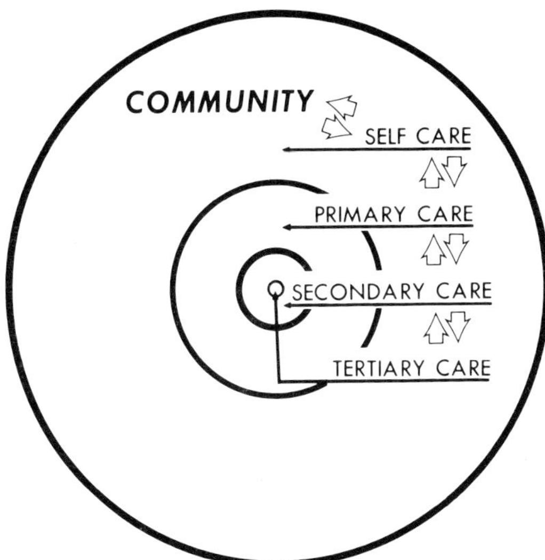

FIG. 1. *Organization of diabetes care.*

up in collaboration with the consumer group. There is, however, a paucity of good randomized trials on diabetics with behavioral modification and follow-up education.

Self care, primary care and shared care

A Swedish model (29) achieves a primary shift by organized instruction in diabetes care for physician/nurse teams in the primary health care groups. We are not informed if this is cost-effective or about the numbers of primary care workers who may have gained a significant increase in their knowledge and effectiveness. From Oxford, UK, fasting blood glucose measurements were used as a discriminatory factor for average blood sugar control over some months (30). In 10 general practices, fasting blood glucose measurements were taken. This paper is important in that it discusses practice nurses working with the general practitioner. Four fasting blood glucose determinations yearly were less expensive than regular urine or blood glucose measurements. Spaulding's editorial (31) again discusses diabetic day care units. He presents no new data but his previous studies showed the effectiveness of specialized day care education units compared with hospital education.

Audit as a function of service

An effective way of monitoring the outcome of any diabetes services is yearly review. This may measure the progress of possible complications, which might suggest a revision of therapy or services. Ideally, a yearly review should be carried out by health workers grouped around primary care physicians working through check lists. The diabetologist is responsible for reviewing audit results. Dietitians and nurse educators can evaluate patient knowledge and understanding, giving an indication for refresher courses or diabetes education classes if patient knowledge is deficient. At annual patient review it is necessary to check the patient's ability to accurately test either urine or blood. Newer test strips (32) provide more reliable estimates of the accurate measurement of glucose concentrations in urine and their use may be helpful in this respect.

A Boston report reviews clinical information from glycosylated hemoglobin assays (33). One should note the sophistication of high-pressure liquid chromatography (HPLC) – certainly not available to most diabetes services – and doubts must remain regarding the cost-effectiveness and accuracy of some glycosylated hemoglobin systems. Regular examinations, including weight, skin thickness or increased fibrosis in the palmar fascia, and examination of the ocular fundi through dilated pupils, of urinary protein, of blood pressure and of the feet are vital, even if financial resources are limited.

Barriers to care occur. Cohen (34) interviewed 103 consecutive patients at a general medical clinic in a city hospital. The physician's behavior was determined by whether the aide had had the patients take off their shoes and socks before being examined. Within any organization there should be a systematic check-list and operating manual for each member of the health care team, setting out their duties. In a review of randomly selected diabetic clinic patients a surprising 40% of younger patients were hypertensive (35). Only 38.7% of diabetics receiving antihypertensive therapy had normal blood pressures.

In a Nottingham trial (36) three different teaching methods and compliance to 7-day food record keeping were assessed by questionnaires. Glycosylated hemoglobin was an end-point of glycemic control. It was shown that an imaginative teaching program may affect the outcome and alter the behavior of those receiving education. There is a paucity of excellent, well-controlled studies as to whether yearly audit and review, an integral part of most diabetes services, is really cost-effective and reduces morbidity and mortality.

Research and evaluation: effectiveness and costs of the organization?

All functional aspects of organizing diabetes care need evaluation. We (37) have already reviewed the necessity for screening for new cases as part of regular primary medical care. There are few good studies evaluating dietary intervention. Rabkin and colleagues (38) rated the differences between two groups of non-insulin-dependent diabetic patients, allocated randomly to either group or individual therapy programs. There was no clear preference for either working with a group or counselling single patients, perhaps because only 40 people were in the trial. A group is more cost-effective in terms of dietitians' salaries utilized. Wales (39) looked at 3-month diet therapy in 182 non-insulin-dependent diabetics attending a routine outpatient clinic. On diet alone, only 20% of these patients achieved normal glucose tolerance. This says little for 'routine' diet therapy given in a diabetes out-patient setting of an English hospital (40).

Similarly, from the Edinburgh Royal Infirmary diabetologists reviewed the dietary education given 178 insulin-dependent diabetics (41). Compliance was rare but if patients understood more facts about the diet (as measured by the questionnaire) they had a lower glycosylated hemoglobin level. Adherence to the diet was poor, with 40% unable to remember dietary prescriptions or to estimate carbohydrate in common foods. If dietary compliance is rare and dietary treatment uncertain, how should the organization present dietary prescription?

Others advocate combining diet and exercise. In the usual organization of a diabetes service, these modalities should be provided. Regrettably, in the study reported by Barnard and co-workers (40), both a Pritikin program of diet together with exercise, were combined in their 60 non-insulin-dependent diabetics so that neither factor can be separately identified.

Mann (42) sums up the present controversy about what an organization for diabetes should recommend. The energy intake should be adjusted to maintain ideal body weight. Insulin-dependent diabetics need regular meal patterns to match injected insulin.

As diabetes education is part of the service, the evaluation of its cost-effectiveness is essential although, as yet, no good study adequately tests this hypothesis. Our unit showed a substantial saving in salaries of primary care district nurses after a home-based patient group had been given education courses in self-injection of insulin (43).

Lieberman and colleagues report from an institutionally-based study of diabetes education services carried out in Florida (44) that the most common problem encountered is lack of trained personnel, educational materials and curriculum development.

Fishbein and colleagues (45) showed the direct total hospitalization cost for insulin-dependent diabetic patients under 30 years of age to be US$ 2200 per patient. Despite an average ten years of duration of diabetes, only 31% of these patients had received more than two hours of diabetes education.

Leichter and colleagues (46) in a larger state-wide investigation into the hospital costs of diabetes in Kentucky showed diabetes to be the leading cause of hospitalization by disease, costing about US$ 100 million alone. Previous estimates of social and economic costs were erroneously low. I believe this paper to be mandatory reading for any person interested in the re-organization of a diabetes service on a major or state-wide basis.

Conclusions

This two-year review of diabetes delivery care systems reports shows a lack of evaluation. Excellent studies from Rhode Island and Kentucky on mortality give a finite end-point as does Connell and Louden's report (2) on under-45 deaths. Few useful studies indicate the cost-effectiveness of introducing reorganization such as the Swedish plan (29), the Danish one for old people (24) or that from New Zealand (10). Morbidity indices such as those developed by Fuller (11), Keen's group (10) or the WHO Multi-National Group (12) need to be used before and after reorganizing a national service.

The functional elements of a diabetes service must be integrated. Most reports, including Sinnock's amputee study (8) and several brief third-world country (16, 23) reports show the enormously high cost of poor education, lack of primary care and lack of self-monitoring. Therefore, any organization in the field of diabetes care should keep pondering the following questions:

- Is our organization and the way it works cost-effective?
- Do our primary services routinely detect increasing intolerance?
- Do our current patient and professional teaching methods and yearly checks save money?

Above all, we need to know whether our scarce resources are most effectively used. Because of potential benefit, nowhere are studies in the cost-effective delivery of services more urgently needed than for measuring the effectiveness of the organization of diabetes care.

References

1. Holman RC, Herron CA, Sinnock P (1983): Epidemiologic characteristics of mortality from diabetes with acidosis or coma. United States, 1970–78. *Am. J. Public Health*, *73*, 1169.
2. Connell FA, Louden JM (1983): Diabetes mortality in persons under 45 years of age. *Am. J. Public Health*, *73*, 1174.
3. Fuller JH, Elford J, Goldblatt P, Adelstein AM (1983): Diabetes mortality: new light on an underestimated public health problem, *Diabetologia*, *24*, 336.
4. Weinstein MC, Stason WB (1977): Foundations of cost-effective analysis for health and medical practices. *N. Engl. J. Med.*, *296*, 716.
5. Siperstein MD (1983): Diabetic microangiopathy and the control of blood glucose. *N. Engl. J. Med.*, *309*, 1577.
6. Czyzyk A (1983): The outpatient clinic in diabetes care. In: *World Book of Diabetes in Practice*, p 190. Editors: L.P. Krall and K.G.M.M. Alberti. Excerpta Medica, Amsterdam.
7. Van der Swaag R, Runyan JW, Davidson JK, Delcher HK, Mainzer I, Baggett HW (1983): A cohort study of mortality in two clinic populations of patients with diabetes mellitus. *Diabetes Care*, *6*, 341.
8. Most RS, Sinnock P (1983): Epidemiology of lower extremity amputations in diabetic individuals. *Diabetes Care*, *6*, 87.
9. National Diabetes Advisory Board (1983): The prevention and treatment of five complications of diabetes: a guide for primary care practitioners. *Diabetes Care*, *6*, 34.
10. Jarrett RJ, McCartney, Keen H (1982): Bedford study: ten year mortality rates in newly diagnosed diabetics, borderline diabetics & normoglycaemic controls & risk indices for coronary heart disease in borderline diabetics. *Diabetologia*, *22*, 79.
11. Fuller JH, Shipley MJ, Rose G, Jarrett RJ, Keen H (1983): Mortality from coronary heart disease and stroke in relation to degree of glycaemia: the Whitehall study. *Br. Med. J.*, *287*, 867.
12. West KM, Ahuja MMS, Bennett PH, Czyzyk A, De Acosta OM, Fuller JH, Grab B, Graubauskas V, Jarrett RJ, Kosaka K, Keen H, Krolewski AS, Miki E, Schliack V, Teuscher A, Watkins PJ, Stober JA (1983): Role of circulating glucose and triglyceride concentrations and their interactions with other 'risk

factors' as determinants of arterial disease in nine diabetic population samples from the WHO multinational study. *Diabetes Care*, *6*, 361.

13. Mogensen CE (1984): Microalbuminuria predicts clinical proteinuria and early mortality in maturity onset diabetes. *N. Engl. J. Med.*, *310*, 1984.
14. Thorn PA, Watkins PJ (1982): ABC of diabetes organisation of diabetic care. *Br. Med. J.*, *285*, 787.
15. Beaven DW (1983): Letter from Yugoslavia, diabetes services in Yugoslavia. *Br. Med. J.*, *287*, 894.
16. Savige J, Martin JIR (1982): Mortality and morbidity of diabetes in Papua, New Guinea. *Diabetologia*, *23*, 136.
17. Sasaki A, Uehara M, Horiuchi N, Hasagawa K (1983): A long-term follow-up study of Japanese diabetic patients: mortality and cause of death. *Diabetologia*, *25*, 309.
18. Wheeler FC, Gollmar CW, Deeb LC (1982): Diabetes and pregnancy in South Carolina: prevalence, perinatal mortality, and neonatal morbidity in 1978. *Diabetes Care*, *5*, 561.
19. Fraser RB (1982): The fate of the pregnant diabetic in a developing country: Kenya. *Diabetologia*, *22*, 21.
20. Keen H, Jarrett RJ, McCartney P (1982): The ten-year follow-up of the Bedford survey (1962-72): glucose tolerance and diabetes. *Diabetologia*, *22*, 73.
21. Zimmet P (1982): Type 2 (non-insulin-dependent) diabetes mellitus – an epidemiological overview. *Diabetologia*, *22*, 399.
22. Krall LP, Alberti KGMM (Eds) (1982): *World Book of Diabetes in Practice 1982*. Excerpta Medica, Amsterdam.
23. Orr DP, Golden MP, Myers G, Marrero DG (1983): Characteristics of adolescents with poorly controlled diabetes referred to a tertiary care centre. *Diabetes Care*, *6*, 170.
24. Agner E, Thorsteinsson B, Eriksen M (1982): Impaired glucose tolerance and diabetes mellitus in elderly subjects. *Diabetes Care*, *5*, 600.
25. Salans LB (1983): Proposed protocol for the clinical trial to assess the relationship between metabolic control and the early vascular complications of type 1 (insulin-dependent) diabetes. *Diabetologia*, *24*, 216.
26. Muir Gray JA (1983): Four box health care: development in a time of zero growth. *Lancet*, *2*, 1185.
27. Rosenstock IM (1974): Historical origins of the health belief model. *Health Educ. Monogr.*, *2*, 328.
28. Beaven DW, Scott RS, Helm AM, Clarkson MJ, Bremer JM, Price M, Taylor LK, Stafford JM (1983): Regional diabetes education centres. A unique New Zealand consumer – health service project. *IDF Bull.*, *28*, 5.
29. Luft R, Rosenqvist U (1982): Diabetes in the primary care: the Swedish model. *Lakartidningen*, *79*, 3452.
30. Muir A, Howe-Davies SA, Turner RC (1982): General practice care of non-insulin-dependent diabetes with fasting blood glucose measurements. *Am. J. Med.*, *73*, 637.
31. Spaulding WB (1983): Diabetic day care units – a must in Utopia? *J. Chronic Dis.*, *36*, 431.
32. Banauch D, Koller PU, Bablok W (1983): Evaluation of diabur-test 5000: a

co-operative study carried out at 12 diabetes centers. *Diabetes Care*, *6*, 213.
33. Nathan DM, Singer DE, Hurxthal K, Goodson JD (1984): The clinical information value of the glycosylated hemoglobin assay. *N. Engl. J. Med.*, *310*, 341.
34. Cohen SJ (1983): Potential barriers to diabetes care. *Diabetes Care*, *6*, 499.
35. Pacy PJ, Dodson PM, Beevers M (1983): The ethnic prevalence of hypertension in a diabetes clinic. *Postgrad. Med. J.*, *59*, 637.
36. McCulloch DK, Mitchell RD, Ambler J, Tattersall RB (1983): Influence of imaginative teaching of diet on compliance and metabolic control in insulin dependent diabetes. *Br. Med. J.*, *287*, 1858.
37. Beaven DW, Scott RS (1982): Diabetes education – Principles in Primary Health Care. In: *Diabetes Mellitus, Primary Health Care Prevention and Control*, pp 69–79. Editors: J. Tuomilheto, P. Zimmet, H. King and M. Pressley. IDF No. 69, Miles Laboratories (Australia) Melbourne, for the International Diabetes Federation.
38. Rabkin SW, Boyko E, Wilson A, Streja DA (1983): A randomised clinical trial comparing behaviour modification and individual counseling in the nutritional therapy of non-insulin-dependent diabetes mellitus: comparison of the effect on blood sugar, body weight and serum lipids. *Diabetes Care*, *6*, 50.
39. Wales JK (1982): Treatment of type 2 (non-insulin-dependent) diabetic patients with diet alone. *Diabetologia*, *23*, 240.
40. Barnard RJ, Lattimore L, Holly RG, Cherny S, Pritikin N (1982): Response of non-insulin-dependent diabetic patients to an intensive program of diet and exercise. *Diabetes Care*, *5*, 370.
41. McCulloch DK, Young RJ, Steel JM, Wilson EM, Prescott RJ, Duncan LJP (1983): Effect of dietary compliance on metabolic control in insulin-dependent diabetics. *Hum. Nutr. Appl. Nutr.*, *37A*, 287.
42. Mann JI (1984): What carbohydrate foods should diabetics eat? *Br. Med. J.*, *288*, 1025.
43. Scott RS, Mountier VM, Brown L, Beaven DW (1983): Utilisation of health services by diabetic patients. 1: The district nursing service. *N. Z. Med. J.*, *96*, 679.
44. Lieberman LS, Rosenbloom AL, O'Malley B (1982): Institutionally based diabetes educational services for patients and their families in Florida. *J. Fl. Med. Assoc.*, *69*, 23.
45. Fishbein HA, Faich GA, Ellis SE (1982): Incidence and hospitalization patterns of insulin-dependent diabetes mellitus. *Diabetes Care*, *5*, 630.
46. Leichter SB, Hernandez C, Fisher A, Collins P, Courtney A (1982): Diabetes in Kentucky. *Diabetes Care*, *5*, 126.

The Diabetes Annual/1
K.G.M.M. Alberti and L.P. Krall, editors

ISBN 0444 90 343 7
$0.85 per article per page (transactional system)
$0.20 per article per page (licensing system)

21 Psychological aspects of diabetes

CLARE BRADLEY

Psychological factors are highly relevant to much of diabetes management but although recently funds have been made available to encourage research into applications of psychology to diabetes management the importance of integrating psychology and medicine has not yet been fully recognized. In 1983, the organizers of the American Diabetes Association asked for abstract submissions from psychologists and other non-medical practitioners. Conference planning, however, separated the psychology from the medicine. Presentations concerned with medical aspects of continuous subcutaneous insulin infusion (CSII), and those dealing with psychosocial aspects of CSII took place at the same time and precluded attendance at both sessions. This lack of appreciation of the importance of interdisciplinary understanding has been noted by other reviewers (1–3).

Recent research developments

In the last 2 years there have been 2 major developments in diabetes-related psychological research: (1) a change of focus away from the unproductive search for the 'diabetic personality' towards greater appreciation of individual differences in beliefs about diabetes; (2) a recognition of the need to evaluate the potential of new technology such as blood glucose monitoring, CSII and newly developed biochemical measures, not only for glycemic control but also for patients' quality of life and general well-being.

Individual differences in beliefs about diabetes and styles of management

The study of attributions is a developing area of psychology which offers a potentially useful framework for understanding motivation – a major concern in diabetes research. Attribution theories are concerned with the attributions or explanations people use to account for events. Attributions

Preparation of this chapter was supported in part by NIH grant number AM28196 to the author.

may be seen to vary along an important dimension from internal (or dispositional) to external (or situational) attributions. Explanations in terms of personality factors or lack of effort are examples of internal attributions which might be used to account for an event such as a period of fluctuating blood glucose levels, but such an event might also be attributed to external factors such as family problems or inappropriate insulin regimen.

Attribution theorists have observed various consistencies in the kinds of attribution made under particular circumstances. The 'actor–observer bias' (4) refers to the tendency for people to differ in their explanations for each other's behavior: 'actors' tend to attribute their own behavior more to situational factors while 'observers' tend to attribute the behavior of actors to those actors' personal dispositions or characteristics. It appears that the lengthy, unproductive search for the 'diabetic personality' is an example of such an attribution bias; researchers and clinicians have overemphasized patients' characteristics such as obsessionality, hypochondriasis, and lack of intelligence in explaining patients' difficulties with diabetes management at the expense of situational explanations which are more likely to be considered by the patient. Recently Skyler (3), Dunn and Turtle (5) and other authors (1, 2, 6–8) have attempted to steer the search for explanations away from the 'myth of the diabetic personality'.

The attributions chosen to explain a person's past successes and failures have important consequences for that person's motives to perform in future. At least 2 further dimensions of attributions have been shown to be important: stable–unstable and controllable–uncontrollable (9). If an individual's performance is attributed to stable personality characteristics, similar performance can be anticipated in future. Unstable attributions to temporary mood states can offer no prediction of future performance. Attributions to luck imply no personal control over similar events in the future, whereas attributions to effort lead to expectations of control over future events.

Although the focus of studies concerned with perceptions of control has so far remained firmly on the patients, attributions, unlike personality characteristics, are more susceptible to environmental influence. Education programs and consultation styles may be designed to facilitate constructive attributions and health beliefs (10). However, there is a need to understand not only the attributions of patients but also those of their advisers. Constructive consultations are more likely to occur when doctors and patients become aware of each other's attributions and can resolve any differences between them.

Commonly used methods of measurement of some aspects of attributions are locus of control measures. The concept of locus of control originated from the work of Rotter (11), who developed a scale to measure generalized expectations of control over outcomes. The Rotter Scale provides a score on a dimension ranging from internal locus of control, where the individual expects to be able to control events, to external locus of control, where the individual has no expectation of personal control. The scale includes items dealing with political, social and personal issues. More recently the Wallstons and their colleagues (12) developed a Health Locus of Control (HLC) scale which is confined to issues concerned with general health and illness. The Multidimensional Health Locus of Control (MHLC) scale was a further development which subdivided external expectancies of control into 'chance' and 'powerful others' (13).

A number of researchers have used a locus of control scale in an attempt to predict differences between patients in level of diabetes control (14–16), but have found mixed support for their expectations that patients with more internal loci of control would be better able to manage their diabetes. In a discussion of contrary findings, Watts (17) suggested that more information was needed concerning the nature of the diabetic regimen and suggested that if patients 'were provided with a system of medical directives, over which they had little control and the usefulness of which they doubted, it is understandable that their response should be poor'. A problem with such studies is that patients' expectations of control over their diabetes may bear little relationship to their generalized expectations of control or even to their general health locus of control.

Bradley and colleagues (18) have recently developed a series of perceived control scales concerned specifically with attributions for diabetes control. These scales were given to 382 insulin-requiring patients participating in a feasibility study of CSII in Sheffield with a view to predicting patients' choice of treatment and the efficacy of different treatment regimens. Preliminary results have shown that the perceived control scales were successful in predicting which patients would choose CSII and which would prefer injection regimens. Those patients who chose CSII were significantly less internal than those who chose either intensified conventional treatment (ICT) or conventional treatment (CT). Thus CSII patients were less likely to feel personal responsibility for outcomes, or to feel in control of outcomes or to believe outcomes were foreseeable, than were patients choosing injection regimens. The results suggested that patients choosing CSII were viewing this treatment as a source of external control of their diabetes rather than as an open loop device which requires active patient involvement to close the loop if normoglycemia is to be attained.

The Health Belief Model Patients who have internal perceptions of control of their diabetes may or may not choose to intensify their treatment regimens. They may differ in the extent to which they believe that the treatment regimens are worthwhile. The Health Belief Model provides a theoretical framework (19, 20), widely used in the general research literature on psychology and medicine, which addresses this issue. The model suggests that 4 major factors are important in determining the extent to which an individual will follow prescribed treatment: beliefs about (1) the benefits of treatment, (2) the barriers to treatment, (3) the severity of the disorder, and (4) vulnerability to the disorder.

Several studies of diabetic patients have employed versions of health belief scales and, although some of the results look promising, support for their hypotheses has been limited and inconsistent (14, 21–24). Most of the studies have modified general health belief scales for use with diabetic individuals, but none has presented data on the reliability of the scales and few have provided sufficient detail about scale contents to allow judgments of face validity. When the measures failed to predict response to treatment, therefore, it was not possible to tell whether the measures were irrelevant or whether they were inadequate for the purpose of the study. Two research groups (18, 25) have recently reported the psychometric properties of diabetes-specific health belief scales allowing for clearer interpretation of future research findings based on scales of known reliability.

It is perhaps not surprising in the light of the actor–observer bias that little attention has been given to the variability and influence of the beliefs of doctors, nurses and other health professionals although a great many studies have been concerned with patients' beliefs.

One study which has examined doctors' beliefs about some aspects of diabetes management is described by Marteau and Baum (26), who compared the beliefs of 104 pediatricians and 119 physicians dealing with adult patients, all of whom were actively involved with diabetes management. Pediatricians underestimated the morbidity and mortality after 30 years of juvenile onset diabetes compared with physicians whose estimates more closely corresponded with the available data. The two groups of doctors differed in their opinions of the optimal target blood glucose levels for children with diabetes: more pediatricians opted for higher values. If pediatricians are unrealistically optimistic about the risks of diabetes and less convinced of a relationship between hyperglycemia and diabetes-related complications, it is likely that their patients' health beliefs and glycemic control will be affected. A combination of correlational and intervention studies would be required to establish the causal relationships between the range of health beliefs of doctors and patients and treatment recommended or followed.

Psychological effects of new techniques in diabetes management

Biochemical developments: C-peptide and GHb measures The use of C-peptide measures of endogenous insulin availability (27) and determination of clinical criteria which may be used in the absence of C-peptide measures for the identification of Type 1 and Type 2 diabetes (28) have important implications for psychophysiological studies of diabetes management. Recent studies controlling for C-peptide levels in examining the association between life events and diabetes control (29, 30) have provided stronger evidence for such relationships than could be shown in earlier studies. Future studies of the effects of acute stress on blood glucose levels will increase our understanding of the mechanisms involved if variance between subjects is reduced by controlling for endogenous insulin availability with C-peptide measures.

The recently developed long-term measures of glycemic control in the form of glycosylated hemoglobin (GHb) has provided a useful tool for both research and treatment. However, the wide availability of this measure has been a mixed blessing. In the same way that psychological tests can be abused if the results are misinterpreted and the limitations of the measures are not appreciated, so too have measures of GHb been misused. GHb has provided a valuable measure in recent studies of the relationship between life events and glycemic control (29, 30) and in a wide range of intervention studies evaluating the effects of new treatment regimens, education programs or specific behavioral interventions. However, in some studies measures of metabolic control have been used as measures of 'compliance' with therapeutic regimens (22). Sulway and colleagues (31) suggested that such 'blind belief in the efficacy of treatment' is unhelpful and listed a number of factors which influence glycemia regardless of patients' 'compliance'. Other authors (31a) have recommended the use of GHb for identifying patients in whom there is a marked discrepancy between diabetes control measured by GHb and diabetes control reflected in urine glucose measurement. In considering the possible mechanisms responsible for discrepant results the authors assumed without question that the patients were fabricating the data. They did not consider other explanations, e.g. the possibility that inaccuracy in the GHb measure might be the source of the discrepancy. Gabbay (32) has documented a number of common conditions which may give rise to falsely abnormal values for GHb. Although there is undoubtedly a small proportion of patients who for various reasons present their physicians with fictitious glucose measures, the actor–observer error may be reflected in the tendency to assume that the patient is responsible for any discrepancies which occur. If constructive, problem-solving alliances with patients are to be achieved, it is essential that both the limitations of GHb assays and the limitations of our own attribution processes be recognized.

Blood glucose monitoring techniques A wide range of rapid home blood glucose monitoring (HBGM) techniques are now available and numerous studies evaluating these techniques have recently appeared (33–35). Several authors have noted differences between patients in the accuracy of measurements obtained using HBGM (33, 34, 36) and have attributed errors of measurement to patient performance. However, laboratory studies of

HBGM performed by researchers themselves or by laboratory staff have indicated other possible explanations for the sources of error, including variable accuracy of the HBGM methods dependent on the range of BG measured (35, 37). Both patient error and technological error may be contributing to observed errors of measurement and both possibilities should be considered in designing and developing HBGM equipment to maximize accuracy and usability (37). It is also important that the limitations of HBGM methods currently in use be recognized in order to ensure appropriate attributions and to allow for effective interventions to reduce or adjust for measurement error.

Essential to the learning and maintenance of any skill is accurate and preferably immediate feedback about performance. Blood glucose monitoring, while offering more accurate and more immediate feedback of blood glucose levels than does urine glucose monitoring, still appears to fall short of ideal as a form of feedback for improving diabetes control. Even if patients can tolerate the inconvenience of multiple daily blood glucose determinations, hypoglycemia may occur without warning and episodes of hyperglycemia may go undetected. It has been suggested (38, 39) that if patients could learn to detect blood glucose levels outside the normoglycemic range, blood testing might be more effectively and economically used to confirm the occurrence of unacceptable fluctuations and allow adjustments to be made. Despite the traditional assumption that all but the most extreme blood glucose levels are asymptomatic, Pennebaker et al. (40) and Cox et al. (41) have demonstrated that 80% of their sample of 30 insulin-requiring adult patients could identify at least one physical symptom which correlated strongly with blood glucose levels. The glucose-related symptoms differed from subject to subject: 9 of the 19 symptoms used in their checklist were associated with high blood glucose for some subjects and with low blood glucose for other subjects.

Feedback has been used to improve detection of various visceral events including heart rate (42), blood pressure (43) and blood alcohol levels (44). A recent report by Gross and colleagues (45) demonstrated that the accuracy of 3 patients in subjective estimation of blood glucose levels was significantly improved during a period of 8–11 days of feedback from measured blood glucose. Although improvements in accuracy were not maintained when feedback was withdrawn, blood glucose levels tended to be lower during periods of feedback. The sample was small and the effects of these changes in blood glucose control on accuracy of estimation were not systematically examined.

The possibilities of training subjects to estimate their blood glucose levels by attending to cues from physical symptoms (46) or from mood states (47) are now being examined.

CSII (continuous subcutaneous insulin infusion) There has been some concern that use of CSII may have negative psychological consequences (48). Recently, small-scale studies (48–50) have found no evidence for deteriorations in psychological state associated with CSII. On the contrary, lower levels of anxiety and depression have been observed in patients after 2 or more months of CSII use (48, 49).

Jacobson and Leibovich (51) pointed out that short-term studies of selected patients have not addressed the psychological experiences of large numbers of patients, evaluated the psychological effects on patients who dropped out, nor examined the association between psychological factors and successful use of therapy. Rodin (52) has suggested that some of the feelings of frustration, depression and helplessness experienced by some individuals with diabetes may be related more to inadequate treatment than to the condition itself, and that improved treatment would be likely to reduce psychological morbidity. Some evidence that psychological problems may sometimes be the result, rather than the cause of diabetic instability has been provided by Lustman and colleagues (53).

Large-scale studies are now underway in which the effects of different treatment regimens, including CSII, on psychological well-being and quality of life are being examined. New psychological measures of quality of life, expectations and experience of treatment, beliefs and attributions, have been designed specifically for people with diabetes (54, 55). The large sample sizes in these studies will permit investigation of differences between patients and the implications of the psychological variables for the metabolic and psychological effects of treatments. Furthermore, psychometric analyses of responses to these scales will be useful in future research.

Overview of other major areas of research into psychological aspects of diabetes

Stress and diabetes onset Several recent reviews have noted the inadequacies of empirical support for the notion that stressful experiences may cause diabetes or precipitate its onset (1, 7, 51, 56). The lack of a conceptual model delineating the mechanism by which psychological factors might influence diabetes onset has also been noted (7), although more recently, Jacobson and Leibovich (51) have offered tentative suggestions for mechanisms by which psychological stress may trigger or cause diabetes. They suggested that stress-induced demands for insulin production by already depleted B-cells may trigger diabetes onset in susceptible individuals, or diabetes may be caused by the effects of psychological stress on immunocompetence. A preliminary report (57) of diabetic/sibling pairs involved in the Barts Windsor Prospective Family Study indicated that severe life events preceding diabetes onset were experienced by 56% of the diabetic subjects but by only 11% of their non-diabetic siblings. Further investigation of such relationships may contribute to the understanding of the etiology of Type 1 diabetes.

The effects of stress on diabetes control Surwit and colleagues (6, 7) have provided useful summaries of the role of the autonomic nervous system in the regulation of carbohydrate metabolism. Although life event research has produced consistent evidence for an association between experiences commonly considered stressful and increases in blood glucose levels (29, 30, 58, 59), the direction of blood glucose change with short-term laboratory stressors has varied between studies. Reviews of this literature (1, 39, 60) concluded that the stressors used had destabilizing effects on diabetes control but that the direction of blood glucose change was not consistent. These studies of acute stressors and metabolism have been criticized on a variety of methodological and conceptual grounds (39, 56, 60, 61). It is now recognized (62) that the assumption that all stressors will have similar physiological effects in healthy subjects is untenable and that the actual and perceived demands on the individual and the individual's actual and perceived ability to cope are important in determining psychophysiological responses. Few of the studies of diabetic individuals established that the supposed stressor was indeed experienced as stressful and some made no attempt to control for the type of diabetes. Future studies may benefit from the availability of C-peptide measures in selecting groups of subjects and from recognizing that the availability of exogenous insulin during experimental sessions will influence the extent and duration of apparent blood glucose changes. Furthermore, consideration of the effects of autonomic neuropathy might well clarify the findings of future studies.

A recent report by Turkat (63) has offered a further method of examining the relationship between stress and diabetes control. Rather than measuring life events or responses to laboratory stressors, Turkat related levels of anxiety (assessed by interview) to GHb levels. In his small sample of patients (16 Type 1 and 1 Type 2), those categorized as high in anxiety had higher GHb levels than patients with moderate or low anxiety. The latter 2 groups did not differ in GHb. This study did not control for between-group differences in sex and the duration of diabetes, and the need for replication of these findings was recognized. Turkat pointed out that while stress management may be appropriate for some patients, it could not be expected to improve diabetes control in people who were not previously anxious.

Stress management Several authors have employed relaxation techniques as a possible means of reducing stress-induced hyperglycemia. Two detailed case reports (64, 65) have demonstrated that insulin requirements were reduced by relaxation training with electromyographic (EMG) biofeedback. In the second of these studies (65) training was terminated when the diabetes became unstable and hypoglycemic symptoms were troublesome. Unlike the subject of the previous case report (64), this subject's diabetes was previously well controlled and no stress-related metabolic disturbances were experienced. It was not clear why relaxation training was thought to be appropriate in such a case.

Surwit and Feinglos (66) have more recently shown that the glucose tolerance of patients with Type 2 diabetes improved with the use of relaxation techniques. Relaxation had no effect on insulin sensitivity or glucose-stimulated insulin secretory activity; findings which led the authors to suggest that the increases in glucose tolerance were mediated by hepatic mechanisms. Similar improvements in glucose tolerance with relaxation have been found in a comparable study of patients with Type 1 diabetes (67). An extensive evaluation of the clinical applications of relaxation techniques to improve control of insulin-requiring diabetes is now underway in Sheffield (68).

Preliminary studies suggest that relaxation techniques may be a valuable aid to diabetes management in cases where stress is causing metabolic instability. Further research will need to determine the optimal methods, the appropriate indications for use of relaxation therapy and the limitations of the techniques.

Psychological issues in the management of complications The lack of knowledge about the mechanisms responsible for the long-term complications of diabetes, our inability to predict which patients will develop complications and which will not, are potential sources of anxiety, helplessness and depression. Most of the few recent papers which consider psychological factors and complications are concerned with impotence associated with diabetes. It has been estimated that between 20% and 60% of men with diabetes will at some time in their lives develop impotence (69). Bancroft (70) has noted that 'the fact that diabetes can cause impotence has led, in the past, to the assumption that impotence in a diabetic man is organic and hence untreatable. We are now taking greater notice of the fact that not only are diabetic men liable to the same psychological problems as non-diabetics, but, more importantly, their psychological reactions to physical impairment may convert what ought to be a trivial problem into total erectile failure'. In a number of recent studies and reviews the relative contributions of psychological, endocrinological, vascular and neuropathic factors in the etiology of diabetic impotence have been examined and the therapeutic options discussed (69, 71, 72). Sex therapy is indicated when psychogenic factors may be the sole or contributory cause of impotence, while sexual counselling may be appropriate in all forms of impotence to aid in exploring alternatives to penovaginal intercourse (72). However, in a study of 54 diabetic men, Smith (73) reported that, of the 26 men who experienced primary impotence and the 9 with secondary impotence, 3 patients had received some limited sexual counselling and that these 3 patients had themselves initiated discussion of impotence and actively sought help. Generally, patients were given no information about impotence and no anticipatory warnings. Smith concluded that the need for sexual counseling for diabetic men was apparent but that adequate help was rarely provided.

Behavioral approaches to enhancing patient self-care Knowledge is a necessary but not a sufficient condition for achieving good diabetes control. Wide discrepancies have been found between the knowledge and behavior of diabetic patients (31) and between knowledge and diabetes control (74). Surwit and colleagues (6, 7) have summarized some of the behavioral strategies that have been used successfully in increasing a variety of self-care behaviors. Some of these strategies are already used routinely in diabetes education programs, e.g. *self-monitoring* behaviors relevant to treatment and *skill training* of new behaviors. Others are rarely used systematically, e.g. *shaping* successive approximations of the desired treatment regimen rather than requiring the patient immediately to adopt a complex new behavior pattern, *contracting* between patient and therapist for desired behavior change, and *reinforcement* of new desired behaviors.

Behavioral approaches have focused on increasing specific self-care behaviors. For instance, a series of studies by Epstein and colleagues demonstrated the use of such approaches in improving both the accuracy in urine glucose determinations by children with diabetes (75) and the percentage of negative urine glucose tests (76). Carney (77) reported improvements in the frequency of blood glucose monitoring. Other behavioral approaches investigating the possibilities of maximizing the value of blood glucose self-monitoring are discussed on page 378. Fisher and colleagues (1) have reviewed a number of studies which successfully used behavioral approaches for dietary regulation and weight loss to which may be added a recent study by Wing (78). Wing found that overweight Type 2 diabetic patients who were assigned to a behavioral weight control program lost significantly more weight than those assigned to nutrition education or a standard care condition. A recent study of the use of sex therapy with men diagnosed as having organic impotence indicated that sexual functioning was improved for 60% of these individuals (79).

Conclusions

Research into psychological aspects of diabetes and the use of psychological approaches in diabetes management is at an early stage. The potential contribution of psychology is gradually being recognized but although progress has been made, psychological methods and approaches are not yet well integrated into diabetes research and treatment. When a more holistic view can be accepted, many of the findings of the studies referred to in this chapter will be seen to be more widely relevant. In this chapter only the most recent developments of the last two years in psychology applied to diabetes have been selected for review. Several important areas, notably the role of the family and interpersonal relationships, have been considered in earlier reviews (1, 2, 8) and have not been dealt with here. It would seem that further improvements in diabetes management may result from more intensive studies which focus on people with diabetes in the wider context of their families and their varied social networks. The need to appreciate the complex interactions between psychological and physical factors is beginning to be understood, particularly in the context of stress management and sexual dysfunction. These psychophysiological relationships provide a useful model for treatment and research in other areas of diabetes management.

References

1. Fisher EB Jr, Delamater AM, Bertelson AD, Kirkley BG (1982): Psychological factors in diabetes and its treatment. *J. Consult. Clin. Psychol.*, *50*, 993.
2. Johnson SB, Rosenbloom AL (1982): Behavioural aspects of diabetes mellitus in childhood and adolescence. *Psychiatr. Clin. North Am.*, *5*, 357.
3. Skyler JS (1981): Psychological issues in diabetes. *Diabetes Care, 4*, 656.
4. Jones EE, Nisbett RE (1982): The actor and the observer: divergent perceptions in the causes of behaviour. In: *Attribution: Perceiving the Causes of Behaviour*, Chapter 5, p. 79. Editors: E.E. Jones, D.E. Kanouse, H.H. Kelly, R.E. Nisbett, S. Valins and B. Weiner. General Learning Press, New Jersey.
5. Dunn SM, Turtle JR (1981): The myth of the diabetic personality. *Diabetes Care*, *4*, 640.
6. Surwit RS, Scovern AW, Feinglos MN (1982): The role of behaviour in diabetes care. *Diabetes Care*, *5*, 337.
7. Surwit RS, Feinglos MN, Scovern AW (1983): Diabetes and behaviour: a paradigm for health psychology. *Am. Psychol.*, *38*, 255.
8. Kosub SM, Cerreto MC (1981): Juvenile diabetes: current trends in psychosocial research. *Soc. Work Health Care*, *6*, 91.
9. Weiner B (1979): A theory of motivation for some classroom experiences. *J. Educ. Psychol.*, *71*, 3.
10. Gillespie C, Bradley C (1984): Motivation and the person with diabetes. *Update J. Postgrad. Gen. Pract.*, in press.
11. Rotter JB (1966): Generalised expectancies for internal versus external control of reinforcement. *Psychol. Monogr.*, *80*, 1.
12. Wallston BS, Wallston K, Kaplan G, Maides S (1976): Development and validation of the health locus of control (HLC) scale. *J. Consult. Clin. Psychol.*, *44*, 580.

13. Wallston KA, Wallston BS, DeVellis R (1978): Development of multidimensional health locus of control (MHLC) scales. *Health Educ. Monogr.*, *6*, 160.
14. Alogna M (1980): Perception of severity of disease and health locus of control in compliant and noncompliant diabetic patients. *Diabetes Care*, *3*, 533.
15. Lowery BJ, DuCette JP (1976): Disease related learning and disease control in diabetics as a function of locus of control. *Nurs. Res.*, *25*, 358.
16. Hamburg BA, Inoff GE (1982): Relationships between behavioural factors and diabetic control in children and adolescents: a camp study. *Psychosom. Med.*, *44*, 321.
17. Watts FN (1982): Attributional aspects of medicine. In: *Attributions and Psychological Change*, Chapter 8, p. 135. Editors: C. Antaki and C.R. Brewin. Academic Press, London.
18. Bradley C, Brewin CR, Gamsu DS, Moses JL (1984): Development of scales to measure perceived control of diabetes mellitus and diabetes related health beliefs. *Diabetic Med.*, *1*, 213.
19. Rosenstock IM (1966): Why people use health services. *Milbank Mem. Fund.*, *44*, 94.
20. Becker MH (1974): The health belief model and personal health behaviour. *Health Educ. Monogr.*, *2*, 324.
21. Bloom Cerkoney KA, Hart LA (1980): The relationship between the health belief model and compliance of patients with diabetes mellitus. *Diabetes Care*, *3*, 594.
22. Harris R, Skyler JS, Linn MW, Pollack L, Tewksbury D (1982): Relationship between the health belief model and compliance as a basis for intervention in diabetes mellitus. *Pediatr. Adolescent Endocrinol.*, *10*, 123.
23. Stevens BJ (1983): Health beliefs, compliance and metabolic control in adolescent diabetics. *Diabetes*, *32*, 37A.
24. La Greca AM, Hanna NC (1983): Diabetes-related health beliefs in children and their mothers: implications for treatment. *Diabetes*, *32*, 17A.
25. Given CW, Given BA, Gallin RS, Condon JW (1983): Development of scales to measure beliefs of diabetic patients. *Res. Nurs. Health*, *6*, 127.
26. Marteau TM, Baum JD (1984): Views on diabetes. *Arch. Dis. Child.*, *59*, 566.
27. Welborn TA, Garcia-Webb P, Bonser A (1981): Basal C-peptide in the discrimination of type 1 from type 2 diabetes. *Diabetes Care*, *4*, 616.
28. Welborn TA, Garcia-Webb P, Bonser A, McCann V, Constable I (1983): Clinical criteria that reflect C-peptide status in idiopathic diabetes. *Diabetes Care*, *6*, 315.
29. Linn MW, Linn BS, Skyler JS, Jensen J (1983): Stress and immune function in diabetes mellitus. *Clin. Immunol. Immunopathol.*, *27*, 223.
30. Cox DJ, Taylor AG, Nowacek G, Holley-Wilcox P, Pohl SL, Guthrow E (1984): The relationship between psychological stress and insulin-dependent diabetic blood glucose control: preliminary investigations. *Health Psychol.*, *3*, in press.
31. Sulway M, Tupling H, Webb K, Harris G (1980): New techniques for changing compliance in diabetes. *Diabetes Care*, *3*, 108.
31a. Citrin W, Ellis GJ, Skyler JS (1980): Glycosylated haemoglobin: a tool in identifying psychological problems. *Diabetes Care*, *3*, 563.

32. Gabbay KH (1982): Glycosylated haemoglobin and diabetes mellitus. *Med. Clin. North Am.*, *66*, 1309.
33. Schiffrin A, Desrosiers M, Belmonte M (1983): Evaluation of two methods of self blood glucose monitoring by trained insulin-dependent diabetic adolescents outside the hospital. *Diabetes Care*, *6*, 166.
34. Fairclough PK, Clements RS, Filer DV, Bell DSH (1983): An evaluation of patient performance of and their satisfaction with various rapid blood glucose measurement systems. *Diabetes Care*, *6*, 45.
35. Nelson J, Woelk MA, Sheps S (1983): Self glucose monitoring: a comparison of the Glucometer, Glucoscan and Hypocount B. *Diabetes Care*, *6*, 262.
36. Pohl SL, Gonder-Frederick L, Cox D (1983): Self measurement of blood glucose concentration: routine correlation with a reference laboratory. *Diabetes*, *32*, 13A.
37. Moses JL, Bradley C (1984): Ergonomics and diabetes. *Ergonomics*, *27*, *Suppl. 1*, 197.
38. Bradley C (1979): Psychophysiological effects of stressful experiences and the management of diabetes mellitus. In: *Research in Psychology and Medicine*, *Vol 1*, p. 133. Editors: D.J. Oborne, M.M. Gruneberg and J.R. Eiser. Academic Press, London.
39. Bradley C (1982): Psychophysiological aspects of the management of diabetes mellitus. *Int. J. Ment. Health*, *11*, 117.
40. Pennebaker JW, Cox DJ, Gonder-Frederick L, Wunsch MG, Evans WS, Pohl S (1981): Physical symptoms related to blood glucose in insulin dependent diabetics. *Psychosom. Med.*, *43*, 489.
41. Cox DJ, Gonder-Frederick L, Pohl S, Pennebaker JW (1983): Reliability of symptom-blood glucose relationships among insulin-dependent adult diabetics. *Psychosom. Med.*, *45*, 357.
42. Brener J, Jones JM (1974): Interoceptive discrimination in intact humans: detection of cardiac activity. *Physiol. Behav.*, *13*, 763.
43. Cinciripini PM, Epstein LH, Martin LE (1979): The effects of feedback on blood pressure discrimination. *J. Appl. Behav. Anal.*, *12*, 345.
44. Lansky D, Nathan PE, Lawson DM (1978): Blood alcohol level discrimination by alcoholics: the role of internal and external cues. *J. Consult. Clin. Psychol.*, *46*, 953.
45. Gross AM, Wojnilower DA, Levin RB, Dale J, Richardson P, Davidson PC (1983): Discrimination of blood glucose levels in insulin-dependent diabetics. *Behav. Modif.*, *7*, 369.
46. Cox DJ, Pennebaker JW, Pohl S, Gonder-Frederick L (1983): Blood glucose determination training with insulin dependent adult diabetics. Paper presented at: The Association for the Advancement of Behavior Therapy, Washington.
47. Bradley C, Moses JL, Gillespie CR (1983): An examination of the possibilities of continuous blood glucose monitoring with minimal blood sampling. *Diabetes*, *32*, 171A.
48. Shapiro J, Wigg D, Charles MA, Perley M (1984): Personality and family profiles of chronic insulin-dependent diabetic patients using portable insulin infusion pump therapy: a preliminary investigation. *Diabetes Care*, *7*, 137–142.

49. Seigler DE, La Greca A, Citrin WS, Reeves ML, Skyler JS (1982): Psychological effects of intensification of diabetic control. *Diabetes Care, 5, Suppl. 1*, 19.
50. Rudolf MC, Ahern JA, Genel M, Bates S, Harding P, Hochstadt J, Quinlan D, Tamborlane WH (1982): Optimal insulin delivery in adolescents with diabetes: impact of intensive treatment on psychosocial adjustment. *Diabetes Care, 5, Suppl. 1*, 53.
51. Jacobson AM, Leibovich JB (1984): Psychological issues in diabetes mellitus. *Psychosomatics, 25*, 7.
52. Rodin GM (1983): Psychosocial aspects of diabetes mellitus. *Can. J. Psychiatry, 28*, 219.
53. Lustman PJ, Skor DA, Carney RM, Santiago JV, Cryer PE (1983): Stress and diabetic control. *Lancet, 1*, 588.
54. Cahill GF (1983): Diabetes control and complications. *Diabetes Care, 6*, 310.
55. Ward JD (1984): Continuous subcutaneous insulin infusion (CSII): therapeutic options. *Diabetic Med., 1*, 47.
56. Johnson SB (1980): Psychosocial factors in juvenile diabetes: a review. *J. Behav. Med., 3*, 95.
57. Robinson N, Fuller JH (1984): Severe life events and their relationship to the aetiology of insulin dependent (Type 1) diabetes mellitus. *Diabetic Med., 1*, 140A.
58. Grant I, Kyle GC, Teichman A, Mendels J (1974): Recent life events and diabetes in adults. *Psychosom. Med., 36*, 121.
59. Bradley C (1979): Life events and the control of diabetes mellitus. *J. Psychosom. Res., 23*, 159.
60. Watts FN (1980): Behavioural aspects of the management of diabetes mellitus: education, self-care and metabolic control. *Behav. Res. Ther., 18*, 171.
61. Lustman P, Carney R, Amado H (1981): Acute stress and metabolism in diabetes. *Diabetes Care, 4*, 658.
62. Cox T (1978): *Stress*. Macmillan, London.
63. Turkat ID (1982): Glycosylated haemoglobin levels in anxious and non anxious diabetic patients. *Psychosomatics, 23*, 1056.
64. Fowler JE, Budzynski TH, VandenBergh RL (1976): Effects of an EMG biofeedback relaxation program on the control of diabetes: a case study. *Biofeedback Self-regul., 1*, 105.
65. Seeburg KN, DeBoer KF (1980): Effects of EMG biofeedback on diabetes. *Biofeedback Self-regul., 5*, 289.
66. Surwit RS, Feinglos MN (1983): The effects of relaxation on glucose tolerance in non-insulin-dependent diabetes. *Diabetes Care, 6*, 176.
67. Surwit RS (1983): Stress, relaxation and the behavioural control of blood glucose. Paper presented at: The Association for the Advancement of Behavior Therapy, Washington.
68. Bradley C (1983): Evaluation of the use of relaxation techniques in the management of insulin requiring diabetes mellitus (abstract). *Biol. Psychol.*, in press.
69. Lehman TP, Jacobs JA (1983): Etiology of diabetic impotence. *J. Urol., 129*, 291.
70. Bancroft J (1982): Erectile impotence – psyche or soma? *Int. J. Androl., 5*, 353.

71. Fairburn CG, Wu FCW, McCulloch DK, Borsey DQ, Ewing DJ, Clarke BF, Bancroft JHJ (1982): The clinical features of diabetic impotence: a preliminary study. *Br. J. Psychiatry*, *140*, 447.
72. Martin LM (1981): Impotence in diabetes: an overview. *Psychosomatics*, *22*, 318.
73. Smith BC (1982): Sexual counselling of diabetic impotence. *Patient Couns. Health Educ.*, *4*, 10.
74. Graber AL, Christman BG, Alogna MT, Davidson JK (1977): Evaluation of diabetes patient-education programs. *Diabetes*, *26*, 61.
75. Epstein LH, Figueroa J, Farkas GM, Beck S (1981): The short-term effects of feedback on accuracy of urine glucose determinations in insulin dependent diabetic children. *Behav. Ther.*, *12*, 560.
76. Epstein LH, Beck S, Figueroa J, Farkas G, Kazdin AE, Daneman D, Becker D (1981): The effects of targeting improvements in urine glucose on metabolic control in children with insulin dependent diabetes. *J. Appl. Behav. Anal.*, *14*, 365.
77. Carney RM, Schecter K, Davis T (1983): Improving adherence to blood glucose testing in insulin-dependent diabetic children. *Behav. Ther.*, *14*, 247.
78. Wing RR (1983): Behaviour weight control for obese type 2 diabetics. Paper presented at: The Association for the Advancement of Behavior Therapy, Washington.
79. Abel G (1983): Behavioural treatment for organic impotence. Paper presented at: The Association for the Advancement of Behavior Therapy, Washington.

The Diabetes Annual/1
K.G.M.M. Alberti and L.P. Krall, editors

ISBN 0444 90 343 7
$0.85 per article per page (transactional system)
$0.20 per article per page (licensing system)

22 Insulin secretion in vitro

JEAN-CLAUDE HENQUIN

Insulin secretion is the outcome of a precise sequence of complex events triggered in B-cells by appropriate secretagogues. Numerous studies published nowadays focus on certain steps of that sequence. Therefore, this review will not be restricted to the narrow limits implied by its title, but will try to cover various aspects of the stimulus-secretion coupling in B-cells. Several topics have been selected for their importance or novelty, selection being dictated in part by space constraints. Certain areas are therefore ignored. In particular the studies using pancreatic tissue from animal models (diabetic, newborn, aged, fasted or partially pancreatectomized), the effects of cytotoxic drugs on the B-cell function and the studies of insulin synthesis and degradation are not covered. An extensive multi-authored review on the stimulus-secretion coupling in B-cells appeared in *Experientia* in October 1984.

Studies on the B-cell function have always been hampered by the limited amount of islet tissue available and by the cellular heterogeneity of islets. During the last two years, increasing efforts have been made to obviate these difficulties. Several types of islet tumors have been used as rich sources of B-cells, but particular interest has been paid to a transplantable rat insulinoma originally induced by X-ray irradiation (1). Cell suspensions or fragments of the tumor failed to release insulin in response to glucose, but a small effect was observed with leucine, glucagon or methylxanthines (2, 3). When the tumor was transplanted under the kidney capsule and the tumor-bearing kidney perfused, insulin secretion could be evoked by glucose, glyceraldehyde or ketoisocaproate (4). However, even under these optimal conditions, high concentrations of the stimulators were required and a paradoxical greater responsiveness to ketoisocaproate than to glucose was observed. Clonal cell lines derived from the same tumor have also been established and certain subclones were found to contain and to release insulin almost exclusively (5). In the most widely used clone (RINm5F), several agents, including glyceraldehyde, increased insulin secretion by 50–100%, but were less effective than a rise of extracellular K^+ (6, 7). In one study, glucose marginally augmented release (by 50%) and its effect was already maximal at the low concentration of 1.4 mmol/l (6). It is thus evident that the parent tumor and the clones derived from it display many abnormal features. Extrapolation of results obtained with these model tissues to the normal B-cell must be made with caution. Human B-cell clones have also been established, which seem to release insulin in response to physiological concentrations of glucose (8).

Separation of the different islet cell types has been achieved in several laboratories by counterflow elutriation (9), by light-scatter flow cytometry (10, 11) or by fluorescence-activated cell sorting (12). The most refined technique has taken advantage of the influence of glucose on the fluorescence of endogenous flavine and nicotinamide adenine dinucleotides to obtain homogenous populations of functionally responsive B-cells (13). Immediately after sorting, B-cell suspensions had a high basal insulin release and did not respond to several secretagogues (11). After 1 day of culture, glucose slightly increased insulin secretion by single B-cells (10, 14); this effect was improved when B-cells were coupled, but remained considerably smaller than in intact islets (14). After 4 days of culture, the insulin-releasing ability of these isolated B-cells was considered to be similar to that of whole islets (11), but it should be noted that the function of the reference islets was clearly impaired by the culture. In contrast to these alterations of insulin release, glucose metabolism was found to be similar in whole islets and in single or reaggregated B-cells (15). Most of these observations suggest that the control of insulin secretion in the intact islet depends on a functional cooperation between B-cells, and perhaps also between B- and non-B-cells.

In this respect, it has been convincingly shown that, in the isolated dog pancreas, somatostatin and glucagon could respectively inhibit and stimulate insulin release at concentrations lower than those present in the pancreatic vein (16). This means that the hormones secreted by the D- and A-cells are unlikely to come in direct contact with their corresponding receptors on the neighboring B-cells. Evidence has also been provided that glucose-induced insulin release by the perfused pancreas is not altered by selective suppression of somatostatin release (17). All these observations cast serious doubts on the physiological relevance of experiments using isolated islets or cultured cells to demonstrate, with antisomatostatin or antiglucagon serum, the paracrine control of insulin secretion.

Islet metabolism

Two laboratories have pursued a detailed investigation of the intricate regulation of glucose metabolism in islet cells. Glucokinase, the enzyme thought to catalyze glucose phosphorylation with a low affinity for the hexose, has been purified from islet and insulinoma cells (18–20). Its characteristics match well the features of glucose and mannose usage by the islets, with the restriction that phosphorylation of the sugars occurs with somewhat lower Km values than expected. Particularly important for hexose metabolism is the higher affinity of glucokinase for the α- than for the β-anomers of glucose and mannose. The conclusion of these investigations (18–20) is that glucokinase may be the glucose-sensor in B-cells. Other studies (21, 22) have discovered that glucose increases the islet content of fructose-2,6-bisphosphate and glucose-1,6-bisphosphate, two powerful activators of phosphofructokinase. Though the increase appears to be simply due to a greater availability of fructose-6-phosphate, the concentration of both activators is sufficient to play a physiological role. It may seem difficult to ascribe the anomeric discrimination of glucose metabolism to phosphofructokinase since it is specific for β-fructose-6-phosphate. However, one of the activators, glucose-1,6-bisphosphate, is formed by the α-stereospecific phosphoglucomutase (23). Obviously the idea that glucokinase functions as the pacemaker of glycolysis in islets is attractive by its simplicity, but the importance of the activators of phosphofructokinase should certainly not be neglected.

The uncertainty as to whether neutral amino acids and 2-keto-acids stimulate insulin release through activation of stereospecific receptors or through their catabolism in B-cells has prompted numerous sophisticated and polemic studies. To make a long story short, it will simply be mentioned that agreement seems imminent (24–28). The effects of leucine, of a non-metabolized analogue, of other neutral amino acids and of various keto-acids can be ascribed either to their own catabolism in B-cells or to their ability to stimulate the catabolism of an exogenous substrate or an endogenous nutrient. Furthermore, it was clearly demonstrated (29) that the catabolism of these endogenous nutrients, in particular amino and fatty acids, substantially contributes to the respiration of the islets, not only in the absence, but also in the presence of physiological concentrations of glucose.

Attention was also paid to the effect of ketone bodies and cationic amino acids. Ketone bodies potentiate insulin release, but the mechanism of this effect remains unclear as it does not correlate well with their rate of oxidation in islet cells (30). Besides arginine, several cationic amino acids induce a Ca-dependent insulin release in the absence or presence of glucose. Their effect is ascribed to the depolarization of the B-cell membrane, which results from their transport as positively charged molecules (31).

Links between metabolism and ionic fluxes

A few years ago, several lines of evidence suggested that a fall in B-cell pH and/or an increased production of reduced nicotinamide nucleotides could be important coupling factors between glucose metabolism and the changes in ionic permeabilities in B-cells. The alterations of glucose-induced electrical activity in B-cells by changes in extracellular Cl^- or HCO_3^- concentrations and by inhibitors of the membrane systems that regulate cellular pH in other tissues have been investigated. Two studies (32, 33) agreed in their conclusion that the increase in electrical activity occurring when the concentration of glucose is raised could be due to the decrease of membrane K^+ permeability caused by a fall in B-cell pH. This interpretation is difficult to reconcile with the evidence, obtained by two different techniques, that glucose does not decrease, but increases the overall pH in islet cells (34, 35). Nevertheless, these techniques do not permit one to rule out that the B-cell pH is heterogeneous and there is little doubt that elucidation of the pH regulatory mechanisms in B-cells will add much to our understanding of the stimulus-secretion coupling. It should also be pointed out that there is, as yet, no evidence that the rise in B-cell pH is important for initiation of insulin release. Thus, omission of extracellular HCO_3^- and CO_2 increases cellular pH (35), but has long been known to depress glucose-induced insulin secretion.

Further support for a role of reduced nicotinamide nucleotides and glutathione in insulin release has been provided (36, 37). These agents could control ionic permeability in B-cells by regulating the thiol:disulfide balance in the plasma membrane. Such a mechanism requires a more reduced state of cytosolic redox couples, and that this occurs during glucose stimulation has been confirmed. Furthermore, aminooxyacetate, an agent which may inhibit the transfer of reducing equivalents from mitochondria to cytosol, impairs the glucose effects on K^+ and Ca^{2+} permeabilities and on insulin release (38). An alternative hypothesis makes of the B-cell mitochondria the primary site of control (39). It proposes that the H^+ supply to the respiratory chain regulates insulin secretion by modulating Ca^{2+} influx into and Ca^{2+} efflux from the mitochondria.

The possible role of mitochondria can also be envisaged from another viewpoint. Thus, it has been confirmed that phosphoenolpyruvate inhibits Ca accumulation by islet mitochondria and further it was shown that this could result from its interaction with the mitochondrial adenine nucleotide translocase (40). Other studies with mitochondria isolated from an insulinoma suggest, however, that the effect of phosphoenolpyruvate is nonspecific (41), and question the possibility that the glycolytic intermediate serves as a physiological means to mobilize intracellular Ca^{2+} during glucose stimulation.

Measurements of $^{86}Rb^+$ efflux from perifused islets prompted the suggestion (42) that glucose increases the Ca^{2+}-sensitive K^+ permeability in B-cells, and does not decrease it as was proposed previously. However, the conclusion may be premature, in particular since extrapolation from ionic fluxes to permeabilities cannot be adequately made without taking the variations in membrane potential into account (43). It has also been shown (44) that the glucose inhibition of $^{86}Rb^+$ efflux from the islets is biphasic. Whether this time-course bears particular significance for the biphasic release of insulin is still unsettled. Finally, the sodium pump of B-cells has been studied with microelectrode techniques: its electrogenic properties have been characterized and its potential role during glucose stimulation clarified (45).

Calcium – calmodulin – magnesium

Two elegant studies (46, 47) have attempted to measure the concentration of cytosolic free Ca^{2+} in clonal insulin-secreting cells (RINm5F) with the fluorescent Ca^{2+} indicator Quin 2. Both estimated a resting Ca^{2+} concentration of about 0.1 μmol/l and showed a verapamil-inhibitable increase in cytosolic Ca^{2+} upon depolarization with high K^+. One report (47) further demonstrated that glyceraldehyde, a weak stimulator of release in these cells, caused an increase in cellular free Ca^{2+}. This observation thus provides support to the idea that certain secretagogues at least trigger insulin release by raising free Ca^{2+} in B-cells. The other report (46) showed that a low concentration of glucose (4 mmol/l) lowered cytosolic Ca^{2+} by about 20%. One could interpret this change as an abnormal feature of these clonal cells, which do not release insulin in response to glucose. The authors favor the alternative explanation that a physiological effect of glucose is to increase calcium sequestration by B-cell organelles. Other data obtained with islets in the same laboratory (48–50) indirectly support that interpretation. Such an effect of glucose would not necessarily exclude that Ca^{2+} triggers exocytosis, but would imply that Ca^{2+} influx has a predominant role.

Much interest has been focused on the mechanisms, besides the Na^+/Ca^{2+} exchange, which contribute to calcium homeostasis in islet cells. Convincing evidence has been presented (51) that a plasma membrane calmodulin-activated Ca^{2+}-ATPase with a high affinity for Ca^{2+} could represent a Ca^{2+}-extrusion pump, able to maintain low levels of free Ca^{2+} in resting B-cells. Endoplasmic reticulum (51, 52) and mitochondria (41) do not seem able to buffer Ca^{2+} at a submicromolar level, but one cannot exclude that they play a role during stimulation. The importance of a mobile Ca^{2+} pool in insulin granules has also been underlined (53–55).

Different laboratories have shown that islet (56–58) and insulinoma (59, 60) cells contain Ca^{2+}-calmodulin-activated protein kinases, which phosphorylate several endogenous proteins. The potential importance of certain of these phosphorylations for insulin release is indicated by a glucose-stimulation in whole islets (58). Identification of the protein kinases and of their substrates is still fragmentary. The best characterized is a myosin light-chain kinase (57, 59), that could phosphorylate myosin during B-cell stimulation, and thereby permit interaction with actin and microfilament contraction. The α and β subunits of tubulin (58) and intermediate filaments of the cytokeratin type (61) are other possible sites of phosphorylation by a calmodulin-dependent protein kinase. It has also been proposed that calmodulin modulates the interaction between insulin granules and the inner face of the plasma membrane (62). Such an effect would be compatible with the phosphorylation of a protein on the granule membrane (63). Finally, preliminary evidence suggests that carboxymethylation of calmodulin (and of other islet proteins) could be involved in the regulation of insulin secretion (64).

A marked influence of glucose on Mg^{2+} fluxes in islet cells has been reported (65). The sugar alters both uptake and efflux of the cation (65), but does not affect total magnesium content of the islets (53). The significance of these changes for stimulus-secretion coupling is still unclear.

Cyclic AMP

The small increase in cAMP brought about by glucose in islet cells has been ascribed to activation of adenylate cyclase by Ca^{2+}-calmodulin. Such an effect was indeed confirmed in rat islets, but could not be observed in mouse islets (66). Since inhibitors of calmodulin do not prevent the effect of glucose on islet cAMP, the mechanisms underlying the glucose stimulation may require reevaluation.

The characteristics of cAMP-dependent protein kinases in islet cells have been established several years ago. It has now been shown that cAMP itself or agents raising cAMP levels induce phosphorylation of a large number of islet proteins (56, 60, 67, 68). One of them has been identified as histone H3 (68), but none of these phosphorylations could as yet be directly related to insulin release.

It has long been considered that cAMP contributes to the rise in cytosolic Ca^{2+} in B-cells exclusively by an effect on calcium stores. However, in agreement with earlier reports, the nucleotide did not exert any effect on Ca^{2+} sequestration by insulinoma mitochondria (41) or by endoplasmic reticulum from islet cells (52). On the other hand, electrophysiological experiments (69, 70) suggested that cAMP augments glucose-induced Ca^{2+} influx in B-cells. Some of these data (70) were obtained with forskolin, an agent which stimulates the adenylate cyclase, and was shown to increase cAMP levels and insulin release in islets (71). These results do not question, however, the notion that cAMP is a potentiator and not an initiator of insulin release.

Phospholipids, arachidonic acid metabolites, protein kinase C

Recent years have seen a marked revival of interest in phospholipid metabolism in pancreatic islets. There is general agreement that glucose and cholinergic agents accelerate phospholipid turnover in islet cells, but the consensus is less complete for several other secretagogues. Both breakdown and synthesis of phospholipids (or resynthesis after breakdown) have been measured (72–78). All studies but one (76) agree that this increased metabolism mainly involves phosphatidylinositol (PI), and particular attention has been paid to the small but probably crucial fraction of polyphosphoinositides (78). This PI turnover is neither necessary nor sufficient to initiate insulin release (73, 77). Its rapidity and time course appear different depending on the experimental design, on the stimulus and on the parameter measured (73–76, 78). PI turnover in islets is decreased in the absence of Ca^{2+}. However, differences in its Ca^{2+}-dependency and in the effect of Ca^{2+}-ionophores have led to variable conclusions. Certain authors consider that initiation of the PI cycle is secondary to the influx of Ca^{2+} or at least to the rise in cellular Ca^{2+} (73, 77, 78). Others (74, 75) acknowledge that one step is Ca^{2+}-dependent, but do not believe that the whole phenomenon is triggered by Ca^{2+} influx. From one of these latter papers (74), it appears that glucose stimulation of PI turnover is much more Ca^{2+}-dependent than the effect of carbamylcholine. This may indicate differences in the nature or in the importance of the phenomenon triggered by two types of secretagogue. It is also important to underline that the subcellular location of the phenomenon is still unsettled. Part of it could occur at intracellular sites rather than in the plasma membrane (79).

Other roles can be envisaged for the PI cycle than the control of Ca^{2+} fluxes. Phospholipid breakdown can release arachidonic acid, which may be metabolized by the cyclooxygenase or the lipoxygenase pathways (76, 80, 81). Glucose causes a rapid release of prostaglandins from the islets (76), but an effect of the sugar on the lipoxygenase pathway has not yet been demonstrated. Exogenous arachidonate increases insulin release (80, 82) and this effect is blocked by inhibitors of the lipoxygenase, but not of the cyclooxygenase pathway. Most of the available evidence is compatible with an inhibitory role of cyclooxygenase products and a stimulatory role of lipoxygenase products, even if certain of these latter can also inhibit secretion (81–83). The release of arachidonic acid has been attributed to a phospholipase A_2, the activity of which increases in glucose-stimulated islets (84). Other studies using inhibitors of the enzyme (mepacrine and p-bromophenacylbromide) have yielded variable results, and adequate controls for the specificity of the effects observed were not provided. The role of a phospholipase A_2 has been challenged (85) and the production of non-esterified arachidonic acid ascribed to the sequential involvement of a phospholipase C and a diacylglycerol lipase.

The activity of a phospholipase C generates diacylglycerol, which might also activate the Ca^{2}- and phospholipid-dependent protein kinase C present in islets as in many other tissues (72). The role of this protein kinase is still unclear, but it could be important for insulin secretion. Thus, protein kinase C is currently considered as a possible receptor protein for tumor-promoting phorbol esters, substances which stimulate insulin release (86–88). The insulinotropic effect of these phorbol esters has also been attributed to an activation of a phospholipase A_2 (86), but the evidence provided was only indirect. On the basis of experiments using a Ca^{2+}-ionophore and a phorbol ester, an attractive model has been proposed (88), which suggests that the first phase of insulin release is due to activation of the Ca^{2+}-calmodulin system, whereas the second phase results mainly from activation of the protein kinase C system.

Insulin granules: characteristics – release – functions

Careful studies have demonstrated that insulin granules possess an inwardly directed, electrogenic, proton-translocating ATPase, the activity of which brings about a difference in membrane potential (inside positive) and lowers intragranular pH to 5–6 (89). These characteristics make a chemiosmotic lysis of the granules (by accumulation of anions and solutes) a possible mechanism for the exocytotic release of insulin. Inhibition of glucose-stimulated secretion by hypertonic solutions, by omission of extracellular Cl^- and by inhibitors of anion transport has been confirmed (90) and thus supports the participation of such a process. However, evidence has been presented (91) that the stimulatory effect of other secretagogues does not exhibit the same Cl^- requirement and that omission of the anion has other effects on B-cell function.

Studies from two laboratories (92, 93) have shown that the pool of insulin granules is not homogenous in the islets. Newly synthesized insulin may be released preferentially to older stored insulin, but the proportions vary with the experimental conditions. Glucose even appears to mark for immediate release insulin granules that are being formed (94). The mechanism of this marking is still unknown, but it is unlikely to involve a change in the granule content, since B-cells appear to release insulin granules at a rate independent of the physicochemical nature of their content (95). It is not clear yet whether this heterogeneity reflects distinct populations of B-cells or distinct populations of granules within each B-cell.

A new function of secretory granules has been proposed. They could transfer somatostatin receptors to the B-cell surface (96), by a mechanism that requires contact between granule and plasma membranes, but not necessarily fission of the granule (and thus insulin release) (97). Experiments evaluating whether the susceptibility of insulin release to somatostatin inhibition varies with the apparent number of receptors will be necessary to ascertain the significance of these observations. Glucose also seems to increase specific binding of muscarinic agonists to islet cells (98), but this change occurs only after several days of culture. Finally, it has been reported that during exocytosis insulin molecules are included in the plasma membrane of B-cells, where they can be recognized by an anti-insulin serum (99). The significance of the phenomenon is completely unknown.

Hypoglycemic and hyperglycemic sulphonamides

It is widely accepted that hypoglycemic sulphonamides stimulate insulin release by facilitating Ca^{2+} influx in B-cells, but the underlying mechanisms are still debated. One hypothesis suggests that they function as Ca^{2+} ionophores, and studies with artificial membrane models have been published in support of that proposal (100). However, experiments from another laboratory have failed to disclose any ionophoretic properties of tolbutamide and glibenclamide (101). The alternative hypothesis ascribes the insulinotropic action of sulphonamides to their ability to decrease K^+ permeability of the B-cell membrane (102). This leads to depolarization and stimulation of Ca^{2+} influx through voltage-dependent Ca-channels. Studies using depolarizing concentrations of K^+ and gliclazide have lent support to that proposal (103). It has also been suggested that in the presence of stimulatory concentrations of glucose, sulphonamides promote Ca^{2+} influx through another pathway (104). As this pathway is very sensitive to verapamil, it would be hazardous to rule out that it corresponds to voltage-dependent Ca-channels. The effect of tolbutamide on the ionic content of single B-cells has been estimated by energy-dispersive X-ray analysis (105). A sharp and transient rise in Ca content was observed without a preceding change in K content. This does not invalidate the second hypothesis. Thus, the depolarization of the B-cell membrane is due to a decrease in K^+ permeability (102) and not at all to an increase in K content as was wrongly discussed (105). Since K^+ influx is also inhibited by tolbutamide (102), no increase in K content must even be expected.

The mechanism whereby diazoxide inhibits insulin secretion has long remained elusive. An interference with islet mitochondrial glycerophosphate-dehydrogenase has been proposed (106). Such an effect could not be confirmed, but inhibition of islet succinate-dehydrogenase has been suggested as an alternative possibility (107). However, this mechanism is unlikely to mediate the effects of diazoxide on insulin release, since tolbutamide also inhibits the enzyme and the effects of both drugs are additive. On the other hand, it has been shown that diazoxide increases K^+ permeability of the B-cell membrane; this leads to hyperpolarization and inhibition of Ca^{2+} influx (102). This mode of action is in complete agreement with the reversal of all diazoxide effects by tolbutamide (102) and with the stimulus-selectivity of its inhibitory effects (108).

Epinephrine – opioid peptides

It has been known for almost 20 years that epinephrine inhibits insulin secretion, but the underlying mechanisms are still unclear. The type of α-adrenergic receptor on islet cells has been characterized with radioligands and found to be of the α_2-subtype (109). Several studies using various agonists and antagonists indeed confirmed that the inhibition of insulin release results from activation of α_2-receptors (110–113). As in many other tissues, α_2-adrenergic agonists inhibited adenylate cyclase in islet cells and the inhibition of insulin release was attributed to the fall in cAMP concentration (110). However, other effects are likely to be important too, since the releasing effect of dibutyryl-cAMP was also inhibited (111). Electrophysiological studies have shown that concentrations of epinephrine sufficient to abolish insulin release altered, but did not suppress glucose-induced electrical activity in B-cells (114, 115). The proposal (115) that epinephrine increases Ca-dependent K^+ permeability in B-cells is probably not correct because this is a typical α_1-effect and because epinephrine was found to decrease and not to increase Rb^+ efflux from islet cells (112). On the other hand, the possibility, already suggested several years ago, that activation of α_2-receptors somehow favors intracellular Ca^{2+} buffering would be compatible with the observed changes in membrane potential and ionic fluxes (112, 114).

Opioid peptides (enkephalins, α-endorphin and dynorphin) failed to initiate insulin release, but potentiated the effect of glucose or glyceraldehyde (116–118), by mechanisms which may involve both a rise in cAMP levels and an increase in Ca^{2+} uptake (116, 117). The effects of these various peptides appear to be mediated by distinct types of opiate receptors.

References

1. Chick WL, Warren S, Chute RN, Like AA, Lauris V, Kitchen KC (1977): A transplantable insulinoma in the rat. *Proc. Natl. Acad. Sci. USA*, *74*, 628.
2. Sopwith AM, Hutton JC, Naber SP, Chick WL, Hales CN (1981): Insulin secretion by a transplantable rat islet cell tumor. *Diabetologia*, *21*, 224.
3. Masiello P, Wollheim CB, Janjic D, Gjinovci A, Blondel B, Praz GA, Renold AE (1982): Stimulation of insulin release by glucose in a transplantable rat islet cell tumor. *Endocrinology*, *111*, 2091.
4. Hoenig M, Ferguson DC, Matschinsky FM (1984): Fuel-induced insulin release in vitro from insulinomas transplanted into the rat kidney. *Diabetes*, *33*, 1.
5. Oie HK, Gazdar AF, Minna JD, Weir GC, Baylin SB (1983): Clonal analysis of insulin and somatostatin secretion and L-dopa decarboxylase expression by a rat islet cell tumor. *Endocrinology*, *112*, 1070.
6. Praz GA, Halban PA, Wollheim CB, Blondel B, Strauss AJ, Renold AE (1983): Regulation of immunoreactive-insulin release from a rat cell line (RINm5F). *Biochem. J.*, *210*, 345.
7. Bhathena SJ, Awoke S, Voyles NR, Wilkins SD, Recant L, Oie HK, Gazdar AF (1984): Insulin, glucagon, and somatostatin secretion by cultured rat islet cell tumor and its clones. *Proc. Soc. Exp. Biol. Med.*, *175*, 35.

8. Matsuba I, Narimiya M, Yamada H, Ikeda Y, Tanese T, Abe M, Ishikawa H (1981): Establishment of clonal strains secreting insulin and somatostatin from human pancreas. *Jikeikai Med. J.*, *28*, 257.
9. Pipeleers DG, Pipeleers-Marichal MA (1981): A method for the purification of single A, B and D cells and for the isolation of coupled cells from isolated rat islets. *Diabetologia*, *20*, 654.
10. Rabinovitch A, Russell T, Shienvold F, Noel J, Files N, Patel Y, Ingram M (1982): Preparation of rat islet B-cell enriched fractions by light-scatter flow cytometry. *Diabetes*, *31*, 939.
11. Fletcher DJ, McLean Grogan W, Barras E, Weir GC (1983): Hormone release by islet B cell-enriched and A and D cell-enriched populations prepared by flow cytometry. *Endocrinology*, *113*, 1791.
12. Nielsen DA, Lernmark A, Berelowitz M, Bloom GD, Steiner DF (1982): Sorting of pancreatic islet cell subpopulations by light scattering using a fluorescence-activated cell sorter. *Diabetes*, *31*, 299.
13. Van de Winkel M, Pipeleers D (1983): Autofluorescence-activated cell sorting of pancreatic islet cells: purification of insulin-containing B-cells according to glucose-induced changes in cellular redox state. *Biochem. Biophys. Res. Commun.*, *114*, 835.
14. Pipeleers D, In 't Veld P, Maes E, Van de Winkel M (1982): Glucose-induced insulin release depends on functional cooperation between islet cells. *Proc. Natl Acad. Sci. USA*, *79*, 7322.
15. Gorus FK, Malaisse WJ, Pipeleers DG (1984): Differences in glucose handling by pancreatic A- and B-cells. *J. Biol. Chem.*, *259*, 1196.
16. Kawai K, Ipp E, Orci L, Perrelet A, Unger RH (1982): Circulating somatostatin acts on the islets of Langerhans by way of a somatostatin-poor compartment. *Science*, *218*, 477.
17. Sorenson RL, Grouse LH, Elde RP (1983): Cysteamine blocks somatostatin secretion without altering the course of insulin or glucagon release. A new model for the study of islet function. *Diabetes*, *32*, 377.
18. Meglasson MD, Trueheart Burch P, Berner DK, Najafi H, Vogin AP, Matschinsky FM (1983): Chromatographic resolution and kinetic characterization of glucokinase from islets of Langerhans. *Proc. Natl Acad. Sci.*, *80*,85.
19. Meglasson MD, Matschinsky FM (1983): Discrimination of glucose anomers by glucokinase from liver and transplantable insulinoma. *J. Biol. Chem.*, *258*, 6705.
20. Meglasson MD, Schinco M, Matschinsky FM (1983): Mannose phosphorylation by glucokinase from liver and transplantable insulinoma. Cooperativity and discrimination of anomers. *Diabetes*, *32*, 1146.
21. Malaisse WJ, Malaisse-Lagae F, Sener A (1982): Glucose-induced accumulation of fructose-2,6-bisphosphate in pancreatic islets. *Diabetes*, *31*, 90.
22. Sener A, Malaisse-Lagae F, Malaisse WJ (1982): Glucose-induced accumulation of glucose-1,6-bisphosphate in pancreatic islets: its possible role in the regulation of glycolysis. *Biochem. Biophys. Res. Commun.*, *104*, 1033.
23. Malaisse-Lagae F, Sener A, Malaisse WJ (1982): Phosphoglucomutase: its role in the response of pancreatic islets to glucose epimers and anomers. *Biochimie*, *64*, 1059.
24. Lenzen S, Formanek H, Panten U (1982): Signal function of metabolism of

neutral amino acids and 2-keto acids for initiation of insulin secretion. *J. Biol. Chem.*, *257*, 6631.
25. Malaisse-Lagae F, Sener A, Garcia-Morales P, Valverde I, Malaisse WJ (1982): The stimulus-secretion coupling of amino acid-induced insulin release. Influence of a nonmetabolized analog of leucine on the metabolism of glutamine in pancreatic islets. *J. Biol. Chem.*, *257*, 3754.
26. Welsh M, Hellerström C, Andersson A (1982): Respiration and insulin release in mouse pancreatic islets. Effects of L-leucine and 2-ketoisocaproate in combination with D-glucose and L-glutamine. *Biochim. Biophys. Acta*, *721*, 178.
27. Malaisse WJ, Sener A, Welsh M, Malaisse-Lagae F, Hellerström C, Christophe J (1983): Mechanism of 3-phenylpyruvate-induced insulin release. Metabolic aspects. *Biochem. J.*, *210*, 921.
28. Lenzen S, Rustenbeck I, Panten U (1984): Transamination of 3-phenylpyruvate in pancreatic B-cell mitochondria. *J. Biol. Chem.*, *259*, 2043.
29. Malaisse WJ, Best L, Kawazu S, Malaisse-Lagae F, Sener A (1983): The stimulus-secretion coupling of glucose-induced insulin release: fuel metabolism in islets deprived of exogenous nutrient. *Arch. Biochem. Biophys.*, *224*, 102.
30. Biden TJ, Taylor KW (1983): Effects of ketone bodies on insulin release and islet-cell metabolism in the rat. *Biochem. J.*, *212*, 371.
31. Charles S, Tamagawa T, Henquin JC (1982): A single mechanism for the stimulation of insulin release and $^{86}Rb^+$ efflux from rat islets by cationic amino acids. *Biochem. J.*, *208*, 301.
32. Eddlestone GT, Beigelman PM (1983): Pancreatic β-cell electrical activity: the role of anions and the control of pH. *Am. J. Physiol.*, *244*, C188.
33. Pace CS, Tarvin JT (1983): pH Modulation of glucose-induced electrical activity in B-cells: involvement of Na/H and HCO_3/Cl antiporters. *J. Membrane Biol.*, *73*, 39.
34. Deleers M, Lebrun P, Malaisse WJ (1983): Increase in CO_3H^- influx and cellular pH in glucose-stimulated pancreatic islets. *FEBS Lett.*, *154*, 97.
35. Lindström P, Sehlin J (1984): Effect of glucose on the intracellular pH of pancreatic islet cells. *Biochem. J.*, *218*, 887.
36. Anjaneyulu K, Anjaneyulu R, Sener A, Malaisse WJ (1982): The stimulus-secretion coupling of glucose-induced insulin release. Thiol: disulfide balance in pancreatic islets. *Biochimie*, *64*, 29.
37. Ammon HPT, Hägele R, Youssif N, Eujen R, El-Amri N (1983): A possible role of intracellular and membrane thiols of rat pancreatic islets in calcium uptake and insulin release. *Endocrinology*, *112*, 720.
38. Lebrun P, Malaisse WJ, Herchuelz A (1983): Impairment by aminooxyacetate of ionic response to nutrients in pancreatic islets. *Am. J. Physiol.*, *245*, E38.
39. Panten U, Zielmann S, Langer J, Zünkler BJ, Lenzen S (1984): Regulation of insulin secretion by energy metabolism in pancreatic B-cell mitochondria. *Biochem. J.*, *219*, 189.
40. Ewart RBL, Yousufzai SYK, Bradford MW, Shrago E (1983): Rat islet mitochondrial adenine nucleotide translocase and the regulation of insulin secretion. *Diabetes*, *32*, 793.

41. Prentki M, Janjic D, Wollheim CB (1983): The regulation of extramitochondrial steady state free Ca^{2+} concentration by rat insulinoma mitochondria. *J. Biol. Chem.*, *258*, 7597.
42. Lebrun P, Malaisse WJ, Herchuelz A (1983): Activation, but not inhibition, by glucose of Ca^{2+}-dependent K^+ permeability in the rat pancreatic B-cell. *Biochim. Biophys. Acta*, *731*, 145.
43. Dawson CM, Croghan PC, Atwater I, Rojas E (1983): Estimation of potassium permeability in mouse islets of Langerhans. *Biomed. Res.*, *4*, 389.
44. Sehlin J, Freinkel N (1983): Biphasic modulation of K^+ permeability in pancreatic islets during acute stimulation with glucose. *Diabetes*, *32*, 820.
45. Henquin JC, Meissner HP (1982): The electrogenic sodium-potassium pump of mouse pancreatic B-cells. *J. Physiol.*, *322*, 529.
46. Rorsman P, Berggren PO, Gylfe E, Hellman B (1983): Reduction of the cytosolic calcium activity in clonal insulin-releasing cells exposed to glucose. *Biosci. Rep.*, *3*, 939.
47. Wollheim CB, Pozzan T (1984): Correlation between cytosolic free Ca^{2+} and insulin release in an insulin-secreting cell line. *J. Biol. Chem.*, *259*, 2262.
48. Gylfe E (1982): Glucose stimulated net uptake of Ca^{2+} in the pancreatic β-cell demonstrated with dual wavelength spectrophotometry. *Acta Physiol. Scand.*, *114*, 149.
49. Hellman B, Honkanen T, Gylfe E (1982): Glucose inhibits insulin release induced by Na^+ mobilization of intracellular calcium. *FEBS Lett.*, *148*, 289.
50. Andersson T (1983): Glucose-induced retention of intracellular ^{45}Ca in pancreatic islets. *Am. J. Physiol.*, *245*, C343.
51. Colca JR, Kotagal N, Lacy PE, McDaniel ML (1983): Comparison of the properties of active Ca^{2+} transport by the islet-cell endoplasmic reticulum and plasma membrane. *Biochim. Biophys. Acta*, *729*, 176.
52. Colca JR, Kotagal N, Lacy PE, McDaniel ML (1983): Modulation of active Ca^{2+} uptake by the islet-cell endoplasmic reticulum. *Biochem. J.*, *212*, 113.
53. Andersson T, Berggren PO, Gylfe E, Hellman B (1982): Amounts and distribution of intracellular magnesium and calcium in pancreatic β-cells. *Acta Physiol. Scand.*, *114*, 235.
54. Hutton JC, Penn EJ, Peshavaria M (1983): Low-molecular-weight constituents of isolated insulin-secretory granules. *Biochem. J.*, *210*, 297.
55. Wolters GHJ, Pasma A, Konijnendijk W (1983): Decreased response of mobile calcium in pancreatic islets of fasted rats to glucose stimulation and calcium manipulation. *Diabetes*, *32*, 235.
56. Harrison DE, Ashcroft SJH (1982): Effects of Ca^{2+}, calmodulin and cyclic AMP on the phosphorylation of endogenous proteins by homogenates of rat islets of Langerhans. *Biochim. Biophys. Acta*, *714*, 313.
57. MacDonald MJ, Kowluru A (1982): Calcium-calmodulin-dependent myosin phosphorylation by pancreatic islets. *Diabetes*, *31*, 566.
58. Colca JR, Brooks CL, Landt M, McDaniel ML (1983): Correlation of Ca^{2+}- and calmodulin-dependent protein kinase activity with secretion of insulin from islets of Langerhans. *Biochem. J.*, *212*, 819.
59. Penn EJ, Brocklehurst KW, Sopwith AM, Hales CN, Hutton JC (1982): Ca^{2+}-calmodulin dependent myosin light-chain phosphorylating activity in insulin-secreting tissues. *FEBS Lett.*, *139*, 4.

60. Schubart UK (1982): Regulation of protein phosphorylation in hamster insulinoma cells. Identification of Ca^{2+}-regulated cytoskeletal and cAMP-regulated cytosolic phosphoproteins by two-dimensional electrophoresis. *J. Biol. Chem.*, *257*, 12231.
61. Schubart UK, Fields KL (1984): Identification of a calcium regulated insulinoma cell phosphoprotein as an islet cell keratin. *J. Cell Biol.*, *98*, 1001.
62. Watkins DT, Cooperstein SJ (1983): Role of calcium and calmodulin in the interaction between islet cell secretion granules and plasma membranes. *Endocrinology*, *112*, 766.
63. Brocklehurst KW, Hutton JC (1983): Ca^{2+}-dependent binding of cytosolic components to insulin-secretory granules results in Ca^{2+}-dependent protein phosphorylation. *Biochem. J.*, *210*, 533.
64. Campillo JE, Ashcroft SJH (1982): Protein carboxymethylation in rat islets of Langerhans. *FEBS Lett.*, *138*, 71.
65. Henquin JC, Tamagawa T, Nenquin M, Cogneau M (1983): Glucose modulates Mg^{2+} fluxes in pancreatic islet cells. *Nature (London)*, *301*, 73.
66. Thams P, Capito K, Hedeskov CJ (1982): Differential effects of Ca^{2+}-calmodulin on adenylate cyclase activity in mouse and rat pancreatic islets. *Biochem. J.*, *206*, 97.
67. Suzuki S, Oka H, Yasuda H, Ikeda M, Cheng PY, Oda T (1983): Effect of glucagon and cyclic adenosine 3′,5′-monophosphate on protein phosphorylation in rat pancreatic islets. *Endocrinology*, *112*, 348.
68. Christie MR, Ashcroft SJH (1984): Cyclic AMP-dependent protein phosphorylation and insulin secretion in intact islets of Langerhans. *Biochem. J.*, *218*, 87.
69. Henquin JC, Meissner HP (1983): Dibutyryl cyclic AMP triggers Ca^{2+} influx and Ca^{2+}-dependent electrical activity in pancreatic B cells. *Biochem. Biophys. Res. Commun.*, *112*, 614.
70. Henquin JC, Schmeer W, Meissner HP (1983): Forskolin, an activator of adenylate cyclase, increases Ca^{2+}-dependent electrical activity induced by glucose in mouse pancreatic B cells. *Endocrinology*, *112*, 2218.
71. Wiedenkeller DE, Sharp GWG (1983): Effects of forskolin on insulin release and cyclic AMP content in rat pancreatic islets. *Endocrinology*, *113*, 2311.
72. Tanigawa K, Kuzuya H, Imura H, Taniguchi H, Baba S, Takai Y, Nishizuka Y (1982): Calcium-activated, phospholipid-dependent protein kinase in rat pancreatic islets of Langerhans. Its possible role in glucose-induced insulin release. *FEBS Lett.*, *138*, 183.
73. Axen KV, Schubart UK, Blake AD, Fleischer N (1983): Role of Ca^{2+} in secretagogue-stimulated breakdown of phosphatidylinositol in rat pancreatic islets. *J. Clin. Invest.*, *72*, 13.
74. Best L, Malaisse WJ (1983): Stimulation of phosphoinositide breakdown in rat pancreatic islets by glucose and carbamylcholine. *Biochem. Biophys. Res. Commun.*, *116*, 9.
75. Best L, Malaisse WJ (1983): Effects of nutrient secretagogues upon phospholipid metabolism in rat pancreatic islets. *Mol. Cell. Endocrinol.*, *32*, 205.
76. Evans MH, Pace CS, Clements RS (1983): Endogenous prostaglandin synthesis and glucose-induced insulin secretion from the adult rat pancreatic islet. *Diabetes*, *32*, 509.

77. Laychock SG (1983): Fatty acid incorporation into phospholipids of isolated pancreatic islets of the rat. Relationship to insulin release. *Diabetes*, *32*, 6.
78. Laychock SG (1983): Identification and metabolism of polyphosphoinositides in isolated islets of Langerhans. *Biochem. J.*, *216*, 101.
79. Dunlop M, Larkins RG (1984): Lipid associated calcium ionophores in islet cell plasma membrane following glucose stimulation. *Biochem. Biophys. Res. Commun.*, *118*, 601.
80. Metz S, Van Rollins M, Strife R, Fujimoto W, Robertson RP (1983): Lipoxygenase pathway in islet endocrine cells. Oxidative metabolism of arachidonic acid promotes insulin release. *J. Clin. Invest.*, *71*, 1191.
81. Yamamoto S, Ishii M, Nakadate T, Nakaki T, Kato R (1983): Modulation of insulin secretion by lipoxygenase products of arachidonic acid. Relation to lipoxygenase activity of pancreatic islets. *J. Biol. Chem.*, *258*, 12149.
82. Falck JR, Manna S, Moltz J, Chacos N, Capdevila J (1983): Epoxyeicosatrienoic acids stimulate glucagon and insulin release from isolated rat pancreatic islets. *Biochem. Biophys. Res. Commun.*, *114*, 743.
83. Metz SA, Murphy RC, Fujimoto W (1984): Effects on glucose-induced insulin secretion of lipoxygenase-derived metabolites of arachidonic acid. *Diabetes*, *33*, 119.
84. Laychock SG (1982): Phospholipase A_2 activity in pancreatic islets is calcium-dependent and stimulated by glucose. *Cell Calcium*, *3*, 43.
85. Schrey MP, Montague W (1983): Phosphatidylinositol hydrolysis in isolated guinea-pig islets of Langerhans. *Biochem. J.*, *216*, 433.
86. Yamamoto S, Nakadate T, Nakaki T, Ishii K, Kato R (1982): Tumor promoter 12-0-tetradecanoylphorbol-13-acetate-induced insulin secretion: inhibition by phospholipase A_2 and lipoxygenase-inhibitors. *Biochem. Biophys. Res. Commun.*, *105*, 759.
87. Malaisse WJ, Lebrun P, Herchuelz A, Sener A, Malaisse-Lagae F (1983): Synergistic effect of a tumor-promoting phorbol ester and a hypoglycemic sulfonylurea upon insulin release. *Endocrinology*, *113*, 1870.
88. Zawalich W, Brown C, Rasmussen H (1983): Insulin secretion: combined effects of phorbol ester and A23187. *Biochem. Biophys. Res. Commun.*, *117*, 448.
89. Hutton JC (1982): The internal pH and membrane potential of the insulin-secretory granule. *Biochem. J.*, *204*, 171.
90. Pace CS, Smith JS (1983): The role of chemiosmotic lysis in the exocytotic release of insulin. *Endocrinology*, *113*, 964.
91. Tamagawa T, Henquin JC (1983): Chloride modulation of insulin release, $^{86}Rb^+$ efflux, and $^{45}Ca^{2+}$ fluxes in rat islets stimulated by various secretagogues. *Diabetes*, *32*, 416.
92. Gold G, Landahl HD, Gishizky ML, Grodsky GM (1982): Heterogeneity and compartmental properties of insulin storage and secretion in rat islets. *J. Clin. Invest.*, *69*, 554.
93. Halban PA (1982): Differential rates of release of newly synthesized and of stored insulin from pancreatic islets. *Endocrinology*, *110*, 1183.
94. Gold G, Gishizky ML, Grodsky GM (1982): Evidence that glucose 'marks' β cells resulting in preferential release of newly synthesized insulin. *Science*, *218*, 56.

95. Halban PA (1982): Inhibition of proinsulin to insulin conversion in rat islets using arginine and lysine analogs. *J. Biol. Chem.*, *257*, 13177.
96. Draznin B, Leitner JW, Sussman KE (1982): Kinetics of somatostatin receptor. Migration in isolated pancreatic islets. *Diabetes*, *31,* 467.
97. Sussman KE, Pollard HB, Leitner JW, Nesher R, Adler J, Cerasi E (1983): Differential control of insulin secretion and somatostatin-receptor recruitment in isolated pancreatic islets. *Biochem. J.*, *214*, 225.
98. Grill V, Östenson CG (1983): Muscarinic receptors in pancreatic islets of the rat. Demonstration and dependence on long-term glucose environment. *Biochim. Biophys. Acta*, *756*, 159.
99. Kaplan DR, Colca JR, McDaniel ML (1983): Insulin as a surface marker on isolated cells from rat pancreatic islets. *J. Cell Biol.*, *97*, 433.
100. Deleers M, Gelbcke M, Malaisse WJ (1983): Transport of Pr^{3+} by hypoglycemic sulfonylureas across liposomal membranes. *FEBS Lett.*, *151*, 269.
101. Gylfe E, Hellman B (1982): Lack of Ca^{2+} ionophoretic activity of hypoglycemic sulfonylureas in excitable cells and isolated secretory granules. *Mol. Pharmacol.*, *22*, 715.
102. Henquin JC, Meissner HP (1982): Opposite effects of tolbutamide and diazoxide on $^{86}Rb^{+}$ fluxes and membrane potential in pancreatic B cells. *Biochem. Pharmacol.*, *31*, 1407.
103. Mathias PCF, Billaudel B, Malaisse WJ (1983): Comparison of the cationic and secretory response of pancreatic islets to gliclazide and/or potassium. *Res. Commun. Chem. Pathol. Pharmacol.*, *42*, 389.
104. Lebrun P, Malaisse WJ, Herchuelz A (1982): Modalities of gliclazide-induced Ca^{2+} influx into the pancreatic B-cell. *Diabetes*, *31*, 1010.
105. Kalkhoff RK, Siegesmund KA, Dragen RF (1983): Tolbutamide perifusion of rat islets. Sequential changes in calcium, phosphorus, sodium, potassium, and chlorine in single beta cells. *J. Clin. Invest.*, *72*, 478.
106. MacDonald MJ (1981): High content of mitochondrial glycerol-3-phosphate dehydrogenase in pancreatic islets and its inhibition by diazoxide. *J. Biol. Chem.*, *256*, 8287.
107. Lenzen S, Panten U (1983): Characterization of succinate dehydrogenase and α-glycerophosphate dehydrogenase in pancreatic islets. *Biochem. Med.*, *30*, 349.
108. Henquin JC, Charles S, Nenquin M, Mathot F, Tamagawa T (1982): Diazoxide and D600 inhibition of insulin release. Distinct mechanisms explain the specificity for different stimuli. *Diabetes*, *31*, 776.
109. Cherksey B, Mendelsohn S, Zadunaisky J, Altszuler N (1982): Demonstration of α_2-adrenergic receptors in rat pancreatic islets using radioligand binding. *Proc. Soc. Exp. Biol. Med.*, *171*, 196.
110. Yamazaki S, Katada T, Ui M (1982): Alpha$_2$-adrenergic inhibition of insulin secretion via interference with cyclic AMP generation in rat pancreatic islets. *Mol. Pharmacol.*, *21*, 648.
111. Nakaki T, Nakadate T, Yamamoto S, Kato R (1983): Inhibition of dibutyryl cyclic AMP-induced insulin release by alpha-2 adrenergic stimulation. *Life Sci.*, *32*, 191.
112. Tamagawa T, Henquin JC (1983): Epinephrine modifications of insulin release and of $^{86}Rb^{+}$ or $^{45}Ca^{2+}$ fluxes in rat islets. *Am. J. Physiol.*, *244*, E245.

113. Ismail NA, El-Denshary ESM, Idahl LA, Lindström P, Sehlin J, Täljedal IB (1983): Effects of alpha-adrenoceptor agonists and antagonists on insulin secretion, calcium uptake, and rubidium efflux in mouse pancreatic islets. *Acta Physiol. Scand.*, *118*, 167.
114. Cook DL, Perara E (1982): Islet electrical pacemaker response to alpha-adrenergic stimulation. *Diabetes*, *31*, 985.
115. Santana de Sa S, Ferrer R, Rojas E, Atwater I (1983): Effects of adrenaline and noradrenaline on glucose-induced electrical activity of mouse pancreatic β cell. *Q. J. Physiol.*, *68*, 247.
116. Green IC, Ray K, Perrin D (1983): Opioid peptide effects on insulin release and c-AMP in islets of Langerhans. *Horm. Metab. Res.*, *15*, 124.
117. Green IC, Perrin D, Penman E, Yaseen A, Ray K, Howell SL (1983): Effect of dynorphin on insulin and somatostatin secretion, calcium uptake, and c-AMP levels in isolated rat islets of Langerhans. *Diabetes*, *32*, 685.
118. Hermansen K (1983): Enkephalins and the secretion of pancreatic somatostatin and insulin in the dog: studies in vitro. *Endocrinology*, *113*, 1149.

The Diabetes Annual/1
K.G.M.M. Alberti and L.P. Krall, editors

ISBN 0444 90 343 7
$0.85 per article per page (transactional system)
$0.20 per article per page (licensing system)

23 C-Peptide and proinsulin

CHRISTIAN BINDER AND OLE FABER

C-PEPTIDE

The discovery of the full biosynthetic pathway of insulin from preproinsulin via proinsulin to insulin and C-peptide was in itself a major breakthrough. The demonstration of equimolar secretion of insulin and C-peptide from the B-cells made C-peptide an attractive quantity to determine with the purpose of evaluating B-cell secretion during insulin treatment. Until the occurrence of C-peptide assays this had been hampered by insulin assays being unable to discriminate between endogenous and exogenous insulin.

Further, in contrast to insulin, C-peptide is not or only to a small extent metabolized by the liver. This makes it possible with certain assumptions to obtain an estimate of the hepatic uptake of insulin from the time course of C-peptide and of insulin concentrations in peripheral plasma.

During the 1970s much work was carried out in the field. This work has recently been comprehensively reviewed (1, 2, 3). The reference lists of these reviews, together with that of the proceedings from 1978 of an international C-peptide research symposium (4), give a very complete cover of the work in the field up to the time of this review.

Methodological aspects

C-peptide and proinsulin are measured radioimmunologically. The interlaboratory differences in ranges of normal values indicate substantial differences among the assays employed. Differences are due to differences in antibodies, in labelled C-peptide, and in standard. Even the same three commercial kits did not show the same mutual correlations of the results obtained in two different laboratories (5, 6). Both works should be consulted before starting an assay. However, in the work of Van Rijn et al. (5), their Figure 1 has misleading units on the x-axis. The scales are logarithmic, and the figures should be 0.3, 1, 10, and 30 ng/ml for the Byk-kit and for the Behringwerke-kit, but 0.03, 0.1, 1.0, and 3.0 ng/ml for the Novo-kit (7).

The instability of C-peptide reactivity in plasma during storage and preventive measures has recently been re-emphasized (8).

There is a great need for an international standardization of C-peptide assays, also because C-peptide measurements are increasingly used in the classification of different types of diabetes mellitus.

The considerable variation in reference ranges of fasting C-peptide (9) is partly due to lack of standardization of assay. However, in normal persons fasting C-peptide correlated significantly with both fasting plasma glucose ($r = 0.312$, $N = 928$) and ideal body weight ($r = 0.438$), where the effect of age was small (9).

The use of urinary C-peptide as an indicator of B-cell secretion under different metabolic conditions has recently had much attention (10–19). About 4% of the total amount secreted per day is found in the urine. Renal clearance is about 16 ml/min, with an increase after a meal (11). There is general agreement about plasma levels correlating with urinary C-peptide. In group comparisons urinary C-peptide seems as sensitive a variable as plasma C-peptide. However, in a comparative study of the intrapatient variation of fasting C-peptide, of the response to glucagon, and of 24-hour excretion of C-peptide in 30 patients with Type 2 diabetes, the following mean relative differences between two consecutive measurements were: 11, 15, and 19% respectively (20). These figures are of the same order of magnitude as the individual figures published by Hoogwerf and Goetz (17).

Twenty-four-hour integrated plasma C-peptide concentrations showed a good correlation with corresponding values of a subsequent day ($r = 0.76$) and with the 24-hour urinary C-peptide content of the same day ($R_s = 0.66$) (12). However, if one calculates the correlation between subsequent 24-hour urinary C-peptide excretions the R_s value is only 0.037.

In conclusion, urinary C-peptide seems to be an acceptable measure of B-cell function, but with a greater intrapatient variability than that of other C-peptide measurements evaluated so far.

B-cell function tests

The differentiation between insulin dependence and non-insulin dependence is made on clinical grounds. Weight loss and proneness to ketosis are clear indicators of insulin dependence. However, in stable-weight patients – normal weight or obese – the physician is frequently in doubt whether the lack of metabolic control is due to low patient compliance or to shortage of endogenous insulin. If the hyperglycemia is caused primarily by insulin resistance as in obesity, insulin treatment may accelerate obesity or hamper weight loss. On the other hand, in cases of decreased insulin secretion a postponement of insulin therapy may accelerate the appearance of diabetic complications.

Recent publications have used basal C-peptide and its response to certain stimuli to predict insulin dependence. The validation of such tests depends critically on the criteria of treatment effects, i.e. the outcome of the various treatment regimens should be based upon defined clinical and biochemical criteria of metabolic control, and compliance with treatment should be carefully monitored. In the case of discontinuation of insulin therapy this should preferably be done under ward conditions.

In a study to test these propositions (21), the maximal C-peptide concentration during an oral glucose tolerance test and an intravenous glucagon test was assessed in obese diabetic patients treated with insulin for years on questionable grounds. Eleven of the 16 patients studied had their insulin discontinued under strict control. Five groups of patients were included as references for the outcome of the tests: (a) 12 non-obese and (b) 12 obese control subjects; (c) 11 non-obese, and (d) 14 obese non-insulin-dependent, and (e) 10 non-obese insulin-dependent patients with classical symptoms at onset and under treatment for at least 2 years. An absent or low response to both tests, comparable to that of the insulin-dependent group was found in 2 out of the 11 non-obese non-insulin-dependent patients. Both showed a rapid increase in plasma ketone bodies and a decrease in bicarbonate after discontinuation of insulin therapy, which had to be resumed. The remaining 9 patients exhibited an appreciable increase in C-peptide during the tests, the response being different from that of the insulin-dependent group. Discontinuation of insulin in these patients led to a slight increase in plasma ketone bodies, no overall change in quality of metabolic control, and a significant weight loss (mean 2.2 kg) during the first 4 weeks off insulin. Thus, in this small series the C-peptide response to glucagon offered a better discrimination of B-cell function than the response to oral glucose.

In another study, 59 patients between 16 and 80 years of age, insulin-treated for 0.2–30 years, and without antecedent episodes of ketoacidosis, were given an intravenous tolbutamide test with C-peptide determinations and subsequent discontinuation of insulin therapy (22). Seventeen patients rapidly developed ketosis, 18 did not, but required supplementary oral hypoglycemic agents for metabolic stabilization, whereas 24 were well controlled on diet alone. All patients with a fasting C-peptide below 1.9 ng/ml (Byk-Mallinkrodt kit; mean (and range) of normal subjects 2.21 (1.05–3.60) ng/ml) (6) needed insulin. When fasting C-peptide was $\geqslant$ 1.9 ng/ml, and the increment 5 minutes after tolbutamide was 20.4 ng/ml the diabetes could be controlled by diet and hypoglycemic drugs in 90% of the cases.

Ninety obese diabetic patients, of whom 55 were insulin-treated, were characterized by the C-peptide and insulin response to an oral glucose load (23). Patients eliciting a peak value of insulin or C-peptide of more than 40 μU/ml and/or 4.0 ng/ml (Byk-Mallinkrodt kit), respectively, were arbitrarily chosen for discontinuation of insulin. The results showed that the increment values which indicated insulin dependence were higher than 60 μU/ml for insulin and 6.0 ng/ml for C-peptide. Similar results were obtained by Rendell (24).

These data confirm earlier observations and indicate that C-peptide measurements can be used not only to delineate patients without or with minimal B-cell function, but also to assist in the other end of the clinical spectrum. However, the test must be simple, short, and convenient, and the interpretation should be possible without computer assistance. Glucagon or sulfonylurea seem the secretagogues of choice (21). The former is more physiological, and its use for the purpose most clearly defined (1, 3, 25). Metoprolol (β_1-adrenergic blocker) (26) and clonidine (27) do not seem to influence the C-peptide response to intravenous glucagon in non-insulin-dependent diabetics.

Further evaluation may even show the outcome of such testing to become part of a revised classification of diabetes mellitus. However, it should be borne in mind that the predictive value of such tests may relate only to the immediate future of the patient's B-cell function. Deterioration of metabolic control without insulin may be due to decline of B-cell function and not necessarily due to low patient compliance.

C-peptide as a quantitative measure of insulin secretion

After the equimolar biosynthesis of insulin and C-peptide in the pancreatic B-cell, the two peptides are secreted into the portal vascular bed together with small amounts of unchanged proinsulin. Before reaching the systemic circulation the peptides have to pass through the liver where approximately 50% of the insulin is extracted. As the fractional hepatic insulin extraction may vary several authors have used peripheral C-peptide concentration for calculation of the insulin secretion rate and hepatic insulin extraction. This indirect method is based on a number of assumptions that are not all adequately validated (28).

The validity of C-peptide measurements as an indicator of B-cell secretion depends on the following assumptions: (1) C-peptide and insulin are *secreted* in equimolar quantities, (2) hepatic extraction of C-peptide is negligible, and (3) the overall kinetics of C-peptide are known under the condition studied.

The equimolar secretion of C-peptide and insulin There is convincing evidence from animal experiments for insulin and C-peptide being synthesized in equimolar amounts and subsequently stored together in the secretory granules of the pancreatic B-cells. The equimolar *secretion* is, however, not definitely proven. In the original studies of C-peptide and insulin release from ^{3}H-leucine incubated rat islets, the authors suggested equimolar secretion even though the ^{3}H-leucine label of the C-peptide fraction was always lower than expected (29). In a recent study of isolated human islets the C-peptide concentration in the culture medium was approximately 10% lower than the insulin concentration over a wide range of insulin concentrations (30).

In dogs the molar ratio between C-peptide and insulin varied between

1.1 and 1.6 in samples taken directly from the portal vein (31). However, an excess of C-peptide may be expected from the study design: thus, in the superior splanchnic vein the molar ratio is approximately 3 while the ratio is supposed to be close to 1 in the pancreatico-duodenal vein. When the blood from these two veins is mixed in the portal vein, the combined molar ratio must exceed 1.

Taken together, these studies support the hypothesis of equimolar secretion. Deviation from equimolarity exceeding 10% is unlikely.

The hepatic extraction of C-peptide Recently, in the in vivo catheterized dog, Polonsky et al. (31) found the overall hepatic extraction of C-peptide indistinguishable from zero, both under basal steady-state conditions (0.3 ± 2.7%) and following stimulation of secretion by intravenous glucose (6.2 ± 4%). However, a significant C-peptide extraction was documented in 3 of the 13 dogs. This may be due to sampling artefacts resulting from streaming of C-peptide in the portal and hepatic veins. Alternatively, significant quantities of C-peptide may be extracted in some animals. Accordingly we found that the C-peptide flux across the pig liver never fell below 12% even after ligation of the hepatic artery (32). Thus, although it cannot be excluded that C-peptide is extracted in the liver, this extraction must be limited and does not seem to exceed 10%.

Kinetics of C-peptide Animal and human studies have consistently shown that the metabolic clearance of C-peptide is lower than that of insulin, and that the principal site of degradation is the kidneys. In normal fasting man the molar concentration of C-peptide is approximately 5 times higher than that of insulin (33). After B-cell stimulation the concentrations of both peptides start to increase simultaneoulsy, but the peak concentration may be observed earlier for insulin than for C-peptide (33). The peak concentration of each peptide is reached at the time when post-hepatic delivery equals degradation. This happens first to insulin because of its lower post-hepatic delivery rate and higher metabolic clearance rate. This difference in timing of the plasma concentration curves also explains the fall in the C-peptide:insulin molar ratio found after B-cell stimulation. For the same reasons insulin concentration returns to its basal level before that of C-peptide.

This implies that a given concentration of one of the peptides may correspond to various concentrations of the other depending on the time of sampling and conditions of the study. This is illustrated schematically in Figure 1. In other words, neither the peripheral venous concentration of insulin or of C-peptide nor their molar ratio, at a specific time point after B-cell stimulation, can be used as quantitative measure of insulin secretion. Kinetic models may solve this problem and have been developed (34, 35). They are currently under evaluation.

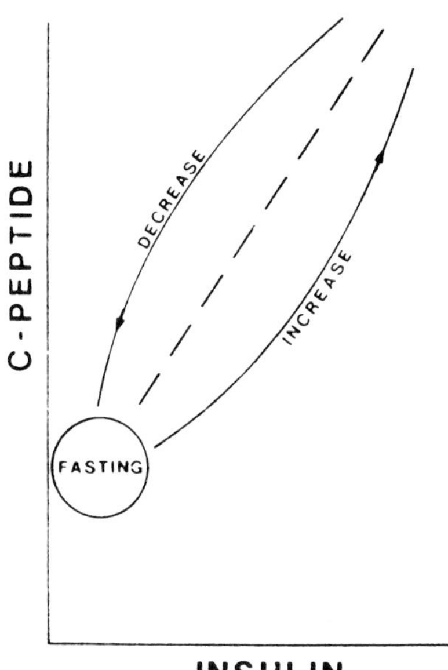

FIG. 1. *The relation between peripheral plasma concentrations of insulin and C-peptide. Due to differences in metabolic clearance, the molar C-peptide concentration will always exceed that of insulin. This also explains why the C-peptide concentration for a given insulin concentration will depend on whether the secretion from the B-cell is increasing or decreasing.*

However, insulin secretion can be evaluated from measurements of peripheral C-peptide concentrations provided the incremental area under the C-peptide curve is used for calculation. Correspondingly, the incremental area under the plasma insulin curve reflects the amount of post-hepatic insulin delivery.

Multiplied by the metabolic clearance rate the incremental area equals secretion rate. The fraction of insulin extracted in the liver is then calculated from the difference between the secreted amounts of C-peptide and insulin divided by the secreted amount of C-peptide. However, these conclusions are only valid if precise knowledge of the overall kinetics and especially of the metabolic clearance of C-peptide is established. Our present knowledge about the metabolic clearance rate of C-peptide in man is scarce because of shortage of human C-peptide. Studies have been carried out in normal subjects as well as in Type 1 diabetics, but only in the fasting state (36). Application of the results to situations other than fasting may be misleading. Furthermore, it is not known whether metabolic clearance in man is dependent on the absolute plasma C-peptide concentration. An infusion study of dog C-peptide infused into dogs (31) suggests that the metabolic clearance is constant at C-peptide concentrations encountered under normal physiological circumstances. In addition, calculations are only valid if the curves are followed until the plasma levels of the peptides return to baseline. When hepatic insulin extraction is compared under different conditions, it is also a prerequisite that the non-hepatic kinetics of the peptides are constant.

Estimation of hepatic insulin extraction based on a single determination of the peripheral concentration of C-peptide and of insulin is not advisable considering the complex relation between the two peptides. However, a sample obtained under steady-state conditions such as after overnight fasting will give useful qualitative information. Thus, estimation of hepatic insulin extraction by this non-invasive indirect method is based on several assumptions that are not all sufficiently validated. Therefore, the results obtained with this technique should be interpreted with some caution. It is, however, of interest that two recent reports both found a reduced C-peptide:insulin molar ratio in obese subjects (37, 38). This suggests that the hyperinsulinemia in obesity may be explained, at least partly, by a decreased clearance of insulin (39).

In comparative studies, where only small differences in insulin secretion are to be expected, similar or identical peripheral insulin levels do not exclude differences in insulin secretion. Thus, Miles et al. found a significant increase in peripheral plasma C-peptide, but unchanged peripheral plasma insulin concentrations in normal subjects after infusion of 3-hydroxybutyrate (40).

B-cell function and metabolic control

The effect of strict glycemic control on B-cell function was evaluated in a controlled study of 15 newly diagnosed Type 1 (IDDM) patients aged 17–37 years (41). The C-peptide response to a test meal was used as the measure of B-cell function and was assessed at 1, 7, 14, 90, and 180 days after initiation of insulin treatment. Intensive treatment was only applied for the initial 10 days after diagnosis. Five days after the end of intensive treatment this group showed a significantly higher B-cell response compared with the control group. However, the effect did not persist at 90 and 180 days. In an uncontrolled study of 10 insulin-dependent patients with longer duration and with no or absolutely minimal B-cell function no effect of 6 months of strict glycemic control was observed (42).

Residual B-cell function as expressed by fasting C-peptide in plasma was inversely and significantly correlated with HbA_{1c} in a prospective study of 131 children (43) and in a study of 27 patients with onset before the age of 30 (44). Postprandial C-peptide correlated weakly but significantly with HbA_{1c} in a study of 177 diabetic children (45). This correlation was not found in another study of 62 children (46). However, this study was retrospective with respect to clinical data which seemingly were compared to actual C-peptide measurements.

Most data favor a metabolic effect of even a minimal B-cell function. This is further supported by a recent short communication demonstrating that insulin-dependent subjects with residual B-cell function (n = 12) showed significantly higher insulin sensitivity compared with an age and sex-matched group without significant B-cell function as measured by fasting C-peptide (47).

Insulin antibodies and B-cell function

It still remains controversial whether the formation of insulin antibodies has a negative effect on B-cell function in the early phases of Type 1 diabetes. Ludvigsson (48) has exposed his data from 50 diabetic children to multiple regression analyses. Age at onset (r = 0.26) and the maximal C-peptide response to a breakfast meal (r = 0.51) were the only variables which correlated with insulin antibody concentration. However, statistical significance is not the same as a cause-and-effect relationship. It is still a hypothesis which demands a large prospective study, or animal experiments with passive transfer of insulin antibodies.

C-peptide in the brain

Previous data indicating that neural structures in the brain synthesize and secrete insulin among other peptides are further supported by the presence of immunoreactive C-peptide in the same nerve cells as insulin (49, 50).

PROINSULIN

Determination of proinsulin in biological fluids has not been widely applied because of cumbersome assay techniques with a need for large sample volumes. Therefore, specific determination of proinsulin has been carried out mostly in pathophysiological conditions characterized by high levels of circulating insulin.

The clinically most important finding was the consistent elevation of proinsulin found in insulinoma patients as emphasized by several authors. This finding has been amply verified, most recently by Heding et al. (51) who, using a highly sensitive and specific double-site radioimmunoassay, found elevated fasting proinsulin concentrations in all of 31 insulinoma patients, irrespective of the prevailing blood glucose concentration. These findings have prompted the use of proinsulin measurement in fasting plasma in patients suspect of organic hyperinsulinemia. If proinsulin is elevated, and other conditions of hyperinsulinemia like hepatic cirrhosis, kidney failure, thyrotoxicosis, obesity, and glucose intolerance have been ruled out, the patient should be strongly suspected of having an insulinoma (52). This approach is limited by a high-quality proinsulin assay not being generally available and by the unknown risk of a false negative and a false positive diagnosis.

The results of recent studies in glucose-intolerant rats (53) and in insulin-dependent diabetic children (54) both suggest an increased proinsulin secretion relative to insulin in support of the hypothesis that increased demands of insulin lead to liberation of immature B-cell granules with an increased relative proinsulin content (55). The finding of relative hyperproinsulinemia in thyrotoxicosis (56) is also in accordance with this concept. Further studies in insulin-dependent diabetic patients without circulating insulin and proinsulin antibodies are, however, needed to confirm this hypothesis.

Pronounced absolute as well as relative hyperproinsulinemia is also found in the rare cases of familial hyperproinsulinemia. These subjects are characterized by defects in the postsynthetic processing of proinsulin. The finding that this dominantly inherited defect is not associated with glucose intolerance re-emphasizes the possibility that proinsulin exerts some biological effects. With the availability of well characterized biosynthetic proinsulin it has been possible to re-examine the biological effect of proinsulin. Thus, Revers et al. (57) have recently found glucose disposal during intravenous infusion of human proinsulin to be 5–10% of that of human insulin. Details of this and of other aspects of proinsulin have recently been extensively reviewed (58).

References

1. Hoekstra JBL, Van Rijn HJM, Erkelens DW, Thijssen JHH (1982): C-peptide. *Diabetes Care*, *5*, 438.
2. Madsbad S (1983): Prevalence of residual B cell function and its metabolic consequences in type 1 (insulin-dependent) diabetes. *Diabetologia*, *24*, 141.
3. Bonser AM, Garcia-Webb P (1984): C-peptide measurement: methods and clinical utility. *CRC Crit. Rev. Clin. Lab. Sci.*, *19*, 297.
4. Binder C, Rubenstein AH (Eds) (1978): Proceedings of an International C-peptide Research Symposium, Copenhagen, 1977. *Diabetes*, *27*, *Suppl. 1*, 145.
5. Van Rijn HJM, Hoekstra JBL, Thijssen JHH (1982): Evaluation of three commercially available C-peptide kits. *Ann. Clin. Biochem.*, *19*, 368.
6. Villaume C, Beck B (1983): C-peptide comparative radioimmunoassays: a study of three commercial kits. *Ann. Biol. Clin. (Paris)*, *41*, 269.
7. Van Rijn HJM (1984): Personal communication.
8. Garcia-Webb P, Bottomley S, Bonser AM (1983): Instability of C-peptide

reactivity in plasma and serum stored at −20 °C. *Clin. Chim. Acta*, *129*, 103.

9. Garcia-Webb P, Bonser A, Whiting D (1982): Importance of fasting plasma glucose concentration and obesity in the interpretation of fasting serum C-peptide values. *Clin. Chim. Acta*, *118*, 323.
10. Landau RL, Rochman H, Blix-Gruber P, Rubenstein AH (1981): The protein-sparing action of protein feeding: absence of relationship to insulin secretion. *Am. J. Clin. Nutr.*, *34*, 1300.
11. Blix PM, Boddie-Willis C, Landau RL, Rochman H, Rubenstein AH (1982): Urinary C-peptide: an indicator of β-cell secretion under different metabolic conditions. *J. Clin. Endocrinol. Metab.*, *54*, 574.
12. Meistas MT, Rendell M, Margolis S, Kowarski AA (1982): Estimation of the secretion rate of insulin from the urinary excretion rate of C-peptide. Study in obese and diabetic subjects. *Diabetes*, *31*, 449.
13. Zick R, Hürter P, Lange P, Mitzkat HJ (1982): Die C-peptidausscheidung im 24 Std-Urin als Indikator der B-Zell-Residualfunktion bei Kindern und Jugendlichen mit Typ-I-Diabetes. *Monatsschr. Kinderheilkd.*, *130*, 209.
14. Matsuda A, Kuzuya T (1982): Urine C-peptide after recovery from diabetic ketoacidosis: an index of insulin dependency. *Diabetes Care*, *5*, 581.
15. Glatthaar C, Beaven DW, Donald RA, Smith JR, Espiner EA (1982): Residual pancreatic function in insulin dependent diabetics. *Aust. NZ J. Med.*, *12*, 43.
16. Aurbach-Klipper J, Sharph-Dor R, Heding LG, Karp M, Laron Z (1983): Residual B cell function in diabetic children as determined by urinary C-peptide. *Diabetologia*, *24*, 88.
17. Hoogwerf BJ, Goetz FC (1983): Urinary C-peptide: a simple measure of integrated insulin production with emphasis on the effects of body size, diet, and corticosteroids. *J. Clin. Endocrinol. Metab.*, *56*, 60.
18. Hoogwerf BJ, Barbosa JJ, Bantle JP, Laine D, Goetz FC (1983): Urinary C-peptide as a measure of beta-cell function after a mixed meal in healthy subjects: comparison of four-hour urine C-peptide with serum insulin and plasma C-peptide. *Diabetes Care*, *6*, 488.
19. Gero L, Korányi L, Tamás G Jr (1983): Residual B-cell function in insulin dependent (type 1) and non-insulin dependent (type 2) diabetics. (Relationship between 24-hour C-peptide excretion and the clinical features of diabetes.) *Diabète Métab.*, *9*, 183.
20. Gjessing HJ, Damsgaard EN, Frøland A, Iversen S, Binder C, Faber OK (1984): Reproducibility of the glucagon test and the 24-hour urine excretion of C-peptide as estimators of B-cell function in patients with NIDDM (Abstract). *Acta Endocrinol. (Copenhagen)*, *105*, *Suppl. 263*, 31.
21. Hoekstra JB, Van Rijn HJM, Thijssen JHH, Erkelens DW (1982): C-peptide reactivity as a measure of insulin dependency in obese diabetic patients treated with insulin. *Diabetes Care*, *5*, 585.
22. Wemeau J-L, Fourlinnie J-Cl, Beuscart R, Vaast D, Romon M, Vie M-Cl, Fossati P (1983): Le dosage du peptide C basal et en réponse au tolbutamide intraveineux dans le dépistage des insulinothérapies abusives (ou abusivement prolongées). *Rev. Méd. Intern.*, *4*, 11.
23. Turkington RW, Estkowski A, Link M (1982): Secretion of insulin or connecting peptide. A predictor of insulin dependence of obsese 'diabetics'. *Arch. Intern. Med.*, *142*, 1102.

24. Rendell M (1983): C-peptide levels as a criterion in treatment of maturity-onset diabetes. *J. Clin. Endocrinol. Metab., 57*, 1198.
25. Garcia-Webb, Bonser A, Welborn TA (1982): Correlation between fasting serum C-peptide and B cell insulin secretory capacity in diabetes mellitus. *Diabetologia*, *22*, 296.
26. Ferlito S, Del Campo F, Damante G, Di Vincenzo S, Patané M, Modica L (1983): The effect of metoprolol on blood glucose, insulin and C-peptide response to glucagon in non-insulin dependent diabetics. *Acta Ther.*, *9*, 53.
27. Ferlito S, Del Campo F, Damante G, Di Vincenzo S, Indelicato G, Raudino M (1983): Influence of clonidine on blood glucose, insulin and C-peptide response to glucagon in non-insulin dependent diabetics. *IRCS Med. Sci.*, *11*, 349.
28. Polonsky KS, Rubenstein AH (1984): C-peptide as a measure of the secretion and hepatic extraction of insulin. *Diabetes*, *33*, 485.
29. Rubenstein AH, Clark JL, Melani F, Steiner DF (1969): Secretion of proinsulin C-peptide by pancreatic β cells and its circulation in blood. *Nature (London)*, *224*, 697.
30. Nielsen JH (1981): Human pancreatic islets in tissue culture. In: *Islet Isolation, Culture and Cryopreservation. International Workshop Giessen 1980, p. 69.* Editor: K. Federlin. Georg Thieme Verlag, Stuttgart-New York.
31. Polonsky J, Jaspan J, Pugh W, Cohen D, Schneider M, Schwartz T, Moossa AR, Tager H, Rubenstein AH (1983): Metabolism of C-peptide in the dog. *J. Clin. Invest.*, *72*, 1114.
32. Kühl C, Faber OK, Hornnes P, Lindkaer Jensen S (1978): C-peptide metabolism and the liver. *Diabetes*, *27*, *Suppl. 1*, 197.
33. Faber OK, Kehlet H, Madsbad S, Binder C (1978): Kinetics of human C-peptide in man. *Diabetes*, *27*, *Suppl. 1*, 207.
34. Eaton RP, Allen RC, Schade DS, Erickson KM, Standefer J (1980): Prehepatic insulin production in man: kinetic analysis using peripheral connecting peptide behavior. *J. Clin. Endocrinol. Metab.*, *51*, 520.
35. Eaton RP, Allen RC, Schade DS (1983): Hepatic removal of insulin in normal man: dose response to endogenous insulin secretion. *J. Clin. Endocrinol. Metab.*, *56*, 1294.
36. Faber OK, Hagen C, Binder C, Markussen J, Naithani VK, Blix PM, Kuzuya H, Horwitz DL, Rubenstein AH, Rossing N (1978): Kinetics of human connecting peptide in normal and diabetic subjects. *J. Clin. Invest.*, *62*, 197.
37. Meistas MT, Margolis S, Kowarski AA (1983): Hyperinsulinemia of obesity is due to decreased clearance of insulin. *Am. J. Physiol.*, *245*, E155.
38. Rossell R, Gomis R, Casamitjana R, Segura R, Vilardell E, Rivera F (1983): Reduced hepatic insulin extraction in obesity: relationship with plasma insulin levels. *J. Clin. Endocrinol. Metab.*, *56*, 608.
39. Faber OK, Christensen K, Kehlet H, Madsbad S, Binder C (1981): Decreased insulin removal contributes to hyperinsulinemia in obesity. *J. Clin. Endocrinol. Metab.*, *53*, 618.
40. Miles JM, Haymond MW, Gerich JE (1981): Suppression of glucose production and stimulation of insulin secretion by physiological concentrations of ketone bodies in man. *J. Clin. Endocrinol. Metab.*, *52*, 34.
41. Madsbad S, Krarup T, Faber OK, Binder C, Regeur L (1982): The transient

effect of strict glycaemic control on B cell function in newly diagnosed type 1 (insulin-dependent) diabetic patients. *Diabetologia*, *22*, 16.

42. Seigler DE, Reeves ML, Skyler JS (1982): Lack of effect of improved glycemic control on C-peptide secretion in patients without residual B-cell function. *Diabetes Care*, *5*, 334.
43. Dahlquist G, Blom L, Bolme P, Hagenfeldt L, Lindgren F, Persson B, Thalme B, Theorell M, Westin S (1982): Metabolic control in 131 juvenile-onset diabetic patients as measured by HbA_{1c}: relation to age, duration, C-peptide, insulin dose, and one or two insulin injections. *Diabetes Care*, *5*, 399.
44. Sjöberg S, Gunnarsson R, Östman J (1983): Residual C-peptide production in type I diabetes mellitus. *Acta Med. Scand.*, *214*, 231.
45. Käär M-L, Åkerblom HK, Huttunen N-P, Knip M, Säkkinen K (1984): Metabolic control in children and adolescents with insulin-dependent diabetes mellitus. *Acta Paediatr. Scand.*, *73*, 102.
46. Koepp P, Kühnau J (1982): Insulinrestsekretion (C-Peptid) und einige andere Parameter für den Langzeitverlauf bei Patienten mit insulinbedürftigem Diabetes mellitus. *Monatsschr. Kinderheilkd.*, *130*, 215.
47. Bonora E, Coscelli C, Butturini U (1983): Residual B cell function and insulin sensitivity in type 1 (insulin-dependent) diabetes mellitus. Letter to the Editor. *Diabetologia*, *25*, 298.
48. Ludvigsson J (1984): Insulin antibodies in diabetic children treated with monocomponent porcine insulin from the onset: relationship to B-cell function and partial remission. *Diabetologia, 26*, 138.
49. Dorn A, Rinne A, Hahn H-J, Bernstein H-G, Ziegler M (1982): C-peptide immunoreactive neurons in human brain. *Acta Histochem. Zeitschr.; Histol. Topochem. (Jena)*, *70*, 326.
50. Dorn A, Bernstein H-G, Rinne A, Ziegler M, Hahn H-J, Ansorge S (1983): Insulin- and glucagon-like peptides in the brain. *Anat. Rec.*, *207*, 69.
51. Heding LG, Faber O, Kasperska-Czyzykowa T, Sestoft L, Turner R (1979): Radioimmunoassay of proinsulin and hyperinsulinemic states. In: S. Baba, T. Kaneko and N. Yanaihara (Eds), *Proinsulin*, *Insulin*, *C-peptide*, *International Congress Series No. 468*, p 254. Excerpta Medica, Amsterdam–Oxford.
52. Faber OK, Kehlet H (1979): Strategy in the diagnosis of insulinoma. *Scand. J. Gastroenterol.*, *14*, *Suppl. 53*, 45.
53. Halban PA, Bonner-Weir S, Weir GC (1983): Elevated proinsulin biosynthesis in vitro from a rat model of non-insulin-dependent diabetes mellitus. *Diabetes*, *32*, 277.
54. Ludvigsson J, Heding L (1982): Abnormal proinsulin/C-peptide ratio in juvenile diabetes. *Acta Diabetol. Lat.*, *19*, 351.
55. Gordon P, Roth J (1969): Plasma insulin: fluctuations in the 'big' insulin component in man after glucose and other stimuli. *J. Clin. Invest.*, *48*, 2225.
56. Sestoft L, Heding LG (1981): Hypersecretion of proinsulin in thyrotoxicosis. *Diabetologia*, *21*, 103.
57. Revers R, Olefsky J, Schmeiser L et al. (1983): The effects of biosynthetic human proinsulin on carbohydrate metabolism. *Clin. Res.*, *31*, 59A (abstract).
58. Robbins DC, Tager HS, Rubenstein AH (1984): Biological and clinical importance of proinsulin. *N. Engl. J. Med.*, *310*, 1165.

The Diabetes Annual/1
K.G.M.M. Alberti and L.P. Krall, editors

ISBN 0444 90 343 7
$0.85 per article per page (transactional system)
$0.20 per article per page (licensing system)

24 Insulin action in vivo

RALPH W. STEVENSON, KURT E. STEINER, NAJI N. ABUMRAD AND ALAN D. CHERRINGTON

In recent years there has been a considerable increase in our knowledge of insulin physiology, advances having been made with regard to its action in control of carbohydrate, fat and protein metabolism. It is the purpose of this review to evaluate the in-vivo role of insulin in each of these areas with particular emphasis on recent findings and issues which are currently controversial. We will begin with consideration of the role of insulin in regulating the disposition of a glucose load and its involvement in the determination of insulin sensitivity. Next, the role of insulin in the in-vivo regulation of ketogenesis and lipolysis will be discussed and lastly we will consider the role that the hormone is thought to play in regulating protein metabolism in vivo.

Insulin and glucose disposition

Oral administration of glucose to man or the dog results in the uptake of glucose by both peripheral and hepatic (or splanchnic) tissues (1–6). However, the relative roles of hyperinsulinemia, hyperglycemia and the route of glucose delivery in promoting these responses has remained controversial.

Hyperinsulinemia and euglycemia

Insulin has long been known to stimulate glucose uptake by the peripheral tissues of the body. Small (20–30 μU/ml) increments in plasma insulin have been shown to increase glucose uptake by the forearm in euglycemic man (7, 8). In addition further studies have shown that when plasma insulin concentration was increased to pharmacological levels by intravenous infu-

---

These investigations were supported by NIH grants AM18243, AM22195 and 5 MO1 RR00095, JDF grant 82R564 and DRTC Grant (NIH) AM20593. R.W.S. is a recipient of a JDF research and career development award. K.E.S. is a recipient of an ADA research and career development award.

sion and euglycemia was maintained by glucose infusion, total body glucose uptake increased to a maximum of 10–12 mg/kg-min (Fig. 1A). However, inhibition of hepatic glucose output was relatively more sensitive to insulin than stimulation of glucose uptake by peripheral tissues (10–12) (Fig. 1A) although one must remember that the portal insulin level is 2–3 times the peripheral level. Although suppression of glucose output by insulin in the postabsorptive animal is almost entirely due to inhibition of hepatic glycogenolysis, it cannot be concluded that gluconeogenesis is unresponsive to insulin (13–16). Indeed the gluconeogenic process is already markedly inhibited after an overnight fast due to the potent effect of low levels of insulin. Basal insulin concentrations inhibit hepatic glycogenolysis by 50% while inhibiting gluconeogenesis by 85%. When the insulin concentration was raised to four times basal, hepatic glycogenolysis was totally suppressed while gluconeogenesis was inhibited by 88%. Much higher insulin levels were required to totally suppress gluconeogenesis, the physiologic significance of which will be discussed later.

It is also apparent from the literature that while pharmacological concentrations of insulin can inhibit hepatic glucose output they cannot stimulate

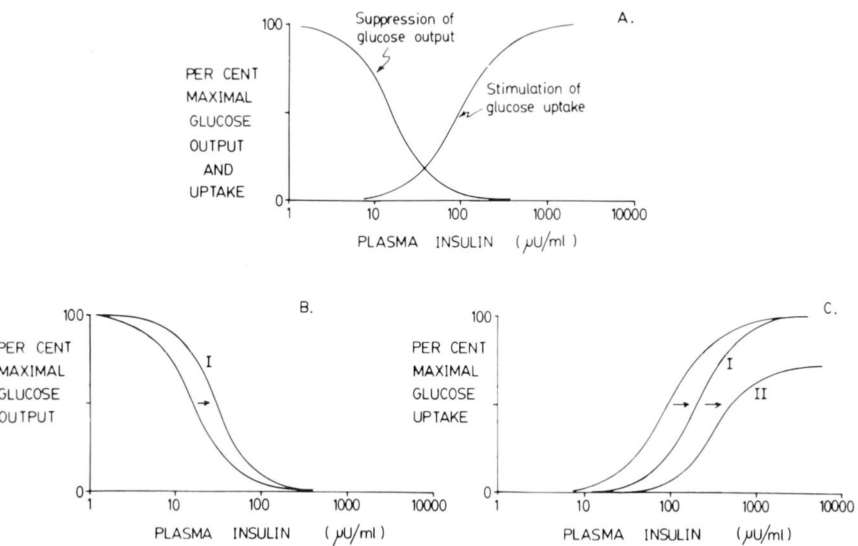

FIG. 1. *A: Normal dose–response characteristics of insulin on glucose output and glucose uptake in man using the euglycemic clamp technique (based on data from refs. 10–12). (Arterial insulin concentrations are depicted.) B and C: Effect of insulin resistance on suppression of glucose output and stimulation of glucose uptake respectively (based on data from ref. 56). I represents the change in the dose–response curves due to decreased receptor number. II represents the change in the dose–response curve due to a post-receptor defect.*

significant uptake of glucose by the splanchnic bed. At insulin concentrations of 400–1,000 μU/ml produced by intravenous insulin infusion during euglycemic conditions in man, splanchnic uptake contributed a maximum of only 8% to total glucose metabolism (9, 10). Similarly, the infusion of insulin at 5 mU/kg-min into the portal circulation of the dog, which resulted in portal vein insulin levels exceeding 500 μU/ml, did not result in any net hepatic glucose uptake under euglycemic conditions (Frizzel and Cherrington, unpublished observation).

Hyperglycemia with normal insulin levels

Hyperglycemia per se, in the presence of basal insulin concentrations, produces a suppression of hepatic glucose output in both man (17) and dog (18). It does not, however, stimulate splanchnic or hepatic uptake of glucose, although it does increase glucose uptake by peripheral tissues due to a mass action effect. In insulin-dependent diabetic subjects receiving a constant infusion of insulin, raising the plasma glucose concentration (76 mg/dl; 4.2 mmol/l) by 2–3 fold resulted in a prompt fall in hepatic glucose production from 1.9 to 0.3 mg/kg-min, despite the unchanged rate of insulin infusion and the absence of a reduction in plasma glucagon or catecholamines (17). The decrease in glucose output which occurred in the dog in response to hyperglycemia, in the presence of fixed basal insulin and glucagon concentrations established using a 'pancreatic clamp', could be accounted for by inhibition of both hepatic glycogenolysis and gluconeogenesis (19).

In the dog, glucose uptake by peripheral tissues increased proportionally with the increase in hyperglycemia so that the metabolic clearance rate of glucose (glucose utilization/[glucose]) remained fairly constant over the range of plasma glucose concentrations tested (100–220 mg/dl) (20). In man, however, the glucose clearance rate tended to decrease as the plasma glucose level increased (for review see ref. 21).

Hyperglycemia and hyperinsulinemia

Contrary to the failure of either hyperglycemia or hyperinsulinemia alone to produce significant uptake of glucose by the liver, the combination of the two does stimulate significant net hepatic glucose uptake in the dog and some net splanchnic glucose uptake in man. However, the human liver appears to take up considerably less glucose than the dog under those conditions.

It was shown many years ago that the addition of insulin to hyperglycemic diabetic dogs immediately converted their livers from glucose producing to glucose consuming organs (22). More recently, Cherrington et al. (23) confirmed that insulin plays a role in regulating net hepatic glucose uptake in normal dogs. When plasma insulin and glucose concentrations were raised to 38 μU/ml and 220 mg/dl (12.2 mmol/l) respectively, in the presence of fixed basal glucagon concentrations, the initial basal glucose output of 2.8 ± 1.2 mg/kg-min was converted to an uptake of 3.4 ± 1.2 mg/kg-min by 60 min. This finding has now been confirmed by Barrett et al. (24) and by Adkins et al. (unpublished observations) (see Table 1) although both of these studies showed somewhat less net hepatic glucose uptake. Since, in the presence of glucose levels in excess of 200 mg/dl, net hepatic glucose uptake was similar (~3–4 mg/kg-min) regardless of whether portal vein insulin was 100 or 400 μU/ml, it would appear that the effect of insulin on hepatic uptake of glucose reaches a maximum at relatively low plasma insulin concentrations. In the presence of these apparently saturating insulin levels, however, it is likely that the glucose concentration becomes rate-limiting as evidenced by the observation that, when the hyperglycemia was maintained at about 150 mg/dl, with portal vein insulin levels of ~180 μU/ml, significantly less hepatic glucose uptake resulted (6) (see Table 1).

When hyperglycemic-hyperinsulinemic clamps were employed in man, however, the contribution of the splanchnic bed to glucose uptake was 0.3–1.6 mg/kg-min, thus the contribution of the liver to total glucose uptake was considerably less than in the dog (2, 10, 25). In either case, the uptake of glucose by the liver in man and dog during hyperinsulinemia and hyperglycemia is insufficient to explain the response to an oral glucose load.

Oral, intraportal and peripheral glucose

It is difficult to compare the relative contribution of the liver and peripheral tissues to the disposal of a glucose load after oral, intraportal, or peripheral glucose administration, since the degree of hyperglycemia and hyperinsulinemia as well as the route of insulin administration has varied between studies. Nevertheless, it appears that hepatic glucose uptake is significantly greater after oral than after peripheral intravenous glucose infusion in both man (1, 2, 26–28) and the dog (Table 1). Although it is well known that oral administration of glucose augments insulin secretion to a greater extent than administration of glucose by other routes, the extra insulin, as noted above, could not account for greater glucose uptake by the liver following oral glucose administration. Initially, DeFronzo et al. (2, 29) suggested that orally consumed glucose caused release of a gut factor which enhanced hepatic uptake of glucose. In order to test this hypothesis, Bergman et al. (3) infused glucose intraportally, albeit in the dog, to mimick the glucose absorption profile after oral administration. They observed that the hepatic uptake of glucose was similar under both conditions (Table 1). This finding has recently been confirmed by Ishida et al. (6) (see Table 1). Intraportal delivery of glucose therefore caused greater hepatic glucose uptake than that observed during peripheral glucose delivery. Thus there is no need to postulate the existence of a gut factor being responsible for stimulating

TABLE 1. *Net hepatic glucose uptake (NHGU; mg/kg-min) by 60 min of peripheral or intraportal venous infusion of glucose, and 60 min after an oral glucose load to conscious dogs. Results are expressed as mean ± SEM. G represents the mean glucose concentration (mg/dl) to which the liver was exposed and I represents the arterial plasma insulin concentration (μU/ml) at 60 min. Portal insulin concentrations can be assumed to be approximately 3-fold higher than arterial concentrations except where noted (82)*

	Route of glucose delivery					
	Peripheral		Oral		Intraportal	
	G/I	NHGU	G/I	NHGU	G/I	NHGU
Bergman et al. (3)	–	–	173/85*	2.3 ± 0.4	182/90*	2.5 ± 0.8
Cherrington et al.	221/43^{+}	1.9 ± 0.2			218/39^{+}	5.0 ± 1.0
Ishida et al. (6)	150/59	0.9 ± 0.8	178/41*	5.4 ± 0.5	194/41*	6.0 ± 1.4
					159/63	5.7 ± 1.2
Barrett et al. (24)	200/250^{++}	3.0 ± 0.7	220/51	4.4 ± 1.3	224/178^{+++}	6.0 ± 1.1
	290/384^{++}	2.8 ± 0.4	203/93	4.2 ± 1.0		

Arterial insulin concentrations result from endogenous secretion except for those achieved by peripheral intravenous infusion^{++} and intraportal insulin infusion^{+++}. The asterisks denote when intraportal infusion was programmed to mimick the glucose absorption profile after an oral glucose load in the same study.
$^{+}$ Adkins and Cherrington, unpublished observations.

uptake of glucose by the liver with the oral route of administration. Rather, it appears that a 'portal factor' is involved in stimulating hepatic glucose uptake in the dog and perhaps in man though the definitive experiment (i.e. intraportal glucose infusion) is technically not feasible in man.

Direct comparison has been made of net hepatic glucose balance during peripheral and intraportal glucose infusion in the same dogs when both the amount of glucose presented to the liver and the portal vein insulin concentrations were fairly similar (6). As shown in Figure 2, portal vein glucose concentrations were maintained at a level of 160–170 mg/dl (8.9–9.4 mmol/l) during both peripheral and intraportal infusion of glucose, while the arterial glucose concentration was at 160–170 mg/dl (8.9–9.4 mmol/l) during peripheral infusion but was significantly reduced to 120–130 mg/dl (6.7–7.2 mmol/l) during intraportal infusion of glucose. About 6-fold more glucose was taken up by the liver during intraportal than peripheral intravenous infusion even though portal vein insulin concentrations were slightly higher in the latter case (~160 μU/ml compared to 120 μU/ml). In addition, more recent studies in our own laboratory showed that when the mean glucose concentration presented to the liver was 220 mg/dl (12.2 mmol/l) and portal vein insulin concentration was about 120 μU/ml (4-fold basal), intraportal administration of glucose produced 2.5-fold more hepatic glucose uptake than peripheral glucose administration (see Table 1). In this study the absolute amount of glucose in the portal vein cannot explain the difference in uptake because the portal glucose concentrations differed by only 9%. Thus, the arterial-portal venous concentration difference of glucose across the liver may be the primary determinant of differing rates of net hepatic glucose uptake.

While, as discussed earlier, the effect of insulin on hepatic glucose uptake was evident during peripheral glucose administration its role during portal or oral administration is unclear. Studies in our own laboratory suggest that

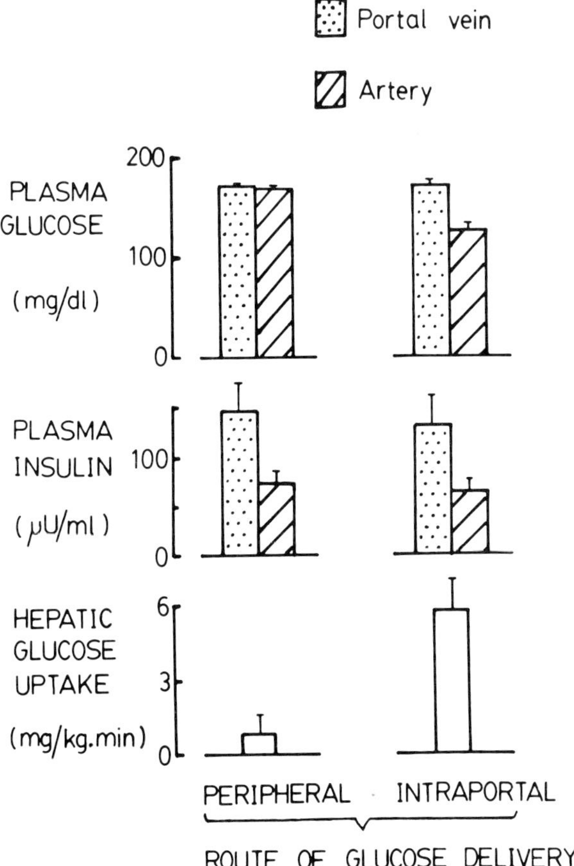

FIG. 2. *Effect of peripheral and intraportal glucose delivery to conscious dogs on portal vein and arterial concentrations of glucose and insulin, and on net hepatic uptake of glucose (based on data from ref. 6). Results are expressed as mean ± SEM.*

insulin does have a role in the disposal of an intraportal glucose load (30). In this instance portal glucose concentrations were maintained in the dog at about 220 mg/dl (12.2 mmol/l) during intraportal and peripheral infusion of glucose, and arterial plasma insulin and glucagon concentrations were fixed at basal levels (7 ± 1 μU/ml and 101 ± 3 pg/ml, respectively) using somatostatin and intraportal hormone replacement. When glucose was infused via the peripheral route, hepatic glucose output was suppressed from 2.2 ± 0.3 to 0.1 ± 0.2 mg/kg-min but no uptake of glucose by the liver could be detected in accordance with other results discussed earlier. Intraportal infusion of glucose, however, did cause hepatic glucose uptake (1.6 ± 0.4 mg/kg-min). When compared with the results obtained with a similar hepatic glucose load in the presence of hyperinsulinemia, it appears that hepatic glucose uptake is impaired during intraportal glucose administration if insulin concentrations are low. Whether this effect of insulin is due to an enhanced peripheral glucose uptake which allowed a greater A–P gradient or a direct effect on the liver is unknown.

In conclusion, it appears that the amount of hepatic glucose uptake following intraportal (and presumably oral) administration of glucose is determined by three factors. Firstly, the glucose level determines the amount of glucose taken up by the liver since, at saturating insulin concentrations, increased hyperglycemia (produced by peripheral glucose administration) resulted in increased hepatic uptake of glucose. Secondly, the arterial-portal vein glucose gradient plays a major role in promoting glucose uptake by the liver since less uptake occurred during peripheral than intraportal glucose administration, regardless of the prevailing insulin concentration. Thirdly, the insulin concentration directly, or indirectly by increasing the arterial-portal vein glucose gradient, affects the amount of hepatic glucose uptake because there was considerably less uptake when insulin levels were fixed at basal rather than elevated levels. The exact interrelationship between these three factors remains to be determined.

Even though there is considerable hepatic glucose uptake following intraportal and oral administration of glucose, it has been shown using isotopic techniques in man (31) and dog (32, 33) that the majority of an ingested glucose load bypasses the liver and there now seems to be general agreement that peripheral tissues (primarily muscle) dispose of most of it (5, 34). Indeed, DeFronzo et al. (5) have now revised their estimate of 50–60% extraction of an oral glucose load by the splanchnic bed in man to less than one third. Since it is known that liver glycogen levels are restored even after intravenous glucose administration (31, 35) and since it is obvious that under this circumstance the carbon for glycogen synthesis could not have come from hepatic glucose uptake, it follows that the source of carbon for glycogen synthesis originates elsewhere. As discussed earlier, physiologic elevations in insulin do not further suppress gluconeogenesis thus glycogen could be formed from gluconeogenic precursors. Therefore, in the absence of carbohydrate in the diet, carnivores would be able to replete their liver glycogen stores.

Glucose disposal and insulin resistance

Suppression of hepatic glucose output and stimulation of glucose uptake by muscle (see Fig. 1A) are both sensitively altered by insulin in normal individuals. However, in insulin-resistant states, the shapes of the insulin dose-response curves change depending on whether the resistance is due to a receptor or a post-receptor defect.

Decreased cellular insulin receptors have been described in non-insulin-dependent (Type 2) diabetes (36–38), obesity (36, 39, 40), acromegaly (41), glucocorticoid excess (42, 43), oral contraceptive therapy (44) and aging (45), and could lead to insulin resistance. However, this relationship is complicated by the existence of 'spare receptors' on cells (46, 47) and by the observation that a maximal response can be achieved by only 10% occupancy of insulin receptors as in stimulation of glucose uptake into isolated adipocytes (46, 48). All the spare receptors are potentially functional and, at least in adipocytes, occupancy of any random 10% would produce a maximum response. However, as receptor loss becomes pronounced (30–50% of original receptor complement) (49) the insulin dose–response curves shift to the right (see Fig. 1C), the extent of the rightward shift being proportional to the decrease in receptors. However, the normal maximal insulin responses will still be possible unless the reduction in insulin receptors is excessive, e.g. to less than 10% of the normal receptor complement in adipocytes. A postreceptor defect such as abnormal coupling between the insulin-receptor complexes and the glucose transport system or an intracellular enzymatic defect results in a decrease in insulin action at all insulin concentrations including maximally effective hormone levels (36, 50, 51) (Figs. 1B and C).

Insulin resistance is a characteristic feature of most patients with Type 2 diabetes (51–53) and it appears that the greater the fasting hyperglycemia or glucose intolerance, the greater the magnitude of insulin resistance (53, 54). In addition, as the degree of carbohydrate intolerance worsens, the frequency of insulin resistance increases (54, 55). As reviewed elsewhere (56), obesity also leads to the development of insulin resistance. Although the vast majority of Type 2 diabetic patients are overweight, the insulin resistance is greater than can be accounted for on the basis of obesity alone. Furthermore, many non-obese Type 2 diabetic patients are also insulin resistant (see ref. 56).

Various methods have been used to assess insulin resistance (57) but the euglycemic insulin clamp technique (58) is the best since it avoids the effects of changes in blood glucose concentration on glucose utilization. In patients with impaired glucose tolerance but normal or mildly abnormal ($<$ 115 mg/dl) fasting plasma glucose concentrations there is a rightward shift in the insulin dose-response curves both with respect to suppression of hepatic glucose output and stimulation of glucose disposal (56), however, the maximal responses are unaffected. These results are consistent with a decrease solely in cellular insulin receptors in both hepatic and peripheral tissues. On the other hand, in overt Type 2 diabetic patients, there is a greater rightward shift in the insulin dose–response curves and a marked decrease in the maximal rate of glucose disposal (56, 59) though maximal suppression of glucose output was still possible (56). Both of the above changes tend to be more pronounced in the obese Type 2 diabetic. The evidence suggests that the primary lesion responsible for the insulin resistant state in overt Type 2 diabetics is a postreceptor defect that occurs only in peripheral tissues. However, decreased receptor numbers in both hepatic and peripheral tissues contribute to the resistance.

Although Type 2 diabetics with fasting hyperglycemia can have normal or elevated basal insulin concentrations, they are uniformly hypoinsulinemic in response to a glucose challenge. Thus, it is conceivable that the insulin resistance resulting from a post-receptor defect is secondary to insulin deficiency. Indeed, recent evidence by Olefsky et al. (60) indicates that intensive insulin treatment for two weeks, to achieve near-normal glycemia, substantially reversed the post-receptor defect in Type 2 diabetic patients. This improvement was indicated by a virtual restoration (72%) of the maximal rate of insulin-stimulated glucose disposal. Furthermore, the decrease in the maximal rate of glucose transport into adipocytes was similarly reversed by intensive insulin therapy (61). However, although basal hepatic glucose output was significantly reduced by insulin treatment, the insulin dose–response curve for insulin-mediated suppression of glucose output during the euglycemic clamp was not significantly changed after insulin treatment i.e. still shifted to the right of normal (60). Therefore, the insulin receptor defect was not corrected by insulin therapy. This is not surprising since circulating insulin levels are known inversely to regulate the number of insulin receptors with the result that insulin treatment could have decreased insulin receptor number in Type 2 diabetics even further. However, in-vitro evidence suggests that receptor loss proceeds only until 30–50% of the original receptor complement is lost, even at pharmacological insulin levels (49). It is conceivable that prolonged intensive insulin therapy will completely abolish the postreceptor defect, i.e. the primary lesion, thus causing a decrease in insulin dosage and a corresponding increase in receptor number.

Another possible means of reversing insulin resistant states may lie in physical exercise. Exercise is known to increase target tissue sensitivity to insulin in normal man (62), and in Type 1 (62) and Type 2 diabetics (63). In addition a regular program of physical exercise enhanced both hepatic and peripheral tissue sensitivity to insulin and ameliorated the hyperinsulinemic response to hyperglycemia in obesity (59).

Insulin resistance can also be a feature of insulin-dependent (Type 1) diabetes. Poorly controlled Type 1 diabetics with long standing disease exhibit reduced glucose disposal even in the presence of normal and high insulin levels (64, 65) though Ginsberg (66) could find no evidence of such a defect in newly diagnosed Type 1 diabetic patients. It appears, therefore, that the abnormality in glucose disposal develops after the onset of the disease and may be a consequence of the diabetic state itself or perhaps insulin therapy per se. It seems likely that this particular insulin resistance involves a postreceptor defect since glucose metabolism has been reported to be reduced in adipocytes isolated from Type 1 diabetic patients (67). As in Type 2 diabetes, the severity of the insulin resistance closely paralleled the degree of hyperglycemia and is largely reversed, at least in alloxan-diabetic dogs by 10–14 days insulin treatment (68).

It appears that hyperglycemia in insulin-dependent diabetes fails to suppress the elevated hepatic glucose production (69–72). However, low infusion rates of insulin readily suppressed the raised hepatic glucose production in insulin-dependent diabetic man (71) and dog (68, 70, 73, 74). The effect of insulin administration on hepatic glucose output is complex since insulin itself acts on the pancreatic A-cell to inhibit glucagon secretion. Indeed, recent results suggest that the insulin-induced fall in plasma glucagon concentrations is the major reason for suppression of the hepatic glucose output in the diabetic dog since re-establishment of the hyperglucagonemic levels by intraportal infusion reversed the fall in glucose output (75). Thus the cause of hepatic glucose overproduction seems to be due to insulin deficiency or glucagon excess rather than hepatic insulin resistance – at least in the dog.

Although euglycemia can readily be achieved in insulin-dependent diabetic man and dog by low-dose infusion of insulin, complete metabolic normalization cannot be achieved using the peripheral route of insulin delivery (73, 76–79). As discussed elsewhere (80), these abnormalities, e.g. subnormal blood glycerol and non-esterified fatty acid concentrations, have been attributed to the hyperinsulinemia associated with peripheral insulin administration. One of the major abnormalities associated with this route of insulin delivery is depressed Cori cycle activity. In insulin-dependent diabetic subjects glucose recycling (i.e. recycling the products of glucose catabolism to glucose) was severely reduced to 6 and 4%, from about 20%, during relatively poor control of blood glucose by subcutaneous insulin injection therapy, and during maintenance of normoglycemia by peripheral intravenous infusion of insulin using the artificial endocrine pancreas respectively (78). This observation was also confirmed in dogs rendered diabetic by alloxan plus streptozotocin (73). Induction of diabetes caused a small increase in glucose recycling from 19 to 24%. However, although hepatic glucose production could be normalized in these diabetic dogs, glucose recycling was reduced to 11%. On the other hand, intraportal infusion of insulin normalized not only glucose production but also glucose recycling. Furthermore, only the portal route of insulin delivery normalized plasma glucose and intermediary metabolite profiles during fasting and during intraduodenal glucose loading (79). The intraportal infusion rate of insulin used to achieve normoglycemia in these diabetic dogs was 350 μU/kg-min, only a little higher than the basal insulin secretion rates (167 to 250 μU/kg-min) found in normal man using C-peptide measurements (81, 82).

Regulation of fat metabolism by insulin

In addition to its role as a crucial regulator of glucose disposal and hepatic glucose production, insulin is an important regulator of fat metabolism in vivo. The net overall changes in fat metabolism caused by insulin are the sum of its stimulatory action on lipogenesis and its inhibitory actions on lipolysis and ketogenesis. The nature of these actions make it the major antagonist of glucagon, epinephrine and norepinephrine all of which can have lipolytic and ketogenic effects under certain circumstances. Not only do basal amounts of insulin potently restrain the lipolysis and ketogenesis which would normally occur in response to these counterregulatory hormones but increments in insulin can virtually abolish both processes.

Effect of selective hyperinsulinemia

Several studies have shown that both the release of non-esterified fatty acids from fat depots and their conversion to ketone bodies in the liver can be affected by relatively small increases in the circulating insulin level. Early studies by Zierler and Rabinowitz (83) in the human forearm showed that an increment of 38 μU/ml in insulin in the brachial artery was sufficient to completely inhibit fatty acid release from the limb. In more recent studies Massi-Benedetti et al. (84) demonstrated the potent antilipolytic and antiketogenic effects of increments in circulating insulin in normal overnight fasted man. When human insulin was infused into a peripheral vein in successive increments creating plasma insulin levels of 30, 40 and 50 μU/ml as compared to basal levels of 9 μU/ml the plasma glycerol level (a good indicator of lipolysis because it must be released from the fat cell following hydrolysis of triglyceride) fell 50, 75 and 80% in response to the 3 insulin levels, respectively. Glucose was infused along with insulin to prevent hypoglycemia and the accompanying stimulation of counterregulatory hormone secretion. The 3-hydroxybutyrate levels fell to a point where they were barely detectable even with the lowest insulin increment. Since changes in plasma non-esterified fatty acid (NEFA) levels were not reported, it is not possible to conclude whether the decline in 3-hydroxybutyrate was due solely to a decline in lipolysis and thus an indirect effect on the liver or a direct inhibitory effect of the hormone on hepatic ketogenesis. Almost identical responses were observed when porcine insulin was used, suggesting that – at least with regard to fat metabolism – the biologic activity of these two molecules is indistinguishable. In insulin-deprived diabetic man Schade and Eaton (85) demonstrated that the antilipolytic and antiketogenic effects of small increments (as little as 7 μU/ml) in insulin were dose dependent, a maximal inhibitory response occurring with increments of 100 μU/ml.

Although a large portion of the antiketogenic effect of increased insulin levels is probably due to a decreased supply of free fatty acids reaching the liver, direct effects of insulin on hepatic ketogenesis have also recently been demonstrated in man. Gerber et al. (86) infused somatostatin in conjunction with replacement infusion of insulin to fix insulin levels at either 10 or 100 μU/ml while an infusion of intralipid and heparin was used to keep non-esterified fatty acid levels fixed. In addition glucose was again infused to preserve euglycemia and prevent counter-regulatory hormone release. Ketone body turnover was measured using labeled acetoacetate. The increase in insulin from 10 to 100 μU/ml was associated with a 66% fall in hepatic production (9.1 ± 1.0 to 3.8 ± 0.8 μmol/kg-min) of ketone bodies even though non-esterified fatty acid levels remained unchanged indicating increments in insulin above basal can have a direct inhibitory effect on hepatic ketogenesis in vivo. In summary, increases in circulating insulin reduce lipolysis and consequently ketogenesis by decreasing the delivery of non-esterified fatty acids to the liver. In addition they can have a direct inhibitory effect on the liver to inhibit ketogenesis.

Effects of acute insulin deficiency

The ability of basal amounts of insulin to inhibit lipolysis and ketogenesis in vivo has also recently been assessed (87–93). Wahren et al. (87) using somatostatin, a potent inhibitor of pancreatic insulin and glucagon release, to create insulin deficiency examined changes in lipolysis and ketogenesis in both postabsorptive and 60-hour fasted normal man. In the overnight fasted subjects both insulin and glucagon levels declined while non-esterified fatty acid levels rose threefold after one hour of somatostatin infusion. Changes in ketone body levels were not measured. In the 60-hour fasted subjects, non-esterified fatty acid levels increased over twofold but 3-hydroxybutyrate levels did not change. Measurements of splanchnic 3-hydroxybutyrate output, however, showed a twofold rise with somatostatin infusion. Since the rise in splanchnic NEFA uptake could account for the rise in ketone production it seems likely that the ketogenic stimulation resulted entirely from increased delivery of non-esterified fatty acids to the liver rather than because of any direct hepatic effects. These changes are probably a conservative indication of the ability of basal insulin to restrain lipolysis and ketogenesis since a fall in glucagon, a ketogenic hormone in vivo during insulin deficiency, accompanied infusion of somatostatin. Metcalfe et al. (88) in 12-hour fasted man have also examined the effects of acute insulin deficiency. In their studies infusion of somatostatin caused a 50% fall in insulin, a 30–40% fall in glucagon and a threefold increase in ketone body levels but the change in non-esterified fatty acid levels was only about twofold. These studies would seem to indicate that unlike those of Wahren et al. (87), insulin deficiency does indeed unveil a direct hepatic effect to stimulate ketone body production. In the dog Keller et al. (89) have shown that if acute insulin deficiency is brought about in the presence of only small changes in glucagon (~20%) rises in glycerol and non-esterified fatty acid levels occur, but that ketone body production increases by 85%. These data indicate that lipolysis was minimally altered by insulin deficiency but that hepatic ketogenesis was significantly augmented.

The antilipolytic and antiketogenic role of basal insulin in insulin-dependent diabetics has also been examined in vivo (90–93) by withdrawing exogenous insulin. Pickup et al. (90) during studies on insulin withdrawal from diabetics observed a progressive rise in 3-hydroxybutyrate levels as free insulin concentrations fell. Even after 9 hours a plateau in 3-hydroxybutyrate levels had not been reached. In similar studies Keller et al. (91) noted a rise in acetoacetate turnover with insulin withdrawal. These results were extended by Miles et al. (92) in studies where insulin-dependent diabetics were deprived of insulin. During the 10 hours that observations were made insulin levels fell from 18 ± 4 to 7 ± 1 μU/ml, glucagon increased from 67 ± 6 to 259 ± 67 pg/ml, while ketone body levels increased 5-fold from 1.4 ± 0.4 mmol/l to 7.2 ± 1.5 mmol/l. Both ketone body production (5.4 ± 1.4 to 18.3 ± 3.9) and utilization (5.5 ± 1.1 to 14.7 ± 2.1 μmol/kg-min) increased in association with a 3-fold rise in the fatty acid levels. Wahren et al. (93) recently reported that increases in fatty acid and ketone body levels occurred following insulin withdrawal, but they noted that even in the presence of a threefold increase in non-esterified fatty acid uptake the fractional extraction of non-esterified fatty acids by the liver was unchanged. Ketone body production was 10-fold higher, indicating that basal levels of insulin have a direct inhibitory effect on hepatic ketogenesis as well as an indirect effect through restraint of lipolysis. The interpretation of this and the previous in-vivo studies in the diabetic, which use somatostatin infusion to create insulin deficiency, is, however, complicated by the fact that glucagon levels rise during insulin withdrawal, and it is difficult to define the changes due solely to insulin deficiency and those due to the rise in glucagon. In fact Gerich et al. (94) have shown that the increases in fatty acid, glycerol and ketone body levels are reduced when glucagon secretion is prevented with somatostatin infusion during insulin withdrawal in insulin-dependent diabetics. The studies summarized in the preceding paragraphs show that basal insulin restrains both lipolysis and ketogenesis but the effectiveness of basal insulin to restrain the lipolytic and ketogenic effects due to increments in glucagon above basal levels is less clear.

Effects of hyperglucagonemia in the presence of basal insulin or insulin deficiency

Studies in overnight fasted man (95, 96) have shown that physiologic increments in glucagon (120–400 pg/ml) in the presence of basal insulin are unable to stimulate ketogenesis. However, during acute insulin deficiency similar increments in glucagon were ketogenic (96, 97). Earlier studies by Gerich et al. (98) also showed that a physiologic increment in glucagon in insulin-deprived diabetics increased both free fatty acid, glycerol and 3-hydroxybutyrate levels. Others (95), however, observed no lipolytic or ketogenic effects of similar increments in glucagon even during acute insulin deficiency in overnight fasted normal man. The above studies indicate that if physiologic increments of glucagon are able to stimulate ketogenesis and/or lipolysis in vivo relative or absolute insulin deficiency is required. Whether the inhibitory effects of basal insulin on lipolysis and ketogenesis could be overcome by a larger physiologic increment in circulating glucagon has not been examined.

Effects of catecholamines in the presence of basal insulin or insulin deficiency

The ability of basal insulin to inhibit the lipolytic and ketogenic effects of increments in catecholamines has also been studied. Several studies (99–101) have used concomitant infusions of somatostatin and epinephrine to determine the role of basal insulin in antagonizing catecholamine-induced ketogenesis. In each case the combined infusion of epinephrine and somatostatin caused a greater increase in ketone body levels than did the infusion of epinephrine alone. Interpretation of these studies is difficult since somatostatin caused both insulin and glucagon deficiency in one study (101) and neither insulin nor glucagon values were reported in the others (99, 100), and ketone production rates were not assessed. More recently, however, Weiss et al. (102) and Gerber et al. (103) have shown that somatostatin-induced insulin deficiency in man enhances the ketogenic and lipolytic effects of epinephrine and norepinephrine respectively. In these studies ketone body production was measured using 3-^{14}C-acetoacetate. However, again neither insulin nor glucagon values were reported and it is likely that somatostatin infusion caused a relative deficiency in both insulin and glucagon levels. In each of the above studies relative glucagon deficiency probably causes an underestimate of insulin's ability to antagonize epinephrine-induced increases in ketone body levels. The roles of norepinephrine and epinephrine in chronically insulin-deficient man have also been investigated (104–106). Epinephrine infusion caused ketone body levels to rise twice as fast in diabetics as in normal individuals (106). The rise in ketone body levels in diabetic man given norepinephrine was more than 50% greater than in normal man given the same amount of the catecholamine (105, 107). Willms et al. (104) saw a similar effect of norepinephrine in diabetics. These data indicate that epinephrine and norepinephrine have a greater ability to augment ketogenesis in the absence of insulin in both the normal and diabetic and provide some measure of the ability of basal insulin to restrain the lipolytic and ketogenic effects of catecholamines.

The potent antilipolytic and antiketogenic effects of insulin in vivo are apparent from the studies cited in this review and are diagrammatically summarized in Figure 3. Under normal conditions the hormone acts as a

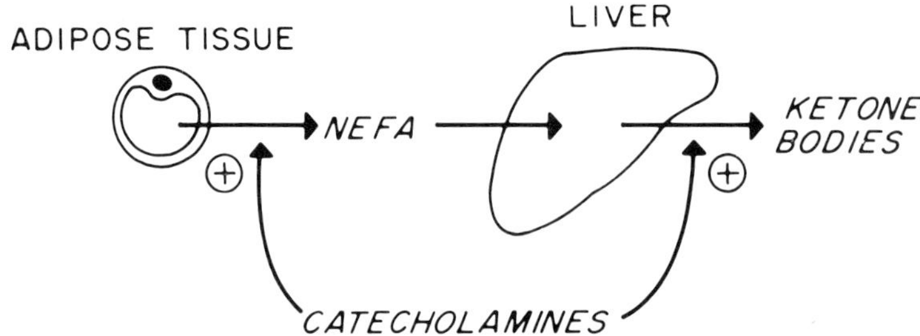

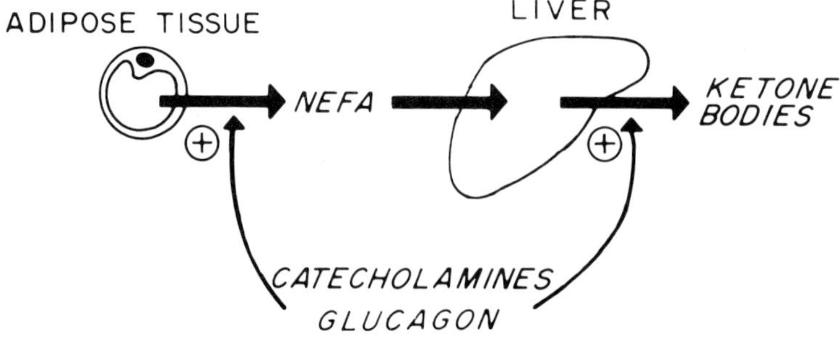

FIG. 3. *The effects of glucagon and catecholamines in the presence of basal insulin and insulin deficiency on lipolysis and ketogenesis in vivo.*

potent restraint on the lipolytic and ketogenic effects of basal glucagon and also of increases in glucagon, epinephrine and norepinephrine. Its absence can lead to large increases in both circulating non-esterified fatty acids and ketone bodies particularly in situations where glucagon and/or catecholamine levels may be increased.

Regulation of protein metabolism by insulin

Complementing its role as a major regulator of carbohydrate and fat homeostasis is the major role insulin plays in the maintenance of nitrogen balance in vivo. The plasma insulin level is probably the most important factor in the regulation of protein and amino acid metabolism. The effect of insulin can be exerted at several sites, the most important of which are the liver and muscle. Both in vitro and in vivo studies showed that insulin stimulates protein synthesis (108) and inhibits protein breakdown (15, 109–113), and simultaneously decreases urea production and the conversion of amino acids to glucose (15, 109, 113). The effects on protein synthesis are mediated by cAMP, while those on protein breakdown are non-cAMP-dependent and require internalization of the insulin–receptor complex (114), which leads – by an as yet unknown mechanism – to the stabilization of lysosomal structure and consequently to a decrease in lysosomal autophagy (109). The action of insulin on amino acid and protein metabolism in muscle has also been extensively documented since this tissue accounts for 80% of body protein. The accumulated evidence suggests that the predominant acute effect of a physiologic rise in insulin is to accelerate amino acid transport into muscle, to inhibit protein degradation at that site and to modulate protein synthesis by increasing the efficiency of ribosomal translation, at the level of peptide chain initiation (115). The long-term effects would involve an additional increase in the capacity for protein synthesis through a rise in the concentration of ribosomes (116).

The relevance of these findings to the physiological situation is currently under intensive investigation. We recently studied the effects of selective changes in plasma insulin (i.e. fixed basal levels of glucagon) on leucine kinetics and protein turnover in vivo using a constant infusion of isotopically labelled leucine (^{3}H- or ^{14}C-) in both conscious dog (117) and man (118). Since leucine is an essential amino acid, in the absence of any exogenous dietary intake its rate of appearance into the plasma compartment provides an estimate of intracellular protein breakdown. Its rate of disappearance from the plasma compartment represents the summation of its individual rates of incorporation into proteins, oxidation, and excretion although the latter component is negligible (117). The contribution of leucine oxidation can be measured independently by determining the appearance of ^{14}C-label in breath CO_2. Our data in the dog indicate that when insulin was selectively withdrawn, by the simultaneous administration of peripheral somatostatin with intraportal replacement of basal glucagon, plasma leucine rose from the basal values of 131 ± 9 to 187 ± 12 μmol/l ($P < 0.005$) by the end of 4 hours (Fig. 4). This was mainly a result of decreased outflow of leucine from the plasma compartment (clearance dropped from basal values of 25 ± 3 to 15 ± 0.3 ml/kg per min by the end of 4 h, $P > 0.005$) without a change in its rate of appearance. Similar studies carried out in overnight fasted normal man (118), showed that insulin withdrawal resulted in an 80% increase in plasma leucine (from 103 ± 4 to 189 ± 6 μmol/l, $P < 0.005$) which was due, as in the dog, to a net decrease in leucine outflow from the plasma compartment (clearance fell from basal values of 17 ± 1 to 10 ± 1 ml/kg-min, $P < 0.005$). In addition, insulin withdrawal resulted in a 60% rise in the rate of leucine oxidation (from 0.27 ± 0.06 to 0.43 ± 0.07 μmol/kg per min, $P < 0.005$). In man as in the dog leucine R_a did not change in response to insulin deficiency. All the changes in concentrations and clearance were reversible when insulin was supplemented to basal levels. Since the rate of leucine disappearance, as calculated by the isotopic method, is equivalent to the sum of the rates of protein synthesis and oxidation, then the decrease in leucine outflow represents the minimum estimate by which protein synthesis is depressed. It is then safe to conclude that acute insulin withdrawal had its major effect on protein synthesis without affecting protein breakdown. On the other hand, a selective but twice basal rise in plasma insulin, resulted simultaneously in decreased entry (R_a dropped from 3.08 ± 0.17 to 2.1 ± 0.14 μmol/kg per min in 4 h, $P < 0.005$) and increased outflow of leucine (clearance increased from basal values of 26 ± 2 to 42 ± 2 ml/kg per min by 4 h, $P < 0.005$). Taken together, these studies indicate a role for insulin in regulating total body protein synthesis in the post-absorptive period without much effect on protein degradation. The latter process was only affected when insulin was raised to twice basal levels, suggesting the presence of a higher threshold for the regulation of protein breakdown in vivo.

Fasting is another condition where low insulin concentrations are presumed to play the major role in regulating protein turnover. It has been suggested that low insulin levels associated with starvation allow for the orderly transfer of amino acids from skeletal muscle to the liver where they are either deaminated, converted to glucose, urea, or fat, or are completely oxidized (119). As a result the essential (E) amino acids, particularly the branched chain amino acids (120) and their corresponding ketoacids (NN Abumrad, unpublished observations), are markedly elevated, while the non-essential (N) amino acids decline resulting in higher E/N ratios (121). Recent observations in our laboratory (122, 123), however, do not totally support this hypothesis. Since the plasma insulin level in the dog fasted 24 or 48 hours does not change significantly while leucine R_a increases in the absence of a change in leucine clearance, our data indicate that the changes

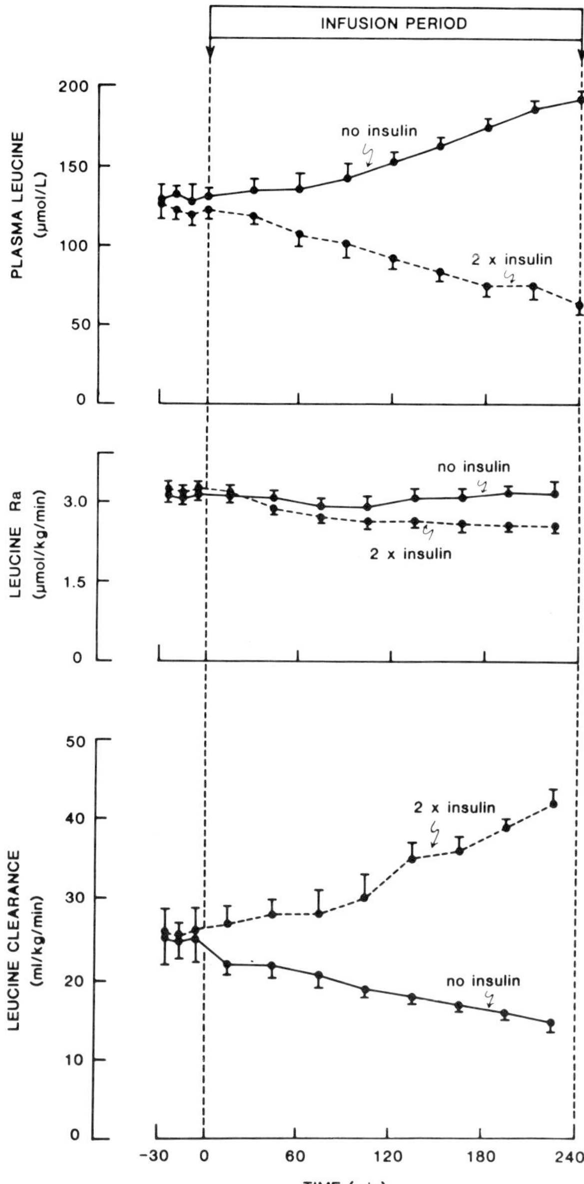

FIG. 4. *Arterial plasma leucine concentration (upper panel), and the rates of leucine appearance (R_a) (middle panel) and leucine clearance (lower panel) in 18-hour fasted conscious dogs maintained on infusions of SRIF (0.8 µg/kg per min) and concurrent intraportal infusions of glucagon (0.65 ng/kg per min) alone (no insulin = solid line) or in combination with insulin (600 µU/kg per min – 2× insulin = broken line). Reproduced from Miller et al. (123), by courtesy of the Editors of Diabetes.*

seen with early fasting (24 and 48 h) can occur independently of changes in plasma insulin levels. Only when fasting is prolonged beyond two days do the changes resemble those seen with insulin deficiency (123). Fasting resulted in a rise in plasma leucine from 116 ± 8 to 147 ± 8 μmol/l ($P < 0.005$). Its rate of appearance also increased (30%, $P < 0.05$) from 3.3 ± 0.2 to 4.4 ± 0.3 μmol/kg-min, while its clearance rate remained unchanged. Acute insulin deficiency brought about by somatostatin and replacement glucagon infusion in 48-h fasted dogs caused an increase in leucine levels by 45% ($P < 0.005$). Leucine R_a rose from 4.3 ± 0.3 to 5.0 ± 0.3 μmol/kg per min ($P < 0.05$) while the metabolic clearance rate fell by 20% in the 48-hour group. In summary, it appears that early (up to 4 days) fasting in the dog and man (unpublished observations) is associated with changes in both rates of protein synthesis and degradation which are not solely related to changes in insulin levels. This complexity in insulin interaction has also been emphasized recently by the observations of Garlick et al. (124) that infusion of insulin to overnight fasted rats so as to achieve levels comparable to those seen with feeding failed to raise the rates of protein synthesis in gastrocnemius muscles to levels seen post-prandially. These data suggest that the response of protein synthesis to both fasting and feeding is complex and involves more than the effects of changing insulin concentrations alone.

The changes in protein turnover which occur with chronic insulin deficiency are less well documented. The accumulated evidence suggests that streptozotocin-induced diabetes is associated with decreased protein synthesis. On the other hand, the effect on protein breakdown is still controversial with some studies showing enhanced (116, 125) and others showing decreased (126) proteolysis. We recently assessed these parameters in four depancreatized dogs (1–3 years' duration) using similar isotopic techniques to those described above. This animal model has the advantage of being similar to human insulin-dependent diabetes mellitus in that there is lack of insulin associated with high circulating glucagon. We measured leucine kinetics after 48 hours of insulin withdrawal and a 24-hour fast. As shown in Figure 5, following two days of insulin withdrawal the rate of leucine appearance into the plasma compartment was at least 65% higher than that seen in the normal post-absorptive dog, suggesting enhanced protein degradation. Thirty minutes after restoration of basal circulating insulin levels by intraportal insulin infusion, plasma leucine began to revert to normal levels as a result of both a decrease in its rate of appearance and an increase in its rate of clearance. Although rates of leucine oxidation were not measured in this study it is reasonable to assume that the effects observed relate to changes in the rates of synthesis and breakdown of protein. Although it is difficult from these studies to identify the tissues involved in this response, these studies are supportive of in-vitro studies which have shown enhanced protein breakdown in skeletal muscle obtained from rats rendered diabetic with streptozotocin (116, 127).

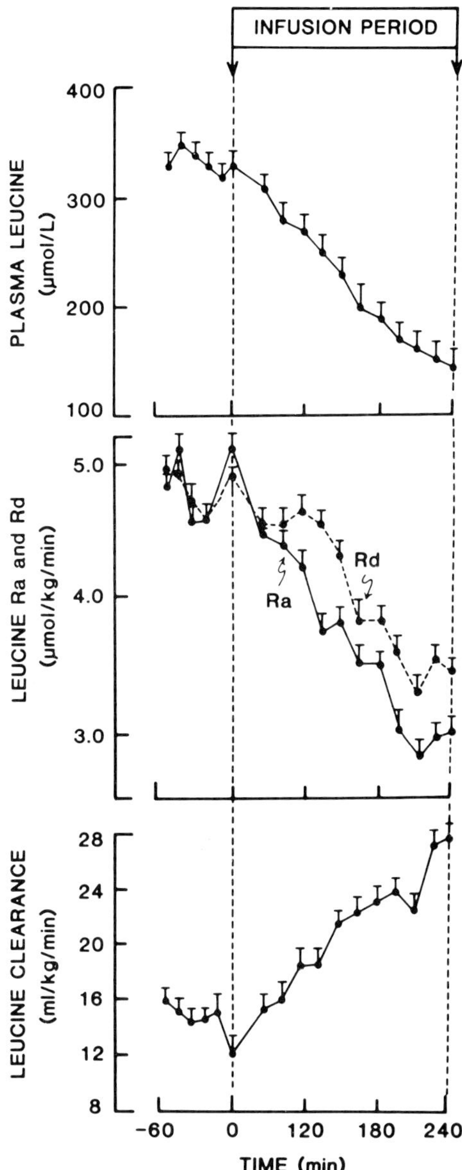

FIG. 5. *Arterial leucine (upper panel), rates of leucine appearance (Ra) and disappearance (Rd) (middle panel) and leucine clearance (lower panel) in 4 depancreatized dogs (1–3 years): the dogs were fasted 24 hours and had insulin withdrawn for 48 hours. During the infusion period, insulin was infused intraportally at 300 µU/ml.*

Conclusions

Insulin is unquestionably a primary regulator of carbohydrate, fat and protein metabolism and its presence is essential in the maintenance of normal control of these metabolic processes. In the past few years its action in vivo has become increasingly well understood. However there are still many aspects of its in-vivo action which remain undefined including the ability of increments in insulin to antagonize the metabolic effects of increases in catecholamines and other counter-regulatory hormones, the interrelationship of insulin with other as yet undefined mechanisms in the regulation of hepatic glucose uptake and the mechanism by which insulin regulates protein turnover during feeding and during a fast. Future studies in these areas should further clarify the role of insulin in vivo while continuing to pose additional new and important questions about the physiologic role of this hormone.

References

1. Felig P, Wahren J, Hendler R (1975): Influence of oral glucose ingestion on splanchnic glucose and gluconeogenic substrate metabolism in man. *Diabetes*, *24*, 468.
2. DeFronzo RA, Ferrannini E, Hendler R, Wahren J, Felig P (1978): Influence of hyperinsulinemia, hyperglycemia, and the route of glucose administration on splanchnic glucose exchange. *Proc. Natl Acad. Sci. USA*, *75*, 5173.
3. Bergman RN, Beir JR, Hourigan PM (1982): Intraportal glucose infusion matched to oral glucose absorption. Lack of evidence for 'gut factor' involvement in hepatic glucose storage. *Diabetes*, *31*, 27.
4. Abumrad NN, Cherrington AD, Williams PE, Lacy WW, Rabin D (1982): Absorption and disposition of a glucose load in the conscious dog. *Am. J. Physiol.*, *242*, E398.
5. Katz LD, Glickman MG, Rapoport S, Ferrannini E, DeFronzo RA (1983): Splanchnic and peripheral disposal of oral glucose in man. *Diabetes*, *32*, 675.
6. Ishida T, Chap Z, Chou J, Lewis R, Hartley C, Entman M, Field JB (1983): Differential effects of oral, peripheral intravenous, and intraportal glucose on hepatic glucose uptake and insulin and glucagon extraction in conscious dogs. *J. Clin. Invest.*, *72*, 590.
7. Zierler KL, Rabinowitz D (1963): Roles of insulin and growth hormone, based on studies of forearm metabolism in man. *Medicine (Baltimore)*, *42*, 385.
8. Pozefsky T, Felig P, Tobin JD, Soeldner JS, Cahill GF Jr (1969): Amino acid balance across tissues of the forearm in post-absorptive man. Effects of insulin at two dose levels. *J. Clin. Invest.*, *48*, 2273.
9. DeFronzo RA, Jacot E, Jequier E, Maeder E, Felber JP (1981): The effect of insulin on the disposal of intravenous glucose: results from indirect calorimetry and hepatic and femoral vein venous catheterization. *Diabetes*, *30*, 1000.

10. DeFronzo RA, Ferrannini E, Hendler R, Felig P, Wahren J (1983): Regulation of splanchnic and peripheral glucose uptake by insulin and hyperglycemia in man. *Diabetes*, *32*, 35.
11. Kolterman OG, Insel J, Saekow M, Olefsky JM (1980): Mechanisms of insulin resistance in human obesity. Evidence for receptor and postreceptor defects. *J. Clin. Invest.*, *65*, 1272.
12. Rizza RA, Mandarino LJ, Gerich JE (1981): Dose-response characteristics for effects of insulin on production and utilization of glucose in man. *Am. J. Physiol.*, *240*, E630.
13. Chiasson JL, Liljenquist JE, Finger FE (1976): Differential sensitivity of glycogenolysis and gluconeogenesis to insulin infusions in dogs. *Diabetes*, *25*, 283.
14. Chiasson JL, Atkinson RL, Cherrington AD (1979): Insulin regulation of gluconeogenesis from alanine in man. *Metabolism*, *29*, 810.
15. Cherrington AD (1981): Gluconeogenesis: its regulation by insulin and glucagon. In: *Diabetes Mellitus*, p. 49. Editor: M. Brownlee. Garland Press, New York.
16. Steiner KE, Williams PE, Lacy WW, Cherrington AD (1981): Effects of the insulin/glucagon molar ratio on glucose production in the dog. *Fed. Proc.*, *40*, 3481.
17. Sacca L, Hendler R, Sherwin RS (1978): Hyperglycemia inhibits glucose production in man independent of changes in glucoregulatory hormones. *J. Clin. Endocrinol. Metab.*, *47*, 1160.
18. Shulman GI, Liljenquist JE, Williams PE, Lacy WW, Cherrington AD (1978): Glucose disposal during insulinopenia in somatostatin-treated dogs. The roles of glucose and glucagon. *J. Clin. Invest.*, *62*, 487.
19. Shulman GI, Lacy WW, Liljenquist JE, Keller U, Williams PE, Cherrington AD (1980): Effect of glucose, independent of changes in insulin and glucagon secretion, on alanine metabolism in the conscious dog. *J. Clin. Invest.*, *65*, 496.
20. Cherrington AD, Williams PE, Harris M (1978): Relationship between the plasma glucose level and glucose uptake in the conscious dog. *Metabolism*, *27*, 787.
21. Gottesman I, Mandarino L, Gerich J (1984): Use of glucose uptake and glucose clearance for the evaluation of insulin action in vivo. *Diabetes*, *33*, 184.
22. Madison LL (1969): Role of insulin in the hepatic handling of glucose. *Arch. Intern. Med.*, *123*, 284.
23. Cherrington AD, Williams PE, AbouMourad N, Lacy WW, Steiner KE, Liljenquist JE (1982): Insulin as a mediator of hepatic glucose uptake in the conscious dog. *Am. J. Physiol.*, *242*, E97.
24. Barrett EJ, Ferrannini E, Gusberg R, Bevilacqua S, DeFronzo RA (1984): Hepatic and extrahepatic splanchnic glucose metabolism in the postabsorptive and glucose fed dog. *Metabolism* (in press).
25. Sacca L, Orofino G, Petrone A, Vigorito C (1984): Differential roles of splanchnic and peripheral tissues in the pathogenesis of impaired glucose tolerance. *J. Clin. Invest.*, *73*, 1683.
26. Scow RO, Cornfield J (1954): Quantitative relationship between the oral and

intravenous glucose tolerance curves. *Am. J. Physiol.*, *179*, 435.
27. Jackson RA, Peters N, Adrani U, Perry G, Rogers J, Brough WH, Pilkington TRE (1973): Forearm glucose uptake during the oral glucose tolerance test in normal subjects. *Diabetes*, *22*, 442.
28. Ferrannini E, Wahren J, Felig P, DeFronzo RA (1980): The role of fractional glucose extraction in the regulation of splanchnic glucose metabolism in normal and diabetic man. *Metabolism*, *29*, 28.
29. DeFronzo R, Ferrannini E, Wahren J, Felig P (1978): Lack of gastrointestinal mediator of insulin action in maturity-onset diabetes. *Lancet*, *2*, 1077.
30. Adkins BA, Myers SR, Williams PE, Cherrington AD (1984): Importance of the route of intravenous glucose delivery to hepatic glucose balance. *Diabetologia*, *27*, 250A.
31. Radziuk J (1982): Sources of carbon in hepatic glycogen synthesis during absorption of an oral glucose load in humans. *Fed. Proc.*, *41*, 110.
32. Steele R, Bjerknes C, Rathgeb I, Altszuler N (1968): Glucose uptake and production during an oral glucose tolerance test. *Diabetes*, *17*, 415.
33. Issekutz TB, Issekutz B Jr, Elahi D (1973): Estimation of hepatic glucose output in non-steady state. The simultaneous use of 2, ^{3}H-glucose and ^{14}C-glucose in the dog. *Can. J. Physiol. Pharmacol.*, *52*, 215.
34. Radziuk J, Inculet R (1983): The effects of ingested and intravenous glucose on forearm uptake of glucose and glucogenic substrate in normal man. *Diabetes*, *32*, 977.
35. Nilsson L H'son, Hultman E (1974): Liver and muscle glycogen in man after glucose and fructose infusion. *Scand. J. Clin. Lab. Invest.*, *33*, 5.
36. Olefsky JM (1976): The insulin receptor: Its role in insulin resistance in obesity and diabetes. *Diabetes*, *25*, 1154.
37. Beck-Nielsen H (1978): The pathogenic role of an insulin receptor defect in diabetes mellitus of the obese. *Diabetes*, *27*, 1175.
38. DeFronzo RA, Diebert D, Hendler R, Felig P (1979): Insulin sensitivity and insulin binding to monocytes in maturity-onset diabetes. *J. Clin. Invest.*, *63*, 939.
39. Kahn CR, Neville DM Jr, Roth J (1973): Insulin-receptor interaction in the obese hyperglycemic mouse. A model of insulin resistance. *J. Biol. Chem.*, *248*, 244.
40. Roth J, Kahn CR, Lesniak MA, Gorden P, DeMeyts P, Megyesi K, Neville DM Jr, Gavin JR III, Soll AH, Freychet P, Goldfine IE, Bar RS, Archer JA (1976): Receptors for insulin, NSILA-s and growth hormone: applications to disease states in man. *Recent Prog. Horm. Res.*, *31*, 95.
41. Muggeo M, Bar RS, Roth J, Kahn CR, Gorden P (1977): The insulin resistance of acromegaly: Evidence for two alterations in the insulin receptor on circulating monocytes. *J. Clin. Endocrinol. Metab.*, *48*, 17.
42. Olefsky JM, Johnson J, Liu F, Jen P, Reaven GM (1975): The effects of acute and chronic dexamethasone administration on insulin binding to isolated rat hepatocytes and adipocytes. *Metabolism*, *24*, 517.
43. Kahn CR, Goldfine ID, Neville DM Jr, DeMeyts P (1978): Alterations in insulin binding induced by changes in vivo in the levels of glucocorticoids and growth hormone. *Endocrinology*, *103*, 1054.

44. Bertoli A, DePirro R, Fusco A, Greco AV, Magnatta R, Lauro R (1980): Differences in insulin receptors between man and menstruating women and influence of sex hormones on insulin binding during the menstrual cycle. *J. Clin. Endocrinol. Metab.*, *55*, 246.
45. Rowe J, Minaker K, Pallotta J, Flier J (1983): Characterization of the insulin resistance of aging. *J. Clin. Invest.*, *71*, 1581.
46. Kono T, Barham FW (1971): The relationship between the insulin-binding capacity of fat cells and the cellular response to insulin: studies with intact and trypsin-treated fat cells. *J. Biol. Chem.*, *246*, 6210.
47. Gliemann J, Gammeltoft S, Vinten J (1975): Time course of insulin-receptor binding and insulin-induced lipogenesis in isolated rat cells. *J. Biol. Chem.*, *250*, 3368.
48. Olefsky JM (1976): Effects of fasting on insulin binding, glucose transport, and glucose oxidation in isolated rat adipocytes: Relationship between insulin receptors and insulin action. *J. Clin. Invest.*, *58*, 1450.
49. Kosmakos RC, Roth J (1980): Insulin-induced loss of the insulin receptor in IM-9 lymphocytes. A biological process mediated through the insulin receptor. *J. Biol. Chem.*, *255*, 9860.
50. Kahn CR (1978): Insulin resistance, insulin insensitivity, and insulin unresponsiveness: a necessary distinction. *Metabolism*, *27*, 1893.
51. Olefsky JM (1981): Insulin resistance and insulin action: An in vitro and in vivo perspective. *Diabetes*, *20*, 148.
52. Harano Y, Ohgaku S, Kosugi K, Yasuda H, Nakano T, Kobayashi M, Hidaka H, Isumi K, Kashiwagi A, Shigeta Y (1981): Clinical significance of altered insulin sensitivity in diabetes mellitus assessed by glucose, insulin, and somatostatin infusion. *Metabolism*, *52*, 982.
53. Kolterman OG, Gray RS, Griffin J, Burstein P, Insel J, Scarlett JA, Olefsky JM (1981): Receptor and post-receptor defects contribute to the insulin resistance in noninsulin dependent diabetes mellitus. *J. Clin. Invest.*, *68*, 957.
54. Olefsky JM, Reaven GM (1977): Insulin binding in diabetes: Relationships with plasma insulin levels and insulin sensitivity. *Diabetes*, *26*, 680.
55. Reaven GM, Bernstein R, Davis B, Olefsky JM (1976): Nonketotic diabetes mellitus: insulin deficiency or insulin resistance. *Am. J. Med.*, *60*, 80.
56. Olefsky JM, Kolterman OG, Scarlett JA (1982): Insulin action and resistance in obesity and noninsulin-dependent type II diabetes mellitus. *Am. J. Physiol.*, *243*, E15.
57. Gerich J, Rizza R, Mandarino L (1982): Assessment of insulin action in humans with observations on the insulin resistance in noninsulin dependent diabetes mellitus. In: *Insulin Update*, p. 74. Editor: J. Skyler. Excerpta Medica, New York.
58. Andres R, Swedloff R, Pozefsky T, Coleman D (1966): Manual feedback technique for the control of blood glucose concentration. In: *Automation in Analytical Chemistry*, p. 486. Editor: L. Skeggs. Mediad, New York.
59. Gerich JE (1984): Assessment of insulin resistance and its role in non-insulin-dependent diabetes mellitus. *J. Lab. Clin. Med.*, *103*, 497.
60. Scarlett JA, Gray RS, Griffin J, Olefsky JM, Kolterman OG (1982): Insulin treatment reverses the insulin resistance of type II diabetes mellitus. *Diabetes Care*, *5*, 353.

61. Scarlett JA, Kolterman OG, Ciaraldi TP, Kao M, Olefsky JM (1983): Insulin treatment reverses the postreceptor defect in adipocyte 3-0-methylglucose transport in type II diabetes mellitus. *J. Clin. Endocrinol. Metab.*, *56*, 1195.
62. Wahren J (1979): Glucose turnover during exercise in healthy man and in patients with diabetes mellitus. *Diabetes*, *28*, *Suppl. 1*, 82.
63. Ruderman WB, Ganda OP, Johanson K (1979): The effect of physical training on glucose tolerance in middle-aged men with chemical diabetes. *Diabetes*, *28*, *Suppl. 1*, 89.
64. DeFronzo R, Hendler R, Simonson D (1982): Insulin resistance is a prominent feature of type 1 (juvenile onset) diabetes mellitus. *Diabetes*, *31*, 795.
65. Proietto J, Nankervis A, Aitken P, Caruso G, Alford F (1983): Glucose utilization in type 1 (insulin-dependent) diabetes: evidence for a defect not reversible by acute elevations in insulin. *Diabetologia*, *25*, 331.
66. Ginsberg HN (1977): Investigation of insulin sensitivity in treated subjects with ketosis-prone diabetes mellitus. *Diabetes*, *26*, 278.
67. Pedersen O, Hjollund E (1982): Insulin receptor binding to fat and blood cells and insulin action in fat cells from insulin dependent diabetics. *Diabetes*, *31*, 706.
68. Caruso G, Proietto J, Calenti A, Alford F (1983): Insulin resistance in alloxan-diabetic dogs: Evidence for reversal following insulin therapy. *Diabetologia*, *25*, 273.
69. Bearn A, Billing B, Sherlock S (1951): Hepatic glucose output and hepatic insulin sensitivity in diabetes mellitus. *Lancet*, *2*, 698.
70. Issekutz B Jr, Issekutz TB, Elahi D, Borkow I (1974): Effect of insulin infusions on the glucose kinetics in alloxan-streptozotocin diabetic dogs. *Diabetologia*, *10*, 323.
71. Brown P, Tompkins C, Juul S, Sonksen P (1978): Mechanism of action of insulin in diabetic patients: a dose-related effect on glucose production and utilization. *Br Med. J.*, *1*, 1239.
72. Davidson MB (1981): Autoregulation by glucose of hepatic glucose balance: permissive effect of insulin. *Metabolism*, *30*, 279.
73. Stevenson RW, Parsons JA, Alberti KGMM (1983): Effect of intraportal and peripheral insulin on glucose turnover and recycling in diabetic dogs. *Am. J. Physiol.*, *244*, E190.
74. Stevenson RW, Parson JA, Alberti KGMM (1981): Comparison of the metabolic responses to portal and peripheral infusions of insulin in diabetic dogs. *Metabolism*, *30*, 745.
75. Stevenson RW, Williams PE, Cherrington AD (1984): Role of glucagon suppression in insulin treatment of the conscious diabetic dog. *Diabetologia*, *27*, 335A.
76. Albisser AM, Leibel BS, Zinman B, Murray FT, Zingg W, Botz CK, Denoga A, Marliss EB (1977): Studies with an artificial endocrine pancreas. *Arch. Intern. Med.*, *137*, 639.
77. Hanna AK, Zinman B, Nakhooda AF, Minuk HL, Stokes EF, Albisser AM, Marliss EB (1980): Insulin, glucagon, and amino acids during glycemic control by the artificial pancreas in diabetic man. *Metabolism*, *29*, 321.
78. Nosadini R, Noy GA, Nattrass M, Alberti KGMM, Johnston DG, Home PD, Orskov H (1982): The metabolic and hormonal response to acute nor-

moglycaemia in type 1 (insulin-dependent) diabetes: studies with a glucose controlled insulin infusion system (artificial endocrine pancreas). *Diabetologia*, *23*, 220.
79. Stevenson RW, Orskov H, Parsons JA, Alberti KGMM (1983): Metabolic responses to intraduodenal glucose loading in insulin-infused diabetic dogs. *Am. J. Physiol.*, *245*, E200.
80. Pickup JC, Stevenson RW (1984): Rate-controlled insulin delivery in normal physiology and in the treatment of insulin-dependent diabetes. In: *Rate-Controlled Drug Administration and Action.* Editor: H.A. Struyker-Bordier, CRC Press, New York, in press.
81. Waldhausl W, Bratusch-Marrain P, Gasic S, Korn A, Nowotny P (1979): Insulin production rate following glucose ingestion estimated by splanchnic C-peptide output in normal man. *Diabetologia*, *17*, 221.
82. Eaton RP, Allen RC, Schade DS, Standefer JC (1980): 'Normal' insulin secretion: The goal of artificial delivery systems. *Diabetes Care*, *3*, 270.
83. Zierler KL, Rabinowitz D (1964): Effect of very small concentrations of insulin on forearm metabolism. Persistence of its action on potassium and free fatty acids without its effect on glucose. *J. Clin. Invest.*, *43*, 950.
84. Massi-Benedetti M, Burrin JM, Capaldo B, Alberti KGMM (1981): A comparative study of the activity of biosynthetic human insulin and park insulin using the glucose clamp technique in normal subjects. *Diabetes Care*, *4*, 163.
85. Schade DS, Eaton RP (1977): Dose response to insulin in man: differential effects on glucose and ketone body regulation. *J. Clin. Endocrin. Metab.*, *44*, 1038.
86. Gerber PPG, Keller U, Stauffacher W (1983): Direct effect of insulin on liver ketogenic capacity in man. *Diabetologia*, *25*, 156.
87. Wahren J, Effendic S, Lift R, Hagenfeldt Z, Bjorkman O, Felig P (1977): Influence of somatostatin on splanchnic glucose metabolism in post-absorptive and 60-hour fasted humans. *J. Clin. Invest.*, *59*, 299.
88. Metcalfe P, Johnston DG, Nosadini R, Orskov H, Alberti KGMM (1981): Metabolic effects of acute and prolonged growth hormone excess in normal and insulin deficient man. *Diabetologia*, *20*, 123.
89. Keller U, Chiasson JL, Liljenquist JE, Cherrington AD, Jennings AS, Crofford OB (1977): The role of insulin, glucagon and free fatty acids in the regulation of ketogenesis in dogs. *Diabetes*, *26*, 1040.
90. Pickup JC, Viberti GC, Bilous RW, Keen H, Alberti KGMM, Home PD, Binder C (1982): Safety of continuous subcutaneous insulin infusion: metabolic deterioration and glycemic autoregulation after deliberate cessation of infusion. *Diabetologia*, *22*, 175.
91. Keller U, Sonnenberg GE, Berger W (1980): Ketone body turnover rates in insulin dependent diabetics following short term withdrawal of a continuous sub-cutaneous infusion of insulin. *Eur. J. Clin. Invest.*, *10*, 18.
92. Miles JM, Rizza RA, Haymond MW, Gerich JE (1980): Effects of acute insulin deficiency on glucose and ketone body turnover in man. *Diabetes*, *29*, 926.
93. Wahren J, Sato Y, Ostmann J, Hagenfeldt L, Felig P (1984): Turnover and splanchnic metabolism of free fatty acids and ketones in insulin dependent diabetics at rest and in response to exercise. *J. Clin. Invest.*, *73*, 1367.

94. Gerich JE, Lorenzi M, Bier DM, Tsalkian E, Schneider V, Karam JH, Forsham PH (1976): Effects of physiologic levels of glucagon and growth hormone on human carbohydrate and lipid metabolism. *J. Clin. Invest.*, *57*, 875.
95. Sonnenberg GE, Stauffacher W, Keller U (1982): Failure of glucagon to stimulate ketone body production during acute insulin deficiency on insulin replacement in man. *Diabetologia*, *23*, 94.
96. Miles JM, Haymond MW, Nissen SL, Gerich JE (1983): Effects of free fatty acid availability, glucagon excess, and insulin deficiency on ketone body production in postabsorptive man. *J. Clin. Invest.*, *71*, 1554.
97. Keller U, Shulman GI (1979): Effect of glucagon on hepatic fatty acid oxidation and ketogenesis in conscious dogs. *Am. J. Physiol.*, *237*, E121.
98. Gerich JE, Lorenzi M, Bier DM, Tsalkian E, Schneider V, Karam JH, Forsham PH (1976): Effects of physiologic levels of glucagon and growth hormone on human carbohydrate and lipid metabolism. *J. Clin. Invest.*, *57*, 875.
99. Johnston DG, Alberti KGMM (1982): Hormonal control of ketone body metabolism in the normal and diabetic state, *Clin. Endocrinol. Metab.*, *11*, 329.
100. Pernet A, Walker M, Gill GV (1980): Ketogenic effect of catecholamines in normal man. *Diabetologia*, *19*, 306.
101. Chideckel EW, Goodner CJ, Kloerker DJ, Johnston DG, Ensick JW (1977): Role of glucagon in mediating metabolic effects of epinephrine. *Am. J. Physiol.*, *232*, E464.
102. Weiss M, Keller U, Brunner S, Stauffacher W (1983): Effect of adrenaline on ketone body kinetics in normal and insulin deficient man. *Diabetologia*, *25*, 203.
103. Gerber PPG, Buehler FR, Keller U (1981): Ketone body kinetics during norepinephrine infusion and insulin deficiency in normal man: A study of mechanisms leading to diabetic ketosis. *Diabetologia*, *21*, 274.
104. Willms B, Bottcher M, Walters V, Sakamoto N, Soling HD (1969); Relationship between fat and ketone body metabolism in obese and nonobese diabetics and nondiabetics during norepinephrine infusion. *Diabetologia*, *5*, 88.
105. Schade D, Eaton RP (1977): The regulation of plasma ketone body concentration by counterregulatory hormones in man. *Diabetes*, *26*, 989.
106. Baker L, Kaye R, Haque N (1969): Metabolic homeostasis in juvenile diabetes mellitus. *Diabetes*, *18*, 421.
107. Schade DS, Eaton RP (1979): The regulation of plasma ketone body concentration by counter-regulatory hormones in man. *Diabetes*, *28*, 5.
108. Jefferson LS, Rannels SL, Munger DG, Morgan HE (1974): Insulin in the regulation of protein turnover in heart and skeletal muscle. *Fed. Proc.*, *33*, 1098.
109. Mortimore GE (1982): Mechanisms of cellular protein catabolism. *Nutr. Rev.*, *40*, 1.
110. Hershko A, Ciechanover A (1982): Mechanisms of intracellular protein breakdown. *Annu. Rev. Biochem.*, *51*, 335.
111. Abumrad NN, Miller B (1983): The physiologic and nutritional significance of plasma free amino acid levels. *J. Parent. Ent. Nutr.*, *7*, 163.

112. Felig P, Wahren J (1971): Influence of endogenous insulin secretion on splanchnic glucose and amino acid metabolism in man. *J. Clin. Invest.*, *50*, 1702.
113. Exton JH, Malette LE, Jefferson LS, Wong EA, Friedman N, Miller TB, Park CR (1970): The hormonal control of hepatic gluconeogenesis. *Rec. Prog. Horm. Res.*, *26*, 411.
114. Draznin B, Trowbridge M (1982): Inhibition of intracellular proteolysis in isolated rat hepatocytes. Possible role of internalized hormone. *J. Biol. Chem.*, *257*, 11988.
115. Jefferson LS, Li JB, Rannels SR (1977): Regulation by insulin of amino acid release and protein turnover in the perfused rat hemicorpus. *J. Biol. Chem.*, *252*, 1476.
116. Pain VM, Albertse EC, Garlick PJ (1983): Protein metabolism in skeletal muscle, diaphragm, and heart of diabetic rats. *Am. J. Physiol.*, *245*, E604.
117. Abumrad NN, Jefferson LS, Rannels SR, Williams PE, Cherrington AD, Lacy WW (1982): The role of insulin in the regulation of leucine kinetics in the conscious dog. *J. Clin. Invest.*, *70*, 1031.
118. Powell CS, Abumrad NN (1982): Effect of basal insulin levels on leucine metabolism in normal man. *Surg. Forum*, *33*, 91.
119. Cahill GF Jr (1971): Physiology of insulin in man. *Diabetes*, *20*, 785.
120. Adibi SA (1976): Metabolism of branched chain amino acids in altered nutrition. *Metab. Clin. Exp. Med.*, *25*, 1287.
121. Swendseid ME, Umezawa CY, Drenick E (1969): Plasma amino acid levels in obese subjects before, during and after starvation. *Am. J. Clin. Nutr.*, *22*, 740.
122. Abumrad NN, Williams PE, Wise KL, Lacy DB, Lacy WW (1981): The effect of starvation on leucine kinetics in the conscious dog. In: *Metabolism and Clinical Implications of Branched Chain Amino and Ketoacids*, p. 355. Editors: M. Walser and J.R. Williamson. Elsevier-North Holland, Amsterdam-New York.
123. Miller B, Buckspan R, Hoxworth B, Lacy WW, Abumrad NN (1984): Insulin's effect on leucine turnover changes during early fasting in the conscious dog. *Diabetes* (in press).
124. Garlick PJ, Fern M, Preedy VR (1983): The effect of insulin infusion and food intake on muscle protein synthesis in post-absorptive rats. *Biochem. J.*, *210*, 669.
125. Dice JF, Walker CD, Byrne B, Cardiel A (1978): General characteristics of protein degradation in diabetes and starvation. *Proc. Natl Acad. Sci. USA*, *75*, 2093.
126. Millward DJ, Garlick PJ, Nnanyelugo DO, Waterlow JC (1976): The relative importance of muscle protein synthesis and breakdown in the regulation of muscle mass. *Biochem. J.*, *156*, 185.
127. Pain VM, Garlick PJ (1974): Effect of streptozotocin-diabetes and insulin treatment on the rate of protein synthesis in tissues of the rat *in vivo*. *J. Biol. Chem.*, *249*, 4510.

The Diabetes Annual/1
K.G.M.M. Alberti and L.P. Krall, editors

ISBN 0444 90 343 7
$0.85 per article per page (transactional system)
$0.20 per article per page (licensing system)

25 Insulin receptors

C. RONALD KAHN

Insulin initiates its action at the cellular level by binding to a specific glycoprotein receptor on the surface of the cell. Since the first direct studies of the insulin receptor published in 1971 (1, 2), there has been an exponential explosion of information in this field. The number of papers published per year has increased to over 300, and as of yet, there is no evidence for a plateau. Not surprisingly, therefore, in the past few years considerable progress has been made, especially in areas of receptor purification, elucidation of the structure of the receptor, studies of receptor biosynthesis and turnover, studies of the protein kinase activity of the receptor, and studies of receptors in disease states. In this chapter, I will attempt to summarize some of the major developments in each of these areas and to analyze some of the areas of continued controversy and investigation.

Structure and purification of the insulin receptor

Like receptors for other hormones and biologically active substances, the insulin receptor serves two functions. The first is to recognize insulin among all the other substances in the blood; this is accomplished by binding insulin with high affinity and specificity. The second is to transmit a transmembrane signal which results in an alteration in intracellular metabolic pathways. Progress in purification of the insulin receptor (3, 4) and studies elucidating the structure of the receptor by both affinity labeling techniques (5–10) and immunoprecipitation (11–13) have helped to explain these two features of the molecule. A working model of the receptor is shown in Figure 1.

After biosynthetic or surface labeling of cells, insulin receptors may be extracted in Triton X-100 and immunoprecipitated using either polyclonal or monoclonal antibodies to the receptor. In both cases, SDS gel electrophoresis of the precipitate reveals two major protein bands: one has an apparent molecular weight of 130,000 to 135,000 and has been termed the α-subunit; the other has a molecular weight of 90,000 to 95,000 and has

This work has been supported in part by NIH grants AM 31036 and AM 33201.

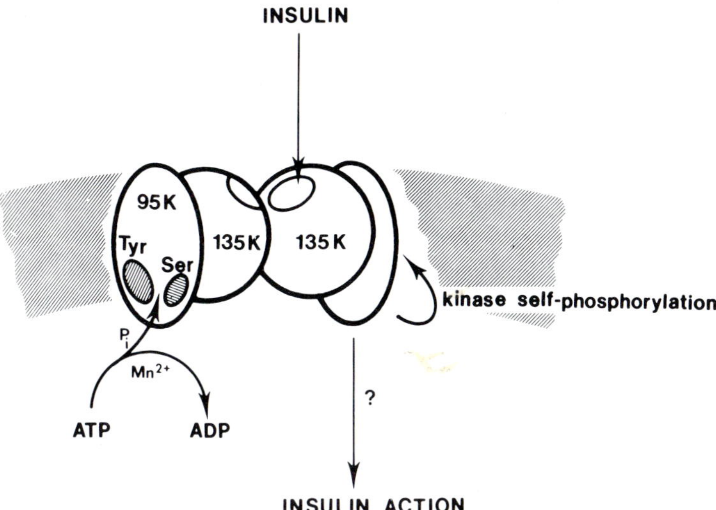

FIG. 1. *A working model of the insulin receptor.*

been termed the β-subunit (11–13). Both are glycoproteins and can be labeled with techniques which label both the amino acids and sugars of the glycoprotein, and both are expressed on the external surface of the cell since they can be labeled using surface labeling techniques. Using various sugars, it has been possible to show that both subunits possess 'complex-type' carbohydrate side chains (12).

Using sequential chromatography on wheat germ-Sepharose and insulin-Sepharose, Fujita-Yamaguchi et al. have succeeded in purifying the receptor from human placenta to near homogeneity (3). Silver-stained SDS gels of the purified receptor have confirmed the presence of only two major subunits (α and β). A minor protein of molecular weight 52,000 is also found in this preparation and is thought to be a degradation product of the β-subunit.

The insulin receptor has been affinity-labeled using iodinated photoreactive insulin analogues (5–7) or by cross-linking ^{125}I-insulin to the receptor using disuccinimidyl suberate (DSS) (8–10). These techniques label the α-subunit, either predominantly or exclusively, indicating that the α-subunit contains the insulin binding site. Both the affinity cross-linking technique and the photoaffinity analogues will also label the β-subunit to a small degree, suggesting that the β-subunit may contribute to the insulin binding site or is at least in close proximity to it. These techniques also label a band with a molecular weight of 40,000 to 45,000. Most investigators believe that this is a degradation product of the β-subunit since it can be increased in amount by treatment of cells or solubilized receptors with certain proteolytic enzymes (9). Yip and Moule, on the other hand, have suggested that these bands represent one or two additional receptor subunits (6). Recently, Chratchko et al. have presented data that this 45K protein may be a component of the major histocompatibility complex non-covalently associated with the receptor (14). Obviously, more work will be needed to clarify this problem.

On non-reducing gels, the subunits of the insulin receptor are disulfide-linked to form high molecular weight oligomers (15, 16). The most frequent model proposed is one consisting of a β–α–α–β structure originally proposed by Massague et al. on the basis of sequential reduction of the receptor after affinity cross-linking (15). This basic model has been further supported by studies of the purified receptor (3) and by studies of the immunoprecipitated receptor (16). Some heterogeneity is observed, however, presumably as a result of proteolytic cleavage of one or both β-subunits to give two species of lower molecular weight. Also, other non-reduced forms of receptor have been observed including α–β heterodimer, α–α homodimer, free α- and β-subunits, and a high molecular form (M_r 520,000) with an unknown number of α- and β-subunits.

Two other models for the receptor have been put forward. One by Yip and Moule consists of two α- and one β-subunit with the two subunits of about 40,000 (6). The other, proposed by Baron and Sonksen consists of two α-, one β-subunit and a δ-subunit of 60,000 MW (17). Neither of these models has been supported by other studies. Studies of receptor structure using radiation inactivation (18, 19) and lectin chromatography (29) had suggested that the insulin receptor was also associated with some type of 'affinity regulatory protein'. Evidence for this protein has continued to occur in functional studies (19), but thus far no structural information has appeared. It is possible that the different disulfide-bonded forms of the receptor have different affinities for insulin (16, 21, 22) and thus may account for the 'apparent affinity regulator'.

In contrast to the previous notion that insulin receptors should be restricted to classical target tissues, direct studies have indicated the receptor is virtually ubiquitous on mammalian cells, occurring in such *unlikely* places as brain (23, 24), circulating erythrocytes (25, 26), vascular endothelial cells (27, 28), and gonadal cells (29). The binding properties of the receptor are very similar in all tissues, suggesting that insulin may have a biological role in almost all tissues. Recent studies, however, have indicated that some microheterogeneity of receptor structure may exist. Thus, the subunits of the insulin receptor in brain tissue are of somewhat lower molecular weight than those in liver or fat and may differ in the degree of glycosylation (24). Possible differences in the nature of the disulfide bonding of subunits (21, 30) and in the state of receptor aggregation (31) in different tissues have also been suggested. Whether these differences indicate receptors specialized for different functions is not yet known. Studies with monoclonal antibodies to the receptor should help detect further differences, if they exist (32, 33).

Little is known of the tertiary structure of the receptor. Functional studies have suggested that the receptors may undergo changes in the state of conformation (34, 35) or aggregation (36, 37) upon binding of insulin. Such changes could provide clues to the early steps in insulin action and need further study.

Biosynthesis and turnover

Like all membrane proteins, the insulin receptor is in a constant state of turnover, i.e. being synthesized and degraded. The insulin receptor appears to be synthesized from a single chain pro-receptor (12, 38–43). The pro-receptor has a molecular weight of 180,000 in a non-glycosylated form (45); however, most studies have focused on a partially glycosylated form with a molecular weight of 190,000. This form of the pro-receptor presumably occurs in the rough endoplasmic reticulum, but contains both subunits in an active form. Thus, the insulin binding site of the pro-receptor can be labeled using affinity techniques (40), a property normally present in the α-subunit of the receptor, and the pro-receptor also undergoes insulin-stimulated autophosphorylation, a property of the β-subunit (42).

Following complete glycosylation, the receptor is cleaved to yield α- and β-subunits and is inserted into the plasma membrane. This whole process requires about 1.5 to 3 hours and can be blocked with the carboxylic ionophore monensin (38, 41). In some ways, the biosynthesis of the insulin receptor resembles that of the insulin molecule which also contains two disulfide-linked chains synthesized as a single chain precursor.

The mature receptor has a half-life of about 7 to 12 hours; that is, every 7 to 12 hours half of all the receptors on the cell are degraded and a new complement is synthesized (43, 45). In a cell with 20,000 receptors, this corresponds to a turnover rate of about 1300 receptors per hour. Just as the subunits are synthesized together, both subunits appear to be degraded simultaneously (44, 46). Exactly how this occurs is uncertain, but in most cells this appears to be linked to a process of receptor-mediated endocytosis (45–49). The fate of the receptor in this process has been difficult to study directly, but based on studies with affinity-labeled receptors (50, 51) and on calculations of insulin internalization rates (52), it appears that only a small fraction of internalized receptors are degraded. Receptor degradation presumably occurs in lysosomes, and is accelerated by exposure of cells to insulin (44, 46, 47, 49, 53) or to anti-receptor antibody (54, 55). This leads to a decrease in the concentration of receptors in cells, a condition termed 'down-regulation' (53), and appears to be an important mechanism for regulation of receptors in physiologic and pathologic states (*vide infra*).

Most internalized receptors escape degradation and are recycled back to the membrane so that a single receptor may make several cycles before being degraded (50–52).

The insulin receptor as a tyrosine-specific protein kinase

In 1982, Kasuga et al. noted that the insulin receptor undergoes insulin-stimulated phosphorylation (56), opening a whole new avenue of insulin receptor research. Since then, considerable evidence has been accumulated that the insulin receptor itself is an insulin-sensitive, tyrosine-specific protein kinase. Protein kinases are enzymes which are involved in the transfer of phosphate groups from high energy phosphate compounds, such as ATP, to amino acid residues of proteins. In the case of the insulin receptor, this leads to an autophosphorylation reaction with incorporation of phosphate groups onto the β-subunit of the receptor, as well as phosphorylation of exogenous substrates.

Insulin receptor phosphorylation was first demonstrated in intact cells prelabeled with ^{32}P-phosphoric acid (56–59), but has been most extensively characterized using receptors extracted from cells with detergents and incubated in a cell-free system with [γ -^{32}P]ATP (60–70). Insulin stimulates phosphorylation of insulin receptors isolated from a wide variety of tissues, and even in receptors purified to near homogeneity (64, 65). In the cell-free system, the phosphorylation occurs predominantly or exclusively on the β-subunit and on tyrosine residues (60). The solubilized insulin receptor will also phosphorylate a variety of exogenous substrates on tyrosine residues including histone (65), casein (66), natural and synthetic peptides containing tyrosine (65, 66, 71), and even synthetic copolymers of tyrosine and glutamic acid (72, 73). The β-subunit of the receptor has been shown to possess an ATP binding site by several affinity-labeling techniques (74–76), suggesting that it is the kinase subunit of the receptor. Further, selective degradation of the β-subunit by proteolytic enzymes results in a loss of receptor kinase activity (77, 78).

In vitro, the receptor kinase activity appears to be regulated by at least two factors: insulin, which increases the V_{max} of the enzyme, and divalent cations, particularly Mn^{++}, which decrease the K_m (69). The insulin effect is maximal within one minute and results in a 10-fold or greater stimulation of autophosphorylation. The kinase activity also appears to be regulated by the state of receptor phosphorylation (79). Thus, pre-incubation of the receptor with ATP and insulin leads to an activation of the receptor kinase activity, which will persist in the absence of continued exposure to insulin.

In addition to insulin, insulin receptor autophosphorylation is stimulated by a number of substances with insulin-like activity on cells. This includes lectins (80), trypsin (81), and vanadate (82). Studies with anti-insulin receptor antibodies have yielded conflicting results. Some workers have shown that anti-receptor antibodies which mimic insulin action stimulate receptor phosphorylation (61, 80, 82), whereas other workers, in some cases using the same antibodies, have found no stimulation (82, 84). This has led Simpson and Hedo to question the role of receptor phosphorylation in insulin action (84). This conclusion is premature since the concentrations of anti-receptor antibody used in these experiments may not have been sufficient, and since it is possible that the antibodies have a different mechanism of action from the normal ligand. Clearly, further studies are needed in this important area.

Comparison of intact and broken cell experiments indicates that receptor phosphorylation is a complex process and probably occurs in at least two steps (56–59). In the broken cell preparation, only tyrosine (or almost only tyrosine) is phosphorylated. In the intact cell, on the other hand, phosphoamino acid analysis reveals sites of serine and threonine phosphorylation, in addition to the tyrosine site (57). This has led to the suggestion that in addition to autophosphorylation on a tyrosine residue, the insulin receptor is also a substrate for some other serine- or threonine-specific protein kinases. The exact relationship of these kinases to the receptor is uncertain, but since serine phosphorylation can be observed in some experiments after solubilization and partial purification of the receptor, some workers believe these kinases are closely linked to the receptor (85, 86).

Although the exact role of the kinase activity of the insulin receptor is unknown, the fact that this activity is intrinsic to the receptor and insulin-stimulated has led to the speculation that this activity is the transmembrane signal leading to the cascade of phosphorylation culminating in insulin's action at the cellular level. Tyrosine protein kinase activity is relatively rare in cells and appears to be a property of proteins which are important in regulation of cellular growth or metabolism. Thus far, the only other known proteins with tyrosine kinase activity are receptors for other growth factors, in particular epidermal growth factor (EGF) (87), platelet-derived growth factor (PDGF) (88), insulin-like growth factor I (IGF-I)/somatomedin-C (89), and the gene products of several of the transforming RNA viruses (90). Although the exact amino acid sequence of the insulin receptor is not yet known, it is likely that it will be homologous to one or more of these other proteins. Recently, the receptor for epidermal growth factor has been cloned and shown to have over 90% sequence homology with an oncogene product from avian erythroblastosis virus, referred to as erb-B (91).

Exactly how activation of a tyrosine kinase might result in signal transduction is uncertain. The most obvious possibility is that the kinase phosphorylates one or more endogenous substrates, perhaps other proteins with kinase or phosphatase activity, leading to a cascade of phosphorylation/dephosphorylation reactions. Attempts to identify an endogenous substrate of the insulin receptor have met thus far with limited success (92).

Insulin receptors in physiological and pathological states

One of the major findings which has come from direct studies of insulin receptors is the realization that the receptor is not a static entity but is regulated in a large number of physiological and pathological states. This regulation may take the form of changes in receptor number and/or affinity, changes in subtle features of insulin binding such as temperature and pH sensitivity, and even changes in receptor kinase activity. A comprehensive summary of this subject is not possible in this chapter, but a review of human studies has been recently published by Grunberger et al. (93) and a list of diseases studied is given in Table 1.

Although insulin receptors in animals may be studied using a wide variety of tissues, only a few cell types are accessible for human studies. The most common cells used in these studies are peripheral blood cells, especially erythrocytes and monocytes. In general, studies using these two cell types show similar changes (94, 95), although there are obvious opportunities for discordance since erythrocytes have little or no protein synthesis and have a very specialized membrane. Recently, it has also become clear that erythrocytes lose insulin receptors during cellular aging (96), and some investigators have suggested correcting studies for red cell age using enzyme

TABLE 1. *Physiological and pathological states in which insulin receptor function in vivo may be altered*

Physiological states	Rabson-Mendenhall syndrome
Age	Lipoatrophic diabetes
Diurnal variation	
Diet	*Insulin-sensitive states*
Exercise	Type 1 diabetes mellitus
Menstrual cycle	Growth hormone deficiency
Pregnancy	Glucocorticoid deficiency
	Anorexia nervosa
Insulin-resistant states	
Obesity	*Other disease states*
Type-2 diabetes mellitus	Insulinoma
Acromegaly	Infants of diabetic mothers
Glucocorticoid excess	Hypoglycemia in childhood
Insulin resistance and acanthosis nigricans, types A and B	Viral infection
Ataxia telangectasia	*Drugs altering insulin binding*
Uremia	Oral hypoglycemic agents
Myotonic dystrophy	Oral contraceptives
Cirrhosis	Glucocorticoids
Leprechaunism	

activity markers (97). Adipocytes have the advantage of allowing direct studies of biological activity, but are less accessible, are subject to a major change in cell size in diseases such as obesity, and also may exhibit different properties when taken from different biopsy sites (98). Possible genetic defects in receptors have also been studied using cultured skin fibroblasts (98–101), B-lymphocytes transformed with Epstein-Barr virus (102), and T-lymphocytes after mitogen stimulation (103). Although these generally agree with studies using freshly isolated cells, some differences have been observed, raising questions about their utility (104).

The most common modification of the receptor is an acquired reduction in receptor number which is observed in a number of hyperinsulinemic states (94, 105, 106). This reduction in receptor number has been termed 'down-regulation', and appears to be the direct result of exposure of cells to high levels of insulin since it can be reproduced in tissue culture (44, 47, 53) or by prolonged administration of insulin to animals (48, 107). Receptor down-regulation occurs in both obesity and Type 2 diabetes mellitus, and in both cases has been thought to contribute to the insulin-resistant state (94, 105–110). The importance of down-regulation of insulin receptors on red cells and monocytes in human obesity and Type 2 diabetes has been questioned because of conflicting data obtained with adipocytes, some investigators finding decreased receptor number (106) and others no change (109, 111). However, a recent study of liver biopsy specimens has confirmed receptor down-regulation in this important tissue in human obesity (112). Thus, the defects in human obesity closely mirror the defect observed in obese rodents (113).

Down-regulation is thought to be the result of an acquired increased receptor degradation (44, 53). Reversal of the hyperinsulinemia by diet or drug treatment results in a return of receptor number toward normal (106, 114). Studies of fibroblasts taken from obese mice (115) and obese humans (100), however, have revealed subtle changes in insulin binding even after several passages in culture. This has raised a question about the possibility of a pre-existing genetic abnormality leading to abnormal receptor regulation.

The role of insulin receptors in the action of oral hypoglycemia agents remains uncertain. Since the initial report by Olefsky and Reaven that chloropropamide increased insulin binding in Type 2 diabetics (116), numerous studies using both sulfonylureas (117–121) and biguanides (121–123) have attempted to explore this phenomenon. Two facts are clear from these studies: first, the effect of the oral hypoglycemic agents is quite variable, and secondly, in many patients, these agents improve glucose tolerance with no change in insulin binding to monocytes or erythrocytes (120, 121, 123).

Studies of cells from patients with rare genetic abnormalities of insulin receptors and insulin action have provided further insights into the molecular nature of the insulin receptor in insulin resistance. The best studied of these syndromes are the syndromes of insulin resistance and acanthosis nigricans Type A and leprechaunism (101, 130–132). The molecular defect in these patients appears to be heterogenous. In most patients studied thus far, the defect consists of a major decrease in insulin binding due to a decrease in receptor number (99, 124). The defect is probably genetic in nature since it is observed in different cells derived from the patient, including freshly isolated erythrocytes and monocytes, and cultured fibroblasts and lymphocytes. In some patients, defects in receptors for insulin-like growth factors also occur (99). In at least one patient with leprechaunism, the binding defect is very subtle and is manifest primarily by abnormalities in the pH and temperature sensitivity of binding (130).

A few patients with the clinical phenotype of the Type A syndrome have totally normal insulin binding. Recently, in two such cases it has been possible to define defects in the receptor kinase activity (126, 127). To do this, it was necessary to develop methods to study receptor phosphorylation using human erythrocytes (67), monocytes (68), and fibroblasts (127). Using these techniques, these patients have been shown to have a marked decrease in receptor kinase activity, despite normal insulin binding. Thus, in these patients, there appears to be a post-binding defect in insulin action located at the level of the receptor kinase. These studies provide further insights into the mechanism of action of insulin, and also provide a potential mechanism for post-binding receptor defects in insulin-resistant states.

References

1. Freychet P, Roth J, Neville DM Jr (1971): Insulin receptors in the liver: Specific binding of ^{125}I-insulin to the plasma membrane and its relation to insulin bioactivity. *Proc. Natl Acad. Sci. USA, 68*, 11833.
2. Cuatrecasas P (1971): Insulin-receptor interactions in adipose tissue cells: Direct measurement of properties. *Proc. Natl Acad. Sci. USA, 68*, 1264.
3. Fujita-Yamaguchi Y, Song C, Sakamoto Y, Itakura K (1983): Purification of insulin receptor with full binding activity. *J. Biol. Chem., 258*, 5045.
4. Jacobs S, Cuatrecasas P (1981): Insulin receptor: Structure and function. *Endocrinol. Rev., 2*, 251.
5. Yip CC. Yeung CWT, Moule ML (1980): Photoaffinity labeling of insulin receptor proteins of liver plasma membrane proteins. *Biochemistry, 19*, 70.
6. Yip CC, Moule ML (1983): Insulin receptor: Its subunit structure as determined by photoaffinity labeling. *Fed. Proc., 42*, 2842.
7. Wisher MH, Baron MD, Jones RH, Sonksen PH, Saunders DJ, Thamm P, Brandenburg D (1980): Photoreactive insulin analogues used to characterize the insulin receptor. *Biochem. Biophys. Res. Commun., 92*, 492.
8. Pilch PF, Czech M (1979): Interaction of cross-linking agents with the insulin

effector system of isolated rat cells. *J. Biol. Chem.*, *254*, 3775.
9. Massague J, Pilch PF, Czech MP (1981): A unique proteolytic cleavage site on the β-subunit of the insulin receptor. *J. Biol. Chem.*, *256*, 3182.
10. Massague J, Czech M (1982): The subunit structures of two distinct receptors for insulin-like growth factors I and II and their relationship to the insulin receptor. *J. Biol. Chem.*, *257*, 5038.
11. Van Obberghen E, Kasuga M, LeCam A, Hedo JA, Itin A, Harrison LC (1981): Biosynthetic labeling of insulin receptor: Studies of subunits in cultured human IM-9 lymphocytes. *Proc. Natl Acad. Sci. USA*, *78*, 1052.
12. Hedo JA, Kasuga M, Van Obberghen E, Roth J, Kahn CR (1981): Direct demonstration of glycosylation of insulin receptor subunits by biosynthetic and external labeling: Evidence for heterogeneity. *Proc. Natl Acad. Sci. USA*, *78*, 4791.
13. Kasuga M, Hedo JA, Yamada KM, Kahn CR (1982): The structure of the insulin receptor and its subunits: Evidence for multiple non-reduced forms and a 210K possible proreceptor. *J. Biol. Chem.*, *257*, 10392.
14. Chratchko Y, Van Obberghen E, Kiger N, Fehlmann M (1983): Immunoprecipitation of insulin receptors by antibodies against class 1 antigens of the murine H-2 major histocompatibility complex. *FEBS Lett.*, *163*, 207.
15. Massague J, Pilch PF, Czech MP (1980): Electrophoretic resolution of three major insulin receptor structures with unique subunit stoichiometries. *Proc. Natl Acad. Sci. USA*, *77*, 7137.
16. Crettaz M, Jialal I, Kasuga M, Kahn CR (1984): Insulin receptor regulation and desensitization in rat hepatoma cells: The loss of the oligomeric forms of the receptor correlates with the change in receptor affinity. *J. Biol. Chem.*, *259*, 11543.
17. Baron MD, Sonksen PH (1983): Elucidation of the quaternary structure of the insulin receptor. *Biochem. J.*, *212*, 79.
18. Harmon JT, Kahn CR, Kempner ES, Schlegel W (1980): Characterization of the insulin receptor in its membrane environment by radiation inactivation. *J. Biol. Chem.*, *225*, 3412.
19. Harmon JT, Hedo JA, Kahn CR (1983): Characterization of a membrane regulator of insulin receptor affinity. *J. Biol. Chem.*, *258*, 6876.
20. Maturo JM III, Hollenberg MD (1978): Insulin receptor: Interaction with non-receptor glycoprotein from liver cell membranes. *Proc. Natl Acad. Sci. USA*, *78*, 3070.
21. Jacobs S, Cuatrecasas P (1980): Disulfide reduction converts the insulin receptor of human placenta to a low affinity form. *J. Clin. Invest.*, *66*, 1424.
22. Maturo JM III, Hollenberg MD, Aglio LS (1983): Insulin receptor: Insulin-modulated interconversion between distinct molecular forms involving disulfide-sulfhydryl exchange. *Biochemistry*, *22*, 2579.
23. Havrankova J, Roth J, Brownstein M (1978): Insulin receptors are widely distributed in the central nervous system of the rat. *Nature (London)*, *272*, 827.
24. Heidenreich KA, Zahniser NR, Berhanu P, Brandenburg D, Olefsky JM (1983): Structural differences between insulin receptors in the brain and peripheral target tissues. *J. Biol. Chem.*, *258*, 8527.
25. Gambhir KK, Archer JA, Bradley CJ (1978): Characteristics of human erythrocyte insulin receptors. *Diabetes*, *27*, 701.

26. Jeong-Hyok I, Meezan E, Rackley CE, Hyun-Dju K (1983): Isolation and characterization of human erythrocyte insulin receptors. *J. Biol. Chem.*, *258*, 5021.
27. King, Gl, Buzney SM, Kahn CR, Hetu N, Buchwald S, MacDonald SG, Rand LI (1983): Differential responsiveness to insulin of endothelial and support cells from micro- and macrovessels. *J. Clin. Invest.*, *71*, 974.
28. Cotlier E, Davidson C (1983): Insulin receptors in calf and human retinal blood vessels. *Ophthalmic Res.*, *15*, 29.
29. Hammond SM, Veldhuis JD, Seale JW, Rechler MM (1982): Intraovarian regulation of granulosa-cell replication. *Adv. Exp. Med. Biol.*, *147*, 341.
30. Schweitzer JB, Smith RM, Jarett L (1980): Differences in the organizational structure of the insulin receptor of rat adipocyte and liver plasma membranes: The role of disulfide bonds. *Proc. Natl Acad. Sci. USA*, *77*, 4692.
31. Lyen KR, Smith RM, Jarett L (1983): Differences in the ability of anti-insulin antibody to aggregate monomeric ferritin-insulin occupied receptor sites on liver and adipocyte plasma membranes. *Diabetes*, *37*, 648.
32. Roth RA, Maddux B, Wong KY, Styne DM, Van Vliet G, Humbel RE, Goldfine ID (1983): Interaction of a monoclonal antibody to the insulin receptor with receptors for insulin-like growth factors. *Endocrinology*, *112*, 1865.
33. Kull, FC Jr, Jacobs S, Ying-Fu S, Svoboda ME, Van Wijk JJ, Cuatrecasas P (1983): Monoclonal antibodies to receptors for insulin and somatomedin C. *J. Biol. Chem.*, *258*, 6561.
34. Harmon JT, Kempner EJ, Kahn CR (1981): Demonstration by radiation inactivation that insulin alters the structure of the insulin receptor in rat liver membranes. *J. Biol. Chem.*, *256*, 7719.
35. Donner DB, Yonkers K (1983): Hormone-induced conformation changes in the hepatic receptor. *J. Biol. Chem.*, *258*, 9413.
36. Schlessinger J, Van Obberghen E, Kahn CR (1980): Insulin and antibodies against the insulin receptor cap on the membrane of cultured lymphocytes. *Nature (London)*, *286*, 729.
37. Kahn, CR, Baird KL, Jarrett DB, Flier JS (1976): Direct demonstration that receptor cross-linking or aggregation is important in insulin action. *Proc. Natl Acad. Sci. USA*, *75*, 4209.
38. Hedo JA, Kahn CR, Hayashi M, Yamada KM, Kasuga M (1983): Biosynthesis and glycosylation of the insulin receptor: Evidence for a single polypeptide precursor of the two major subunits. *J. Biol. Chem.*, *258*, 10020.
39. Ronnett GV, Knutson VP, Kohanski RA, Simpson TI, Lane MD (1984): Role of glycosylation in the processing of newly translated insulin proreceptor in 3T3-L1 adipocytes. *J. Biol. Chem.*, *259*, 4566.
40. Detusch PJ, Wang CF, Rosen OM, Rubin CS (1983): Latent insulin receptors and possible receptor precursors in 3T3-L1 adipocytes. *Proc. Natl Acad. Sci. USA*, *80*, 133.
41. Jacobs S, Kull FC Jr, Cuatrecasas P (1983): Monensin blocks the maturation of receptors for insulin and somatomedin C: Identification of receptor precursors. *Proc. Natl Acad. Sci. USA*, *80*, 1228.
42. Rees-Jones RW, Hedo JA, Zick Y, Roth J (1983): Insulin-stimulated phosphorylation of the insulin receptor precursor. *Biochem. Biophys. Res. Commun.*, *116*, 417.

43. Ronnett GV, Knutson VP, Kohanski RA, Simpson TL, Lane MD (1984): Role of glycosylation in the processing of the newly translated insulin proreceptor in 3T3-L1 adipocytes. *J. Biol. Chem.*, *259*, 4566.
44. Kasuga M, Kahn CR, Hedo JA, Van Obberghen E, Yamada KM (1981): Insulin-induced receptor loss in cultured lymphocytes is due to accelerated receptor degradation. *Proc. Natl Acad. Sci. USA*, *78*, 6917.
45. Marshall S (1983): Kinetics of insulin receptor biosynthesis and membrane insertion. Relationship to cellular function. *Diabetes*, *32*, 319.
46. Simpson IA, Hedo JA, Cushman SW (1984): Insulin-induced internalization of the insulin receptor in the isolated rat adipose cell: Detection of both major receptor subunits following their biosynthetic labeling in culture. *Diabetes*, *33*, 13.
47. Knutson VP, Ronnett GV, Lane MD (1983): Rapid, reversible internalization of cell surface insulin receptors. Correlation with insulin-induced down-regulation. *J. Biol. Chem.*, *258*, 12139.
48. Lopez S, Desbuquois B (1983): Changes in the subcellular distribution of insulin receptors in rat liver induced by acute endogenous hyperinsulinemia. *Endocrinology*, *113*, 783.
49. Krupp M, Lane MD (1981): On the mechanism of ligand-induced down-regulation of insulin receptor level in the liver cell. *J. Biol. Chem.*, *256*, 1689.
50. Fehlmann M, Carpentier JL, Van Obberghen E, Preychet P, Thamm P, Saunders D, Brandenburg D, Orci L (1982): Internalized insulin receptors are recycled to the cell surface in rat hepatocytes. *Proc. Natl Acad. Sci. USA*, *79*, 5921.
51. Heidenreich KA, Berhanu P, Brandenburg D, Olefsky JM (1983): Degradation of insulin receptors in rat adipocytes. *Diabetes*, *32*, 1001.
52. Marshall S, Olefsky JM (1983): Separate intracellular pathways for insulin receptor recycling and insulin degradation in isolated rat adipocytes. *J. Cell. Physiol.*, *117*, 195.
53. Gavin JR III, Roth J, Neville DM Jr, DeMeyts P, Buell DN (1974): Insulin-dependent regulation of insulin-receptor concentration. *Proc. Natl Acad. Sci. USA*, *71*, 84.
54. Roth RA, Maddux BA, Cassell DJ, Goldfine ID (1983): Regulation of the insulin receptor by a monoclonal anti-receptor antibody. Evidence that receptor down-regulation can be independent of insulin action. *J. Biol. Chem.*, *258*, 12094.
55. Taylor SI, Marcus-Samuels B (1984): Anti-receptor antibodies mimic the effect of insulin to down-regulate insulin receptors in cultured human lymphoblastoid (IM-9) cells. *J. Clin. Endocrinol. Metab.*, *58*, 182.
56. Kasuga M, Karlsson FA, Kahn CR (1982): Insulin stimulates the phosphorylation of the 95,000-Dalton subunit of its own receptor. *Science*, *215*, 185.
57. Kasuga M, Zick Y, Blithe DL, Karlsson FA, Haring HU, Kahn CR (1982): Insulin stimulation of phosphorylation of the β-subunit of the insulin receptor: Formation of both phosphoserine and phosphotyrosine. *J. Biol. Chem.*, *257*, 9891.
58. Haring HU, Kasuga M, Kahn CR (1982): Insulin receptor phosphorylation in intact adipocytes and in a cell-free system. *Biochem. Biophys. Res. Commun.*, *108*, 1538.

59. Plehwe WE, Williams PF, Caterson ID, Harrison LC, Turtle JR (1983): Calcium-dependence of insulin receptor phosphorylation. *Biochem. J., 214*, 361.
60. Kasuga M, Zick Y, Blithe DL, Crettaz M, Kahn CR (1982): Insulin stimulates tyrosine phosphorylation of the insulin receptor in a 'cell-free' system. *Nature (London), 298*, 667.
61. Petruzelli LM, Ganguly S, Smith CJ, Cobb MH, Rubin CS, Rosen OM (1982): Insulin activates tyrosine-specific protein kinase in extracts of 3T3-L1 adipocytes and human placenta. *Proc. Natl Acad. Sci. USA, 79*, 6792.
62. Avruch J, Nemenoff RA, Blackshear PJ, Pierce MW, Osathanondh R (1982): Insulin-stimulated tyrosine phosphorylation of the insulin receptor in detergent extracts of human placental membranes. *J. Biol. Chem., 257*, 15162.
63. Zick Y, Kasuga M, Kahn CR, Roth J (1983): Characterization of insulin-mediated phosphorylation of the insulin receptor in a cell-free system. *J. Biol. Chem., 258*, 75.
64. Kasuga M, Fujita-Yamaguchi Y, Blithe DL, Kahn CR (1983): Tyrosine-specific protein kinase activity is associated with the purified insulin receptor. *Proc. Natl Acad. Sci. USA, 80*, 2137.
65. Kasuga M, Fujita-Yamaguchi Y, Blithe DL, White MF, Kahn CR (1983): Characterization of the insulin receptor kinase purified from human placental membranes. *J. Biol. Chem., 258*, 10973.
66. Zick Y, Whittaker J, Roth J (1983): Insulin stimulated phosphorylation of its own receptor. Activation of a tyrosine-specific protein kinase that is tightly associated with the receptor. *J. Biol. Chem., 258*, 3431.
67. Grigorescu F, White MF, Kahn CR (1983): Insulin binding and insulin-dependent phosphorylation of the insulin receptor solubilized from human erythrocytes. *J. Biol. Chem., 258*, 13708.
68. Grunberger G, Zick Y, Roth J, Gorden P (1983): Protein kinase activity of the insulin receptor in human circulating and cultured mononuclear cells. *Biochem. Biophys. Res. Commun., 115*, 560.
69. White M, Haring HU, Kasuga M, Kahn CR (1984): Kinetic properties and sites of autophosphorylation of the partially purified insulin receptor from hepatoma cells. *J. Biol. Chem., 259*, 255.
70. Haring HU, Kasuga M, White MF, Crettaz M, Kahn CR (1984): Phosphorylation and dephosphorylation of the insulin receptor: Evidence against an intrinsic phosphatase activity. *Biochemistry, 23*, 3298.
71. Stadtmauer LA, Rosen OM (1983): Phosphorylation of exogenous substrates by the insulin receptor-associated protein kinase. *J. Biol. Chem., 258*, 6682.
72. Grunberger G, Zick Y, Roth J, Gorden P (1983): Protein kinase activity of the insulin receptor in human circulating and cultured mononuclear cells. *Biochem. Biophys. Res. Commun., 115*, 560.
73. Braun S, Raymond WE, Racker E (1984): Synthetic tyrosine polymers as substrates and inhibitors of tyrosine-specific protein kinases. *J. Biol. Chem., 259*, 2051.
74. Roth R, Cassell DJ (1983): Insulin receptor: Evidence that it is a protein kinase. *Science, 219*, 299.
75. Shia MA, Pilch PF (1983): The β subunit of the insulin receptor is an insulin-activated protein kinase. *Biochemistry, 22*, 717.

76. Van Obberghen E, Rossi B, Kowalski A, Gazzano H, Ponzio G (1983): Receptor-mediated phosphorylation of the hepatic insulin receptor: Evidence that the M(r) 95,000 receptor subunit is its own kinase. *Proc. Natl Acad. Sci. USA*, *80*, 945.
77. Roth RA, Mesirow ML, Cassell DJ (1983): Preferential degradation of the beta subunit of purified insulin receptor. Effect of insulin binding and protein kinase activities of the receptor. *J. Biol. Chem.*, *258*, 14456.
78. Shia MA, Rubin JB, Pilch PF (1983): The insulin receptor protein kinase. Physiochemical requirements for activity. *J. Biol. Chem.*, *258*, 14450.
79. Rosen OM, Herrera R, Olowe Y, Petruzzelli LM, Cobb MH (1983): Phosphorylation activates the insulin receptor tyrosine protein kinase. *Proc. Natl Acad. Sci. USA*, *80*, 3237.
80. Roth RA, Cassell DJ, Maddux BA, Goldfine ID (1983): Regulation of insulin receptor kinase activity by insulin mimickers and an insulin antagonist. *Biochem. Biophys. Res. Commun.*, *115*, 245.
81. Tamura S, Fujita-Yamaguchi Y, Larner J (1983): Insulin-like effect of trypsin on the phosphorylation of rat adipocyte insulin receptor. *J. Biol. Chem.*, *258*, 14749.
82. Tamura S, Brown TA, Whipple JH, Fujita-Yamaguchi Y, Dubler RE, Cheng K, Larner J (1984): A novel mechanism for the insulin-like effect of vanadate on glycogen synthase in rat adipocytes. *J. Biol. Chem.*, *259*, 6650.
83. Zick Y, Rees-Jones RW, Taylor SI, Gorden P, Roth J (1984): The role of anti-receptor antibodies in stimulating phosphorylation of the insulin receptor. *J. Biol. Chem.*, *259*, 4396.
84. Simpson IA, Hedo JA (1984): Insulin receptor phosphorylation may not be a prerequisite for acute insulin action. *Science*, *223*, 1301.
85. Zick Y, Grunberger G, Podskalny JM, Moncada V, Taylor SI, Gorden P, Roth J (1983): Insulin stimulates phosphorylation of serine residues in soluble insulin receptors. *Biochem. Biophys. Res. Commun.*, *116*, 1129.
86. Gazzano H, Kowalski A, Fehlmann M, Van Obberghen E (1983): Two different protein kinase activities are associated with the insulin receptor. *Biochem. J.*, *216*, 575.
87. Cohen S, Carpentėr G, King L Jr (1980): Epidermal growth factor-receptor-protein kinase interactions: Co-purification of receptor and epidermal growth-enhanced phosphorylation activity. *J. Biol. Chem.*, *255*, 4834.
88. Ek B, Heldin CH (1982): Characterization of a tyrosine-specific kinase activity in human fibroblast membranes stimulated by platelet-derived growth factor. *J. Biol. Chem.*, *257*, 10486.
89. Jacobs S, Kull FC Jr, Earp HS, Svoboda MF, Van Wyk JJ, Cuatrecasas P (1983): Somatomedin-C stimulates the phosphorylation of the β-subunit of its own receptor. *J. Biol. Chem.*, *258*, 9581.
90. Weiss R (Ed) (1982): RNA tumor viruses. *Cold Spring Harbor Symposium*, Cold Spring Harbor.
91. Downward J, Yarden Y, Mayes E, Scarce G, Totty N, Stockwell P, Ullrich A, Schlessinger J, Waterfield MD (1984): Close similarity of epidermal growth factor receptor and v-erb-B oncogene protein sequences. *Nature (London)*, *307*, 521.

92. Rees-Jones RW, Quarum M, Taylor SI (1984): An endogenous substrate for the insulin receptor-associated tyrosine kinase. *Diabetes, 33, Suppl. 1*, 7A.
93. Grunberger G, Taylor SI, Dons RF, Gorden P (1983): Insulin receptors in normal and disease states. *Clin. Endocrinol. Metab., 12*, 191.
94. Dons RF, Ryan J, Gorden P, Washslicht-Rodbard H (1981): Erythrocyte and monocyte insulin-binding in man. A comparative analysis in normal and disease states. *Diabetes, 30*, 896.
95. Spanheimer RG, Bar RS, Ginsberg BH, Peacock ML, Martino I (1982): Comparison of insulin binding to cells of fed and fasted obese patients: Results in erythrocytes and monocytes. *J. Clin. Endocrinol. Metab., 54*, 40.
96. Dons RF, Corash LM, Gorden P (1981): The insulin receptor is an age-dependent integral component of the human erythrocyte membrane. *J. Biol. Chem., 256*, 2982.
97. Camagna A, De Pirro R, Tardella L, Rossetti L, Lauro R, Caprari P, Samoggia P, Salvo G (1983): Red blood cell age, pyruvate kinase activity, and insulin receptors. Evidence that monocytes and RBCs may behave differently. *Diabetes, 32*, 1017.
98. Bolinder J, Engfeldt P, Ostman J, Arner P (1983): Site differences in insulin receptor binding and insulin action in subcutaneous fat of obese females. *J. Clin. Endrocinol. Metab., 57*, 455.
99. Podskalny JM, Kahn CR (1982): Cell culture studies on patients with extreme insulin resistance. I. Receptor defects on cultured fibroblasts. *J. Clin. Endocrinol. Metab., 54*, 261.
100. Mott DM, Howard BV, Savage PJ, Nagulesparan M (1983): Altered insulin binding to monocytes and diploid fibroblasts from obese donors. *J. Clin. Endrocrinol. Metab., 57*, 1.
101. Massague J, Freidenberg GF, Olefsky JM, Czech MP (1983): Parallel decreases in the expression of receptors for insulin and insulin-like growth factor I in a mutant human fibroblast line. *Diabetes, 32*, 541.
102. Taylor SI, Samuels B, Roth J, Kasuga M, Hedo JA, Gorden, P, Brasel DE, Pokora T, Engel RR (1982): Decreased insulin binding in cultured lymphocytes from two patients with extreme insulin resistance. *J. Clin. Endocrinol. Metab., 54*, 919.
103. Helderman JH, Pietri AO, Raskin P (1983): In vitro control of T-lymphocyte insulin receptors by in vivo modulation of insulin. *Diabetes, 32*, 712.
104. Taylor SI, Underhill LH, Hedo JA, Roth J, Serrano-Rios M, Blizzard RM (1983): Decreased insulin binding to cultured cells from a patient with the Rabson-Mendenhall syndrome: dichotomy between studies with cultured lymphocytes and cultured fibroblasts. *J. Clin. Endocrinol. Metab., 56*, 856.
105. Kahn CR (1982): Insulin receptors and syndromes of insulin resistance. *Diabetes Care, 5, Suppl. 2*, 98.
106. Olefsky JM, Kolterman OG (1981): Mechanisms of insulin resistance in obesity and non-insulin dependent (Type II) diabetes. *Am. J. Med., 70*, 151.
107. Kahn CR (1978): Insulin resistance, insulin insensitivity and insulin unresponsiveness: A necessary distinction. *Metabolism, 27, Suppl. 2*, 1893.
108. Schulz B, Doberne L, Greenfeld M, Reaven GM (1983): Insulin receptor binding and insulin-mediated glucose uptake in Type II diabetics. *Exp. Clin. Endocrinol., 81*, 49.

109. Lonnroth P, Digirolamo M, Krotkiewski M, Smith U (1983): Insulin binding and responsiveness in fat cells from patients with reduced glucose tolerance and type II diabetes. *Diabetes*, *32*, 748.
110. Rizza RA, Mandarino LJ, Gerich JE (1981): Mechanisms of insulin resistance in man. Assessment using the insulin dose-response curve in conjunction with insulin receptor binding. *Am. J. Med.*, *70*, 169.
111. Bolinder J, Ostman J, Arner P (1983): Influence of aging on insulin receptor binding and metabolic effects of insulin on human adipose tissue. *Diabetes*, *32*, 959.
112. Arner P, Einarsson K, Backman L, Nilsell K, Lerea KM, Livingston JN (1983): Studies of liver insulin receptors in non-obese and obese human subjects. *J. Clin. Invest.*, *72*, 1729.
113. Soll AH, Kahn CR, Neville DM Jr, Roth J (1983): Insulin receptor deficiency in genetic and acquired obesity. *J. Clin. Invest.*, *56*, 769.
114. Bar RS, Gorden P, Roth J, Kahn CR, De Meyts P (1976): Fluctuations in the affinity and concentration of insulin receptors on circulating monocytes of obese patients: Effects of starvation, feeding, and dieting. *J. Clin. Invest.*, *58*, 1123.
115. Raizada MK, Tan G, Fellows RE (1980): Fibroblastic culture from the diabetic db/db mouse. Demonstration of decreased insulin receptors and impaired responses to insulin. *J. Biol. Chem.*, *255*, 9149.
116. Olefsky JM, Reaven GM (1976): Effects of sulfonylurea therapy on insulin binding to mononuclear leukocytes of diabetic patients. *Am. J. Med.*, *60*, 89.
117. Nowak SM, McCaleb ML, Lockwood DH (1983): Extrapancreatic action of sulfonylureas: Hypoglycemic effects are not dependent on altered insulin binding or inhibition of transglutaminase. *Metabolism*, *32*, 398.
118. Dolais-Kitabgi J, Alengrin F, Freychet P (1983): Sulfonylureas in vitro do not alter insulin binding or insulin effects on amino acid transport in rat hepatocytes. *Diabetologia*, *224*, 441.
119. Hjollund E, Richelsen B, Beck-Nielsen H, Pedersen O (1983): The effect of glibenclamide on insulin receptors in normal man: Comparative studies of insulin binding to monocytes and erythrocytes. *J. Clin. Endocrinol. Metab.*, *57*, 1257.
120. Marchand E, Grigorescu F, Buysschaert M, De Meyts P, Ketelslegers JM, Brems H, Nathan MC, Lambert AE (1983): The hypoglycemic effect of a sulfonylurea (gliclazide) in moderate type II diabetes and glucose intolerance is not accompanied by changes in insulin action and insulin ending to erythrocytes. *Mol. Physiol.*, *4*, 83.
121. Prager R, Schernthaner G (1983): Insulin receptor binding to monocytes, insulin secretion, and glucose tolerance following metformin treatment. Results of a double-blind cross-over study in type II diabetics. *Diabetes*, *32*, 1083.
122. Trischitta V, Gullo D, Pezzino V, Vigneri R (1983): Metformin normalizes insulin binding to monocytes from obese nondiabetic subjects and obese type II diabetic patients. *J. Clin. Endocrinol. Metab.*, *57*, 713.
123. Lord JM, White SI, Bailey CJ, Atkins TW, Fletcher RF, Taylor KG (1983): Effect of metformin on insulin receptor binding and glycaemic control in type II diabetes. *Br. Med. J.*, *286*, 830.

124. Kahn CR, Flier JS, Bar RS, Archer JA, Gorden P, Martin MM, Roth J (1976): The syndromes of insulin resistance and acanthosis nigricans: Insulin receptor disorders in man. *N. Engl. J. Med.*, *294*, 739.
125. Bar RS, Muggeo M, Kahn CR, Gorden P, Roth J (1980): Characterization of the insulin receptor in patients with syndromes of insulin resistance and acanthosis nigricans. *Diabetologia*, *18*, 209.
126. Grunberger G, Zick Y, Gorden P (1984): Defect in phosphorylation of insulin receptors in cells from an insulin-resistant patient with normal insulin binding. *Science*, *223*, 932.
127. Grigorescu F, Flier JS, Kahn CR: A defect in receptor phosphorylation ion erythrocytes and fibroblasts associated with severe insulin resistance. *J. Biol. Chem.*, in press.
128. Dons RF, Havlik R, Taylor SI, Baird KL, Chernick SS, Gorden P (1983): Clinical disorders associated with autoantibodies to the insulin receptor. Stimulation by passive transfer of immunoglobulins to rats. *J. Clin. Invest.*, *72*, 1072.
129. Rudiger HW, Dreyer M, Kuhnau J, Bartelheimer H (1983): Familial insulin-resistant diabetes secondary to an affinity defect of the insulin receptor. *Hum. Genet.*, *64*, 407.
130. Taylor SI, Leventhal S (1983): Defect in cooperativity in insulin receptors from a patient with a congenital form of extreme insulin resistance. *J. Clin. Invest.*, *71*, 1676.
131. Kobayashi M, Olefsky JM, Elders J, Mako ME, Given BD, Schedwie HK, Fiser RH, Hintz RL, Horner JA, Rubenstein AH (1978): Insulin resistance due to a defect distal to the insulin receptor: Demonstration in a patient with leprechaunism. *Proc. Natl Acad. Sci. USA*, *75*, 3469.
132. Schilling EE, Rechler MM, Grunfeld C, Rosenbert AM (1979): Primary defect of insulin receptors in skin fibroblasts cultured from an infant with leprechaunism and insulin resistance. *Proc. Natl Acad. Sci. USA*, *76*, 5872.

The Diabetes Annual/1
K.G.M.M. Alberti and L.P. Krall, editors

ISBN 0444 90 343 7
$0.85 per article per page (transactional system)
$0.20 per article per page (licensing system)

26 Plasma lipoproteins in human diabetes mellitus

JOHN D. BRUNZELL, ALAN CHAIT, AND EDWIN L. BIERMAN

Abnormalities of plasma lipids in diabetes have long attracted attention due to the association between hyperlipidemia and atherosclerosis (see refs. 1–7). Hypertriglyceridemia is known to be highly prevalent in the untreated diabetic patient, usually accompanied by a decrease in high-density lipoprotein (HDL) cholesterol. The hypertriglyceridemia associated with diabetes improves during therapy with insulin or oral sulfonylureas. Whether or not diabetes affects low-density lipoprotein (LDL) levels has been less clear. The effect of therapy for hyperglycemia on lipid and lipoprotein levels has been clouded by inadequate attention to modalities and efficacy of therapy. Common conditions that affect lipoprotein metabolism such as obesity, renal disease and use of diuretic agents and beta adrenergic blocking drugs, are particularly prevalent in the diabetic patient. In addition, the type of patients in a diabetic population under study can be strongly influenced by the specific interests of the investigator; for instance, those followed in lipid clinics and by cardiologists are more likely to have hyperlipidemia.

During the past few years epidemiological studies have put the prevalence of lipoprotein abnormalities in diabetes into perspective. The effect that treatment of the diabetes has on lipoprotein levels has been clarified to some extent by the increased attention that has been given to the role of tight glycemic control of lipoprotein metabolism. Further, it has been suggested that the effects of concomitant other disease, of body fat content, and of diet on lipoproteins are important determinants of the form of hyperlipidemia present in the treated individual with diabetes. Finally, the pathogenic mechanisms accounting for the changes in individual lipoprotein levels, and in lipoprotein composition, have been the subject of increased interest.

Epidemiology of lipids and lipoproteins in diabetes

The frequency of hyperlipidemia, especially hypertriglyceridemia in diabetes mellitus has long been known to be increased, but the exact prevalence in different studies varies greatly. This is in part due to differences in selection criteria for these studies, which has resulted in marked heterogeneity of patients and which reflects the interests of the investigators. To obviate these biases, a population-based study was recently undertaken which evaluated the prevalence of hyperlipidemia in diabetes in an American suburban population (8). Hypertriglyceridemia was observed in association with diabetes which represented an unbiased sampling of diabetics in this population. The increase in plasma triglyceride was independent of age and relative body weight. Total plasma cholesterol levels were not found to be elevated. Measurement of lipoprotein levels in a random sample of non-insulin dependent diabetic individuals in this population (9), revealed that very low-density lipoprotein (VLDL) cholesterol levels were elevated and HDL cholesterol levels were decreased. No abnormality in LDL was noted. In the much larger WHO Multinational Study of Vascular Disease in Diabetes, serum triglyceride and cholesterol levels were measured in 5 of the 14 national samples of patients (10). Ischemic heart disease was more strongly associated with plasma triglyceride than with cholesterol. Several risk factors for coronary artery disease, such as hypertriglyceridemia, hypertension and obesity, have been noted to cluster in diabetic patients (11), in part due to the probability that the obesity seen in non-insulin dependent diabetes (NIDD) is inherited as part of the diabetic syndrome (12).

The predominant lipoprotein defect in diabetes is an increase in VLDL levels, often in association with decreased levels of HDL. Although elevated LDL has been noted, most studies still report LDL as the density fraction 1.006 to 1.063 g/ml, which also includes the intermediate density lipoprotein (IDL) composed largely of remnants of triglyceride-rich lipoprotein catabolism. When studies are performed to separate IDL (1.006–1.019 g/ml) from LDL (1.019–1.063 g/ml) (13), most of the elevation in total LDL is due to an increase in IDL. Indeed, a strong correlation between increases in VLDL and IDL has been noted (14).

Effect of diabetic treatment on lipoproteins

Insulin-dependent diabetes mellitus

It is widely acknowledged that mild to moderate hypertriglyceridemia occurs in the untreated insulin-dependent diabetic patient. Many studies have been performed in the last few years to assess the relation between degree of control of hyperglycemia and abnormalities in lipoprotein levels in insulin-dependent diabetes (IDD). Insulin-dependent diabetics who are poorly controlled have elevated levels of total triglyceride, VLDL cholesterol, and LDL cholesterol as compared to non-diabetics or to insulin-dependent diabetics in fair to good control (15, 16). Poor diabetic control also has been associated with decreased HDL cholesterol levels (16). Further evidence that glycemic control determines lipid levels is provided by the observation that glucosylated hemoglobin and/or fasting glucose levels correlate with elevated triglyceride (16–19), VLDL triglyceride (16, 18) and LDL cholesterol levels (6). HDL cholesterol levels have been inversely correlated to the degree of glycemia in some (16, 20) but not other (15, 17, 18) studies. In a group of patients with IDD followed for one year, changes in glycosylated hemoglobin were associated with changes in plasma and VLDL triglyceride and LDL cholesterol levels, but not with changes in HDL cholesterol (21). Thus, in IDD the major lipoprotein abnormality appears to be an elevation in VLDL level leading to hypertriglyceridemia, which appears to be related to degree of control of plasma glucose.

LDL and HDL levels in treated IDD are often within the normal range for these lipoproteins, but LDL may be increased in those diabetics with the greatest hyperglycemia. Apoprotein AI, the major apoprotein of HDL, has been noted to be decreased (22) and normal (23) in IDD. When HDL subfractions have been examined, an increase in HDL_3 (24) or in HDL_{2a} (25) has been noted. HDL_{2b}, i.e. the fraction that best predicts risk for atherosclerosis, is often normal and is inversely related to plasma triglyceride levels (25, 26). It is conceivable that HDL may be influenced by factors other than blood glucose levels. These factors need to be considered in the evaluation of lipoprotein levels in IDD. Thus, the observation that in IDD the level of HDL cholesterol or apoprotein AI and AII is correlated positively (27) or negatively (23) to the dose of insulin administered, raises the possibility that insulin may affect HDL other than via glucose control. Subtle alterations in renal function may also be important. Among diabetic patients with normal renal function and without gross proteinuria (28), it was noted that those with albuminuria in excess of 216 mg/day had higher plasma triglyceride and apoprotein B levels, as well as elevated LDL and decreased HDL cholesterol levels, when compared to subjects with less proteinuria. IDD patients with 58–216 mg per day protein in their urine had higher plasma apoprotein B levels than those with less than 58 mg per day. Diet also may influence plasma lipoproteins in IDD. The continued use of carbohydrate restricted, high fat diets, recommended in the past, may still be a cause of elevated LDL cholesterol and perhaps apoprotein levels in some diabetics (29).

A number of studies have been performed to assess the effects of normalization of glucose levels on plasma lipoproteins in patients with IDD by the use of continuous subcutaneous insulin infusions or with multiple insulin injections per day. Almost all studies demonstrate a decrease in triglyceride levels after near normalization of glucose levels (30–35). Changes in LDL and HDL levels were variable. Even though LDL levels did not exceed the normal range in most patients while on conventional therapy, they nonetheless fell in response to intensive insulinization. The degree of glycemic control prior to the commencement of intensified therapy also influences the lipoprotein response. When the diabetic subjects were divided into groups by degree of control (34), patients with the worst glycemic control had a decrease in their LDL cholesterol and an increase in their HDL cholesterol levels within two to three weeks of intensive insulin therapy; no change in these lipoproteins was noted with treatment in the group who previously had been in better control. The duration of intensive insulin therapy may help explain the lack of change in HDL cholesterol in some studies. Short durations of intensive therapy may not be associated with changes in HDL (31, 33); however, HDL is higher after a longer duration of intensive therapy (32, 36). The relationship between diabetic control and these metabolic changes has been put into perspective by a study in which a group of children were entered into a multistaged program of intensification of diabetes therapy. The greatest metabolic improvement was noted after early routine measures to improve diabetic control rather than later after intensive adjustment of insulin dosage (37). Dietary factors also may be important. The use of a diet with reduced fat and increased carbohydrate content, with an increase in the ratio of polyunsaturated to saturated fat, led to improvement in glucose control, but no changes in lipoprotein levels over a 6-week period (38).

Non-insulin-dependent diabetes mellitus

It is relatively easy to assess the effect of treatment on lipoprotein levels in IDD since all patients are treated with insulin at the onset of their illness. However, in NIDD, evaluation of the effects of treatment on plasma lipoprotein levels is more difficult due to heterogeneity of therapy used in this disease. Patients with NIDD who have never been treated with insulin or oral sulfonylureas, often have elevated plasma triglyceride and decreased HDL cholesterol levels (39, 40). The elevated triglyceride can be correlated with glycemic control as assessed by glucosylated hemoglobin (41, 42); this correlation is improved when the effects of relative body weight are taken into account (42).

The use of insulin to lower blood glucose levels in previously untreated patients with NIDD is associated with a decrease in triglyceride, a drop in LDL cholesterol, and an increase in HDL cholesterol (40). Weight gain often occurs with insulin or oral sulfonylurea therapy in NIDD. Nevertheless, plasma triglyceride levels usually improve as blood glucose levels fall (42). Improved glycemic control in previously treated patients, even when glycemic control is so poor that insulin therapy is required, leads to much less noticeable changes in lipoprotein levels in NIDD (40). A residual effect of previous oral sulfonylurea 3 to 4 months after they are discontinued may explain the lack of effect on lipoproteins of retreatment with other oral sulfonylureas (43) or insulin (40).

In chronically treated patients with NIDD, elevated levels of plasma triglyceride or VLDL triglyceride (22, 41, 44, 45), and decreased levels of HDL cholesterol (22, 27, 44–49) are often seen. Some of the decrease in HDL cholesterol can be accounted for by substitution of triglyceride for cholesterol in the core of the HDL particles. However, even after correction for this phenomenon, HDL cholesterol levels are still decreased in NIDD (44, 46). Diet therapy leading to successful loss of weight is associated with a decrease in glycemia, plasma and VLDL triglyceride levels, and an increase in HDL cholesterol (50–52). Specific lipid lowering treatment with bezafibrate lowers VLDL levels and raises HDL cholesterol levels without changing the level of LDL cholesterol (53).

Pathophysiology of lipoprotein abnormalities in diabetes

Very low-density lipoproteins

Hypertriglyceridemia in the diabetic has been reported previously to be associated with both increased VLDL synthesis and impaired VLDL and chylomicron catabolism (1–7). Increased VLDL synthesis has been demonstrated in patients with NIDD who have never received insulin or oral sulfonylurea therapy and who have fasting plasma glucose levels below 200 mg/dl (11.1 mmol/l) (54). Subjects with mild to moderate diabetes and mild hypertriglyceridemia have a decreased fractional catabolic rate of VLDL in addition. In most other studies also, the predominant abnormality accounting for the hypertriglyceridemia was an increase in VLDL synthesis (55–58). A decrease in the fractional catabolic rate for VLDL was often seen, presumably in part due to the effect of expanded VLDL pool size on limiting the rate of VLDL catabolism. In some subjects the decreased VLDL catabolism found in the presence of normal VLDL synthesis must represent a VLDL removal defect. The effect of prior oral sulfonylurea treatment on VLDL metabolism in most (56) or some (55, 57–59) patients in these studies is unknown, but residual effects of oral sulfonylurea therapy may last for months. The Pima Indians may be unique since in these diabetics with moderate obesity the mild hypertriglyceridemia was due to defective VLDL catabolism (59).

In the treated patient with NIDD, or subjects with mild untreated fasting hyperglycemia, the major defect associated with hypertriglyceridemia is likely to be increased VLDL synthesis due to increased free fatty acids presented to the liver, particularly in the presence of obesity and other causes of insulin resistance. The change in plasma and VLDL triglyceride levels seen with intensive improvement in glycemic control appears to be related to a decrease in VLDL synthesis (60), presumably related to a decrease in free fatty acid mobilization from adipose tissue. In moderately to severely hyperglycemic, untreated patients with NIDD on the other hand, insulin deficiency is present in addition to concomitant insulin resistance. Such individuals might be expected to have abnormalities in lipoprotein lipase activity since insulin is needed for the maintenance of this enzyme (61).

Not all diabetics have decreased lipoprotein lipase activity (1, 42). Chronically treated patients with either IDD or NIDD appear to have normal lipoprotein lipase activity, the level of which is independent of the degree of hyperglycemia (62). Subjects with impaired glucose tolerance or mild untreated NIDD also have normal lipoprotein lipase activity. The previous use of sulfonylurea agents might render lipoprotein lipase activity normal due to some residual effect of these agents. On the other hand, untreated insulin dependent diabetics have low lipoprotein lipase activity both in adipose tissue and in plasma. Other studies indicate that some non-insulin dependent subjects also have low lipoprotein lipase activity, especially those who have never previously been treated or who have symptomatic diabetes with moderate to marked hyperglycemia associated with moderate insulin deficiency (1, 39, 42, 63). Treatment of the hyperglycemia is associated with correction of the lipoprotein lipase abnormality after several weeks to months (42, 62) and improvement of the lipid abnormality. The relative roles of increased VLDL synthesis and decreased VLDL catabolism in the untreated, severely hyperglycemic patient with NIDD still need to be resolved. One would expect the decrease of lipoprotein lipase levels seen in the untreated diabetic to play some role in the hypertriglyceridemia, since lipoprotein lipase activity correlates with measures of VLDL catabolism in a number of clinical settings (62, 64).

For many years hyperinsulinism due to insulin resistance has been suggested to be the mediator through which hypertriglyceridemia can occur. Increased hepatic VLDL production was thought to be the mechanism by which this occurred by some (1, 7), and decreased VLDL removal via lipoprotein lipase by others (26, 65). This disagreement is confounded by the observation that hypertriglyceridemia can in itself lead to insulin resistance both in tissue culture (66) and in vivo (67, 68). Hypertriglyceridemia-induced insulin resistance may explain the increase in glucosylated hemoglobulin levels seen in non-diabetic patients with hypertriglyceridemia (69), rather than the previously postulated role of impaired glucose tolerance leading to hypertriglyceridemia. Attempts to study the effect of insulin on VLDL synthesis in vitro have been performed with primary cultured hepatocytes (70–72). In this system, insulin could not be demonstrated to increase VLDL synthesis, in part due to limited free fatty acid availability. More importantly, insulin does not seem to have a direct effect on fatty acid utilization, but has an anti-glucagon effect (73) and thus the effect of insulin in culture would only be expected to occur in the presence of glucagon.

Low-density lipoproteins

The metabolism of LDL has also been examined in detail in NIDD. In many population studies of LDL levels in diabetes alluded to earlier, the density cuts chosen resulted in the inclusion of IDL in the LDL fraction. Metabolic studies of LDL in diabetes, however, have evaluated LDL without IDL, since IDL is reported to be elevated in diabetes (13, 14). When LDL kinetic parameters were assessed in untreated patients with mild NIDD, both an increase in LDL synthesis and removal in association with normal LDL levels have been observed (74). In untreated NIDD patients with moderate hyperglycemia, LDL synthesis was normal, while a mild defect in LDL catabolism was associated with a slight increase in LDL levels (74). This catabolic defect is compatible with the finding that glucosylated LDL is removed from plasma more slowly than normal LDL when injected into guinea pigs (75). The increase in LDL catabolism in normal men during a euglycemic hyperinsulinemic clamp (76) or in non-diabetics during hyperinsulinemia associated with total parenteral nutrition (77) suggests that insulin can stimulate LDL catabolism in vivo, perhaps by receptor-mediated degradation (78), and might explain the reduction in LDL levels in poorly controlled subjects with IDD when they undergo intensive insulin therapy.

High-density lipoproteins

Several excellent reviews detail the pathophysiological abnormalities associated with the changes seen in HDL cholesterol in diabetes (3, 26). Subsequent studies have shed further light on the changes in HDL levels. Low HDL cholesterol levels occur in both untreated IDD (79) and NIDD (39, 40, 52), and increase during therapy with insulin (39, 40, 49), weight loss (52), or oral sulfonylureas (80). Some of this increase in HDL cholesterol is associated with lowering of VLDL levels and replacement of triglyceride in the core of HDL with cholesterol. Additionally, HDL cholesterol might increase due to improvement in VLDL catabolism, with provision of VLDL surface components to HDL via lipoprotein lipase action on LDL (26). This transfer of unesterified cholesterol to HDL seems to slow ›wn the catabolism of the HDL apoproteins AI and AII, with a resultant ıncrease in HDL levels (64). In the well-treated patient with either IDD or NIDD an inverse relation still exists between VLDL and HDL cholesterol levels (44, 81). HDL cholesterol levels appear to be independent of glucosylated hemoglobin and fasting glucose levels (17–19, 21, 27, 46, 49) with few exceptions (16, 20, 41). In fact, glucosylation of HDL, in contrast to glucosylation of LDL, might accelerate its rate of catabolism (82).

It has been suggested that obesity plays a major role in explaining the variability in HDL cholesterol levels in treated diabetic patients (83). Many patients with IDD are of low relative body weight (12), which could account for the increase in HDL often seen in IDD (26), while obese NIDD might have low HDL cholesterol levels on this basis. This would be compatible with the finding of low HDL levels in NIDD patients compared to control subjects (27, 39, 46). When HDL subfractions are assessed in IDD patients (24), it appears that HDL_2 cholesterol varies with the level of VLDL, while HDL_3 cholesterol accounts for the increase in HDL.

Lipoprotein interactions in diabetes

Lipoprotein interactions with cells are discussed fully in chapter 19. Interactions between lipoproteins have been studied recently. When plasma from normal individuals was incubated with normal cultured fibroblasts, net transport of unesterified cholesterol to lipoproteins was demonstrated, with subsequent esterification, and finally transfer of the cholesteryl ester to VLDL, IDL, and LDL (84). In patients with NIDD several differences in this in vitro phenomenon were demonstrated. These include reversal of net unesterified cholesterol transport from plasma to the cultured fibroblasts and decreased cholesteryl ester transfer from HDL to VLDL and LDL (84). These changes were suggested to be secondary to unesterified cholesterol enrichment of VLDL and LDL in NIDD (85). This would block cholesteryl ester uptake and provide unesterified cholesterol to be transported to the cells. Insulin therapy of the patient or removal of apoprotein E containing particles from the VLDL–LDL spectrum was found to reverse these in vitro abnormalities, presumably by removing old VLDL or 'remnant' particles which accumulate in plasma in the diabetic state (13, 14). While the authors demonstrated unesterified cholesterol enrichment of VLDL and LDL (85), others have not found increased unesterified cholesterol in LDL in treated diabetic patients whether normolipidemic or hypertriglyceridemic (86) or during poor control, or after intensive therapy which resulted in lower glucose and triglyceride levels (87). Some of these variations in LDL composition may be related to the observation that two subpopulations of LDL may be present in diabetic patients, one more dense than normal LDL and one less dense than normal (88), or may be due to triglyceride enrichment and cholesterol depletion of LDL described in hypertriglyceridemic states (89). The significance of these findings will need to await further studies.

The human insulin gene, hypertriglyceridemia, and atherosclerosis

The human insulin gene is on the short arm of chromosome 11 (90). The 5′-end of the gene is a highly variable region, characterized by insertions of different lengths. Polymorphism in this region has been suggested to be associated with non-insulin dependent diabetes mellitus (91, 92), but this has not been confirmed by others (90, 93). Two different reasons have been proposed to reconcile these differences. First, large insertions in the 5′ flanking region were found in non-insulin-dependent diabetic patients who were hypertriglyceridemic, but not in normolipidemic diabetics (94). Second, although another group initially thought that the large polymorphism found in the 5′-end was associated with NIDD (92), it was later suggested that this association was due to the presence of macrovascular atherosclerotic disease and not to NIDD. This association was not mediated by known risk factors for arteriosclerosis, including lipoproteins (95). The ultimate relationships between polymorphisms in the human insulin gene and NIDD, hypertriglyceridemia, and atherosclerosis needs further study.

The genes for the lipoproteins apoprotein AI and apoprotein CIII are also found on chromosome 11, but at too great a distance from the insulin gene to expect a great interaction.

The chylomicronemia syndrome

Massive hypertriglyceridemia (plasma triglyceride over 2000 mg/dl) with chylomicronemia occurs with increased frequency in diabetes. The chylomicronemia is associated with a constellation of symptoms and signs, such as abdominal pain, impaired memory, objective dyspnea, paresthesiae of the extremities, hepatomegaly and eruptive xanthomata (96, 97), which clear with lowering of plasma triglyceride levels. Perhaps as many as 50% of individuals with the chylomicronemia syndrome have diabetes (98). The marked hypertriglyceridemia also interferes with many laboratory determinations (96, 99).

It was originally believed that the marked degree of hypertriglyceridemia seen in the chylomicronemia syndrome in IDD (diabetic lipemia) could be completely accounted for by the severe insulin deficiency that was present. In the subjects seen by our group, an additional familial form of hypertriglyceridemia is required to manifest this degree of triglyceride elevation, even in those with IDD (96). This would explain the relative rarity of the chylomicronemia syndrome in diabetes clinics as opposed to lipid clinics (79, 96).

The treatment of the chylomicronemia syndrome requires the use of insulin or sulfonylureas for the hyperglycemia. 'Diet alone' is an inappropriate form of therapy, especially since the regain of weight may lead to massive elevations in plasma triglycerides. When associated with pancreatitis, the patient can be treated conservatively as with other forms of pancreatitis, and with clofibrate or one of its analogs. Rarely, if ever, are extremes of therapy such as plasmapheresis necessary (100), although total parenteral nutrition is one way of avoiding exogenous dietary fat during pregnancy associated with chylomicronemia and pancreatitis (101).

Conclusions

1. In untreated diabetes mellitus, the primary lipoprotein abnormalities are an increase in VLDL and a decrease in HDL.
2. Treatment of the hyperglycemia is associated with correction of the abnormalities in VLDL and HDL toward normal.
3. Elevated low-density lipoprotein levels reported in the past may be due to several factors other than the diabetic state: (a) in some studies, intermediate density lipoproteins were included in LDL; (b) microalbuminuria can be associated with increased LDL; and (c) some elevation in LDL may have been related to a high saturated fat intake with the carbohydrate restricted diet.
4. In the untreated insulin deficient patient with NIDD and moderately severe symptomatic hyperglycemia with hypertriglyceridemia, a defect in lipoprotein lipase and VLDL catabolism can be seen, similar to that found in the untreated patient with IDD. In most other circumstances, the increase in VLDL appears to be due to accelerated VLDL synthesis.
5. Variations in HDL cholesterol in diabetes are related in part to the degree of control of the hyperglycemia, in part to the degree of concomitant hypertriglyceridemia, and in part to changes in body composition related to body fat content.
6. The chylomicronemia syndrome occurs relatively commonly in diabetes, is usually easy to treat, and should be entirely preventable.
7. The role of alterations of lipids and lipoproteins in the pathogenesis of atherosclerosis in diabetes, although undoubtedly important, is still not entirely clear. Thus, what are the relative roles of elevated VLDL levels, decreased HDL levels, and increased IDL and possibly LDL levels? What role do changes in the composition of lipoproteins, in particular LDL and HDL, play in the predisposition for atherosclerosis? How do the lipoprotein abnormalities interact with other risk factors, in particular smoking and hypertension, and with other components of the blood and arterial wall?

For further details of work accomplished prior to the time of this review, see the references 1–7.

References

1. Brunzell JD (1981): Obesity, diabetes and hypertriglyceridemia. In: *Recent Advances in Obesity Research: III*, Chapter 33, pp. 239–247. Editors: P.

Bjorntorp, M. Cairella and A.N. Howard. John Libbey and Co., London.
2. Dunn FL (1982): Hyperlipidemia and diabetes. *Med. Clin. North Am.*, *77*, 1347.
3. Eder HA, Bergman M (1983): Metabolism of plasma lipids and lipoproteins. In: *Diabetes Mellitus, Theory and Practice, 3rd Ed.*, Chapter 3, pp. 61–76. Editors M. Ellenberg and H. Rifkin. Medical Examination Publishing Co., New Hyde Park, N.Y.
4. Ganda OP (1980): Pathogenesis of macrovascular disease in the human diabetic. *Diabetes*, 29, 931.
5. Goldberg RB (1981): Lipid disorders in diabetes. *Diabetes Care*, *4*, 561.
6. Gries FA, Koschinsky T, Berchtold P (1979): Obesity, diabetes, and hyperlipoproteinemia. In: *Atherosclerosis Reviews*, *Vol. 4*, pp. 7–95. Editors: R. Paoletti and A.M. Gotto, Jr. Raven Press, New York.
7. Reaven GM, Greenfield MS (1981): Diabetic hypertriglyceridemia: evidence for three clinical syndromes. *Diabetes*, *30*, 66.
8. Barrett-Connor E, Grundy SM, Holdbrook MJ (1982): Plasma lipids and diabetes mellitus in an adult community. *Am. J. Epidemiol.*, *115*, 657.
9. Barrett-Connor E, Witztum JL, Holdbrook M (1983): A community study of high density lipoproteins in adult noninsulin-dependent diabetics. *Am. J. Epidemiol.*, *117*, 186.
10. West KM, Ahuja MMS, Bennett PH, Czyzyk A, Mateo de Acosta O, Fuller JH, Grab B, Grabauskas V, Jarrett RJ, Kosaka K, Keen H, Krolewski AS, Miki E, Schliack V, Teuscher A, Watkins PJ, Stober JA (1983): The role of circulating glucose and triglyceride concentrations and their interactions with other 'risk factors' as determinants of arterial disease in nine diabetic population samples from the WHO multinational study. *Diabetes Care*, *6*, 361.
11. Wingard DL, Barrett-Connor E, Criqui MH, Suarez L (1983): Clustering of heart disease risk factors in diabetic compared to nondiabetic adults. *Am. J. Epidemiol.*, *117*, 19.
12. Brunzell JD (1984): Obesity and coronary heart disease: a targeted approach. *Arteriosclerosis*, *4*, 180.
13. Gabor J, Spain M, Kalant N (1980): Composition of serum very-low-density and high-density lipoproteins in diabetes. *Clin. Chem.*, *26*, 1261.
14. Hughes TA, Cone JT, Fairclough P (1983): Effect of insulin therapy on the lipoprotein profile of NIDDM. *Diabetes*, *32*, *Suppl. 1*, 63A.
15. Sosenko JM, Breslow JL, Miettinen OS, Gabbay KH (1980): Hyperglycemia and plasma lipid levels: a prospective study of young insulin-dependent diabetic patients. *New Engl. J. Med.*, *302*, 650.
16. Lopes-Virella MF, Wohltmann HJ, Loadholt CB, Buse MG (1981): Plasma lipids and lipoproteins in young insulin-dependent diabetic patients: relationship with control. *Diabetologia*, *21*, 216.
17. Glasgow AM, August GP, Hung W (1981): Relationship between control and serum lipids in juvenile-onset diabetes. *Diabetes Care*, *4*, 76.
18. Andersen GE, Christiansen JS, Mortensen HB, Christiansen KM, Pedersen-Bjergaard L, Kastrup KW, Vestermark S (1983): Serum lipids and lipoproteins in 157 insulin dependent diabetic children and adolescents in relation to metabolic regulation, obesity and genetic hyperlipoproteinemia. *Acta Paediatr. Scand.*, *72*, 361.

19. Bachem MG, Paschen K, Strobel B, Jastram HU, Janssen EG, Dati F (1982): Correlations between lipoproteins and glycosylated hemoglobins in juvenile diabetes mellitus. *Klin. Wochenschr.*, *60*, 497.
20. Carvajal F, Quesada X, Gonzalez P (1983): High density lipoprotein cholesterol in insulin-dependent diabetic children. *Acta Diabetol. Lat.*, *20*, 289.
21. Sosenko JM, Breslow J, Miettinen OS, Gabbay KH (1982): Hyperglycemia and plasma lipid levels: covariations in insulin-dependent diabetes. *Diabetes Care*, *5*, 40.
22. Briones ER, Mao SJT, Palumbo PJ, O'Fallon WM, Chenoweth W, Kottke BA (1984): Analysis of plasma lipids and apolipoproteins in insulin-dependent and noninsulin-dependent diabetics. *Metabolism*, *33*, 42.
23. Eckel RH, Albers JJ, Cheung MC, Wahl PW, Lindgren FT, Bierman EL (1981): High density lipoprotein composition in insulin-dependent diabetes mellitus. *Diabetes*, *30*, 132.
24. Durrington PN (1982): Serum high density lipoprotein cholesterol subfractions in Type I (insulin-dependent) diabetes mellitus. *Clin. Chim. Acta*, *120*, 21.
25. Mattock MB, Salter AM, Fuller JH, Omer T, Gohart R-E, Redmond SD, Keen H (1982): High density lipoprotein subfractions in insulin-dependent diabetic and normal subjects. *Atherosclerosis*, *45*, 67.
26. Nikkila EA (1981): High density lipoproteins in diabetes. *Diabetes*, *30*, *Suppl. 2*, 82.
27. Schernthaner G, Kostner GM, Dieplinger H, Prager R, Mühlhauser I (1983): Apolipoproteins (A-I, A-II, B), Lp(a) lipoprotein and lecithin:cholesterol acyltransferase activity in diabetes mellitus. *Atherosclerosis*, *49*, 277.
28. Vannini P, Ciavarella A, Flammini M, Bargossi AM, Forlani G, Borgnino LC, Orsoni G (1984): Lipid abnormalities in insulin-dependent diabetic patients with albuminuria. *Diabetes Care*, *7*, 151.
29. Blanc MH, Ganda OP, Gleason RE, Soeldner JS (1983): Improvement of lipid status in diabetic boys: the 1971 and 1979 Joslin Camp lipid levels. *Diabetes Care*, *6*, 64.
30. Tamborlane WV, Sherwin RS, Genel M, Felig P (1979): Restoration of normal lipid and amino acid metabolism in diabetic patients treated with a portable insulin-infusion pump. *Lancet*, *2*, 1258.
31. Pietri A, Dunn FL, Raskin P (1980): The effect of improved diabetic control on plasma lipid and lipoprotein levels: a comparison of conventional therapy and continuous subcutaneous insulin infusion. *Diabetes*, *29*, 1001.
32. Dunn FL, Pietri A, Raskin P (1981): Plasma lipid and lipoprotein levels with continuous subcutaneous insulin infusion in Type I diabetes mellitus. *Ann. Intern. Med.*, *95*, 426.
33. Hershcopf R, Plotnick LP, Kaya K, Benedict GW, Hadji-Georgopoulos A, Margolis S, Kowarski AA (1982): Short term improvement in glycemic control utilizing continuous subcutaneous insulin infusion: the effect on 24-hour integrated concentrations of counterregulatory hormones and plasma lipids in insulin-dependent diabetes mellitus. *J. Clin. Endocrinol. Metab.*, *54*, 504.
34. Lopes-Virella MF, Wohltmann HJ, Mayfield RK, Loadholt CB, Colwell JA (1983): Effect of metabolic control on lipid, lipoprotein, and apolipoprotein levels in 55 insulin-dependent diabetic patients. *Diabetes*, *32*, 20.

35. Vlachokosta FV, Asmal AC, Ganda OP, Aoki TT (1983): The effect of strict control with the artificial β-cell on plasma lipid levels in insulin-dependent diabetes. *Diabetes Care*, *6*, 351.
36. Falko JM, O'Dorisio TM, Cataland S (1982): Improvement of high-density lipoprotein-cholesterol levels. Ambulatory Type I diabetics treated with the subcutaneous insulin pump. *J. Am. Med. Assoc.*, *247*, 37.
37. Daneman D, Epstein LH, Siminerio L, Beck S, Farkas G, Figueroa J, Becker DJ, Drash AL (1982): Effects of enhanced conventional therapy on metabolic control in children with insulin-dependent diabetes mellitus. *Diabetes Care*, *5*, 472.
38. Taskinen M-R, Nikkilä EA, Ollus A (1983): Serum lipids and lipoproteins in insulin-dependent diabetic subjects during high-carbohydrate, high-fiber diet. *Diabetes Care*, *6*, 224.
39. Taskinen M-R, Nikkilä EA, Kuusi T, Harno K (1982): Lipoprotein lipase activity and serum lipoproteins in untreated type 2 (insulin-independent) diabetes associated with obesity. *Diabetologia*, *22*, 46.
40. Rabkin SW, Boyko E, Streja DA (1983): Changes in high density lipoprotein cholesterol after initiation of insulin therapy in non-insulin dependent diabetes mellitus: relationship to changes in body weight. *Am. J. Med. Sci.*, *285*, 14.
41. Schmitt JK, Poole JR, Lewis SB, Shore VG, Maman A, Baer RM, Forsham PH (1982): Hemoglobin A_1 correlates with the ratio of low- to high-density-lipoprotein cholesterol in normal weight type II diabetics. *Metabolism*, *31*, 1084.
42. Pfeifer MA, Brunzell JD, Best JD, Judzewitsch RG, Halter JB, Porte D Jr. (1983): The response of plasma triglyceride, cholesterol, and lipoprotein lipase to treatment in non-insulin-dependent diabetic subjects without familial hypertriglyceridemia. *Diabetes*, *32*, 525.
43. Greenfield MS, Doberne L, Rosenthal M, Vreman HJ, Reaven GM (1982): Lipid metabolism in non-insulin-dependent diabetes mellitus: effect of Glipizide Therapy. *Arch. Intern. Med.*, *142*, 1498.
44. Biesbroeck RC, Albers JJ, Wahl PW, Weinberg CR, Bassett ML, Bierman EL (1982): Abnormal composition of high density lipoproteins in non-insulin-dependent diabetics. *Diabetes*, *31*, 126.
45. Jialal I, Joubert SM, Asmal AC (1982): Cholesterol, triglyceride and high-density lipoprotein cholesterol levels in non-insulin-dependent diabetes in the young. *S. Afr. Med. J.*, *61*, 393.
46. Taylor KG, John WG, Matthews KA, Wright AD (1982): A prospective study of the effect of 12 months treatment on serum lipids and apolipoproteins A-I and B in type 2 (non-insulin-dependent) diabetes. *Diabetologia*, *23*, 507.
47. Lee S-C, Chen D, Tsai WJ, Chen M-L, Ding Y-A, Li Y-B (1982): Lipid profiles of plasma lipoproteins in normal Chinese and in patients with hypertension and diabetes mellitus, *Chin. Med. J.*, *29*, 234.
48. Shoukry M, Jayyab AKA (1983): Plasma HDL in non-insulin-dependent diabetes and the effect of various types of treatment. *Atherosclerosis*, *49*, 333.
49. Agardh C-D, Nilsson-Ehle P, Schersten B (1982): Improvement of the

plasma lipoprotein pattern after institution of insulin treatment in diabetes mellitus. *Diabetes Care*, *5*, 322.

50. Barnard RJ, Massey MR, Cherny S, O'Brien LT, Pritikin N (1983): Long-term use of a high-complex-carbohydrate, high-fiber, low-fat diet and exercise in the treatment of NIDDM patients. *Diabetes Care*, *6*, 268.
51. Weisweiler P, Drosner M, Schwandt P (1982): Dietary effects on very low-density lipoproteins in type 2 (non-insulin-dependent) diabetes mellitus. *Diabetologia*, *23*, 101.
52. Kennedy L, Walshe K, Hadden DR, Weaver JA, Buchanan KD (1982): The effect of intensive dietary therapy on serum high density lipoprotein cholesterol in patients with type 2 (non-insulin-dependent) diabetes mellitus: a prospective study. *Diabetologia*, *23*, 24.
53. Prager R, Schernthaner G, Kostner GM, Mühlhauser I, Zechner R, Dorda W (1982): Effect of bezafibrate on plasma lipids, lipoproteins, apolipoproteins AI, AII and B and LCAT activity in hyperlipidemic, non-insulin-dependent diabetics. *Atherosclerosis*, *43*, 321.
54. Kissebah AH, Alfarsi S, Evans DJ, Adams PW (1982): Integrated regulation of very low density lipoprotein triglyceride and apolipoprotein-B kinetics in non-insulin-dependent diabetes mellitus. *Diabetes*, *31*, 217.
55. Greenfield M, Kolterman O, Olefsky J, Reaven GM (1980): Mechanism of hypertriglyceridaemia in diabetic patients with fasting hyperglycaemia. *Diabetologia*, *18*, 441.
56. Ginsberg H, Grundy SM (1982): Very low density lipoprotein metabolism in non-ketotic diabetes mellitus: effect of dietary restriction. *Diabetologia*, *23*, 421.
57. Abrams JJ, Ginsberg H, Grundy SM (1982): Metabolism of cholesterol and plasma triglycerides in nonketotic diabetes mellitus. *Diabetes*, *31*, 903.
58. Dunn FL, Raskin P, Bilheimer DW, Grundy SM (1984): The effect of diabetic control on very low-density lipoprotein-triglyceride metabolism in patients with type II diabetes mellitus and marked hypertriglyceridemia. *Metabolism*, *33*, 117.
59. Howard BV, Reitman JS, Vasquez B, Zech L (1983): Very-low-density lipoprotein triglyceride metabolism in non-insulin-dependent diabetes mellitus. *Diabetes*, *32*, 271.
60. Pietri AO, Dunn FL, Grundy SM, Raskin P (1983): The effect of continuous subcutaneous insulin infusion on very-low-density lipoprotein triglyceride metabolism in type I diabetes mellitus. *Diabetes*, *32*, 75.
61. Brunzell JD, Schwartz RS, Eckel RH, Goldberg AP (1981): Insulin and adipose tissue lipoprotein lipase activity in humans. *Int. J. Obesity*, *5*, 685.
62. Brunzell JD, Porte D Jr, Bierman EL (1979): Abnormal lipoprotein lipase mediated plasma triglyceride removal in untreated diabetes mellitus associated with hypertriglyceridemia. *Metabolism*, *28*, 897.
63. Lopes-Virella MF, Mordes D, Harstine L, Colwell JA (1983): Plasma hepatic and lipoprotein lipase activities after prolonged infusion of heparin in type II diabetic females. *Clin. Res.*, *31*, 851A.
64. Magill P, Rao SN, Miller NE, Nicoll A, Brunzell J, St. Hilaire J, Lewis B (1982): Relationships between the metabolism of high density and very-low-density lipoproteins in man: studies of apolipoprotein kinetics and adipose

tissue lipoprotein lipase activity. *Eur. J. Clin. Invest.*, *12*, 113.
65. Bazelmans J, Nestel PJ, Nolan C (1983): Insulin-induced glucose utilization influences triglyceride metabolism. *Clin. Sci.*, *64*, 511.
66. Steiner G (1979): Insulin and hypertriglyceridemia. In: *Diabetes. Proceedings of the 10th Congress of the International Diabetes Federation, Vienna, Austria, September 9–14, 1979*, pp. 590–593. Editor: W.K. Waldhäusl. Excerpta Medica, Amsterdam.
67. Steiner G, Morita S, Vranic M (1980): Resistance to insulin but not to glucagon in lean human hypertriglyceridemics. *Diabetes*, *29*, 899.
68. Brunzell JD (1981): Endogenous hypertriglyceridemia: A splanchnic defect, hyperinsulinism or both? *Metabolism*, *30*, 836.
69. Fedele D, Lapolla A, Cardone C, Baldo G, Crepaldi G (1983): Glycosylated hemoglobin in endogenous hypertriglyceridemia. *Acta Diabetol. Lat.*, *20*, 303.
70. Patsch W, Franz S, Schonfeld G (1983): Role of insulin in lipoprotein secretion by cultured rat hepatocytes. *J. Clin. Invest.*, *71*, 1161.
71. Durrington PN, Newton RS, Weinstein DB, Steinberg D (1982): Effects of insulin and glucose on very low density lipoprotein triglyceride secretion by cultured rat hepatocytes. *J. Clin. Invest.*, *70*, 63.
72. Patsch W, Tamai T, Schonfeld G (1983): Effect of fatty acids on lipid and apoprotein secretion and association in hepatocyte cultures. *J. Clin. Invest.*, *72*, 371.
73. McGarry JD, Foster D (1983): Ketogenesis. In: *Diabetes Mellitus, Theory and Practice, 3rd ed.*, Chapter 29, pp. 611–619. Editors: M. Ellenberg and H. Rifkin. Medical Examination Publishing Co., New Hyde Park, New York.
74. Kissebah AH, Alfarsi S, Evans DJ, Adams PW (1983): Plasma low density lipoprotein transport kinetics in noninsulin-dependent diabetes mellitus. *J. Clin. Invest.*, *71*, 655.
75. Steinbrecher UP, Witztum JL (1984): Glucosylation of low-density lipoproteins to an extent comparable to that seen in diabetes slows their catabolism. *Diabetes*, *33*, 130.
76. Mazzone T, Foster D, Chait A (1984): *In vivo* stimulation of low-density lipoprotein degradation by insulin. *Diabetes*, *33*, 333.
77. Chait A, Foster D, Miller DG, Bierman EL (1981): Acceleration of low density lipoprotein catabolism in man by total parenteral nutrition. *Proc. Soc. Exp. Biol. Med.*, *168*, 97.
78. Chait A, Bierman EL, Albers JJ (1979): Low density lipoprotein receptor activity in cultured human skin fibroblasts: Mechanism of insulin-induced stimulation. *J. Clin. Invest.*, *64*, 1309.
79. Soltesz G, Molnar D, Klujber L, Kardos M (1982): Relationship between metabolic control and plasma lipoprotein level in diabetic children. *Acta Paediatr. Acad. Sci. Hung.*, *23*, 75.
80. Paisley R, Elkeles RS, Hambley J, Magill P (1978): The effect of chlorpropamide and insulin on serum lipids, lipoproteins, and fractional triglyceride removal. *Diabetologia*, *15*, 81.
81. Beach KW, Brunzell JD, Conquest LL, Strandness DE (1979): The correlation of arteriosclerosis obliterans with lipoproteins in insulin-dependent and non-insulin-dependent diabetes. *Diabetes*, *28*, 836.

82. Witztum JL, Fisher M, Pietro T, Steinbrecher UP, Elam RL (1982): Nonenzymatic glucosylation of high-density lipoprotein accelerates its catabolism in guinea pigs. *Diabetes. 31*, 1029.
83. Harno K, Nikkilä EA, Kuusi T (1980): Plasma HDL-cholesterol and postheparin plasma hepatic endothelial lipase (HL) activity: Relationship to obesity and non-insulin dependent diabetes (NIDDM). *Diabetologia, 19*, 281.
84. Fielding CJ, Reaven GM, Fielding PE (1982): Human non-insulin-dependent diabetes: identification of a defect in plasma cholesterol transport normalized in vivo by insulin and in vitro by selective immunoadsorption of apoliprotein E. *Proc. Natl Acad. Sci. USA, 79*, 6365.
85. Fielding CJ, Reaven GM, Liu G, Fielding PE (1984): Increased free cholesterol in plasma low and very low density lipoproteins in non-insulin-dependent diabetes mellitus: its role in the inhibition of cholesterol ester transfer. *Proc. Natl Acad. Sci. USA, 81*, 2512.
86. Hiramatsu K, Bierman EL, Chait A (1984): Metabolism of low density lipoprotein from patients with diabetic hypertriglyceridemia by cultured human skin fibroblasts. *Diabetes*, in press.
87. Lopes-Virella MF, Sherer GK, Lees AM, Wohltmann H, Mayfield R, Sagel J, LeRoy EC, Colwell JA (1982): Surface binding, internalization and degradation by cultured human fibroblasts of low density lipoproteins isolated from type 1 (insulin-dependent) diabetic patients: changes with metabolic control. *Diabetologia, 22*, 430.
88. Kraemer FB, Chen Y-DI, Cheung RMC, Reaven GM (1982): Are the binding and degradation of low density lipoprotein altered in type 2 (non-insulin-dependent) diabetes mellitus? *Diabetologia, 23*, 28.
89. Deckelbaum RJ, Granot E, Oschry Y, Rose L, Eisenberg S (1982): Plasma triglyceride determines structure-composition in low and high density lipoproteins. *Arteriosclerosis, 4*, 225.
90. Bell GI, Karam JH, Rutter WJ (1981): Polymorphic DNA region adjacent to the 5′ end of the human insulin gene. *Proc. Natl Acad. Sci. USA, 78*, 5758.
91. Rotwein PS, Chirgwin J, Province M, Knowler WC, Pettitt DJ, Cordell B, Goodman HM, Permutt MA (1983): Polymorphism in the 5′ flanking region of the human insulin gene: a genetic marker for non-insulin-dependent diabetes. *N. Engl. J. Med., 308*, 65.
92. Owerbach D, Billesbølle P, Schroll M, Johansen K, Poulsen S, Nerup J (1982): Possible association between DNA sequences flanking the insulin gene and atherosclerosis. *Lancet, 2*, 1291.
93. Ullrich A, Dull TJ, Gray P, Phillips JA, Reser S (1982): Variation in the sequence and modification state of the human insulin gene flanking regions. *Nucleic Acids Res., 10*, 2225.
94. Jowett NI, Williams LG, Hitman GA, Galton DJ (1984): Diabetic hypertriglyceridaemia and related 5′ flanking polymorphism of the human insulin gene. *Br. Med. J., 288*, 96.
95. Mandrup-Poulsen T, Mortensen SA, Meinertz H, Owerbach D, Johansen K, Sørensen H (1984): DNA sequences flanking the insulin gene on chromosome 11 confer risk of atherosclerosis. *Lancet, 1*, 250.
96. Brunzell JD, Bierman EL (1982): Chylomicronemia syndrome: interaction of genetic and acquired hypertriglyceridemia. *Med. Clin. North Am., 66*, 455.

97. Ditzel J (1984): Clinical significance and management of diabetic lipemia. *Pract. Cardiol.*, *10*, 155.
98. Chait A, Brunzell JD (1983): Severe Hypertriglyceridemia: role of familial and acquired disorders. *Metab. Clin. Exp.*, *32*, 209.
99. Lawlor J (1982): Hyperlipidemia interference in radioimmunoassays. *Clin. Chem.*, *28*, 2326.
100. Gerard A, Schooneman F, Guine JM, Roche G, Canton P, Dureux JB, Janot C, Streiff F (1982): Treatment by plasma exchange of a patient with hyperlipidemia and diabetic ketoacidosis with lesional pulmonary edema and acute pancreatitis. *Vox Sang.*, *43*, 147.
101. Weinberg RB, Sitrin MD, Adkins GM, Lin CC (1982): Treatment of hyperlipidemic pancreatitis in pregnancy with total parenteral nutrition. *Gastroenterology*, *83*, 1300.

The Diabetes Annual/1
K.G.M.M. Alberti and L.P. Krall, editors

ISBN 0444 90 343 7
$0.85 per article per page (transactional system)
$0.20 per article per page (licensing system)

27 Glucagon in diabetes

ROGER H. UNGER

Physiology and pathophysiology

Glucagon was discovered by Murlin and Kimball within a year of the discovery of insulin but was not recognized as a true hormone for almost half a century. Even after its hormonal status had been accepted, recognition of the vital nature of its physiologic mission and of its deleterious role in the pathophysiology of diabetes was slow in coming. Evidence gathered within the past decade indicates that glucagon is secreted in tightly coupled coordination with insulin *and* plays an essential role as a regulator of hepatic production of glucose and ketone bodies, the two fuels utilized by the brain (see refs. 1 and 2 for reviews). Two-thirds of the basal hepatic glucose production is glucagon-mediated (3). Since the brain accounts for three-fifths of basal glucose utilization, the glucagon-mediated component of hepatic glucose production is essential to prevent fasting hypoglycemia and neuroglucopenia (4) which occur in glucagon deficiency (5). Glucagon also helps prevent hypoglycemia during exercise (6) and during the ingestion of carbohydrate-free meals (7). When insulin is deficient as in diabetes, glucagon causes the hepatic glucose and ketone body overproduction that characterizes poorly controlled diabetes (8). When glucagon is experimentally suppressed (9) or blocked (10), glucose and ketone production by the liver remain normal even in the total absence of insulin (11). Thus, diabetes meets the clinical definition of IDDM only if glucagon is present; in the absence of glucagon insulin lack causes only mild fasting and postprandial hyperglycemia but the catabolic cascade and ketoacidosis that define the IDDM syndrome does not occur. In a sense the absence of glucagon converts the IDDM syndrome into a mild NIDDM syndrome.

Glucagon biosynthesis

Glucagon is a 29-amino acid polypeptide synthesized in pancreatic alpha cells. Their initial gene product, pre-proglucagon, is a 180-amino acid pro-

This work has been supported by VA Institutional Research Support grant 549-8000-01 and National Institutes of Health grant AM-02700-25.

tein with five components (12): a signal peptide, an N-terminal 'glicentin-related pancreatic peptide' (GRPP) (13), glucagon (14), glucagon-like peptide-1 (GLP-1), and glucagon-like peptide-2 (GLP-2) (12). GRPP consists of 30 amino acid residues identical to the sequence of glicentin 1 through 30 (13). The proglucagon molecule is called glicentin or GLI-1 and is made up of 69 amino acid residues (14, 15). It contains the full glucagon sequence with a GRPP sequence connected to the N-terminus of glucagon by a lysine–arginine pair and a hexapeptide connected to the C-terminus of glucagon by an arginine–arginine pair. These amino acid pairs are the sites of the tryptic cleavage that generates glucagon. The pre-proglucagon gene contains 3 intervening sequences: one that codes for the signal peptide and part of the GRPP molecule, a second that codes for the remainder of GRPP plus glucagon and its C-terminal hexapeptide and a third that codes for GLP-1 and GLP-2 (12).

Peak 2 glucagon-like immunoreactivity (GLI-2, enteroglucagon, oxyntomodulin) is the carboxyterminal section of glicentin, i.e. it contains glucagon, the arg-arg pair and the C-terminal hexapeptide. It binds to glucagon receptors and activates adenylate cyclase in hepatic plasma membranes with 10–20% of the potency of glucagon (16, 17). It stimulates adenylate cyclase in plasma membrane fractions of the oxyntic mucosa of the stomach and inhibits gastric acid secretion and is therefore also called oxyntomodulin (18, 19).

The secretory granules of pancreatic A-cells consist of a central core that contains the glucagon and a halo of the granule that contains glicentin (21). The material secreted by the pancreas consists of glucagon with traces of glicentin-like immunoreactivity. By contrast, the homogeneous secretory granules of the intestinal L-cells contain only glicentin material distributed evenly throughout the granules and are negative when stained for glucagon. They presumably lack the tryptic enzymes required to process proglucagon to glucagon. If L-cells are exposed to tryptic digestion, they then react positively when exposed to antiglucagon serum. L-cells probably secrete both GLI peak 1 which has a molecular weight comparable to glicentin, and GLI peak 2. GLI-1 increases after intraduodenal glucose (22, 23).

It is reported that the GLI polypeptides can be converted to true glucagon after entering the circulation (24). They may therefore constitute a source of circulating glucagon following total pancreatectomy, perhaps accounting for the normal glucagon levels in such patients (25). However, true glucagon-containing cells have been described in the human gut (26).

Molecular biology – glucagon actions

Glucagon interacts with its receptor on the surface of hepatocytes, acts to increase cAMP and is internalized (27). Residues 1 to 6 on the hydrophilic

N-terminal region of the glucagon molecule reportedly stimulate the liver adenylate cyclase system with an activity of about five orders of magnitude less than that of the intact hormone and were originally thought to be the active portion of the molecule (28). However, Frandsen et al. report that deletion of the first four amino acids from glucagon does not abolish binding to its receptor (29), while C-terminal extension of the glucagon molecule prevents both its binding and biologic activity. The latter observations point to the importance of the C-terminal region in glucagon action. The apparent discrepancy has prompted Rodbell (30) to suggest that both portions of the glucagon molecule are required for its action and that the receptor is composed of two subunits, one of which reacts with the hydrophilic 1–6 region to give glucagon action, while the other subunit reacts with the hydrophobic residues to anchor the molecule. This would be consistent with the estimate by target analysis (31) that in its active state the glucagon receptor has a molecular weight of approximately 100,000 daltons, whereas the affinity labelled receptor is estimated at 58,000 daltons (32), perhaps reflecting two or more subunits for the receptor (29).

Once the interaction between glucagon and its receptor has occurred, the receptor communicates with a pair of homologous guanine nucleotide binding regulatory proteins or G-proteins, one of which, G_s, mediates the stimulation of adenylate cyclase activity and the other of which, G_i, inhibits the enzyme. The G-proteins control the activity of the catalyst of adenylate cyclase. (For a brief review, see ref. 33.) The inhibitory guanine nucleotide binding protein is detected because it binds the islet activating protein produced by *Bordetella pertussis* (34). Within moments after glucagon is administered, cAMP concentrations rise in the liver as a consequence of increased adenylate cyclase activity relative to that of phosphodiesterase, the degrading enzyme for cAMP.

Biochemistry of glucagon action (Fig. 1)

The cAMP in the cytosol of hepatocytes binds to the inactive dimeric form of the cAMP-dependent protein kinase. Activation of this enzyme induces all of the known actions of glucagon in the liver through phosphorylation events that alter the activity of the key enzymes involved in glycogenolysis, glycogen synthesis, gluconeogenesis and glycolysis and, indirectly, in lipogenesis.

Phosphorylation of phosphorylase, the rate-limiting enzyme of glycogenolysis, converts it to the active *a*-form whereas phosphorylation of glycogen synthase changes it to the inactive *b*-form. These events enhance glycogenolysis and reduce glycogenesis. Insulin can oppose this action of glucagon if its concentration rises proportionately with that of glucagon. While this may in part be via activation of phosphodiesterase, it more probably reflects inhibition of the cAMP-dependent protein kinase (35). Consequently, when kinase activity is low, as when glucagon is suppressed, insulin can have little or no effect on these pathways (36, 37). This explains why the total absence of insulin does not cause hyperglycemia or ketoacidosis when glucagon is deficient (9, 38, 39) or when its action is blocked by glucagon antagonists (10).

A second consequence of glucagon-induced activation of cAMP-dependent protein kinase is phosphorylation of a key bifunctional enzyme that determines the level of fructose-2,6-bisphosphate, the potent regulator of

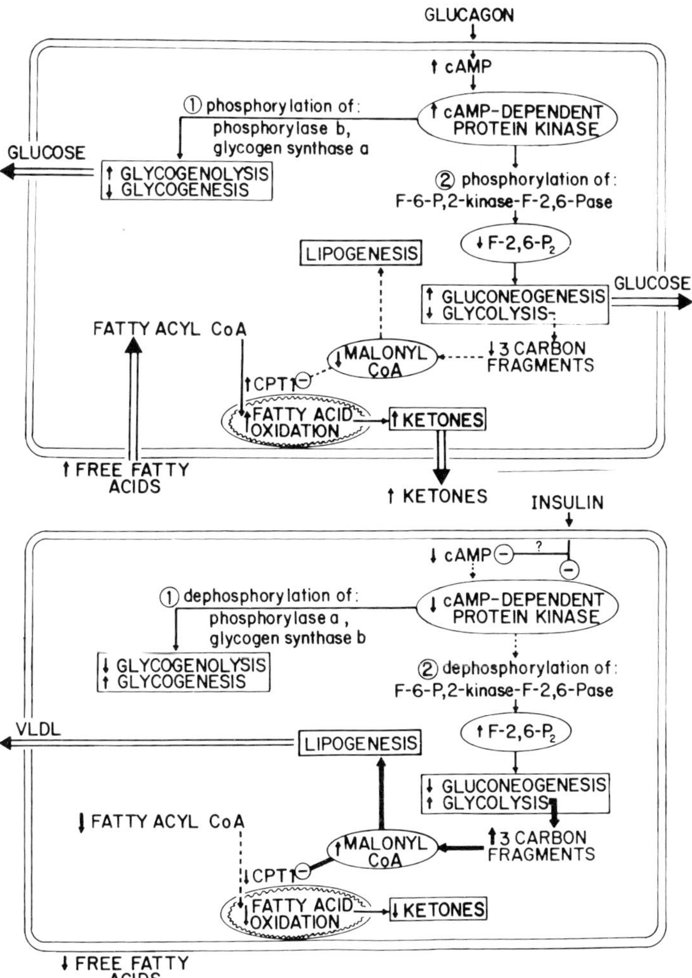

FIG. 1. *The biochemical basis for insulin-glucagon interactions on fuel metabolism in the liver (see text for details). Modified from R.H. Unger and D.W. Foster in: Williams Textbook of Endocrinology, 6th Edition. WB Saunders, Philadelphia 1985.*

glycolysis and gluconeogenesis (40–42). When this enzyme is phosphorylated, as would be the case when glucagon is high relative to insulin, it acts as a fructose-bis-phosphatase-2 and reduces hepatic fructose-2,6-bisphosphate levels. When insulin is high relative to glucagon, the enzyme is dephosphorylated and it acts as a phosphofructokinase-2 raising fructose-2,6-bisphosphate levels. Fructose-2,6-bisphosphate allosterically catalyzes phosphofructokinase-1 activity, the key enzyme in glycolysis. The resulting enhancement of the flow of 3-carbon fragments down the glycolytic pathway provides increased substrate for lipogenesis by the liver. The newly synthesized fatty acids are esterified to triglycerides and secreted as very low-density lipoprotein (VLDL), in which form fat is transported to adipocytes for storage. The increased lipogenesis increases the intrahepatic levels of malonyl-CoA, the first committed intermediate in lipogenesis. Malonyl-CoA is a powerful inhibitor of the enzyme carnitine palmitoyl transferase-1 (CPT-1) which transesterifies fatty acyl-CoA to fatty acyl carnitine, the form in which it can traverse the outer leaflet of the mitochondrial membrane to enter the mitochondrion, where it undergoes beta-oxidation to ketones (43). When insulin is low, free fatty acids are released from adipocytes in increased quantities and reach the liver where they are now able to cross into mitochondria for oxidation to ketones. Thus the increase in fructose-2,6-bisphosphate ultimately is responsible for increasing carbohydrate-derived VLDL production and inhibiting ketogenesis. The work of Van Schaftingen et al. (40), Richards and Uyeda (41), and Pilkis et al. (42) on fructose-2,6-bisphophate, and that of McGarry and Foster on the control of ketogenesis (43) provide the basis for the unifying scheme depicted in Figure 1. (See ref. 44 for review.)

When glucagon is high relative to insulin as in starvation or diabetes, fructose-2,6-bisphosphate levels drop (45). This is observed even at 10^{-13} molar glucagon, which is well below the detection limit of most radioimmunoassays (46). Thus, even minute quantities of glucagon, if unopposed by insulin, are capable of important catabolic and antianabolic effects on the liver. These facts readily explain why depancreatized humans with glucagon levels in a low-normal range (47) exhibit overproduction of glucose and ketones in the absence of insulin. (In the total absence of glucagon this does not occur (48).)

Islet morphology

The glucagon-secreting A-cells are linked both anatomically and functionally to the insulin-secreting B-cells (49) in a manner believed to make possible their coordinated secretion. In this way the bihormonal mixture of insulin and glucagon may, through the previously discussed biochemical mechanisms, set hepatic metabolism at a level appropriate for the fuel needs of the organism at a particular moment. In the rat islet A-cells are peripherally located to form a cortex. In the human islet they form the outer layer of multiple pseudolobules. Between the A-cells, which comprise approximately 25% of the endocrine pancreas, and the B-cells, which comprise over 60%, are somatostatin-containing D-cells which make up close to 10% of the population (50). In the posterior portion of the head of the human pancreas pancreatic polypeptide-containing F-cells replace the glucagon cells (51). Gap junctions between islet cells, both of the same and of different types, form discrete synctitial domains within the pancreas (52). While the functional significance of these membrane differentiations is uncertain, it is known that small molecules such as nucleotides can pass via these channels from one cell to another.

Islet physiology

Insulin, glucagon and somatostatin each influence the secretory activity of A-, B- and D-cells. Insulin inhibits insulin (53), glucagon (54) and somatostatin (55) secretion; glucagon stimulates insulin (56) and somatostatin (57) secretion, but inhibits glucagon secretion (58); somatostatin inhibits insulin (59), glucagon (60) and somatostatin secretion (61). The contiguity of these cells has suggested that the hormones might influence the secretory activity of the endocrine pancreas via a direct paracrine route through the interstitial space (62). Perhaps the most persuasive evidence in support of this hypothesis has been the studies of Asplin et al. (63). On the other hand, in the isolated perfused rat pancreas an arterial concentration of somatostatin that is only 10–20% of that in the venous effluent inhibits both insulin and glucagon secretion; this suggests that the somatostatin receptors on A- and B-cells are in a somatostatin-poor compartment separated from the far higher somatostatin concentrations that are present at the secretory pole of the somatostatin-secreting cells (64). Morphologic evidence for separate 'arterial' and 'venous' capillaries has also recently been reported (65). The demonstration by Bonner-Weir and Orci (66) that arterial blood flows first to the B-cells of the rat islet and subsequently reaches the A-cell-rich cortical regions of the rat islet is consistent with the recent report that anti-insulin serum perfused in a non-recirculating isolated rat pancreas system causes an immediate increase in glucagon secretion (67) before the antibody could have left the circulation of the islets. This suggests that insulin has a continuing suppressive effect on glucagon secretion that is transmitted via the capillaries within the islet rather than via the interstitium.

Neurotransmitted signals may be extremely important in islet cell response both to feeding and to stressful circumstances. (See ref. 68 for review.) Cholinergic signals may be involved in the early anticipatory response of glucagon and insulin secretion to meals and may help prevent wide postprandial fluctuations in nutrient concentration (69). Far more important to survival is the sympathetic control of insulin and glucagon secretion during exercise, stressfull illness and hypoglycemia. Prevention of hypoglycemia during exercise permits increased glucose consumption by muscle without reducing glucose delivery to the brain. Similarly, whenever cerebral blood flow is jeopardized by a reduction in blood volume, as in cardiogenic or hemorrhagic shock, traumatic or thermal injury or sepsis, stress hyperglycemia may compensate for diminished cerebral blood flow. Together with catecholamines glucagon plays an important role by enhancing glucose production through increased glycogenolysis, gluconeogenesis and ketogenesis via the biochemical mechanisms described above.

In the above circumstances the glucagon response may in large part be mediated by neutrotransmitted norepinephrine and circulating catecholamines which stimulate glucagon secretion (70). These sympathetic effects on the islets are generally considered to originate in the central nervous system in the ventral medial nucleus of the hypothalamus (71). However, recent evidence suggests that the glucagon response to glucopenia may be locally regulated by nerve endings within the pancreas. Glucopenia causes norepinephrine release from the isolated canine pancreas (72) and the concomitant increase in glucagon secretion caused by glucopenia in the isolated perfused rat pancreas can be in large part blocked by alpha-adrenergic blockade (67). Thus, neuroglucopenia may elicit a discharge of catecholamine from adrenergic nerve endings. In the pancreas such a discharge would stimulate the release of glucagon and reduce secretion of insulin.

In addition to glucagon and by catecholamines acting directly on the liver, other stress hormones may also contribute to stress hyperglycemia in various ways. β-Endorphin (73), growth hormone (74) and vasopressin (75) all stimulate glucagon secretion.

In Type 1 diabetes the glucagon response to stress is exaggerated but the response to hypoglycemia, which together with catecholamines is responsible for recovery from insulin-induced hypoglycemia (see 76 for review), may be markedly attenuated (77). This defect is independent of loss of B-cells or insulin (78).

References

1. Unger RH (1981): The milieu interieur and the islets of Langerhans. *Diabetologia*, *20*, 1.
2. Unger RH, Orci L (1981): Glucagon and the A-cell. Physiology and pathophysiology. *N. Engl. J. Med.*, *304*, 1518 and 1575.
3. Chiasson JL, Cherrington AD (1979): Glucagon and liver glucose output. In: *Glucagon I, Handbook of Experimental Pharmacology 66/1*, p. 361, Editor: P.J. Lefebvre. Springer-Verlag, Berlin.

4. Rizza RA, Cryer PE, Gerich JE (1979): Role of glucagon, catecholamines and growth hormone in human counterregulation. *J. Clin. Invest.*, *64*, 62.
5. Vidnes J, Oyasaeter S (1977): Glucagon deficiency causing severe neonatal hypoglycemia in a patient with normal insulin secretion. *Pediatr. Res.*, *11*, 943.
6. Issekutz B, Vranic M (1980): Role of glucagon in the regulation of glucose production in exercising dogs. *Am. J. Physiol.*, *238*, E13.
7. Cherrington AD, Vranic M (1973): Effect of arginine on glucose turnover and plasma free fatty acids in normal dogs. *Diabetes*, *22*, 577.
8. Unger RH, Orci L (1975): The essential role of glucagon in the pathogenesis of diabetes mellitus. *Lancet*, *1*, 14.
9. Gerich JE, Lorenzi M, Bier DM, Schneider V, Tsalikian E, Karam JH, Forsham PH (1975): Prevention of human diabetic ketoacidosis by somatostatin: Evidence for an essential role of glucagon. *N. Engl. J. Med.*, *292*, 985.
10. Johnson DG, Goebel CU, Hruby VJ, Bregman MD, Trivedi D (1982): Hyperglycemia of diabetic rat decreased by a glucagon receptor antagonist. *Science*, *215*, 1115.
11. Cherrington AD, Lacy WW, Chiasson JL (1978): Effect of glucagon on glucose production during insulin deficiency in the dog. *J. Clin. Invest.*, *62*, 664.
12. Bell GI, Sanchez-Pescador R, Laybourn PJ, Najarian RC (1983): Exon duplication and divergence in the human pre-proglucagon gene. *Nature (London)*, *304*, 368.
13. Thim L, Moody AJ (1982): Porcine glicentin-related pancreatic peptide (GRPP): Purification and chemical characterization of glicentin-related pancreatic peptide (proglucagon fragment). *Biochim. Biophys. Acta*, *703*, 134.
14. Moody AJ, Frandsen EK, Jacobson H, Sundby F, Orci L (1976): The structural and immunologic relationship between gut GLI and glucagon. *Metabolism*, *25*, *Suppl. 1*, 1336.
15. Thim L, Moody AJ (1981): The primary structure of porcine glicentin (proglucagon). *Regulatory Peptides*, *2*, 139.
16. Kaneko T, Cheng PY, Toda G, Oka H, Yanaihara N, Yanaihara C, Mihara S, Nishida T, Kaise N, Shin S, Imagawa K (1979): Biologic and binding actions of synthetic possible C-terminal fragments of glicentin in rat liver plasma membrane. In: *Gut Peptide Secretion, Function and Clinical Aspects*, p. 157. Editor: A. Miyoshi. Elsevier North-Holland, Amsterdam.
17. Bataille D, Coudray AM, Carquist M, Rosselin G, Mutt V (1982): Isolation of glucagon 37 (bioactive enteroglucagon/oxyntomodulin) from pork jejuno-ileum. Isolation of the peptide. *FEBS Lett.*, *146*, 73.
18. Bataille D, Gespach C, Coudray AM, Rosselin G (1981): Enteroglucagon: A specific effect on gastric glands isolated from the rat fundus. Evidence for an 'oxyntomodulin' action. *BioSci. Rep.*, *1*, 151.
19. Moody AJ, Thim L (1983): Glucagon, glicentin and related peptides. In: *Glucagon I, Handbook of Experimental Pharmacology 66/1*, p. 139. Editor: P.J. Lefebvre. Springer-Verlag, Berlin.
20. Kirkegaard P, Moody AJ, Holst JJ, Laud FB, Skov Olsen P, Christensen J (1982): Glicentin inhibits gastric acid secretion in the rat. *Nature*, *297*, 156.
21. Ravazzola M, Orci L (1980): Glucagon and glicentin immunoreactivity are

topographically segregated in the a-granule of the human pancreatic cell. *Nature*, *284*, 66.
22. Valverde I, Ghiglione M, Matensanz R, Casado S (1979): Chromatographic pattern of gut glucagon-like immunoreactivity (GLI) in plasma before and during glucose absorption. *Horm. Metab. Res.*, *11*, 343.
23. Ghatei MA, Bloom SR (1981): Enteroglucagon in man. In: *Gut Hormones*, p. 332. Editors: S.R. Bloom and J.M. Polak. Churchill-Livingstone, Edinburgh.
24. Koranyi F, Peterfy F, Szabo J, Torok A, Guoth M, Tamas GY (1981): Evidence for transformation of glucagon-like immunoreactivity of gut into pancreatic glucagon in vivo. *Diabetes*, *30*, 792.
25. Holst JJ, Holst-Pedersen J, Baldissera F, Stadil F (1983): Circulating glucagon after total pancreatectomy in man. *Diabetologia*, *25*, 396.
26. Garaud JC, Eloy R, Moody AJ, Stock C, Grenier F (1980): Glucagon- and glicentin-immunoreactive cells in the lumen of the digestive tract. *Cell Tissue Res.*, *213*, 121.
27. Gorden P, Carpentier JL, Freychet P, Orci L (1980): Internalization of polypeptide hormones. Mechanism, intracellular localization and significance. *Diabetologia*, *18*, 263.
28. Wright DE, Rodbell M (1979): Glucagon 1–6 binds to the glucagon receptor and activates adenylate cyclase. *J. Biochem.*, *254*, 268.
29. Frandsen EK, Gronvald FC, Heding LG, Johansen NL, Lundt BF, Moody AJ, Markusen J, Volund AA (1981): Glucagon: Structure-function relationships investigated by sequence deletions. *Hoppe-Seylers Z. Physiol. Chem. (Berlin)*, *362*, 665.
30. Rodbell M (1983): The actions of glucagon at its receptor: Regulation of adenylate cyclase. In: *Glucagon I, Handbook of Experimental Pharmacology 66/I*, p. 284. Editor: P.J. Lefebvre. Springer-Verlag, Berlin.
31. Houslay MD, Ellory JC, Smith GA, Hesketh TR, Stein JM, Warren GP, Metcalf JC (1977): Exchange of partners in glucagon receptor adenylate cyclase complexes: Physical evidence for the independent mobile receptor model. *Biochim. Biophys. Acta*, *467*, 208.
32. Johnson GL, Macandrew VI, Pilch PF (1981): Identification of the glucagon receptor in rat liver membranes by photoaffinity cross-linking. *Proc. Natl Acad. Sci. USA*, *78*, 875.
33. Gillman AG (1984): Guanine nucleotide binding regulatory proteins and dual control of adenylate cyclase. *J. Clin. Invest.*, *73*, 1.
34. Northrup JK, Sternweis PC, Gilman AC (1983): The subunits of the stimulatory regulatory component of adenylate cyclase. Resolution, activity and properties of the 35,000 dalton (B) subunit. *J. Biol.-Chem.*, *258*, 11361.
35. Gabbay RA, Lardy HA (1984): Site of insulin inhibition of cAMP-stimulated glycogenolysis. cAMP-dependent protein kinase is affected independent of cyclic-AMP changes. *J. Biol. Chem.*, *259*, 6052.
36. Hue L, Van de Werve G (1981): *Short-term Regulation of Liver Metabolism*. Elsevier North-Holland, Amsterdam.
37. Boyd ME, Albright EB, Foster DW, McGarry JD (1981): In vitro reversal of the fasting state of liver metabolism in the rat. *J. Clin. Invest.*, *68*, 142.
38. Dobbs RE, Sakurai H, Faloona GR, Valverde I, Baetens D, Orci L, Unger

RH (1975): Glucagon: Role in the hyperglycemia of diabetes mellitus. *Science, 187*, 544.

39. Nakabayashi H, Dobbs RE, Unger RH (1978): The role of glucagon deficiency in the Houssay phenomenon of dogs. *J. Clin. Invest., 61*, 1355.
40. Van Schaftingen E, Hue L, Hers HG (1980): Fructose-2,6-bisphosphate, the probable structure of the glucose- and glucagon-sensitive stimulator of phosphofructokinase. *Biochem. J., 192*, 892.
41. Richards CS, Uyeda K (1980): Changes in the concentration of activation factor for phosphofructokinase in hepatocytes in response to glucose and glucagon. *Biochem. Biophys. Res. Commun., 97*, 1535.
42. Pilkis SJ, El-Maghrabi MR, Pilkis J, Claus TH (1981): Fructose-2,6-bisphosphate. A new activator of phosphofructokinase. *J. Biol. Chem., 256*, 3171.
43. McGarry JD, Foster DW (1979): In support of the roles of malonyl-CoA and carnitine acyl-transferase I in the regulation of hepatic fatty acid metabolism. *J. Biol. Chem., 254*, 8163.
44. McGarry JD, Foster DW (1983): Glucagon and ketogenesis. In: *Glucagon I, Handbook of Experimental Pharmacology 66/I*, p. 383. Editor: P.J. Lefebvre. Springer-Verlag, Berlin.
45. Neely P, El-Maghrabi MR, Pilkis SJ, Claus TH (1981): Effect of diabetes, insulin, starvation and refeeding on the level of rat hepatic fructose-2,6-bisphosphate. *Diabetes, 30*, 1062.
46. Richards CS, Yokoyama M, Furuya E, Uyeda K (1982): Reciprocal changes in fructose-2,6-phosphate,2-kinase and fructose-2,6-bisphosphatase activity in response to glucagon and epinephrine. *Biochem. Biophys. Res. Commun., 104*, 1073.
47. Boden G, Master RW, Rezvani I, Palmer JP, Lobe TE, Owen OE (1980): Glucagon deficiency and hyperaminoacidemia after total pancreatectomy. *J. Clin. Invest., 65*, 706.
48. Santeusanio F, Massi-Benedetti M, Angeletti G, Calabrese G, Bueti A, Brunetti P (1981): Glucagon and carbohydrate disorder in a totally pancreatectomized man (a study with the aid of an artificial endocrine pancreas). *J. Endocrinol. Invest., 4*, 93.
49. Orci L, Malaisse-Lagae F, Amherdt M, Ravazzola M, Weiss-Wange A, Dobbs R, Perrelet A, Unger RH (1975): Cell contacts in human islets of Langerhans. *J. Clin. Endocrinol. Metab., 41*, 841.
50. Orci L, Baetens D, Rufener C, Amherdt M, Ravazzola M, Studer P, Malaisse-Lagae F, Unger RH (1976): Hypertrophy and hyperplasia of somatostatin-containing D-cells in diabetes. *Proc. Natl Acad. Sci. USA, 73*, 1338.
51. Malaisse-Lagae F, Stefan Y, Cox J, Perrelet A, Orci L (1979): Identification of a lobe in the adult human pancreas rich in pancreatic polypeptide. *Diabetologia, 17*, 361.
52. Meda P, Cohen E, Cohen C, Rabinovitch A, Orci L (1982): Direct communication of homologous and heterologous endocrine islet cells in culture. *J. Cell Biol., 92*, 221.
53. Liljenquist JE, Horwitz DL, Jennings AS, Chiasson JL, Keller U, Rubenstein AH (1978): Inhibition of insulin secretion by exogenous insulin in normal man as demonstrated by C-peptide assay. *Diabetes, 27*, 563.

54. Samols E, Tyler JM, Marks V (1973): Glucagon-insulin interrelationships. In: *Glucagon. Molecular Physiology, Clinical and Therapeutic Implications*, p. 151. Editors: P.J. Lefebvre and R.H. Unger. Pergamon Press, Oxford.
55. Gerber PPG, Trimble ER, Wollheim CB, Renold AE (1981): Effect of insulin on glucose- and arginine-stimulated somatostatin secretion from the isolated perfused rat pancreas. *Endocrinology*, *109*, 279.
56. Samols E, Marri G, Marks V (1965): Promotion of insulin secretion by glucagon. *Lancet*, *2*, 415.
57. Patton GS, Dobbs RE, Orci L, Vale W, Unger RH (1976): Stimulation of pancreatic immunoreactive somatostatin (IRS) release by glucagon. *Metabolism*, *25*, *Suppl. 1*, 1499.
58. Kawai K, Unger RH (1982): Inhibition of glucagon secretion by exogenous glucagon in the isolated perfused dog pancreas. *Diabetes*, *31*, 512.
59. Alberti KGMM, Christensen NJ, Christensen SE, Handsen AAP, Iversen J, Lundbaek K, Seyer-Hansen K, Orskov H (1973): Inhibition of insulin secretion by somatostatin. *Lancet*, *2*, 1299.
60. Koerker BJ, Ruch W, Chideckel E, Palmer J, Goodner CJ, Ensinck J, Gale CC (1974): Somatostatin: Hypothalamic inhibitor of the endocrine pancreas. *Science*, *184*, 482.
61. Ipp E, Rivier J, Dobbs RE, Brown M, Vale W, Unger RH (1979): Somatostatin analogs inhibit somatostatin release. *Endrocrinology*, *104*, 1270.
62. Unger RH, Orci L (1977): Hypothesis: The possible role of the pancreatic D-cell in the normal and diabetic states. *Diabetes*, *26*, 241.
63. Asplin CM, Paquette TL, Palmer JP (1981): In vivo inhibition of glucagon secretion by paracrine beta cell activity in man. *J. Clin. Invest.*, *68*, 314.
64. Kawai K, Ipp E, Orci L, Perrelet A, Unger RH (1982): Circulating somatostatin acts on the islets of Langerhans by way of a somatostatin-poor compartment. *Science*, *218*, 477.
65. Bonner-Weir S (1984): Morphological evidence for B-cell polarity within the islet of Langerhans in the rat. *Diabetes*, *33*, *Suppl. 1*, 81A.
66. Bonner-Weir S, Orci L (1982): New perspectives on the microvasculature of the islets of Langerhans in the rat. *Diabetes*, *31*, 883.
67. Hisatomi A, Maruyama H, Starke A, Vasko M, Orci L, Grodsky GM, Unger RH (1984): Mechanisms of the glucagon (IRG) response to hypoglycemia and its loss in diabetes. *Diabetes*, *33*, *Suppl. 1*, 79A.
68. Palmer JP, Porte D Jr (1983): Neural control of glucagon secretion. In: *Glucagon II. Handbook of Experimental Pharmacology 66/I*, p. 114. Editor: P.J. Lefebvre. Springer-Verlag, Berlin.
69. Bloom S, Vaughan N, Russell R (1974): Vagal control of glucagon release in man. *Lancet*, *2*, 546.
70. Bloom S, Edwards A, Vaughan N (1974): The role of autonomic innervation in the control of glucagon release during hypoglycemia in the calf. *J. Physiol.*, *236*, 611.
71. Frohman LA, Bernardis LL (1971): Effect of hypothalamic stimulation on plasma glucose, insulin and glucagon levels. *Am. J. Physiol.*, *221*, 1596.
72. Christensen NJ, Iversen J (1973): Release of large amounts of noradrenaline from the isolated perfused canine pancreas during glucose deprivation. *Diabetologia*, *9*, 396.

73. Ipp E, Schusdziarra V, Harris V, Unger RH (1980): Morphine-induced hyperglycemia: Role of insulin and glucagon. *Endrocrinology*, *107*, 461.
74. Tai TY, Pek S (1976): Direct stimulation by growth hormone of glucagon and insulin release from isolated rat pancreas. *Endocrinology*, *99*, 69.
75. Dunning BE, Moltz JH, Fawcett CP (1984): Actions of neurohypophysial peptides on pancreatic hormone release. *Am. J. Physiol.*, *246*, E108.
76. Cryer PE (1981): Glucose counterregulation in man. *Diabetes*, *30*, 261.
77. Gerich JE, Langlois M, Noacco C, Karam J, Forsham PH (1973): Lack of a glucagon response to hypoglycemia in diabetes: Evidence for an intrinsic pancreatic alpha cell defect. *Science*, *182*, 171.
78. Bolli G, De Feo P, Perriello G, De Cosmo S, Compagnucci P, Santeusanio F, Brunetti P, Unger RH (1984): Mechanisms of glucagon secretion during insulin-induced hypoglycemia in man. Role of the beta cell and arterial hyperinsulinemia. *J. Clin. Invest.*, *73*, 917.

The Diabetes Annual/1
K.G.M.M. Alberti and L.P. Krall, editors

ISBN 0444 90 343 7
$0.85 per article per page (transactional system)
$0.20 per article per page (licensing system)

28 Possible animal models for diabetes mellitus: syndromes involving toxic or immune etiology

ALBERT E. RENOLD

It will soon be one hundred years since Minkowski and von Mehring established that diabetes mellitus can be caused by total pancreatectomy in the dog. A likely pathogenetic link between the islets of Langerhans and human diabetes has been accepted ever since, culminating in 1921 in the isolation of the anti-diabetic hormone, insulin, from pancreatic tissue by Banting and Best. The latter discovery was based on an animal model, the pancreatectomized dog, for estimating the biological effect of the various pancreatic fractions from which insulin was extracted.

As discussed elsewhere in this Annual, it has become evident that human diabetes is better understood if it is considered a heterogeneous and multifactorial disorder. The large number of observations presently available has resulted in acceptance of a classification in which *Type 1 diabetes*, insulin-dependent and more frequent in the young, is distinguished from *Type 2 diabetes*, non-insulin-dependent, more frequent in the elderly and the obese. In Type 1 diabetes, an early dysfunction of the islets of Langerhans, especially its insulin-producing B-cells, is a characteristic feature, whereas insulin deficiency is a much later event in Type 2 diabetes, in which additional pathogenetic features include decreased effectiveness of insulin at its target tissues. As discussed in other chapters and by Fajans (1), Albin and Rifkin (2) and in the volumes edited by Köbberling and Tattersall (3) and by Melish, Hanna and Baba (4), the clear recognition of two major types of diabetes is likely to represent just the beginning of an etiologically much more complex and diverse heterogeneity. In recognizing the existence of such a heterogeneity of a human disease, diabetes mellitus, we must also accept our indebtedness to the discovery of diabetes in animals, and to the even earlier realization that the etiology of spontaneous diabetes in animals is clearly heterogeneous as well. Much of what was known in 1981 about animal models of diabetes was reviewed in the Proceedings of the Task Force appointed by the Diabetes Mellitus Coordinating Committee of the National Institutes of Health to report on animal models of diabetes mellitus and its complications (5). Additional reviews were published in 1982 and 1983 (6–8) and a comprehensive report of recent information is included in a volume published in autumn 1984 (9). The references in this chapter will therefore include primarily the most recent ones, selected from the last 2 to 3 years.

Whenever reviewing information on diabetes, emphasis may be given either to endocrine B-cell damage and its etiology, or to the many defects secondary to dysfunction of the islets of Langerhans. This chapter will be concerned principally with the pathogenesis and nature of B-cell damage, whether of exogenous or endogenous origin. It should be clearly understood that the use of the word 'model' never suggests identity between an etiology or pathogenetic factor in animals and a similar, established or presumed, event in man. What we suggest at this time is simply that the multiplicity of animal disorders associated with hyperglycemia confirms the increasingly accepted notion that human, as well as animal diabetes, is extremely heterogeneous.

Chemical agents with specific cytotoxicity for pancreatic B-cells

A number of chemicals exist that exert significantly greater cytotoxicity on pancreatic B-cells than on any other tissue. It would be clearly of interest to have detailed understanding of the message implied, i.e. the structural and chemical particularities of the insulin-producing cells that make them uniquely sensitive to the agents involved. The topic was reviewed extensively in 1981 (10) and well summarized quite recently (8). The principal B-cytotoxic diabetogenic agents are *alloxan* (a pyrimidine with structural similarities to uric acid and glucose), *streptozotocin* (a 2-deoxymethyl-nitrosourea-glucopyranose) and *Vacor*®, a rodenticide with the active ingredient N-3-pyridylmethyl-N′-*p*-nitrophenyl urea. The diabetogenic properties of alloxan were discovered in 1943, a major though serendipitous discovery recently described by McLetchie who, as a medical student, participated in its discovery in Glasgow (11). It was studied as a putative metabolite of uric acid. The diabetogenic activity of streptozotocin was observed during routine testing of potential antibiotics from *Streptomyces achromogenes* by the Upjohn Company, and the rodenticide Vacor was observed to be diabetogenic in man because it was used for attempted suicide both in Korea and in California. It may well be that, as suggested by Karam et al. (12) a structural similarity exists between all three diabetogenic agents and thus the possibility for a common cytotoxic mechanism (Fig. 1). It is worth mentioning that a more stable derivative of alloxan, dehydrouramil hydrate hydrochloride, that may also be a metabolite of uric acid, may be the alloxan-like compound most favorable for in-vitro use (13) because of its greater stability. Vacor cannot be used as an experimental tool in vivo in rodents because of its general toxicity: it is lethal before it is diabetogenic. Although these three agents differ in a number of respects (14), evidence has accumulated to indicate that they are similar in exerting at least part of their cytotoxic effect through the generation of superoxide and, especially, hydroxyl radicals. The evidence is much the strongest for alloxan (15–19) but the studies on the protective effects of the enzyme superoxide dismutase also concerned streptozotocin and Vacor in vitro (20), as well as streptozotocin in vivo (20–22). Other hydroxyl radical – or peroxide – scavengers, or modifiers, have been shown similarly to affect some aspects of streptozotocin toxicity (23–25).

For *alloxan*, Malaisse and his collaborators have reviewed comprehensively the information supporting his present hypothesis of alloxan B-cytotoxicity (16). This review is especially informative because it deals in detail with the many prior studies having been considered in the light of different hypotheses, and attempts to resolve many of the apparent contradictions. Taken together, present evidence favors both rapid alloxan entry into pancreatic B-cells and tissue-specific B-cell sensitivity to superoxide radicals (16, 26). Glucose and mannose (but not fructose or galactose) as well as some other nutrients exert a protective effect on alloxan-induced damage. This protection is probably related to the capacity to generate reducing equivalents and thus to increase the $NADH/NAD^+$ and $NADPH/NADP^+$ ratios. Generation of such reducing equivalents would serve to decrease the levels of superoxides during alloxan recycling through dialuric acid. In support of this general view of the nature of at least part of the B-cytotoxicity of alloxan, an important observation is that pretreatment of pancreatic islets with other auto-oxidizing (and superoxide-generating) compounds, such as dihydroxyfumarate, causes dose-related inhibition of glucose-stimulated insulin release (27).

In the vigorous defense of his hypothesis (16) Malaisse argues plausibly that other lesions proposed as primary by other investigators (e.g. primary

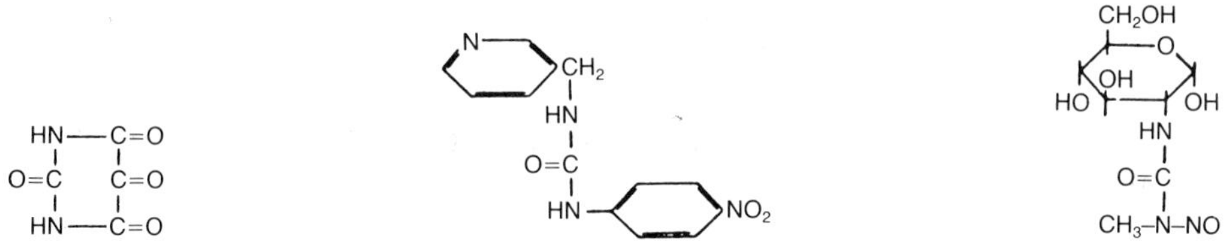

ALLOXAN

N-3-PYRIDYMETHYL N′-p-NITROPHENYL UREA (RH-787)

STREPTOZOTOCIN

FIG. 1. *Chemical structures of alloxan, of the active component of Vacor, and of streptozotocin. Modified from Mordes et al. (14).*

interaction with plasma membrane, with adenylate cyclase, or with reduced thiols) might well be secondary to the early (2 to 5 min) generation of highly active hydroxyl radicals facilitated by the rapid penetration of alloxan into pancreatic B-cells. He is particularly successful in arguing that all suppressors of alloxan cytotoxicity could be effective as a consequence either of decreased production or enhanced scavenging of peroxide radicals, or of interference with the early cellular uptake of the pyrimidine.

The great potential interest of detailed understanding of the intimate biochemical events involved in pancreatic B-cytotoxicity results not only from the occurrence of similar substances in our environment (12, 28) but also from the possible relevance of their action to pathogenetic mechanisms of B-cell damage. Thus, it has long been known that nicotinamide prevents the B-cytotoxicity of alloxan and streptozotocin when administered before or with either drug. When administered immediately *after* alloxan, nicotinamide is inactive, whereas it retains its full B-cell 'protective' activity when administered 10 minutes after streptozotocin, about half of that protective activity 30 minutes after streptozotocin, and even some protective activity after two hours (29).

Recent studies by Okamoto and his associates have clearly established that both alloxan and streptozotocin act in part by inducing islet DNA strand breaks (presumably as a result of peroxide radical action) with consequent activation of poly(ADP-ribose) synthetase and a precipitous fall (within 20 minutes) in islet cell NAD. This sequence of events may be interrupted either by providing hydroxyl radical scavenging activity or by inhibiting poly(ADP-ribose) synthetase with such agents as aminophylline, nicotinamide and 3-amino benzamide HCl (25, 30–33). It is noteworthy that inhibition of poly(ADP-ribose) synthetase, without hydroxyl radical scavengers, prevents diabetogenic damage and may thus represent an obligatory link for the hydroxyl radical toxicity. Finally, very recent evidence is compatible with an ameliorating effect of poly(ADP) synthetase inhibitors on hyperglycemia in rats, an amelioration possibly associated with facilitation of islet B-cell regeneration (34).

In the next section it will be seen that streptozotocin-associated toxicity may also be involved in an induced model of autoimmune damage to the islets of Langerhans.

Pancreatic B-cytotoxicity associated with insulitis and the induction of autoimmune reactions

In the preceding section, the possible similarities in the B-cytotoxic action of streptozotocin with those of alloxan were emphasized. Thus, both drugs act in part through generation of active peroxide and hydroxyl radicals, their toxic actions being similarly, although not identically, modulated by agents or conditions decreasing the net production or facilitating the scavenging of these highly bioactive forms of oxygen. Both drugs may also be selectively drawn to insulin-producing cells through the special capacity of such cells to recognize and metabolize glucose rapidly: structurally alloxan is somewhat glucose-like (see also ref. 35) and streptozotocin is glucose with a highly reactive side chain. It would therefore also seem reasonable that some transportable sugars interfere with the toxicity of both agents, even though they are not metabolized (16, 35).

Differences between alloxan and streptozotocin must also, however, be considered. Evidence of irreversible alloxan damage occurs in the range of 2 to 5 minutes and is structurally grossly evident within one hour. The evidence for streptozotocin is by contrast for the occurrence of irreversible damage between 30 minutes and two hours. The glucose and glucose analogues capable of protecting from streptozotocin differ significantly from those effective against alloxan. Nicotinic acid is fully active in suppressing the diabetogenic activity of alloxan, but inactive in affecting streptozotocin (29). Finally, nicotinamide retains considerable protective activity when injected as late as 30 minutes to 2 hours *after* streptozotocin, but has *no* such post-alloxan action (29).

The most important difference between streptozotocin and alloxan is the ability of doses of the former which are insufficient to produce an immediate (after 2 days) hyperglycemic response, to produce later and progressive (from 1-2 weeks onward) hyperglycemia in susceptible species and strains. This was first described in mice after the intraperitoneal administration of 5 daily subdiabetogenic doses of 40 mg/kg each, the fully diabetogenic dose being 200 mg/kg (36). Such an additive as well as delayed effect is pharmacologically unusual, especially for an unstable substance. It proved to be associated with lymphocytic infiltration of the pancreatic islets (insulitis). Since both the hyperglycemia and the insulitis could be prevented by rabbit antisera against mouse lymphocytes (37) participation in this process of an autoimmune component was strongly suspected. Further examination of this hypothesis during recent years has produced full confirmation, and established the obligatory participation of T-cell mediated autoimmune mechanisms (38–40). By contrast, B-lymphocytes are not involved (41).

Susceptibility to autoimmune activation by streptozotocin of inbred mice of different genetic background is greatly influenced by genotypic variations. This was first reported by Rossini (42) and the available data were recently and comprehensively summarized (43). Present evidence suggests that susceptibility or resistance to progressive hyperglycemia induced by several low doses of streptozotocin is strongly influenced by at least two separate genes, at least one of which is located within the major mouse histocompatibility complex H-2, and one or more outside the complex (43, 44). It is still unclear whether the insulitis is at the origin of the B-cell destruction or rather its consequence. Similarly the mechanism by which the streptozotocin effect is enhanced in males and potentiated by androgens remains elusive, as does the precise identity of the lymphocytes or macrophages required for a full streptozotocin-induced autoimmune response (45–49).

Although the standard procedure for eliciting autoimmune pancreatic B-cytotoxicity and insulitis in mice uses 5 daily injections of a clearly subdiabetogenic dose of streptozotocin, it has also been observed that when the hydroxyl radical-mediated toxicity of a single fully diabetogenic dose of the drug is attenuated by a hydroxyl radical scavenger, dimethyl-urea, early diabetogenic activity and cell death may be prevented, yet delayed hyperglycemia associated with insulitis may occur instead (50). Indeed, pretreatment of repeated low-dose streptozotocin injected mice with dimethyl-urea has been reported to protect against even delayed hyperglycemia, but not against insulitis. Even repeated subdiabetogenic dose treatment results in a significant decrease in pancreatic insulin content (51) and it would seem that the interrelation between decreased B-cell mass, autoimmune response and insulitis is indeed a complex one, about which much remains to be learned. It is worth noting that workers from East Germany have recently reported that low-dose streptozotocin diabetes may be produced in dogs, but only after partial pancreatectomy (52). Finally, mention should be made of another report that even a single, intermediate but still subdiabetogenic dose of streptozotocin in mice may result in delayed (about 4 weeks) hyperglycemia and insulitis, together with circulating antibodies to nucleic acids (53). Pertussis vaccine administered i.p. or i.v. 3 days prior to streptozotocin completely suppressed hyperglycemia, nucleic acid antibodies and insulitis (54). The interpretation tentatively proposed is that enterobacterial endotoxins may modulate T-cell proliferation by helper or suppressor lymphocytes (54), a suggestion that may be related to the recent report of enhanced autoimmune activation in mice using a lipopolysaccharide polyclonal activator from *Escherichia coli* (55).

Spontaneous diabetes with evidence for immune etiology in animals

Mononuclear infiltrates in the islets of Langerhans (insulitis) have been described by pathologists examining autopsy specimens of patients having died with acute diabetes before the beginning of this century and thus well before the discovery of insulin. Gepts first drew attention to the high frequency of insulitis in diabetic subjects who would now be classified as Type 1 (IDDM) and who were autopsied within a year or less of the onset of their disease. Experimentally induced insulitis in animals was first observed in cows (56), sheep (57) and rabbits (58) having undergone prolonged immunization with homologous or heterologous (both imperfectly pure) insulin in adjuvants. Starting in the early 1970's, increasing recognition of the probable importance of circulating antibodies to islet cells in Type 1 diabetes (for review see ref. 59) and that of HLA antigens coded for by the major histocompatibility gene complex on Chromosome 6 (reviewed in ref. 3), resulted in acceptance of an etiologic role for autoimmunity in Type 1 diabetes. Acceptance of the general validity of this etiology was further accelerated by the recognition, in 1977, of the first model of autoimmune diabetes in the rat (60). Evidence for autoimmune participation in the pathogenesis of diabetes in animal models now concerns the following major syndromes.

The spontaneously diabetic BB rat

This is probably the most important animal 'model' for Type 1 diabetes and one which has already greatly contributed to a better understanding of possible pathogenetic mechanisms of autoimmunity in islet cell damage, even to possible directions for its prevention. First recognized in 1977 (60, 61) BB diabetic rats were shown to present both the abrupt onset of hyperglycemia (most often between 60 and 120 days of age) with striking evidence of lymphocytic infiltration, and subsequent destruction, of the islets of Langerhans. The characteristics of these animals were reviewed in 1982 (62), and extensively in a workshop published as a separate supplement (63). Genetic studies suggest that the disease is inherited as an autosomal recessive with incomplete penetrance (64), possibly involving three separate genes (65), certainly two (66). One gene determines the T-cell lymphopenia, the second is associated with RT_1, the major histocompatibility complex of the rat. Under conditions of partial inbreeding, between 40 and 60% of diabetes-prone animals become diabetic (62) and both sexes are equally affected. The rats are lean, ketosis-prone, and require insulin for survival.

Coincidence of diabetes and pancreatic insulitis suggests participation of a cell-mediated immune pathogenesis. The supportive evidence is impressive: passive transfer of insulitis was achieved into the nude mouse (67) and passive transfer of diabetes accomplished by means of concanavalin-A stimulated lymphocytes (68); in addition, circulating autoantibodies to islet cells and lymphocytes have been observed (69–71). In addition diabetes may be prevented by total lymphoid irradiation (72); by immunosuppressive agents such as antilymphocyte serum (73) and cyclosporin A (74); and by immune modulations such as neonatal thymectomy (75) or neonatal bone marrow grafts (76, 77). Finally, transfusion of diabetes-prone BB/W rats with whole blood from diabetes-resistant BB/W rats was effective in preventing diabetes as well as insulitis and some anomalies of circulating lymphocytes (78). This effect could be clearly traced to the T-lymphocytes of blood from diabetes-resistant BB/W rats (79).

Many features of the spontaneous diabetes of BB rats are comparable to similar anomalies typical of human Type 1 diabetes. The probably obligatory association with generalized lymphopenia, however, does not seem to have an equally marked counterpart in the human. The lymphopenia in the BB rat precedes the clinical disorder, involves primary and secondary lymphoid tissues and is most marked for T-helper lymphocytes (80). The T-cell immuno-incompetence appears to be post-thymic, possibly a peripherally acquired maturational defect (81). Because of the suspected (but still to be defined) role of circulating autoantibodies to islet cell surface antigens in human diabetes, development and correlation with insulitis and/or diabetes have been carefully studied for 157 days in BB/Worcester diabetes-prone and diabetes-resistant rats, and in similar animals derived from the related BB/Ontario strain (82, 83). Such auto-antigens were clearly more frequent and more abundant in diabetes-prone than in diabetes-resistant animals, and they were always present at weaning in all animals from diabetes-prone litters, and thus preceded, often by many weeks, the onset of either insulitis or hyperglycemia (83). The development of insulin-dependent diabetes in BB rats was thus often preceded by or associated with these auto-antibodies, but was *not* dependent upon them (83). Other studies have suggested a tighter correlation between the beginning of mononuclear infiltration and the onset of diabetes (84), as well as a seemingly more direct relation between the appearance of complement-fixing antibodies to islet cell surface and clear evidence for pancreatic islet destruction (85).

The general importance of the many similarities between human Type 1 diabetes and the diabetic BB rat derives especially from two aspects. First, the BB rat model makes it possible to study intensively the silent period separating genetic predisposition and clinical onset in the search for a reliable marker for the approaching active phase of pancreatic B-cell destruction. Second, the availability of the model may ultimately allow for the planning of human intervention studies through detailed analysis of environmental influences that may exert an activating or preventive action on the pathogenetic sequence of events leading to clinical expression of diabetes. Thus, the observation that the earliest autoantibodies found in *both* man and BB rats may be directed against a probable B-cell membrane-specific 64-kilodalton protein (86), well before the appearance of anti-B-cytoplasmic antibodies, suggests that further related work in the BB rat model may indeed advance our knowledge about the 'prediabetic' silent period in human diabetes. On the other hand, observations such as that the onset of BB rat diabetes is strongly influenced by the protein content of the diet (87) or by cyclosporin administration (74), may soon provide us with rational and testable strategies for prevention programs directed toward at least some forms of diabetes in man.

The non-obese diabetic (NOD) mouse

Starting from a spontaneously glycosuric female mouse of the CTS strain, Tochino and collaborators (88, 89) obtained through inbreeding for some 20 generations a strain of mice characterized by insulitis beginning at 4–5 weeks of age. The lymphocytic infiltration is progressively and selectively associated with pancreatic B-cell destruction, diabetes occurring between 13 and 30 weeks, with hyperglycemia, ketonuria and, in some instances, absolute requirement of insulin. Although diabetes is more frequent in females (80–90% by 30 weeks) than in males (20%), lymphocytic infiltration occurs by 5 weeks in both sexes (females 82%, males 58%). The lymphocytes have the appearance of T-lymphocytes (89) and the insulitis is remarkable in that the lymphocyte infiltration is massive (90) and primarily surrounds the islets even though the morphological evidence for B-cell alteration occurs throughout the islet. Cells histochemically labelled for somatostatin, glucagon or pancreatic polypeptide are unaffected. Lymphopenia and antilymphocyte antibodies are present from 3 weeks of age (91–93), islet cell surface antibodies occur at 6 weeks and reach maximal prevalence (50%) between 12 and 18 weeks. Immunohistochemical typing of the peri-insular lymphocytes suggests predominantly B-lymphocytes and smaller numbers of helper and cytotoxic T-lymphocytes, and also some natural killer (NK) cells (93). Indeed, the lymphocytic infiltration exhibits clear elements of lymphoid tissue structure and this syndrome, unlike that in the BB rat, may be partly related to B-lymphocyte function, at least locally. Although the information accumulated is as yet sparse, the existence of a second syndrome combining insulitis, abnormal production of lymphocytes and insulin-dependent diabetes is of extraordinary importance and promise. Thus, a monoclonal antibody to islet cell surface antigen has already been produced through hybridization of spleen lymphocytes from NOD mice (94).

Other hyperglycemic syndromes in which an autoimmune component has been suggested

The general interest aroused by the three preceding syndromes, has led to re-evaluation of autoimmune contributions to other animal models, even those more closely resembling Type 2 diabetes (NIDD). Space prevents more than a very brief discussion of the interesting results that have been added recently.

Dogs: Evidence has been found for participation of pancreatic-B-cytotoxic or inhibitory lymphocytes or serum activities in six insulinopenic dogs (95) that may well be representative of the IDD or Type 1 syndrome in that species. Only one pancreas could be examined post-mortem and did not exhibit insulitis. The paper includes an excellent analysis of available information in that species that brings the 1982 review (96) up-to-date.

Monkeys: The endocrine pancreatic lesion in spontaneous diabetes in *Macaca nigra* is predominantly amyloidosis (97). A majority (91%) of 43 monkeys with mild to severe insulinopenia or hyperglycemia exhibited islet-cell antibodies, as compared with 13% of non-diabetic controls. Islet amyloidosis was found at biopsy or autopsy in 35 monkeys, of which 30 (86%) had islet-cell antibodies (98). It is possible that in this species autoimmune damage could be involved in the genesis of deposition of amyloid. (See ref. 99 for a more extensive review of diabetes in non-human primates.)

Mice: As already reviewed by Coleman (100) reduced cellular immunity has been reported both in obese (*ob/ob*) and diabetes (*db/db*) mouse mutants, although the question of primary or secondary (environmental) T-lymphocyte anomaly was left open. Debray-Sachs et al. (101) have recently and intensively re-investigated the problem in C57Bl/KsJ *db/db* mice and observed clear evidence for anti-islet immunity and thymic dysfunction. The observation is convincing although it remains to be seen what relation, if any, exists between the *db* gene and the suggested autoimmunity. In this context it must be remembered that the phenotypic expression of the *db* or *ob* genes is entirely conditioned by the remainder of the genome and, in particular, by the H-2 haplotype (102). It is of further interest that Kolb et al. (103) have suggested that spontaneous autoimmune reactions against pancreatic islets (with insulitis) occur frequently in mouse strains with generalized autoimmune disease as, for example, in NZB (New Zealand Black) mice. This observation, however, remains totally unconfirmed (104). Indeed even in the closely related NZO (New Zealand Obese) strain, there *is* evidence for kidney-directed, but *no* evidence for islet-directed autoimmunity (105).

References

1. Fajans SS (1982): Classification and natural history of diabetes mellitus. In: *Diabetes Mellitus and Obesity*, Chapter 39, p 349. Editors: B.N. Brodoff and S.J. Bleicher. Williams & Wilkins, Baltimore–London.
2. Albin J, Rifkin H (1982): Etiologies of diabetes mellitus. *Med. Clin. N. Am.*, *66*, 1209.
3. Köbberling J, Tattersall RL (Eds) (1982): *The Genetics of Diabetes Mellitus. Proceedings of the Serono Symposium, Freiburg, West Germany, April 9-11, 1981, Vol. 47*, 293 pp. Academic Press, London.
4. Melish JS, Hanna J, Baba S (Eds) (1982): *Genetic Environmental Interaction in Diabetes Mellitus. Proceedings of the Third Symposium on Diabetes Mellitus in Asia and Oceania, Honolulu, February 6-7, 1981*, 437 pp. Excerpta Medica, Amsterdam-Oxford-Princeton.
5. Salans LB, Graham BJ (Eds) (1984): Proceedings of a Task Force on Animals

Appropriate for Studying Diabetes Mellitus and its Complications – 1982. *Diabetes*, *31*. *Suppl. 1*.

6. Coleman DL, Brodoff BN (1982): Spontaneous diabetes and obesity in rodents. In: *Diabetes Mellitus and Obesity*, Chapter 32, p 283. Editors: B.N. Brodoff and S.J. Bleicher. Williams & Wilkins, Baltimore–London.
7. Dulin WE, Gerritsen GC, Chang AY (1982): Experimental and spontaneous diabetes in animals. In: *Diabetes Mellitus*, *Vol. 3*, p 361. Editors: M. Ellenberg and H. Rifkin. McGraw-Hill, New York.
8. Bell RH Jr, Hye RJ (1983): Animal models of diabetes mellitus: physiology and pathology. *J. Surg. Res.*, *35*, 433.
9. Shafrir E, Renold AE (Eds) (1984): *Lessons from Animal Diabetes.* John Libbey Co., London.
10. Cooperstein SJ, Watkins D (1981): Action of toxic drugs on islet cells. In: *The Islets of Langerhans*, p 416. Editors: S.J. Cooperstein and D. Watkins. Academic Press, London.
11. McLetchie NGB (1982): Alloxan diabetes: The sorcerer and his apprentice. *Diabetologia*, *23*, 72.
12. Karam JH, Lewitt PA, Young CW, Nowlain RE, Frankel BJ, Fujiya H, Freedman ZR, Grodsky GM (1980): Insulinopenic diabetes after rodenticide (Vacor) ingestion. A unique model of acquired diabetes in man. *Diabetes*, *29*, 971.
13. Tait SPC, Poje M, Rocic B, Ashcroft SJH (1983): Diabetogenic action of alloxan-like compounds: The effect of dehydrouramil hydrate hydrochloride on isolated islets of Langerhans of the rat. *Diabetologia*, *25*, 360.
14. Mordes JP, Muller WA, Rossini AA (1982): Experimental and spontaneous diabetes in animals. In: *Diabetes Mellitus and Obesity*, Chapter 31, p 273. Editors: B.N. Brodoff and S.J. Bleicher. Williams & Wilkins, Baltimore–London.
15. Heikkila RE, Winston B, Cohen G, Barden H (1976): Alloxan-induced diabetes: evidence for hydroxyl radical as a cytotoxic intermediate. *Biochem. Pharmacol.*, *25*, 1085.
16. Malaisse WJ (1982): Alloxan toxicity to the pancreatic B-cell. A new hypothesis. *Biochem. Pharmacol.*, *31*, 3527.
17. Täljedal I-B (1981): On insulin secretion. *Diabetologia*, *21*, 1.
18. Grankvist K, Marklund S, Sehlin T, Täljedal I-B (1979): Superoxide dismutase, catalase and scavengers of hydroxyl radical protect against the toxic action of alloxan on pancreatic islet cells in vitro. *Biochem. J.*, *182*, 17.
19. Asayama K, English D, Slonim A, Burr IM (1984): Chemiluminescence as an index of drug-induced free radical production in pancreatic islets. *Diabetes*, *33*, 160.
20. Gandy SE, Buse MG, Crouch RK (1982): Protective role of superoxide dismutase against diabetogenic drugs. *J. Clin. Invest.*, *70*, 650.
21. Robbins MJ, Sharp RA, Slonim AE, Burr IM (1980): Protection against streptozotocin-induced diabetes by superoxide dismutase. *Diabetologia*, *18*, 55.
22. Marklund S, Grankvist K (1981): Polyethyleneglycol-superoxide dismutase (PEG-SOD) protect against streptozotocin-induced diabetes in mice. *Acta Endocrinol. (Copenhagen)*, *98*, *Suppl. 245*, 43 (abstract).

23. Sandler S, Andersson A (1982): The partial protective effect of the hydroxyl radical scavenger dimethyl urea on streptozotocin-induced diabetes in the mouse in vivo and in vitro. *Diabetologia*, *23*, 374.
24. Slonim AE, Surber ML, Page DL, Sharp RA, Burr IM (1983): Modification of chemically induced diabetes in rats by vitamin E. Supplementation minimizes and depletion enhances development of diabetes. *J. Clin. Invest.*, *71*, 1282.
25. Sandler S, Welsh M, Andersson A (1983): Streptozotocin-induced impairment of islet B-cell metabolism and its prevention by a hydroxyl radical scavenger and inhibitors of poly(ADP-ribose) synthetase. *Acta Pharmacol. Toxicol.*, *53*, 392.
26. Malaisse WJ, Malaisse-Lagae F, Sener A, Pipeleers DC (1982): Determinants of the selective toxicity of alloxan to the pancreatic B cell. *Proc. Natl Acad. Sci. USA*, *79*, 927.
27. Fischer LJ, Hamburger SA (1981): Impaired insulin release after exposure of pancreatic islets to autooxidizing dihydroxyfumarate. *Endocrinology*, *108*, 2331.
28. Helgason T, Jonasson MR (1981): Evidence for a food additive as cause of ketosis-prone diabetes. *Lancet*, *2*, 716.
29. Stauffacher W, Burr I, Gutzeit A, Beaven D, Veleminsky J, Renold AE (1970): Streptozotocin diabetes: Time course of irreversible B-cell damage; further observations on prevention by nicotinamide. *Proc. Soc. Exp. Biol. Med.*, *133*, 194.
30. Yamamoto H, Uchigata Y, Okamoto H (1981): Streptozotocin and alloxan induce DNA strand breaks and poly(ADP-ribose) synthetase in pancreatic islets. *Nature (London)*, *294*, 284.
31. Uchigata Y, Yamamoto H, Kawamura A, Okamoto H (1982): Protection by superoxide dismutase, catalase, and poly(ADP-ribose) synthetase inhibitors against alloxan- and streptozotocin-induced islet DNA strand breaks and against the inhibition of proinsulin synthesis. *J. Biol. Chem.*, *257*, 6084.
32. Uchigata Y, Yamamoto H, Nagai H, Okamoto H (1983): Effect of poly-(ADP-ribose) synthetase inhibitor administration to rats before and after injection of alloxan and streptozotocin on islet proinsulin synthesis. *Diabetes*, *32*, 316.
33. Fischer LJ, Falany J, Fisher R (1983): Characteristics of nicotinamide and Nsub 1-methylnicotinamide protection from alloxan diabetes in mice. *Toxicol. Appl. Pharmacol.*, *70*, 148.
34. Yonemura Y, Takashima T, Miwa K, Miyazaki I, Yamamoto H, Okamoto H (1984): Amelioration of diabetes mellitus in partially depancreatized rats by poly(ADP-ribose) synthetase inhibitors: evidence of islet B-cell regeneration. *Diabetes*, *33*, 401.
35. Virji MA, Steffes MW, Estensen RD (1984): Concanavalin A and alloxan interactions on glucose-induced insulin secretion and biosynthesis from islets of Langerhans. *Diabetes*, *33*, 164.
36. Like AA, Rossini AA (1976): Streptozotocin-induced pancreatic insulitis: new model of diabetes mellitus. *Science*, *193*, 415.
37. Rossini AA, Williams RM, Appel MC, Like AA (1978): Complete pro-

tection from low-dose streptozotocin-induced diabetes in mice. *Nature (London)*, *276*, 182.
38. Paik SG, Fleischer N, Shin S (1980): Insulin dependent diabetes mellitus induced by subdiabetogenic doses of streptozotocin: obligatory role of cell-mediated autoimmune processes. *Proc. Natl Acad. Sci. USA*, *77*, 6129.
39. Paik SG, Blue M-L, Fleischer N, Shin S (1982): Diabetes susceptibility of BALB/cBOM mice treated with streptozotocin. Inhibition by lethal irradiation and restoration by splenic lymphocytes. *Diabetes*, *31*, 808.
40. Nedergaard M, Egeberg J, Kromann H (1983): Irradiation protects against pancreatic islet degeneration and hyperglycaemia following streptozotocin treatment of mice. *Diabetologia*, *24*, 382.
41. Blue M-L, Shin S (1984): Diabetes induction by subdiabetogenic doses of streptozotocin in BALB/cBOM mice: noninvolvement of host B-lymphocyte functions. *Diabetes*, *33*, 105.
42. Rossini AA, Appel MC, Williams RM, Like AA (1977): Genetic influence of streptozotocin-induced insulitis and hyperglycemia. *Diabetes*, *26*, 916.
43. Wolf J, Lilly F, Shin S (1984): The influence of genetic background on the susceptibility of inbred mice to streptozotocin-induced diabetes. *Diabetes*, *33*, 567.
44. Kiesel U, Falkenberg FW, Kolb H (1983): Genetic control of low-dose streptozotocin-induced autoimmune diabetes in mice. *J. Immunol.*, *130*, 1719.
45. Leiter EH, Beamer WG, Shultz LD (1983): The effect of immunosuppression on streptozotocin-induced diabetes in C57BL/KsJ mice. *Diabetes*, *32*, 148.
46. Leiter EH (1982): Multiple low-dose streptozotocin-induced hyperglycaemia and insulitis in C57BL mice: Influence of inbred background, sex, and thymus. *Proc. Natl Acad. Sci. USA*, *79*, 630.
47. Paik SG, Michelis MA, Kim YT, Shin S (1982): Induction of insulin-dependent diabetes by streptozotocin. Inhibition by estrogens and potentiation by androgens. *Diabetes*, *31*, 724.
48. Kromann H, Christy M, Lernmark Å, Nedergaard M, Nerup J (1982): The low dose streptozotocin murine model of type 1 (insulin-dependent) diabetes mellitus: Studies in vivo of the modulating effect of sex hormones. *Diabetologia*, *22*, 194.
49. Kiesel U, Kolb H (1983): Suppressive effect of antibodies to immune response gene products on the development of low-dose streptozotocin-induced diabetes. *Diabetes*, *32*, 869.
50. Sandler S (1984): Protection by dimethyl urea against hyperglycaemia, but not insulitis, in low-dose streptozotocin-induced diabetes in the mouse. *Diabetologia*, *26*, 386.
51. Bonnevie-Nielsen V, Steffes MW, Lernmark Å (1981): A major loss in islet mass and B-cell function precedes hyperglycemia in mice given multiple low doses of streptozotocin. *Diabetes*, *30*, 424.
52. Freyse EJ, Von Dorsche HH, Fischer U (1983): Low dose streptozotocin diabetes after partial pancreatectomy in dogs. Histological findings in a new type of experimental diabetes. *Acta Biol. Med. Germ.*, *41*, 1203.
53. Huang S-W, Taylor GE (1981): Immune insulitis and antibodies to nucleic acids induced with streptozotocin in mice. *Clin. Exp. Immunol.*, *43*, 425.

54. Huang S-W, Taylor GE (1982): Pertussis vaccine inhibits immune insulitis induced with streptozotocin. *Clin. Exp. Immunol.*, *48*, 375.
55. Flechner I, Muntefering H, Smadja Y, Laron Z (1984): Polyclonal activation and streptozotocin-induced diabetes in mice. In: *Lessons from Animal Diabetes*, p 305. Editors: E. Shafrir and A.E. Renold. John Libbey and Co., London.
56. LeCompte PM, Steinke J, Soeldner JS, Renold AE (1966): Changes in the islets of Langerhans in cows injected with heterologous and homologous insulin. *Diabetes*, *15*, 586.
57. Federlin K, Renold AE, Pfeiffer EF (1968): Antigen-binding leucocytes in patients and in insulin-sensitized animals with delayed insulin allergy. In: *Proceedings, Fifth International Symposium on Mechanisms of Inflammation Induced by Immune Reactions, Punta Ala (Italy), June 1967.* Editors: P. Miescher and P. Grabar. Schwabe and Co, Basel–Stuttgart and Grune and Stratton, Inc., New York.
58. Toreson WE, Lee JC, Grodsky GM (1968): The histopathology of immune diabetes in the rabbit. *Am. J. Pathol.*, *52*, 1099.
59. Bottazzo GF (1984): B-cell damage in diabetic insulitis: are we approaching a solution? *Diabetologia*, *26*, 241.
60. Nakhooda AF, Like AA, Chappel CI, Murray FT, Marliss EB (1977): The spontaneously diabetic Wistar rat. Metabolic and morphologic studies. *Diabetes*, *26*, 100.
61. Nakhooda AF, Like AA, Chappel CI, Wei C-N, Marliss EB (1978): The spontaneously diabetic rat (the 'BB' rat). *Diabetologia*, *14*, 199.
62. Like AA, Butler L, Williams RM, Appel MC, Weringer EJ, Rossini AA (1982): Spontaneous autoimmune diabetes mellitus in the BB rat. *Diabetes*, *31*, *Suppl. 1*, 7.
63. Marliss EB (Ed) (1983): The Juvenile Diabetes Foundation Workshop on the Spontaneously Diabetic BB Rat: its Potential for Insight into Human Juvenile Diabetes. Banff, Alberta, Canada, September 8-10, 1982. *Metab. Clin. Exp.*, *32*, *Suppl. 1*, 166 pp.
64. Butler L, Guberski DL, Like AA (1983): Genetic analysis of the BB/W diabetic rat. *Can. J. Genet. Gynecol.*, *25*, 7.
65. Guttmann RD, Colle E, Michel F, Seemayer T (1983): Spontaneous diabetes mellitus syndrome in the rat. II. T lymphopenia and its association with clinical disease and pancreatic lymphocytic infiltration. *J. Immunol.*, *130*, 1732.
66. Buse JB, Ben-Nun A, Klein KA, Eisenbarth GS, Seidman JG, Jackson RA (1984): Specific class II histocompatibility gene polymorphism in BB rats. *Diabetes*, *33*, 700.
67. Nakhooda AF, Sima AAF, Poussier P, Marliss EB (1981): Passive transfer of insulitis from the 'BB' rat to the nude mouse. *Endocrinology*, *109*, 2264.
68. Koevary S, Rossini AA, Stoller W, Chick W, Williams RM (1983): Passive transfer of diabetes in the BB/W rat. *Science*, *220*, 727.
69. Dyrberg T, Nakhooda AF, Baekkeskov S, Lernmark Å, Poussier P, Marliss EB (1982): Islet cell surface antibodies and lymphocyte antibodies in the spontaneously diabetic BB Wistar rate. *Diabetes*, *31*, 278.
70. Elder M, Maclaren N, Riley W, Connell T (1982): Gastric parietal and other autoantibodies in the BB rat. *Diabetes*, *31*, 313.

71. Like AA, Appel MC, Rossini AA (1982): Autoantibodies in the BB/W rat. *Diabetes*, *31*, 816.
72. Rossini AA, Slavin S, Woda BA, Geisberg M, Like AA, Mordes JP (1984): Total lymphoid irradiation prevents diabetes mellitus in the Bio-Breeding/ Worcester (BB/W) rat. *Diabetes*, *33*, 543.
73. Like AA, Rossini AA, Appel MC, Guberski DL, Williams RM (1983): Spontaneous diabetes mellitus: reversal and prevention in the BB/W rat with antiserum to rat lymphocytes. *Science*, *206*, 1421.
74. Laupacis A, Stiller CR, Gardell C, Keown P, Dupré J, Wallace AC, Thibert P (1983): Cyclosporin prevents diabetes in BB Wistar rats. *Lancet*, *1*, 10.
75. Like AA, Kislauskis E, Williams RM, Rossini AA (1982): Neonatal thymectomy prevents spontaneous diabetes mellitus in the BB/W rat. *Science*, *216*, 644.
76. Naji A, Silvers WK, Bellgrau D, Anderson AO, Plotkin S, Barker CF (1981): Prevention of diabetes in rats by bone marrow transplantation. *Ann. Surg.*, *194*, 328.
77. Naji A, Silvers WK, Kimura H, Bellgrau D, Markham JF, Barker CF (1983): Analytical and functional studies on the T-cells of untreated and immunologically tolerant diabetes-prone BB rats. *J. Immunol.*, *130*, 2168.
78. Rossini AA, Mordes JP, Pelletier AM, Like AA (1983): Transfusions of whole blood prevent spontaneous diabetes mellitus in the BB/W rat. *Science*, *219*, 975.
79. Rossini AA, Faustman D, Woda BA, Like AA, Szymanski I, Mordes JP (1984): Lymphocyte transfusions prevent diabetes in the biobreeding/Worcester rat. *J. Clin. Invest.*, *74*, 39.
80. Poussier P, Nakhooda AF, Falk JA, Lee C, Marliss EB (1982): Lymphopenia and abnormal lymphocyte subsets in the 'BB' rat: relationship to the diabetic syndrome. *Endocrinology*, *110*, 1825.
81. Elder ME, Maclaren NK (1983): Identification of profound peripheral T lymphocyte immuno-deficiencies in the spontaneously diabetic BB rat. *J. Immunol.*, *130*, 1723.
82. Dyrberg T (1984): Islet cell surface autoantibodies prior to the development of diabetes in the BB rat. In: *Lessons from Animal Diabetes*. p 273. Editors: E. Shafrir and A.E. Renold. John Libbey and Co., London.
83. Dyrberg T, Poussier P, Nakhooda AF, Marliss EB and Lernmark Å (1984): Islet cell surface and lymphocyte antibodies often precede the spontaneous diabetes in the BB rat. *Diabetologia*, *26*, 159.
84. Logothetopoulos J, Valiquette N, Madura E, Cvet D (1984): The onset and progression of pancreatic insulitis in the overt, spontaneously diabetic, young adult BB rat studied by pancreatic biopsy. *Diabetes*, *33*, 33.
85. Martin DR, Logothetopoulos J (1984): Complement-fixing islet cell antibodies in the spontaneously diabetic BB rat. *Diabetes*, *33*, 93.
86. Baekkeskov S, Dyrberg T, Lernmark Å (1984): Autoantibodies to a 64-kilodalton islet cell protein precede the onset of spontaneous diabetes in the BB rat. *Science*, *224*, 1348.
87. Elliott RB, Martin JM (1984): Dietary protein: a trigger of insulin-dependent diabetes in the BB rat? *Diabetologia*, *26*, 297.
88. Makino S, Kunimoto K, Muraoka Y, Mizushima Y, Katagiri K, Tochino Y

(1980): Breeding of a non-obese, diabetic strain of mice. *Exp. Anim. (Tokyo)*, *29*, 1.

89. Fujita T, Yui R, Kusomoto Y, Serizawa Y, Makino S, Tochino Y (1982): Lymphocyte insulitis in a 'non-obese diabetic (NOD)' strain of mice: an immunohistochemical and electron microscope investigation. *Biomed. Res.*, *3*, 429.
90. Taniguchi H, Fujii S, Ejiri K, Ishihara K, Baba S (1984): Profuse infiltration of lymphocytes in islets of spontaneously developed non-obese (NOD) mice. In: *Lessons from Animal Diabetes*, p 290. Editors: E. Shafrir and A.E. Renold. John Libbey and Co., London.
91. Toyota T, Goto Y, Kataoka S, Fujiya H, Sato J, Oya K, Shintani S, Kumagai K (1984): Immunologic studies on NOD mice as a model of IDDM. In: *Lessons from Animal Diabetes*, p 308. Editors: E. Shafrir and A.E. Renold, John Libbey and Co., London,
92. Kataoka S, Satoh J, Fujiya H, Toyota T, Suzuki R, Itoh K, Kumagai K (1983): Immunologic aspects of the nonobese diabetic (NOD) mouse. Abnormalities of cellular immunity. *Diabetes*, *32*, 247.
93. Kanazawa Y, Komeda K, Sato S, Mori S, Akanuma K, Takadu F (1984): Non-obese-diabetic (NOD) mice: Immune-mechanisms of pancreatic beta-cell destruction. *Diabetologia* (in press).
94. Yokono K, Shii K, Hari J, Yaso S, Imamura Y, Ejiri K, Ishihara K, Fujii S, Kazumi T, Taniguchi H, Baba S (1984): Production of monoclonal antibodies to islet cell surface antigens using hybridization of spleen lymphocytes from non-obese diabetic mice. *Diabetologia*, *26*, 379.
95. Sai P, Debray-Sachs M, Jondet A, Gepts W, Assan R (1984): Anti-beta-cell immunity in insulinopenic diabetic dogs. *Diabetes*, *33*, 135.
96. Engerman RL, Kramer JW (1982): Dogs with induced or spontaneous diabetes as models for the study of human diabetes mellitus. *Diabetes*, *31*, *Suppl. 1*, 26.
97. Howard CF, Jr (1978): Insular amyloidosis and diabetes mellitus in Macaca nigra. *Diabetes*, *27*, 357.
98. Howard CF,. Jr and Fang T-Y (1984): Islet cell cytoplasmic antibodies in Macaca nigra. *Diabetes*, *33*, 219.
99. Howard CF, Jr (1982): Nonhuman primates as models for the study of human diabetes mellitus. *Diabetes*, *31*, *Suppl. 1*, 37.
100. Coleman DL (1982): Diabetes-obesity syndromes in mice. *Diabetes*, *31*, *Suppl 1*, 1.
101. Debray-Sachs M, Dardenne M, Sai P, Savino W, Quiniou M-C, Boillot D (1983): Anti-islet immunity and thymic dysfunction in the mutant diabetic C57BL/KsJ *db/db* mouse. *Diabetes*, *32*, 1048.
102. Leiter EH, Coleman DL, Hummel KP (1981): The influence of genetic background on the expression of mutations at the diabetes locus in the mouse. III. Effect of H-2 haplotype and sex. *Diabetes*, *30*, 1029.
103. Kolb H, Freytag G, Kiesel U, Kolb-Bachofen V (1980): Spontaneous autoimmune reactions against pancreatic islets in mouse strains with generalized autoimmune disease. *Diabetologia*, *19*, 216.
104. Seemayer TA, Colle E (1984): Pancreatic cellular infiltrates in autoimmune-prone New Zealand black mice. *Diabetologia*, *26*, 310.

105. Melez KA, Harrison LC, Gilliam JN, Steinberg AD (1980): Diabetes is associated with autoimmunity in the New Zealand Obese (NZO) mouse. *Diabetes*, *29*, 835.

Subject index